Springer Proceedings in Mathematics & Statistics

Volume 353

Springer Proceedings in Mathematics & Statistics

This book series features volumes composed of selected contributions from workshops and conferences in all areas of current research in mathematics and statistics, including operation research and optimization. In addition to an overall evaluation of the interest, scientific quality, and timeliness of each proposal at the hands of the publisher, individual contributions are all refereed to the high quality standards of leading journals in the field. Thus, this series provides the research community with well-edited, authoritative reports on developments in the most exciting areas of mathematical and statistical research today.

More information about this series at http://www.springer.com/series/10533

Marie Wiberg • Dylan Molenaar • Jorge González
Ulf Böckenholt • Jee-Seon Kim
Editors

Quantitative Psychology

The 85th Annual Meeting of the Psychometric Society, Virtual

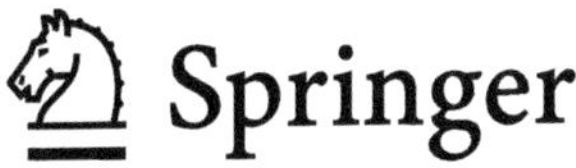

Editors
Marie Wiberg
Department of Statistics, USBE
Umeå University
Umeå, Västerbottens Län, Sweden

Jorge González
Facultad de Matemáticas
Pontificia Universidad Católica de Chile
Santiago, Chile

Jee-Seon Kim
Department of Educational Psychology
University of Wisconsin-Madison
Madison, WI, USA

Dylan Molenaar
Department of Psychology
University of Amsterdam
Amsterdam, The Netherlands

Ulf Böckenholt
Kellogg School of Management
Northwestern University
Evanston, IL, USA

ISSN 2194-1009 ISSN 2194-1017 (electronic)
Springer Proceedings in Mathematics & Statistics
ISBN 978-3-030-74774-9 ISBN 978-3-030-74772-5 (eBook)
https://doi.org/10.1007/978-3-030-74772-5

This Springer imprint is published by the registered company Springer Nature Switzerland AG
The registered company address is: Gewerbestrasse 11, 6330 Cham, Switzerland

Preface

This volume represents presentations given at the 85th annual meeting of the Psychometric Society, that due to the pandemic of covid-19 was held virtually. This is the first IMPS meeting held only over internet and it was given during July 14-17, 2020. There were 230 abstracts submitted (154 oral presentations, 89 posters, and 3 symposia). The virtual meeting attracted 378 participants, 54 of whom also participated in the virtual short course pre-conference workshop. There were three keynote presentations, three invited presentations, eight spotlight speaker presentations, and one dissertation award presentation.

Since the 77th meeting in Lincoln, Nebraska, Springer publishes the proceedings volume from the annual meeting of the Psychometric Society to allow presenters at the annual meeting to spread their ideas quickly to the wider research community, while still undergoing a thorough review process. This is especially important now as meeting in person was difficult in 2020. The previous eight volumes of the meetings were received successfully, and we expect these proceedings to be successful as well.

The authors were asked to use their presentation at the meeting as the basis of their chapters, possibly extended with new ideas or additional information. The result is a selection of 42 stateof- the-art chapters addressing a diverse set of psychometric topics, including but not limited to item response theory, factor analysis, test equating, cognitive diagnostic models, response time, IRT as well as psychometric applications within different fields.

Umeå, Västerbottens Län, Sweden — Marie Wiberg

Amsterdam, The Netherlands — Dylan Molenaar

Santiago, Chile — Jorge González

Evanston, IL, USA — Ulf Böckenholt

Madison, WI, USA — Jee-Seon Kim

Contents

A Rotation Criterion That Encourages a Hierarchical Factor Structure

Chen Tian and Yang Liu

1 Introduction

In Yung, Thissen, and McLeod's terminology (1999), a hierarchical factor model may have several layers of factors: Each manifest variable loads on exactly one of the factors in each layer. Hierarchical factor structures are common in educational and psychological testing. For example, the big five personality traits can be divided into many aspects, and each aspect can further be divided into facets (e.g., Allen & DeYoung, 2017). These relationships between personality traits, aspects, facets, and manifest variables can be represented and analyzed using the higher-order factor model, a special case of hierarchical factor model with proportionality constraints. Another example is the testlet effect: Both the construct and the testlet factors contribute to the observed responses in a compensatory fashion. In addition to explaining the correlated errors, testlets may also explicitly represent higher-order facets within the hierarchy of interested constructs (Cooke et al., 2007).

Despite the wide-spread usage in theorizing constructs, it remains challenging to directly obtain hierarchical structures in Exploratory Factor Analysis (EFA) since there lacks a suitable rotation criterion. Rotation to a partially specified target may be used, but it requires fully specifying the positions of zero loadings in the target matrix (Browne, 1972, 2001). For circumstances where we have limited prior knowledge on the exact pattern of factor-item dependencies, Jennrich and Bentler (2011) discussed rotation criterions that encourage a bifactor structure which is the simplest hierarchical model with one general factor and one layer of specific factors. A rotation criterion function measures the discrepancy from an exact bifactor structure, which requires each item to load on at most one specific

C. Tian (✉) · Y. Liu
University of Maryland, College Park, MD, USA
e-mail: ctian1@terpmail.umd.edu

M. Wiberg et al. (eds.), *Quantitative Psychology*, Springer Proceedings in Mathematics & Statistics 353, https://doi.org/10.1007/978-3-030-74772-5_1

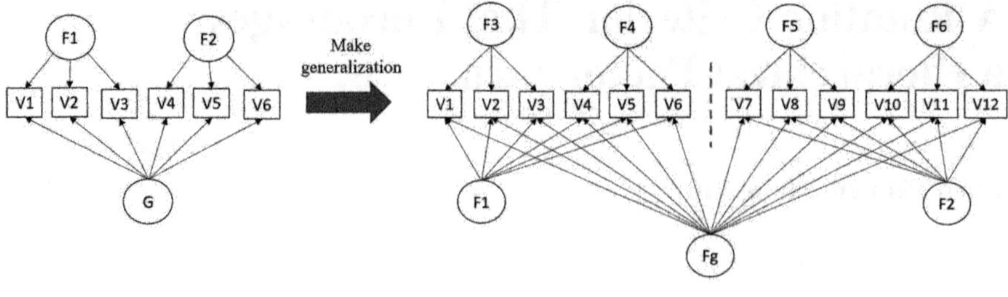

Fig. 1 Generalizing the rotation cretirion from a bi-factor structure to a hierarchical structure

factor. One example from Jennrich and Bentler (2011) is to apply the quartimin rotation criterion to the specific factors: $\sum_{i=1}^{p}\sum_{r=2}^{k}\sum_{s=r+1}^{k}\lambda_{ir}^2\lambda_{is}^2$, where λ_{ir} is the loading of item i on factor r, p is the number of items, and k is the number of factors.

Inspired by Jennrich and Bentler's exploratory bifactor analysis using the quartimin rotation criterion, the goal of this study is to propose a generalized rotation criterion for a two-layer hierarchical structures in EFA. Fig. 1 displays an example of such a structure: The corresponding factor loading matrix is expressed as eq. (1), in which asterisks denote non-zero loading entries, and the columns from left to right represent F_g and F1-F6. In the sequel, we say that a higher level factor is the parent of an adjacent lower level factor if all the items loading on the lower level factor also load on the higher level factor, and that two lower level factors having the same parent are sibling factors. In Fig. 1, F1 is the parent of F3 and F4, and F2 is the parent of F5 and F6.

$$\Lambda = \left(\begin{array}{cc|cc|ccc} * & * & 0 & * & 0 & 0 & 0 \\ * & * & 0 & * & 0 & 0 & 0 \\ * & * & 0 & * & 0 & 0 & 0 \\ * & * & 0 & 0 & * & 0 & 0 \\ * & * & 0 & 0 & * & 0 & 0 \\ * & * & 0 & 0 & * & 0 & 0 \\ * & 0 & * & 0 & 0 & * & 0 \\ * & 0 & * & 0 & 0 & * & 0 \\ * & 0 & * & 0 & 0 & * & 0 \\ * & 0 & * & 0 & 0 & 0 & * \\ * & 0 & * & 0 & 0 & 0 & * \\ * & 0 & * & 0 & 0 & 0 & * \end{array}\right) \qquad (1)$$

2 Methods

2.1 Proposed Rotation Criterion Function

The proposed rotation criterion function should first be able to encourage a simple structure within each layer, and this can be achieved by summing up the quartimin criterion applied to different layers. In our case with F1 and F2 in the first level, there is only one pair to constrain, so the corresponding term is $\sum_{i=1}^{p} \lambda_{i1}^2 \lambda_{i2}^2$. Minimizing this non-negative term encourages either λ_{i1}^2 or λ_{i2}^2 in the F1-F2 pair to be close to 0. With four factors in the second level, F3-F6, there are $\binom{4}{2} = 6$ pairs of factors, and the corresponding quartimin term is $\sum_{i=1}^{p} \lambda_{i3}^2 \lambda_{i4}^2 + \lambda_{i3}^2 \lambda_{i5}^2 + \lambda_{i3}^2 \lambda_{i6}^2 + \lambda_{i4}^2 \lambda_{i5}^2 + \lambda_{i4}^2 \lambda_{i6}^2 + \lambda_{i5}^2 \lambda_{i6}^2$. Summing up those terms from two layers allows us to simplify the within-layer structure simultaneously for the two layers.

The rotation criterion should also be able to constrain the between-layer relationship to avoid items being loaded on the same second-level factor but different first-level factors. Ideally, this constraint on the parent-child relationship can be achieved using indicator functions. In the hierarchical structure shown in eq. (1), we consider the product of two sums for each child factor. If F3 is a child of F1, as shown in Fig. 1 and Eq. (1), for all the items loading on F1, the sum of their squared loadings on F3, $\sum_{i=1}^{p} I\left(\lambda_{i1}^2 \neq 0\right) \cdot \lambda_{i3}^2$, should be non-zero; for all the items loading on F2, the sum of their squared loadings on F3, $\sum_{i=1}^{p} I\left(\lambda_{i2}^2 \neq 0\right) \cdot \lambda_{i3}^2$, should be zero. Taking the product of these two sums encourages F3 to be the child of either F1 or F2: In other words, it penalizes the case when F3 is the child of both F1 and F2. Similarly, we can encourage that F1 is the only parent of F4, and F2 is the only parent of F5 and F6.

The proposed rotation criterion function designed for a two-layer binary-split hierarchical structure can be written in the following equation:

$$\begin{aligned} P(\Lambda) = &\sum_{i=1}^{p} \left(\lambda_{i1}^2 \lambda_{i2}^2 + \lambda_{i3}^2 \lambda_{i4}^2 + \lambda_{i3}^2 \lambda_{i5}^2 + \lambda_{i3}^2 \lambda_{i6}^2 + \lambda_{i4}^2 \lambda_{i5}^2 + \lambda_{i4}^2 \lambda_{i6}^2 + \lambda_{i5}^2 \lambda_{i6}^2\right) \\ &+ \left(\sum_{i=1}^{p} I\left(\lambda_{i1}^2 = 0\right) \cdot \lambda_{i3}^2\right) \times \left(\sum_{i=1}^{p} I\left(\lambda_{i2}^2 = 0\right) \cdot \lambda_{i3}^2\right) \\ &+ \left(\sum_{i=1}^{p} I\left(\lambda_{i1}^2 = 0\right) \cdot \lambda_{i4}^2\right) \times \left(\sum_{i=1}^{p} I\left(\lambda_{i2}^2 = 0\right) \cdot \lambda_{i4}^2\right) \\ &+ \left(\sum_{i=1}^{p} I\left(\lambda_{i1}^2 = 0\right) \cdot \lambda_{i5}^2\right) \times \left(\sum_{i=1}^{p} I\left(\lambda_{i2}^2 = 0\right) \cdot \lambda_{i5}^2\right) \\ &+ \left(\sum_{i=1}^{p} I\left(\lambda_{i1}^2 = 0\right) \cdot \lambda_{i6}^2\right) \times \left(\sum_{i=1}^{p} I\left(\lambda_{i2}^2 = 0\right) \cdot \lambda_{i6}^2\right) \end{aligned} \quad (2)$$

The first seven terms constrain the within-layer relationship between factors in the same level, and the others consider the parent-child relationship between two layers of factors. As indicated by the notation, the proposed rotation criterion assumes the position of parent and children factors in the loading matrix: The second and third columns should be the parent factors F1 and F2, and the fourth to seventh columns should be the child factors F3 to F6. This rotation criterion can be generalized to cases where one parent has more than two children by adding more terms that control the relationship between a low-level factor and all other high-level factors. For example, if we have three first-level factors, the between-layer term for F3 can be generalized to $\left(\sum_{i=1}^{p} I\left(\lambda_{i1}^2=0\right)\cdot\lambda_{i3}^2\right)\times\left(\sum_{i=1}^{p} I\left(\lambda_{i2}^2=0\right)\cdot\lambda_{i3}^2\right)+\left(\sum_{i=1}^{p} I\left(\lambda_{i1}^2=0\right)\cdot\lambda_{i3}^2\right)\times\left(\sum_{i=1}^{p} I\left(\lambda_{i3}^2=0\right)\cdot\lambda_{i3}^2\right)+\left(\sum_{i=1}^{p} I\left(\lambda_{i2}^2=0\right)\cdot\lambda_{i3}^2\right)\times\left(\sum_{i=1}^{p} I\left(\lambda_{i3}^2=0\right)\cdot\lambda_{i3}^2\right)$, which ensures that F3 has only one parent. It can also be generalized beyond two layers of factors by adding another collection of terms constraining the children-grandchildren relationship.

2.2 Computational Techniques

The non-continuous indicator function was approximated by the smooth exponential function such that the criterion function is differentiable as required by the optimization algorithm. The exponential function used in this simulation is $y = e^{-\alpha x}$, with $\alpha = 1{,}000{,}000$.

The Riemannian trust-region algorithm (Liu, 2020) was used to perform the orthogonal rotation, a second-order optimization algorithm for numerical search on the orthogonal group, i.e., the space of rotation matrices. It converges much faster than the gradient projection algorithm (Jennrich, 2001) with fewer iterations.

As the criterion function is sensitive to starting values and may converge to local minima, we used multiple random starts and chose the best as the final solution. It is a common practice for rotation criterions that are sensitive to starting values (e.g., Kiers, 1994; Rozeboom, 1992). In this study, we used 30 random starts and pick the solution with the minimum resulted function value from all 30 solutions.

2.3 Simulation Design

To understand the tolerance of the criterion function to the non-perfect and diverse EFA practices, three design factors were manipulated in the simulation study: loading matrices having (a) different numbers of rows/items; (b) magnitude of small errors replacing zeros; and (c) equal/unequal numbers of manifest variables among sibling factors. This study considers hierarchical structures with binary split: The numbers of items are 16, 32, and 64. To generate a scenario that is more realistic than the condition with exact hierarchical patterns, slight departures from the exact structure were generated by substituting exact zero loadings with random variates independently sampled from Uniform [−0.05, 0.05] or Uniform [−0.1, 0.1]. The non-zero loadings were simulated from Uniform [0.3, 1]. For the third factor involving the balancing condition of items loading on sibling factors, we considered three levels: balanced loading matrices with 50:50 items loading on sibling factors (*balanced*), unbalanced loading matrices with 35:65 items loading on sibling factors (*unbalanced 1*), and unbalanced loading matrices with 20:80 items loading on sibling factors (*unbalanced 2*). Note that F3 and F4 are siblings because their parent is F1, and F3 and F5 are not siblings because they do not have the same parent. For the unbalanced conditions, we may have non-integer numbers of items per factor (e.g. 16×0.2=3.4), and those numbers were rounded to the closest integers.

An initial loading matrix with an unrecognizable structure, which mimics the result of EFA, was the matrix to be rotated using the proposed rotation criterion. We need to make sure the initially unrecognizable matrix is finally recognizable. Therefore, the initial matrix was created by randomly rotating the true loading matrix. Thirty replications were done for each of the 3×3×3 conditions. The convergence tolerance was set to 10^{-5}. To evaluate the results, we calculate the scaled Frobenius-norm error between the true matrix and the rotated loading matrix averaged across 30 replications:

$$\frac{1}{\sqrt{pk}}\left\|\hat{\Lambda}-\Lambda\right\|_F=\sqrt{\frac{\sum_{i=1}^{p}\sum_{j=1}^{k}\left(\hat{\lambda_{ij}}-\lambda_{ij}\right)^2}{pk}}, \tag{3}$$

where k is the total number of factors or columns in the complete loading matrix Λ and p is the number of items.

3 Results

For the 30 replications of each of the 3×3×3 conditions, all the final solutions converged, and the mean of minimized criterion function values over 30 replications are summarized in Table 1. The results show that when the true loading matrix has some errors, the function value will be greater than 0 because the true value itself is greater than 0. Holding the error range and the extent of balance constant, the more items we have, the larger the minimized function value; holding the number of items and the error range constant, the more balanced the true loading matrix, the larger the minimized function value.

The scaled Frobenius-norm error was summarized in Table 2 and depicted in Fig. 2. The values in Table 2 reflect the estimated error per entry and can be seen as the "averaged distance" between true and estimated loading matrices, considering the size of the matrices. Table 2 shows that holding the error range and the number of items constant, the more unbalanced the true matrix is, the larger the distances

Table 1 The mean of minimized criterion function values over 30 replications for all conditions

		Balanced (50%)	Unbalanced 1 (35%)	Unbalanced 2 (20%)
16 items	0 errors	0	0	0
	Unif (−0.05, 0.05)	0.007	0.006	0.005
	Unif (−0.1, 0.1)	0.023	0.018	0.008
32 items	0 errors	0	0	0.001
	Unif (−0.05, 0.05)	0.019	0.019	0.016
	Unif (−0.1, 0.1)	0.071	0.069	0.033
64 items	0 errors	0	0	0
	Unif (−0.05, 0.05)	0.043	0.043	0.043
	Unif (−0.1, 0.1)	0.174	0.163	0.11

Table 2 The scaled Frobenius-norm error averaged across 30 replications for all conditions

		Balanced (50%)	Unbalanced 1 (35%)	Unbalanced 2 (20%)
16 items	0 errors	0	0	0.042
	Unif (−0.05, 0.05)	0.057	0.081	0.258
	Unif (−0.1, 0.1)	0.180	0.241	0.327
32 items	0 errors	0	0	0.017
	Unif (−0.05, 0.05)	0.035	0.044	0.172
	Unif (−0.1, 0.1)	0.114	0.223	0.335
64 items	0 errors	0	0	0
	Unif (−0.05, 0.05)	0.034	0.035	0.047
	Unif (−0.1, 0.1)	0.079	0.123	0.328

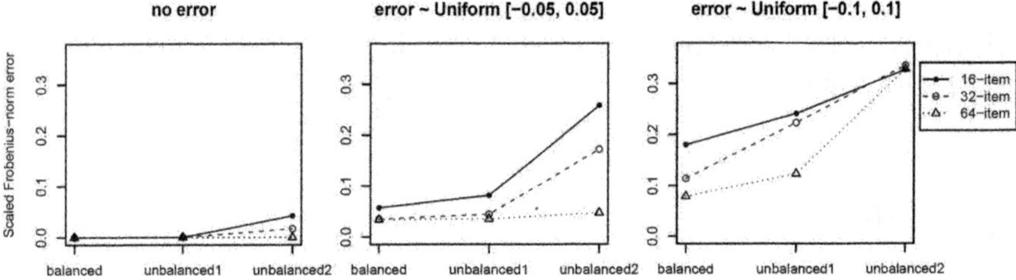

Fig. 2 The scaled Frobenius-norm error averaged across 30 replications for all conditions

between true and estimated loading matrix. Holding the balance extent and the number of items constant, the larger the errors, the larger the distances. Holding the balance extent and the error range constant, the more items we have, which means more pieces of information, the smaller the distances are.

4 Discussions

This proposed function is a generalization of Jennrich and Bentler's exploratory bifactor analysis to a two-layer hierarchical structure, which facilitates recovering and testing of a more complicated hierarchical structure in EFA with limited prior knowledge about item-factor dependency. Starting from an initial matrix with an unrecognizable structure, we can find a rotation matrix such that the rotated matrix is as close to a matrix with the hierarchical structure as possible. Our simulation results suggest that the proposed criterion function is generally robust to realistic scenarios when slight to moderate departures from a perfect hierarchical structure are present and when the matrix is moderately unbalanced. We also observe that parameter recovery is worsened by the magnitude of imperfect factor structure and the unbalancedness while improved as the number of items increases (Fig. 2). When the error ranges from -0.1 to 0.1, given that the meaningful loading value ranges from 0.3 to 1, we may have a too-small signal-to-noise ratio to recover the true hierarchical loading matrix. The negative effect of errors was intensified when we also have a severely unbalanced true matrix.

There are some limitations of the current study. First, the proposed rotation criterion requires us to know exactly how many factors we have at each layer and locks the positions of factors of a specific layer. In other words, the criterion function implicitly assumes that the general factor lies in the first column, the two first-level factors lie in the second and third columns, and the four second-level factors lie in the fourth to seventh columns. The problem is that, if we reorder the columns of a loading matrix with a perfect hierarchical structure in some ways, say, let the general factor lie in the fourth column and a second-level factor lie in the first column, then the function value is not zero, even though the re-ordered matrix has a perfect hierarchical structure. An ideal criterion function should always give a zero for matrices with the perfect hierarchical structure regardless of the ordering of columns, which is not satisfied by the current criterion function. In our numerical experiments, we observed local minima for the simpler bifactor structure as well, but not as severe as the two-layer structure which has more constrains to the column-wise relationships. Second, the proposed criterion function has many local minima. Some initial matrices may be easily rotated to a point which does not give a zero function value, then be further distorted when forcing the function value to be zero. Using random starts is only a heuristic solution, and more investigation is needed.

References

Allen, T. A., & DeYoung, C. G. (2017). Personality neuroscience and the five factor model. In *Oxford handbook of the five factor model* (pp. 319–352). Oxford University Press.

Browne, M. (1972). Orthogonal rotation to a partially specified target. *British Journal of Mathematical and Statistical Psychology, 25*(1), 115–120.

Browne, M. W. (2001). An overview of analytic rotation in exploratory factor analysis. *Multivariate Behavioral Research, 36*(1), 111–150.

Cooke, D. J., Michie, C., & Skeem, J. (2007). Understanding the structure of the psychopathy checklist–revised: An exploration of methodological confusion. *The British Journal of Psychiatry, 190*(S49), s39–s50.

Jennrich, R. I. (2001). A simple general procedure for orthogonal rotation. *Psychometrika, 66*(2), 289–306.

Jennrich, R. I., & Bentler, P. M. (2011). Exploratory bi-factor analysis. *Psychometrika, 76*(4), 537–549.

Kiers, H. A. L. (1994). SIMPLIMAX: Oblique rotation to an optimal target with simple structure. *Psychometrika, 59*, 567–579.

Liu, Y. (2020). Riemannian Newton and trust-region algorithms for analytic rotation in exploratory factor analysis. *British Journal of Mathematical and Statistical Psychology*.

Rozeboom, W. W. (1992). The glory of suboptimal factor rotation: Why local minima in analytic optimization of simple structure are more blessing than curse. *Multivariate Behavioral Research, 27*, 585–599.

Yung, Y. F., Thissen, D., & McLeod, L. D. (1999). On the relationship between the higher-order factor model and the hierarchical factor model. *Psychometrika, 64*(2), 113–128.

Comparison Between Different Estimation Methods of Factor Models for Longitudinal Ordinal Data

Silvia Bianconcini and Silvia Cagnone

1 Introduction

In recent years, common statistical applications have dealt with multivariate longitudinal data with the purpose of measuring changes in constructs over time, such as attitudes, opinions, performances and abilities. In this context, both the multifaceted nature of the data and the longitudinal evolution of the underlying constructs have to be studied jointly, and Generalised Linear and Latent Variable Models (GLLVMs) (Dunson, 2003; Cagnone et al., 2009) represent a useful framework. GLLVMs assume that the entire set of the responses given by an individual to a certain number of items at different occasions, called the response pattern, can be expressed as a function of one or more latent variables and random effects through a monotone differentiable link function.

A potential barrier to the application of these latent variable models is the computational challenge presented by typically large datasets. Panel studies usually have several thousands of respondents which, when combined with multiple waves of measurement and a large choice set, renders unfeasible existing estimation approaches (likelihood-based and Bayesian one). Even when cross-sectional models are used, if the observed variables are of different nature, continuous and discrete, the estimation of these models is cumbersome. It can be carried out using a full information maximum likelihood method via either the EM algorithm or direct maximisation, but, in both cases, the integrals involved in the likelihood computation have no analytical solutions and need to be approximated. This problem is more evident in presence of longitudinal data since the number of latent variables and random effects increases proportionally to the number of observed items. In

S. Bianconcini (✉) · S. Cagnone
Department of Statistical Sciences, University of Bologna, Bologna, Italy
e-mail: silvia.bianconcini@unibo.it; silvia.cagnone@unibo.it

M. Wiberg et al. (eds.), *Quantitative Psychology*, Springer Proceedings in Mathematics & Statistics 353, https://doi.org/10.1007/978-3-030-74772-5_2

presence of multidimensional longitudinal data, classical quadrature techniques, such as the adaptive Gauss Hermite, that represents the gold standard in the GLLVM framework, is already unfeasible when four items are observed at three different time points. Alternatively, the widely applied Laplace approximation is known to provide inaccurate estimates in presence of discrete data.

Alternative methods that can be used to produce estimators with desired statistical properties and that, in addition, simplify the estimation process, are greatly needed. The most popular method that offers reduction in estimation complexity is the composite likelihood approach, introduced by Lindsay in 1988 (Lindsay, 1988) and further discussed, among the others, by Varin and Vidoni (2005). The composite likelihood estimator is obtained by maximising the univariate and/or bivariate likelihood products that contain the greatest quantity of model parameter information. The immediate effect of the composite likelihood estimation is the reduction of the number of integrations required in the likelihood computation.

Another approach that has been recently proposed in the literature is the dimension-wise quadrature, developed by Bianconcini et al. (2017). It consists in reducing the dimension of the multidimensional integrals by truncating the Taylor series expansion of the integrand. This makes the computation feasible also when the number of latent variables is large. The proposed approach provides a higher order approximation than the Laplace one but does not require any derivative computation, hence it is very simple to implement. Furthermore, the corresponding estimators are asymptotically as accurate as the adaptive Gauss Hermite estimators.

This paper investigates the use of pairwise likelihood methods and dimension-wise quadratures for estimating latent variable models for multivariate longitudinal ordinal data. A simulation study is carried out to compare the performance of these estimators under different common empirical scenarios, and their behaviour is also highlighted through a real data example.

2 Generalized Linear Latent Variable Models for Longitudinal Ordinal Data

Let $y_{t1}, y_{t2}, \ldots, y_{tp}$ be a vector of p ordinal observed variables at time $(t,\ t = 1, \ldots, T)$ each of them with $c_j, j = 1, \ldots, p$, categories, and $z_1, z_2, \ldots, z_T$ a latent variable that accounts for the associations among the p items at each time point. Let $u_1, u_2, \ldots, u_p$ be p random effects that account for the associations of the same item at different time points. We consider the Generalized Linear Latent Variable Models (GLLVM) approach for longitudinal data that has been discussed by Dunson (2003) for mixed observed variables, and by Cagnone et al. (2009) in the specific case of ordinal data. According to the GLLVM approach, we define the joint density of the observed variables as

$$f(\mathbf{y}) = \int_{R^q} g(\mathbf{y} \mid \mathbf{z}, \mathbf{u}) h(\mathbf{z}, \mathbf{u}) d\mathbf{z} d\mathbf{u}$$

where $g(\mathbf{y} \mid \mathbf{z}, \mathbf{u})$ is referred to as measurement part of the model and $h(\mathbf{z}, \mathbf{u})$ as structural part of the model. The dimension of the integral depends on the number of observed variables and the number of time points, that is $q = p + T$.

The measurement part of the model is defined as a generalized linear model with random component given by

$$g(\mathbf{y}|\mathbf{z}, \mathbf{u}) = \prod_{t=1}^{T} \prod_{j=1}^{p} g(y_{tj}|z_t, u_j) = \tag{1}$$

$$= \prod_{t=1}^{T} \prod_{j=1}^{p} \prod_{r=1}^{c_j} (\gamma_{tj(r)}(z_t, u_j) - \gamma_{tj(r-1)}(z_t, u_j))^{y_{tj(r)}}, r = 1, \ldots, c-1$$

where the first equality comes from the conditional independence assumption between items and over time. Each conditional marginal density $g(y_{tj}|z_t, u_j)$ follows a multinomial distribution of parameter $\gamma_{tj(r)}(z_t, u_j)$ that is the cumulative probability that an individual responds to item j at time t up to category r. $y_{tj(r)}$ is a dummy variable that assumes value 1 up to category r.

The systematic component defines the linear predictor

$$\eta_{tj(r)} = \tau_{tj(r)} - \lambda_{tj} z_t - u_j$$

where $\tau_{tj(r)}$'s are item, time and category-dependent thresholds and λ_{tj}'s are item and time-dependent factor loadings. The link between the systematic component and the conditional means of the random component distributions is $\eta_{tj(r)} = \nu_{tj(r)}(\gamma_{tj(r)}(z_t, u_j))$ where $\nu_{tj(r)}$ is the link function which can be any monotonic, differentiable function. We consider the logit link function.

As for the structural part of the model, we consider the specification given by Cagnone et al. (2009), that is we assume that the latent variables follow an autoregressive no stationary process of first order as follows

$$z_t = \phi z_{t-1} + \delta_t, \tag{2}$$

where ϕ is the autoregressive coefficient, $\delta_t \sim N(0, 1)$ and $z_1 \sim N(0, \sigma_1^2)$.

Moreover, the joint density $h(\mathbf{z}, \mathbf{u}) \sim N(\mathbf{0}, \boldsymbol{\Psi})$ where

$$\boldsymbol{\Psi} = \begin{bmatrix} \boldsymbol{\Gamma} & 0 \\ 0 & \boldsymbol{\Omega} \end{bmatrix}.$$

$\boldsymbol{\Omega} = diag_{j=1,\ldots,p}\{\sigma_{uj}^2\}$ and the inverse of $\boldsymbol{\Gamma}$ has a well known special pattern whose expression can be found in Cagnone et al. (2009).

3 Model Estimation

Model estimation is usually performed by using a full maximum likelihood method. Given a sample of size n, the log-likelihood is given by:

$$L(\boldsymbol{\theta}) = \sum_{i=1}^{n} \log f(\mathbf{y}_i, \boldsymbol{\theta}) = \sum_{i=1}^{n} \log \int_{R^q} g(\mathbf{y}_i \mid \mathbf{z}_i, \mathbf{u}_i) h(\mathbf{z}_i, \mathbf{u}_i) d\mathbf{z}_i d\mathbf{u}_i \tag{3}$$

where $\boldsymbol{\theta}$ is the vector of parameters to be estimated. A problem related to the maximization of the log-likelihood is that, in general, the multidimensional integral in (3) is not solvable analytically.

Among the remedies proposed in the literature, numerical quadrature-based methods represent a widespread solution to this problem and, among them, the adaptive Gauss Hermite quadrature is considered the gold standard approach (Rabe-Hesketh et al., 2005; Schilling & Bock, 2005). Alternatively, the Laplace approximation avoids the integral computation and represents the easiest method to implement (Liu & Pierce, 1994; Huber et al., 2004). The adaptive Gauss Hermite quadrature provides more accurate estimates than the Laplace approximation, but it is computationally unfeasible as the number of latent variables and random effects increases. To overcome these limitations, recent solutions proposed for factor models for longitudinal ordinal data are the pairwise likelihood approach (Vasdekis et al., 2012) and the dimension-wise quadrature method (Bianconcini et al., 2017).

3.1 *Pairwise Likelihood Approach*

The pairwise likelihood estimator is obtained by maximizing bivariate likelihood products that contain the greatest quantity of model parameter information (Lindsay, 1988; Cox & Reid, 2004). The immediate effect of the pairwise likelihood estimation is the reduction of the number of integrations in the expression of the likelihood (3). Indeed, the contribution of any given individual to the pairwise log-likelihood is given by

$$pl(\theta; \mathbf{y}) = \sum_{i=1}^{n} pl(\theta; \mathbf{y}_i) \tag{4}$$

with $pl(\theta; \mathbf{y}_i) = \sum_{t,t',j,j'} \log f(y_{tji}, y_{t'j'i}; \theta)$. In particular, for the factor model for longitudinal ordinal data described in Sect. 2, the bivariate density for a pair of responses $(y_{tji}, y_{t'j'i})$ is given by

$$f(y_{tji}, y_{t'j'i}; \theta) = \int_{-\infty}^{+\infty} \int_{-\infty}^{+\infty} \int_{-\infty}^{+\infty} \int_{-\infty}^{+\infty} f(y_{tji}, y_{t'j'i}, z_{ti}, z_{t'i}, u_{ji}, u_{j'i}) dz_{ti} dz_{t'i} du_{ji} du_{j'i}$$

$$= \int_{-\infty}^{+\infty}\int_{-\infty}^{+\infty}\int_{-\infty}^{+\infty}\int_{-\infty}^{+\infty} f(y_{tji}|z_{ti}, u_{ji}) f(y_{t'j'i}|z_{t'i}, u_{j'i}) \times \tag{5}$$

$$\times h(z_{ti}, z_{t'i}, u_{ji}, u_{j'i}) dz_{ti} dz_{t'i} du_{ji} du_{j'i}.$$

The dimensional of the integrals involved in the expression of the likelihood components is four and if $j = j'$ or $t = t'$ it reduces to three. Thus, the three/four-dimensional integral can be easily approximated using a the Gauss Hermite quadrature method.

The resulting estimators are generally consistent and asymptotically normally distributed (Varin & Vidoni, 2005).

3.2 Dimension-Wise Quadrature Method

Let $\mathbf{b} = (\mathbf{z}, \mathbf{u})$ denote the vector of latent variables and random effects and consider the following representation of the marginal density function

$$\begin{aligned} f(\mathbf{y}; \theta) &= \int_{R^q} \frac{\prod_{j=1}^{p} g(y_j|\mathbf{b}) h(\mathbf{b})}{\phi(\mathbf{b}; \mathbf{b}_{mo}, \mathbf{\Sigma}_{mo})} \phi(\mathbf{b}; \mathbf{b}_{mo}, \mathbf{\Sigma}_{mo}) d\mathbf{b} = \\ &= |\mathbf{C}_{mo}| \int_{R^q} \frac{\prod_{j=1}^{p} g(y_j|\mathbf{C}_{mo}\mathbf{b}^* + \mathbf{b}_{mo}) h(\mathbf{C}_{mo}\mathbf{b}^* + \mathbf{b}_{mo})}{\phi(\mathbf{b}^*; \mathbf{0}, \mathbf{I})} \phi(\mathbf{b}^*; \mathbf{0}, \mathbf{I}) d\mathbf{b}^* = \\ &= |\mathbf{C}_{mo}| \int_{R^q} m(\mathbf{b}^*) \phi(\mathbf{b}^*; \mathbf{0}, \mathbf{I}) d\mathbf{b}^* = \\ &= |\mathbf{C}_{mo}| E_{\phi}[m(\mathbf{b}^*)] \end{aligned} \tag{6}$$

where $\mathbf{b}_{mo}$ is the maximum of the integrand $g(\mathbf{y} \mid \mathbf{z}, \mathbf{u})h(\mathbf{z}, \mathbf{u})$ and $\mathbf{\Sigma}_{mo} = \mathbf{C}_{mo}\mathbf{C}'_{mo}$ is minus the inverse of the corresponding Hessian matrix evaluated in the mode $\mathbf{b}_{mo}$. $\phi(\cdot)$ the normal density function.

The dimension-wise method is applied to the expected value $E_{\phi}[m(\mathbf{b}^*)]$. It is based on the Taylor expansion of $m(\mathbf{b}^*)$ around 0 up to the s term as follows

$$\hat{m}(\mathbf{b}^*) = \sum_{w=1}^{s} t_w \tag{7}$$

where each component t_w considers all the derivatives of $m(\mathbf{b}^*)$ taken with respect to w latent factors, that is

$$t_w = \sum_{j_1, j_2, \ldots, j_w} \sum_{k_1 < k_2 < \ldots < k_w} \frac{1}{j_1! j_2! \ldots j_w!} \frac{\partial^{j_1+j_2, \ldots, +j_w} m}{\partial b_{k_1}^{*j_1} \partial b_{k_2}^{*j_2} \ldots \partial b_{k_w}^{*j_w}} (\mathbf{0}) b_{k_1}^{*j_1} b_{k_2}^{*j_2} \ldots b_{k_w}^{*j_w} \tag{8}$$

The approximated function $\hat{m}(\mathbf{b}^*)$ admits the following equivalent representation (Bianconcini et al., 2017)

$$\hat{m}(\mathbf{b}^*) = \sum_{l=0}^{s}(-1)^l \binom{q-s+l-1}{l} m_{s-l}(\mathbf{b}^*) \tag{9}$$

where $m_{s-l}(\mathbf{b}^*) = m(0, \cdots, b^*_{k_1}, 0 \cdots, 0, b^*_{k_{s-l}}, 0, \cdots, 0)$. Thus, m_{s-l} is a function of just $s-l$ variables being all the remaining fixed to 0. Replacing Eq. (9) in Eq. (6), we obtain the approximate density function

$$f_a(\mathbf{y};\theta) = |\mathbf{C}_{mo}| \left[\sum_{l=0}^{s-1}(-1)^l \binom{q-s+l-1}{l} \int_{R^{s-l}} \sum_{k_1<\ldots<k_{s-l}} m_{s-l}(\mathbf{b}^*)\times \right. \tag{10}$$

$$\left. \phi(b^*_{k_1}) \cdots \phi(b^*_{k_{s-i}}) db^*_{k_1}..db^*_{k_{s-l}} \right].$$

The dimension of the integrals in expression (10) depends on the choice of s. If $s = 1$, we obtain a linear combination of unidimensional integrals, if $s = 2$, we obtain a linear combination of uni- and bi-dimensional integrals and so on. For small values of s, the integrals can be easily approximated using the Gauss Hermite quadrature method. In the extreme cases of $s = 0$ and $s = q$ the solution is equivalent to the classical Laplace and to the adaptive Gauss-Hermite quadrature ones, respectively.

The dimension-wise quadrature estimators share the same accuracy as the adaptive Gauss-Hermite method (Bianconcini et al., 2017), but avoiding the main computational limitations of the latter.

4 Simulation Study

The performance of the two approximation methods are compared through a simulation study.

We consider a first scenario where the number of factors is fixed to four, that is we assume to have observed two items at two different occasions ($q = 4, p = 2, T = 2$). This simple scenario allows us to also consider the Adaptive Gauss Hermite (AGH) quadrature that is feasible with number of quadrature points nq equal to 8 (AGH8) and 15 (AGH15). The AGH with 15 quadrature points can be considered the benchmark providing an almost exact representation of the function (Bianconcini et al., 2017). In this scenario, the AGH corresponds to the dimension-wise method (DWM) with $s = 4$. We also estimate the classical Laplace approximation, that corresponds to DWM with $s = 0$. Finally, we consider the dimension-wise quadrature with $s = 1, 2$, and 3. We set sample sizes equal to $n = 200$ and 1000, and, as suggested by Vasdekis et al. (2012), we consider 100 replications for each condition of the study.

Table 1 reports the bias and Root Mean Square Error (rmse) of the parameter estimates in the case of $n = 200$. The first loading is fixed to 1 for identification reasons and measurement invariance of thresholds and loadings over time is assumed.

As known, the Laplace approximation produces strongly biased estimates but with generally lower rmse than AGH15. The accuracy of the DWM estimates improves as s increases, and with similar results to AGH15 when $s = 3$.

The pairwise method also produces similar estimates to those of AGH15. Thus, for finite samples ($n = 200$), the pairwise method and the dimension-wise with $s = 3$ perform similarly. The main differences in the performance of the pairwise and dimension-wise methods are evident in larger samples, that is for $n = 1000$.

Figures 1 and 2 show the density estimates for λ_2 and ϕ, respectively.

The Laplace estimator is very inaccurate whereas the DWM estimator based on $s = 3$ is the closest to the AGH15 one. The pairwise behaves in between DWM with $s = 2$ and DWM with $s = 3$. It is interesting to notice that even if DWM with $s = 1$ is less accurate than the same method with higher values of s and pairwise, it is far superior to the Laplace estimator. The parameter estimators not shown here have a similar performance.

Table 1 Results for the 4-factor model, $n = 200$

	Pairwise		*Laplace* $s = 0$		*DWM* $s = 1$		*DWM* $s = 2$		*DWM* $s = 3$	
True	Bias	rmse	Bias	rmse	Bias	rmse	Bias	rmse	Bias	rmse
$\lambda_1 = 1$										
$\lambda_2 = 1.61$	0.00	0.70	−0.67	0.67	−0.35	0.83	−0.15	0.87	0.06	0.82
$\phi = 0.8$	−0.02	0.19	0.11	0.12	0.01	0.15	0.00	0.17	−0.05	0.18
$\sigma_1^2 = 2$	0.51	1.29	0.69	1.39	1.10	2.84	0.92	2.26	0.59	1.50
$\sigma_{u_1}^2 = 1$	−0.12	0.71	−0.96	1.11	−0.76	1.06	−0.46	0.99	−0.13	0.75
$\sigma_{u_2}^2 = 1.5$	0.19	0.95	−0.44	0.92	−0.52	1.22	0.20	1.28	0.50	1.62
	AGH8 $s = 4$		*AGH15* $s = 4$							
True	Bias	rmse	Bias	rmse						
$\lambda_1 = 1$										
$\lambda_2 = 1.61$	0.03	0.76	0.05	0.78						
$\phi = 0.8$	−0.02	0.17	−0.02	0.17						
$\sigma_1^2 = 2$	0.59	1.58	0.57	1.58						
$\sigma_{u_1}^2 = 1$	−0.10	0.84	−0.14	0.81						
$\sigma_{u_2}^2 = 1.5$	0.34	1.25	0.48	1.59						

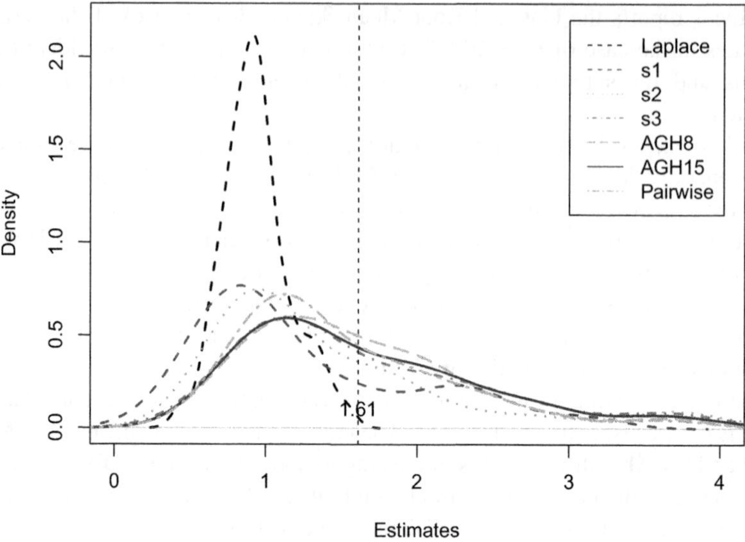

Fig. 1 Densities estimation of λ_2 (true value: 1.61) for the 4-factor model, $n = 1000$

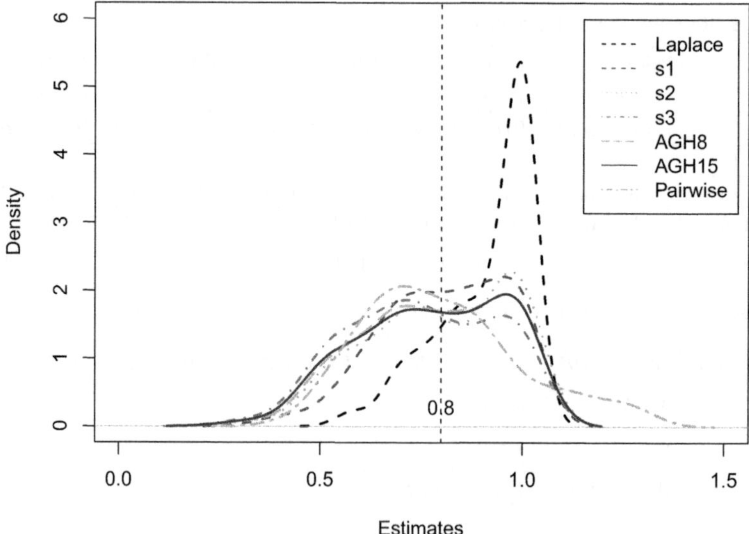

Fig. 2 Densities estimation of ϕ (true value: 0.8) for the 4-factor model, $n = 1000$

In Fig. 3 the values of the log-likelihood for an increasing number of quadrature point nq, that is 3, 5, 8, 11, and 15 are reported for the analyzed methods. We can observe that in all the cases pairwise performs worse than AGH, DWM with $s = 2$ and $s = 3$, whereas the log-likelihood values based on DWM with $s = 3$ and AGH

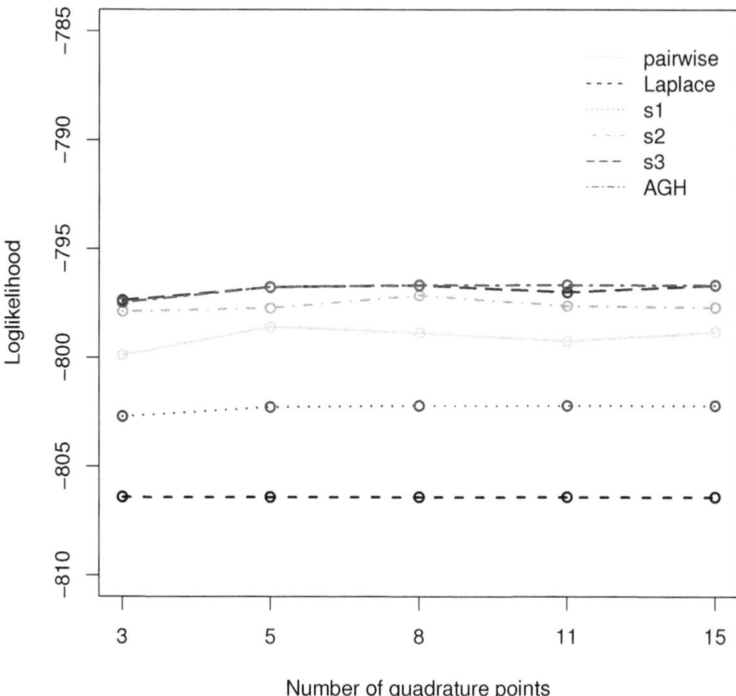

Fig. 3 Log-likelihood for increasing number of quadrature points, 4-factor model, $n = 1000$

are almost identical, independently on the number of quadrature points used in the integral approximations.

In the second simulation scenario we consider a factor model with seven factors, that is we assume to observe three items at four different occasions ($q = 7, p = 3, T = 4$). In this setting the AGH is not feasible. As before, we consider sample sizes equal to 200 and 1000, and 100 replications for each condition of the study.

The results are reported in Tables 2 and 3 for $n = 200$ and $n = 1000$, respectively. It is interesting to notice that, in this scenario, for both small and large sample sizes, even DWM with $s = 2$ outperforms the pairwise method in terms of bias as well as rmse. The pairwise performs more similarly to DWM with $s = 1$.

5 Real Data Analysis

Lastly, the two different approximation techniques considered through this research are compared using a real dataset, taken from the British Household Panel Survey

Table 2 Results for the 7-factor model, $n = 200$

	Pairwise		*Laplace* $s = 0$		*DWM* $s = 1$		*DWM* $s = 2$		*DWM* $s = 3$	
True	Bias	rmse	Bias	rmse	Bias	rmse	Bias	rmse	Bias	rmse
$\lambda_1 = 1$										
$\lambda_2 = 1.61$	0.23	0.39	−0.32	0.35	−0.15	0.34	−0.03	0.25	0.03	0.29
$\lambda_3 = 0.66$	0.05	0.20	−0.06	0.15	−0.10	0.17	−0.01	0.15	0.00	0.16
$\phi = 0.4$	−0.04	0.11	0.08	0.13	0.02	0.11	0.00	0.01	−0.01	0.10
$\sigma_1^2 = 2$	0.01	0.59	−0.29	0.44	−0.20	0.41	−0.03	0.11	0.00	0.33
$\sigma_{u_1}^2 = 1$	0.17	0.33	−0.32	0.50	−0.21	0.47	0.00	0.22	0.08	0.52
$\sigma_{u_2}^2 = 1.5$	0.38	0.61	−0.18	0.51	−0.07	0.49	0.03	0.26	0.05	0.52
$\sigma_{u_3}^2 = 2$	0.19	0.57	0.32	0.86	0.45	1.09	0.16	0.60	0.14	0.75

Table 3 Results for the 7-factor model, $n = 1000$

	Pairwise		*Laplace* $s = 0$		*DWM* $s = 1$		*DWM* $s = 2$	
True	Bias	rmse	Bias	rmse	Bias	rmse	Bias	rmse
$\lambda_1 = 1$								
$\lambda_2 = 1.61$	0.28	0.31	−0.33	0.33	−0.19	0.22	−0.05	0.12
$\lambda_3 = 0.66$	0.04	0.10	−0.06	0.09	−0.10	0.12	−0.01	0.07
$\phi = 0.4$	−0.05	0.07	0.09	0.10	0.03	0.06	0.01	0.11
$\sigma_1^2 = 2$	−0.08	0.25	−0.29	0.33	−0.20	0.25	−0.03	0.05
$\sigma_{u_1}^2 = 1$	0.28	0.31	−0.37	0.40	−0.26	0.32	−0.06	0.06
$\sigma_{u_2}^2 = 1.5$	0.42	0.47	−0.21	0.30	−0.11	0.24	−0.01	0.23
$\sigma_{u_3}^2 = 2$	0.14	0.28	0.17	0.37	0.26	0.46	0.05	0.31

(BHPS). The data are composed of an annual nationally representative sample of approximately 10,000 individuals (5000 households) aged 16 years and over. The main objective of the BHPS is to study social and economic changes in Britain at individual and household levels. To analyze the data, five waves were selected (1992, 1994, 1996, 1998, 2000), as well as three ordinal items that indicate social and political attitudes. After eliminating the missing values, we are left with a sample size of 3784 individuals. The manifest items that are to be analyzed are taken from the section on values and opinions and indicate respondents views on responsibility of the private sector, Government and trade unions for labor conditions. The items are:

1. Private enterprise is the best way to solve the UKs economic problems [Enterp].
2. It is the Governments responsibility to provide a job for everyone who wants one [Govern].

3. Strong trade unions are needed to protect the working conditions and wages of employees [TrUnion].

Permitted responses to these questions were agree strongly (AS), agree (A), not agree/disagree (Neither A nor D), disagree (D), disagree strongly (DS). Due to the fact that a small proportion of respondents fall into the first and last item categories, the first two and last two categories have been collapsed; thus leaving us with three categories for each item. Finally, the response categories of item Enterp have been reversed.

A one factor model is fitted with the time-dependent factors (latent variables) as an AR(1) autoregressive model. Previously, Vasdekis et al. (2012) analyzed the same data by allowing all model item parameters that are associated with the measurement model (thresholds and slopes) to vary across time points. The analysis proceeded with the fitting of the models, exclusively with: equal thresholds, equal loadings, and, finally, equal thresholds and loadings. The model with equal loadings, but not thresholds, across time was the preferred, and we quote here the results for this model. The model is estimated using the pairwise likelihood method and by applying the diwension-wise quadrature with different levels of approximation (s ranging from 0 to 3). The choice of s in the dimension-wise quadrature has been done by increasing its value until the mean of the relative absolute differences in parameter estimates ($Av(\Delta)$) was sufficiently small (order 10^{-3}). The stability in the estimated parameters is achieved with $s = 3$. Hence, Table 4 gives the estimated model parameters using the pairwise likelihood method and the dimension-wise quadrature with s set equal to three.

As observed in the simulation study, the two methods provide similar results. Loadings are all found to be positive and close to one-another. The large estimated variances for the random effects are indicative of the presence of a large amount of heterogeneity in the responses within each item over time. Heterogeneity that clearly could not be entirely accounted for by the autoregressive model was fitted upon the time-dependent latent variables. The latter are characterised by a strong correlation between subsequent time-dependent factors, which is judged by the large estimated autoregressive parameter ϕ equal to 0.83, with an estimated standard error equal to 0.002, for the pairwise method, and equal to 0.896 (with standard error equal to 0.005) for the dimension-wise quadrature.

Table 4 Estimated factor loadings with standard errors in brackets for the non-stationary model with time-specific latent variables and estimated variances for the item-specific random effects based on pairwise likelihood and dimension-wise quadrature ($s = 3$) methods

	Pairwise		*DWM*	
Item	λ_j	σ_{u_j}	λ_j	σ_{u_j}
Enterp	1.00	3.65 (0.21)	1.00	3.30 (0.15)
Govern	1.30 (0.07)	6.67 (0.37)	1.29 (0.04)	6.64 (0.33)
TrUnion	1.27 (0.07)	5.80 (0.40)	1.05 (0.03)	6.36 (0.71)

6 Discussion

The estimation of models for longitudinal data with random components, such as latent variable models, involve multidimensional integrations. A way to avoid the high dimensional integrations is to base the estimation and inference on lower data dimensions such as bivariate or trivariate. It is found that composite likelihood estimation, using the bivariate marginal likelihoods, and dimension-wise quadratures for a latent variable model with longitudinal ordinal responses, produce estimates with desirable properties. These results are endorsed by the simulation studies. In presence of multidimensional longitudinal data, these approximate likelihood estimation methods also allow the fit of more realistic models to data sets with many items and a few factors on each time dimension.

Both the simulation results and the real data application have shown the similar performance of the pairwise approach and the dimension-wise quadrature with $s = 3$. However, the latter is more advantageous than the pairwise likelihood method, since its implementation is straightforward and does not depend on the specified model. On the other hand, the pairwise approach becomes unfeasible in a longitudinal setting where the latent variable model has more than one factor at each occasion, and the matrix of the factor loadings does not have a simple structure.

Further work needs to be done to corroborate the findings of this study. The properties of the dimension-wise based and pairwise estimators should be investigated and compared theoretically. Furthermore, more efficient versions of the pairwise likelihood estimation based on weighted estimators should be also considered. The real application from the British Household Panel study has shown the potential of the proposed methodologies to the analysis of real data sets. More complex models for the structural part of the model and the inclusion of covariates in the measurement model are useful additions.

References

Bianconcini, S., Cagnone, S., & Rizopoulos, D. (2017). Approximate likelihood inference in generalized linear latent variable models based on the dimension-wise quadrature. *Electronic Journal of Statistics, 11*, 4404–4423.

Cagnone, S., Moustaki, I., & Vasdekis, V. (2009). Latent variable models for multivariate longitudinal ordinal responses. *British Journal of Mathematical and Statistical Psychology, 62*, 401–415.

Cox, D. R., & Reid, N. (2004). A note on pseudolikelihood constructed from marginal densities. *Biometrika, 91*, 729–737.

Dunson, D. (2003). Dynamic latent trait models for multidimensional longitudinal data. *Journal of the American Statistical Association, 98*, 555–563.

Liu, Q., & Pierce, D.A. (1994). A note on Gauss-Hermite quadrature. *Biometrika, 81*, 624–629.

Lindsay, B. (1988). Composite likelihood methods. In N. U. Prabhu (Ed.), *Statistical inference from stochastic processes* (pp. 221–239). Providence: American Mathematical Society.

Huber, P., Ronchetti, E., & Victoria-Feser, M. P. (2004). Estimation of generalized linear latent variable models. *Journal of the Royal Statistical Society, Series B, 66*, 893–908.

Rabe-Hesketh, S., Skrondal, A., & Pickles, A. (2005). Maximum likelihood estimation of limited and discrete dependent variable models with nested random effects. *Journal of Econometrics, 128*, 301–323.
Schilling, S., & Bock, R. D. (2005). High-dimensional maximum marginal likelihood item factor analysis by adaptive quadrature. *Psychometrika, 70*, 533–555
Varin, C., & Vidoni, P. (2005). A note on composite likelihood inference and model selection. *Biometrika, 92*, 519–528.
Vasdekis, V., Cagnone, S., & Moustaki, I. (2012). A pairwise likelihood inference in latent variable models for ordinal longitudinal responses. *Psychometrika, 77*, 425–441.

An Efficient Scheduling Algorithm for Parallel Planar Rotations of Factors

Yiu-Fai Yung and W. Clay Thompson

1 Factor Rotation and Planar Rotations

1.1 General Factor Rotation Problem

A factor analysis postulates a set of latent factors that explains the correlations among a much larger set of observed variables (Harman, 1976; Lawley & Maxwell, 1971). It usually produces an initial factor solution with a set of orthogonal factors that define the factor space. To enhance the interpretability of factors, factor rotation is often applied to the initial solution.

A factor rotation can be described as a process that finds a transformation of the initial pattern matrix **A** to yield a rotated pattern matrix **B** that has a "simple structure"—that is,

$$\mathbf{B} = \mathbf{AT} \tag{1}$$

where **A** and **B** are both $p \times m$ factor pattern matrices for p variables and m factors, and **T** is an $m \times m$ transformation matrix that is chosen to optimize a simplicity function (or criterion). Various definitions of simplicity functions have been proposed. For example, the varimax criterion (Kaiser, 1958) is popular. The generalized Crawford-Ferguson (GCF) family of rotations (Jennrich, 1973, Eq. 48) subsumes varimax, quartimax (see Harman, 1976) and many other rotation criteria as special cases.

Y.-F. Yung (✉) · W. C. Thompson
SAS Institute Inc., Cary, NC, USA
e-mail: Yiu-Fai.Yung@sas.com; Clay.Thompson@sas.com

M. Wiberg et al. (eds.), *Quantitative Psychology*, Springer Proceedings in Mathematics & Statistics 353, https://doi.org/10.1007/978-3-030-74772-5_3

Although closed-form analytic solutions for **T** are available for some classes of rotations (for example, PROMAX, see Hendrickson & White, 1964), they are not available for the GCF family of rotations (and, in particular, the varimax rotation). Rather, the GCF rotations require iterative steps for obtaining an optimal **T**. Theoretically, standard constrained optimization techniques such as Newton-Raphson, conjugate gradient, and so on, can carry out these iterative steps. For example, the gradient projection method (Jennrich, 2001, 2004) is such a method. However, this approach has not been widely used and has been found to be inferior to the planar rotation method (Jennrich, 2001).

1.2 Factor Rotation via Component Planar Rotations

The planar rotation method (see, e.g., Jennrich, 1970) refers to an algorithm that optimizes the simplicities of component factor planes successively in iterative cycles. Each component planar rotation focuses on a specific pair of factors (say, i and j, which are both between 1 and m) and rotates the corresponding (i, j)-plane according to the specified simplicity criterion. Analytic solutions are usually available for rotating a component plane for two factors (Clarkson & Jennrich, 1988). A cycle of the planar orthogonal rotation consists of rotations of all $m(m-1)/2$ distinct component planes. The cycles of planar rotations repeat until the simplicity function value cannot be improved any further (with respect to a prespecified convergence criterion). The final rotated factor pattern is thus obtained by accumulating component planar rotations in cycles.

The remaining of the paper is organized as follows. Section 2 describes the problem of using parallel processing for orthogonal planar rotations. An efficient scheduling algorithm, which is shown to be justified by the theory of 1-factorizations of complete graphs, is proposed for dealing with any numbers of factors and threads for computations. Some properties of the proposed algorithm are discussed. Then, Sect. 3 demonstrates the practical performance of the proposed scheduling algorithm and is followed by some conclusions.

2 Scheduling Parallel Orthogonal Planar Rotations

We limit ourselves to orthogonal planar rotations and use examples to demonstrate the issues associated with scheduling parallel planar rotations. For an orthogonal rotation of six factors, a cycle of component planar rotation maximizes the simplicity of 15 component factor planes in sequence, as depicted schematically by the following list:

```
(2,1)
(3,1),(3,2)
(4,1),(4,2),(4,3)
(5,1),(5,2),(5,3),(5,4)
(6,1),(6,2),(6,3),(6,4),(6,5)
```

After each component planar rotation, the associated pairs of factor columns in the factor pattern matrix would be updated for the next rotation. To the best of our knowledge, all planar rotations in existing factor analysis software are carried out one plane at a time. In contrast, multithreaded computation rotates several factor planes simultaneously to improve efficiency. For example, the (2,1)-plane and the (4–3)-plane can be rotated simultaneously by two processing units or threads.

But to take advantage of parallel processing, one must carefully schedule the component planar rotations in batches to avoid potential conflicts. For example, if the (2,1)-plane is scheduled to be rotated, then no other planes in the same batch of parallel rotations should involve factors 1 or 2 (e.g., (3,1) or (3,2)); otherwise, there would be a conflict in using and updating the same column of the factor pattern matrix.

One approach that could be used to address this issue is resource serialization via semaphores. Each factor is associated with a locking resource that indicates when it is "in use." A list of all possible pairs of factors (planes) is enqueued for processing, and these tasks are dispatched by multiple processing threads. For each plane, the thread must obtain exclusive access to two semaphores (one for each factor), compute the planar rotation, and then release the semaphores. If a semaphore cannot be obtained (because the factor is already in use) a thread can search through the list of planes to find the first available rotation.

To demonstrate the use of semaphores, assume the planar rotations are ordered: (2,1),(3,1),(3,2),(4,1),. . .,(6,1),(6,2),(6,3),(6,4),(6,5). The first processing thread obtains the (2,1) pair. Then second processing thread obtains the (4,3) pair, because this is the next pair in the list for which neither factor is in use. Finally, the third processing thread obtains the (6,5) pair. After this initial batch is complete,[1] the first processing unit obtains the (3,1) pair, while the second processing unit obtains the (4,2) pair. However, the third processing unit must remain idle, because the only remaining pair that can be obtained, (6,5), has already been processed.

[1]When semaphores are used, it is not necessary to synchronize the processing threads into batches. The discussion remains qualitatively accurate as long as the time required for a component planar rotation exceeds the time required to manage the semaphores. This will certainly be the case for large factor patterns.

This processing schedule is summarized by the following schematic:

```
(2,1),(4,3),(6,5)
(3,1),(4,2),idle
(3,2),(4,1),idle
(5,1),(6,2),idle
(5,2),(6,1),idle
(5,3),(6,4),idle
(5,4),(6,3),idle
```

Thus, 7 batches of parallel processes are required to complete a cycle. Because each of the last 6 batches contain an idle thread, this scheduling method does not utilize the computational resources efficiently.

An efficient scheduling method should use the minimum possible number of batches of parallel planar rotations and at the same time satisfies the following two requirements:

Requirement 1. In any given batch of parallel rotations, each component planar rotation should involve distinct factors.

Requirement 2. Each of the component planes is rotated exactly once in a rotation cycle.

The proposed scheduling algorithm, which is described in Sects. 2.2, 2.3, 2.4, and 2.5, satisfies these two requirements by generating an efficient schedule of batches of parallel planar rotations:

```
(6,1),(2,5),(3,4)
(6,2),(3,1),(4,5)
(6,3),(4,2),(5,1)
(6,4),(5,3),(1,2)
(6,5),(1,4),(2,3)
```

The next few sections describe the rationale and the deterministic steps of the proposed scheduling algorithm.

2.1 1-Factorizations of Complete Graphs

This section illustrates the theory behind the proposed scheduling algorithm. The crucial analogy is to a complete (undirected) graph. A complete graph is a graph in which every node is directly connected to every other node by a single edge. To demonstrate, the left panel in Fig. 1 shows a complete graph K_6 with 6 nodes and 15 edges (solid lines).

Consider each factor in a factor solution to be represented by a node in an undirected graph. A pairing of two factors for a planar rotation is represented by

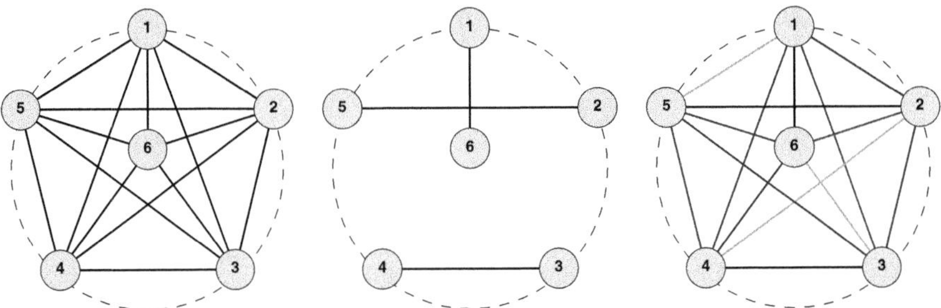

Fig. 1 The complete graph K_6 (left) with a 1-factor (middle) and a 1-factorization (right)

an edge connecting two nodes. Thus the set of all possible pairs of factors for planar rotation is represented by the complete graph. Hence, the complete graph K_6 in Fig. 1 represents all 15 planar rotations for 6 factors in a cycle of iterative rotations.

A subset of these edges can be identified so that every node in the graph is incident to exactly one edge. This is defined as a *1-factor* of a graph. The edges of a 1-factor correspond to a batch of planar rotations that can be computed simultaneously without any risk of resource conflict. For example, the middle panel in Fig. 1 shows a 1-factor, which is associated with a batch of 3 parallel planar rotations. This graph (batch) satisfies **Requirement 1** for scheduling parallel orthogonal planar rotations—that is, because no node in the middle panel is associated with more than one edge, each component planar rotation in this batch involves distinct factors.

Now consider dividing up all the edges of the complete graph into disjoint 1-factors. Such a decomposition is called a 1-factorization. For example, by mentally rotating the edges of the middle panel in Fig. 1 about the center repeatedly generates a 1-factorization that is shown as an edge-coloring of K_6 in the right panel of Fig. 1. This 1-factorization corresponds to 5 color-coded batches of parallel rotations of component planes for 6 factors.

Clearly, the right panel of Fig. 1 has the same number of distinct edges as the left panel—both are complete graphs that represent all 15 component planar rotations in a rotation cycle. Hence, the right panel satisfies **Requirement 2** for scheduling parallel orthogonal planar rotations—that is, each of the 15 component planes is rotated exactly once in a rotation cycle. In addition, similar to what has been explained for the middle panel that represents a single batch of parallel rotations, each of the 5 color-coded batches (1-factors) in the right panel also satisfies **Requirement 1**.

Essentially, the 1-factorization of a complete graph (Trick, 2004) just illustrated in the right panel of Fig. 1 represents the batches of parallel rotations of the proposed scheduling algorithm. For theoretical details of complete graphs, see Suksompong (2016), Trick (2004), and the references therein. Sections 2.2, , 2.3, 2.4, and 2.5 describe the deterministic steps of the proposed scheduling algorithm.

2.2 The Proposed Scheduling Algorithm

Without loss of generality, assume that a factor solution contains an even number of factors, $m = 2r$. If it does not, then a single 'dummy factor' can be added. In addition, suppose for the moment that r processing threads are available for parallel planar rotations. Cases for an odd number of factors and different number of processing threads are covered in Sects. 2.3, 2.4, and 2.5.

The first batch of parallel rotations consists of the planes

$$(2r, 1), (2, 2r - 1), (3, 2r - 2), \ldots, (r, r + 1). \tag{2}$$

To obtain the next batch of planes for parallel rotations,

1. Replace $2r - 1$ with 0
2. Add 1 (mod $2r - 1$) to each index except $2r$.

This process is repeated until $2r - 1$ batches of parallel planar rotation have been created.

The scheduling algorithm proposed here is considered to be an adaptation from the theory of 1-factorizations of complete graphs, which is discussed in Sect. 2.1. For the 6-factor ($m = 6, r = 3$) example in Sect. 2, we apply the proposed algorithm to obtain those 5 ($2r - 1$) batches of parallel rotations that complete a cycle of planar rotations efficiently.

Define $s = m/2$ if the number of factors, m, is even and $s = (m - 1)/2$ if m is odd. The next three sections extend the algorithm to different cases:

- More than s processing threads
- Less than s processing threads
- m being an odd number

2.3 Case with More Than s Processing Threads

Theoretically, the maximum number of processing threads that you can use to gain computational advantage is s. Even if there are more than s processing threads available for use, the proposed scheduling algorithm should still use only s threads.

The reason is that s is the maximum number of planes that can be constructed from m factors such that each plane involves two *distinct* factors. Adding more planes beyond s is necessarily a violation of **Requirement 1**.

2.4 Case with Less than s Processing Threads

With q ($q < s$) processing threads for parallel rotations, the proposed algorithm begins with the schedule for s threads. The component pairs are then grouped (in reading order) into batches of size q. The number of batches needed for completing a cycle of rotation is $m(m-1)/(2q)$ if this quotient is a whole number and $\lfloor m(m-1)/(2q)\rfloor+1$ otherwise.

This case is best illustrated by using the 6-factor example with 2 processing threads. The algorithm begins with the same table of pairings as seen previously. It then forms 8 (= $\lfloor 6\times5/(2\times2)\rfloor+1$) batches of parallel rotations of 2 independent factor planes:

```
(6,1),(2,5)
(3,4),(6,2)
(3,1),(4,5)
(6,3),(4,2)
(5,1),(6,4)
(5,3),(1,2)
(6,5),(1,4)
(2,3),idle
```

An idle component rotation is appended at the last batch. Both **Requirements 1** and **2** are still satisfied.

2.5 *Case with an Odd Number of Factors*

For cases with an odd number of factors (m), a dummy factor denoted by an asterisk (*) is added to make the total number of factors even. The batches of parallel rotations are first constructed as usual with $(m+1)/2$ threads. Once the sequence of component planar rotations is determined, those pairs with the dummy factor are ignored. Then the sequence of planar rotations can be fed to any number of threads that is strictly less than $(m+1)/2$.

For example, for an orthogonal rotation with 7 factors, an 8-factor scheduling for 4 threads is first constructed as in the following:

```
(*,1),(2,7),(3,6),(4,5)
(*,2),(3,1),(4,7),(5,6)
(*,3),(4,2),(5,1),(6,7)
(*,4),(5,3),(6,2),(7,1)
(*,5),(6,4),(7,3),(1,2)
(*,6),(7,5),(1,4),(2,3)
(*,7),(1,6),(2,5),(3,4)
```

The first column involves dummy factors and therefore is ignored. The resultant scheduling is immediately applicable to a parallel rotation with 3 threads (or more). For cases with fewer than 3 threads, apply the serialization method described in Sect. 2.4. Both **Requirements 1** and **2** would still be satisfied.

2.6 Practical Considerations

In practice, the proposed scheduling algorithm will not improve computational efficiency linearly in the number of threads. There are two main reasons for this. First, the management of parallel computations, which includes distribution of tasks, integration of results, and memory management in threads, can offset parts of the advantage of parallel rotations. When the number of factors or variables is small, parallel rotations might not improve and might even degrade computational performance. Second, because the integration of component rotation results must be done after all threads finish, the computing time to finish a batch of parallel rotations is determined by the slowest thread.

3 Simulated and Real Examples

3.1 A Simulated Text Mining Example

A motivation of the current research was to meet the challenge of a simulated text mining problem raised by our colleague. The rotation problem involved 155,467 features (variables) and 300 topics (factors), which is not atypical in the field of text mining.

Table 1 shows the computing time to finish a varimax rotation of a factor pattern for different numbers of threads. A Unix machine was used for computations (in February 2020) and the FACTOR procedure of SAS/STAT (SAS Institute Inc, 2018) was used for factor rotation. Because the same sequence of component planar rotations in cycles was used in all threaded conditions (including the 1-thread condition), all consumed 102 cycles of planar rotations to converge to the same result.

Under the single-thread condition, which represents the traditional application of the planar rotation algorithm without threading, the computing time (real or CPU) was about 5 h. With the proposed scheduling algorithm for parallel rotations, the real time reduced approximately by half with 4 or 8 threads. Therefore, while it is a notable performance improvement, the improvement is clearly not linear in the number of threads.

Note that the CPU time was calculated by adding up the computing time in threads in which parallel computations were carried out. Thus, the CPU time was usually greater than that of the corresponding real time in the multithreading conditions.

Table 1 Computing time for varimax rotation of a large factor pattern matrix

	1-Thread	4-Thread	8-Thread
Real time	4 h 57 m 28 s	2 h 26 m 17 s	2 h 17 m 58 s
CPU time	4 h 58 m 24 s	5 h 40 m 07 s	6 h 25 m 13 s

3.2 A Real Data Example About Human Activity Recognition by Smartphones

Anguita, Ghio, Oneto, Parra, and Reyes-Ortiz (2013) collected data about human activity recognized by using smartphones. Combining the training and test samples, the data set contains 10,299 observations and 563 variables, measured or transformed, for measuring movements. The data were factor-analyzed under 12 levels of threading (1–12), with the proposed scheduling algorithm for parallel factor rotations. The following conditions were also included:

- Number of factors (4 levels): 65, 81, 104, and 124, which were determined by using the following factor extraction criteria, respectively: 90% common variance explained, MAP-2 (Minimum average partial with second power; see Glorfeld, 1995; Horn, 1965), 95% common variance explained, and MAP-4.
- Rotation criterion (2 levels): quartimax and varimax.

The MAP-2 and MAP-4 criteria explain, respectively, 92% and 97% of common variance. The real time for completing factor rotations in various conditions was recorded. To average out random computational noise, the computing time reported here was an average of 10 trials. A Unix machine with six physical cores was used to carry out all computations (in February 2020) and the FACTOR procedure of SAS/STAT (SAS Institute Inc, 2018) was used for factor extraction and rotation.

To make the threading conditions comparable, the single-threaded rotations used the same component planar rotation sequence as that of the multithreaded rotations. Consequently, given the same number of factors and the same rotation criterion, the numbers of cycles to achieve rotational convergence with different numbers of threads were the same. For the quartimax rotation, 51, 50, 92, and 34 cycles, respectively, were used for 65, 81, 104, and 124 factors. For the varimax rotation, 58, 40, 37, and 23 cycles, respectively, were used for 65, 81, 104, and 124 factors.

Figure 2 shows four plots of rotation time for different numbers of factors. Within each plot, curves for varimax and quartimax rotations across different number of threads are shown. A very clear pattern is shown in all curves. Parallel rotations with multithreading reduce the computing time more dramatically with 2 or 3 threads. However, after 4 or 5 threads, the curves flatten out, showing no additional improvement of computational performance.

4 Conclusions

The proposed scheduling algorithm enables parallel planar rotations of factors. Theoretically, it allows for a *performance improvement that is linear in the size of the matrix to be rotated*, up to a maximum improvement of $\lfloor m/2 \rfloor$-fold. Practically, performance is also determined by other factors so that linear improvement cannot be expected.

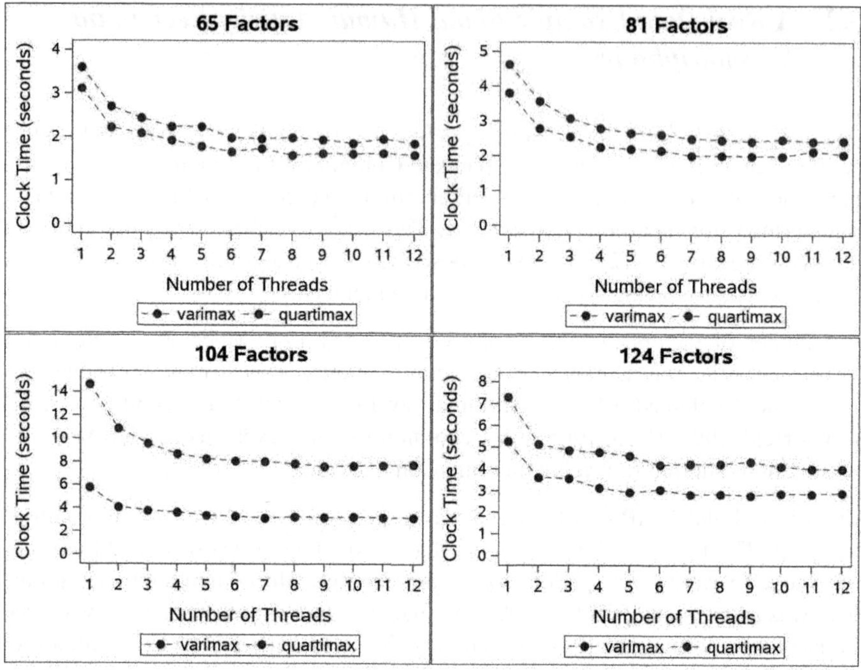

Fig. 2 Computing time for factor rotations

So far, only orthogonal rotation was discussed. Oblique rotation requires a few minor additions to the algorithm. First, oblique rotation requires planar rotations over all *ordered* pairs of factors. This can be accomplished by generating batches of parallel planar rotations exactly as described above, then repeating the batches with the factor orderings reversed (i.e., (i, j) becomes (j, i)). Also, after each batch of oblique rotations, the factor covariance matrix must be updated (Clarkson & Jennrich, 1988).

Rotation of dimensions has not only been used in factor analysis, but it has also been used for rotating components in principal component analysis, canonical variates in canonical correlation analysis, and topics in text analytics. Therefore, the proposed scheduling algorithm applies directly to these areas too.

References

Anguita, D., Ghio, A., Oneto, L., Parra, X., & Reyes-Ortiz, J. L. (2013). A public domain dataset for human activity recognition using smartphones. In *21th European symposium on artificial neural networks, computational intelligence and machine learning, ESANN 2013*, Bruges, 24–26 Apr.

Clarkson, D. B., & Jennrich, R. I. (1988). Quartic rotation criteria and algorithms. *Psychometrika, 53*, 251–259. https://doi.org/10.1007/BF02294136

Glorfeld, L. W. (1995). An improvement on horn's parallel analysis methodology for selecting the correct number of factors to retain. *Educational and Psychological Measurement, 55*, 377–393. https://doi.org/10.1177/0013164495055003002

Harman, H. H. (1976). *Modern factor analysis* (3rd ed.). Chicago: University of Chicago Press.

Hendrickson, A. E., & White, P. O. (1964). Promax: A quick method for rotation to oblique simple structure. *British Journal of Statistical Psychology, 17*, 65–70. https://doi.org/10.1111/j.2044-8317.1964.tb00244.x

Horn, J. L. (1965). A rationale and test for the number of factors in factor analysis. *Psychometrika, 30*, 179–185. https://doi.org/10.1007/BF02289447

Jennrich, R. I. (1970). Orthogonal rotation algorithms. *Psychometrika, 35*, 229–235. https://doi.org/10.1007/BF02291264

Jennrich, R. I. (1973). Standard errors for obliquely rotated factor loadings. *Psychometrika, 38*, 593–604. https://doi.org/10.1007/BF02291497

Jennrich, R. I. (2001). A simple general procedure for orthogonal rotation. *Psychometrika, 66*, 289–306. https://doi.org/10.1007/BF02294840

Jennrich, R. I. (2004). Derivative free gradient projection algorithms for rotation. *Psychometrika, 69*, 475–480. https://doi.org/10.1007/BF02295647

Kaiser, H. F. (1958). The varimax criterion for analytic rotation of factor analysis. *Psychometrika, 23*, 187–200. https://doi.org/10.1007/BF02289233

Lawley, D., & Maxwell, A. (1971). *Factor analysis as a statistical method* (2nd ed.). New York: American Elsevier Publishing Company, Inc.

SAS Institute Inc. (2018). *SAS/STAT 15.1 user's guide*. Cary, NC: Author.

Suksompong, W. (2016). Scheduling asynchronous round-robin tournaments. *Operations Research Letters, 44*, 96–100. https://doi.org/10.1016/j.orl.2015.12.008

Trick, M. (2004). Scheduling court-constrained sports tournaments. In *Fifth Conference on the Practice and Theory of Automated Timetabling*. http://www.patatconference.org/patat2004/proceedings/371.pdf

Explanatory Response Time Models

Daniella Rebouças-Ju and Ying Cheng

1 Introduction

Response times have recently grown in popularity in educational assessment and, to a lesser degree, in the psychological assessment context. Psychological testing can provide a deeper understanding of one's profile as well as a diagnosis to a pathology. Hence, in low-stakes as well as high-stakes contexts, those diagnoses are given in part based on the individual's self-report item response data. In those instances, data quality assurance and methods to detect aberrant response behavior become essential to the validity of scores and consequently, of the diagnosis.

Additionally, response times (e.g., total or per page) have been proposed as an alternative source that can be used to detect careless response behavior (Meade & Craig, 2012). Understanding the underlying mechanisms that affect one's working speed, whether due to person's or to item's characteristics, is a crucial step to obtain precise estimates of the working speed and allow further application of response time modeling, such as methods to flag aberrant response behavior (e.g., Hong et al., 2021).

In the psychological assessment context, there may a relationship between how quickly the individual works through the survey, that is, their *working speed*, and some item or person characteristics. From the subject's side, response times may depend on the participant's reading ability, processing speed, experience with computerized surveys, etc. On the item's side, there are likely differences, for instance, due to the sentiment of the item (e.g. reverse-coded or negatively worded items).

D. Rebouças-Ju (✉) · Y. Cheng
University of Notre Dame, Notre Dame, IN, USA
e-mail: drebouca@alumni.nd.edu

M. Wiberg et al. (eds.), *Quantitative Psychology*, Springer Proceedings in Mathematics & Statistics 353, https://doi.org/10.1007/978-3-030-74772-5_4

Given the relations between response times and person and item characteristics, and the work previously developed in the field of explanatory item response theory (De Boeck et al., 2011, 2016), in this study, we propose an explanatory framework for modeling response times, where either person or item properties may be used as covariates in a model predicting response times at the item level.

2 Explanatory Response Time Models

2.1 Descriptive-Only Response Time Model

Let t_{ip} be the item response times given by person p, with $p = 1, ..., N$, to item i, with $i = 1, ..., M$. The log-transformed response times are modeled as follows:

$$\ln t_{ip} = \beta_i - \tau_p + \varepsilon_{ip}, \tag{1}$$

$$\tau_p \sim N(0, \sigma_\tau^2), \text{ and } \varepsilon_{ip} \sim N(0, \sigma_\varepsilon^2), \tag{2}$$

where τ_p is the *working speed* a respondent exhibits during the course of the assessment, β_i is the *time-intensity* parameter corresponding to the consumption of time by item i, and ε_{ip} is the measurement error for person p and item i with (homogeneous) variance σ_ε^2. Note that this model is a simplified version of the lognormal model (van der Linden, 2006), where the time discrimination parameters are all fixed equal to $1/\sigma_\varepsilon^2$.

In terms of a mixed-effects model, the model in Equation 1 is a random intercept-only model with indicator variables X_{ik} for K covariates, with $k = 1, ..., K$:

$$\ln t_{ip} = \tau_{p0} X_{i0} + \Sigma_{k=1}^{K} \beta_i X_{ik} + \varepsilon_{ip}, \tag{3}$$

where $X_{i0} = -1$ for all items. $X_{ik} = 1$ if $i = k$, and $X_{ik} = 0$ otherwise, with $K = M$, that is, there are as many indicators as the number of items. In this model, τ_{p0} is a random effect with $\tau_{p0} \sim N(0, \sigma_\tau^2)$ and the β_i's are fixed effects. Thus, each subject has its own intercept, but the slopes (item parameters) are the same for all subjects.

2.2 Person-Explanatory Response Time Model

The person-explanatory model includes predictors of person properties, which may account for differences in response times given, for example, biological sex, ethnic/racial groups, or response styles. Following the descriptive model defined in Equation 1 and considering J person predictors Z_{pj}, $j = 1, ..., J$, the person-explanatory response time model is

$$\ln t_{ip} = \beta_i - \tau_{p0} + \varepsilon_{ip}, \ \varepsilon_{ip} \sim N(0, \sigma_\epsilon^2) \quad (4)$$

$$\text{with } \tau_{p0} = \Sigma_{j=1}^J \eta_j Z_{pj} + \delta_p, \ \ \delta_p \sim N(0, \sigma_\delta^2), \quad (5)$$

where η_j are the fixed effects for each person covariate, σ_δ^2 is the person-specific residual variance, and σ_ε^2 is the residual variance. This is a *latent regression model*, where the random intercepts τ_{p0} are partly random and partly predicted by person properties. Note that the descriptive model is recovered if $\eta_1 = \eta_2 = ... = \eta_J = 0$, and therefore $\sigma_\delta^2 = \sigma_\tau^2$.

Similarly to the descriptive-only model, the person-explanatory response time model can be expressed in the framework of a mixed-effects model, with Z_{pj} as level-2 predictors, and σ_δ^2 as the between-person variance.

2.3 Item-Explanatory Response Time Model

Following the parameters defined in Equation 1 and considering K predictors of the item parameters, the item-explanatory response time model is

$$\ln t_{ip} = \beta_i' - \tau_p + \varepsilon_{ip}, \quad \varepsilon_{ip} \sim N(0, \sigma_\epsilon^2), \quad (6)$$

$$\tau_p \sim N(0, \sigma_\tau^2), \quad (7)$$

$$\text{and } \beta_i' = \Sigma_{k=1}^K \gamma_k X_{ik} + \zeta_i, \text{ with } \zeta_i \sim N(0, \sigma_\zeta^2), \quad (8)$$

where γ_k are the fixed effects for each item covariate. Thus the item parameters' expected value corresponds to the part of Equation 8 with the item predictors, while some error is allowed in the prediction.

Just as before, this model can be expressed in the framework of a mixed-effects model. The item-explanatory model is a multilevel model with two levels, where the item parameters are predicted by a set of K, $K < M$, covariates:

$$\ln t_{ip} = \tau_p X_{i0} + \beta_i' + \varepsilon_{ip}, \text{ with } \beta_i' = \Sigma_{k=1}^K \gamma_k X_{ik} + \zeta_i, \quad (9)$$

where $X_{i0} = -1$ for all items, X_{ik} are the covariates predictors of item properties, with ζ_i as the errors in such a prediction. Note that the latent working speed is a random effect, as well as β_i' are random effects that account for between-item variability.

Model Estimation. The model parameters can be estimated through a restricted maximum likelihood (REML) approach (Verbeke & Molenberghs, 2001). An alternate choice is to estimate the models in a Bayesian framework (van der Linden, 2006). For the sake of simplicity, we will use a frequentist approach in this study.

Model Comparison. Model fit indices will be used for the purposes of model comparison. For comparing the descriptive and the person-explanatory model, we will also use the likelihood-ratio test (LRT). Because the descriptive-only and item-explanatory models are not nested, the LRT is not appropriate in that case. The traditional AIC and BIC measures may be used for comparison of non-nested models, but they are not appropriate for mixed-effects models. Therefore, for comparison between the descriptive and the person-explanatory models we will use the conditional AIC (cAIC; Vaida & Blanchard, 2005; Säfken et al., 2018), which is recommended when the focus of comparison is on the clusters (persons), and the degrees of freedom are adjusted for a finite sample. In addition, we will use the adjusted BIC (aBIC; Cho & De Boeck, 2018; Delattre et al., 2014), where the number of observations is equal to the number of subjects (N), since the models have only person-related random effects. For comparison between the descriptive and the item-explanatory models, we will use the marginal AIC (mAIC; Vaida & Blanchard, 2005), which is recommended when the focus of comparison is on the population, and the aBIC, where the number of observations for the item-explanatory model is equal to the number of subjects times the number of items (NM), since the model has both item- and person-related random effects.

In the next section, we present a motivating example for the use of the person-explanatory and the item-explanatory models.

3 Real Data Example

We apply the descriptive-only, the person- and the item-explanatory response time models to a sample of high school students responding to the second Big-Five Inventory (BFI-2) of personality (Soto & John, 2017). Students in this sample ranged from ages 16 to 18, and were asked to fill the survey on a desktop computer in class or on a tablet/smartphone at home. Demographic background questions were asked at an earlier point of data collection, including questions about biological sex, ethnicity/race, school membership, etc. For the purposes of this illustration, we excluded a respondent's data if their data were missing for any item's response times or for the predictors' data. The final sample size was $N = 205$, with about 50% of the sample Female.

Time stamps for each selected answer as well as item order presented and observed were recorded at the item level. These time stamps were converted into response times by recording the elapsed time between two response selections. Note that students were allowed to change their answer selection if they changed their mind, for example, from "Strongly Agree" to simply "Agree." If there were any answer changes, the response times associated with that item were summed up to report one observed response time per item for each person.

All models were fit using the function `lmer` from the package `lme4` (Bates et al., 2015) in R (R Core Team, 2020). The estimates were obtained using REML.

3.1 Descriptive-Only Model

The descriptive model included one fixed effect for each item on the questionnaire, for a total of 60 item effects β_i, and one random effect, that is, variance term for person σ_τ^2, and the residual variance σ_ε^2.

3.2 Person-Explanatory Model and Covariates

We first fit the person-explanatory model with several predictors: biological sex, free/reduced-lunch status, device (desktop or mobile), and some process data such as number of clicks on a page, and similarity measures QSI and normalized length of longest common sub-sequence (NLLCS). Similarity measures are used to express the distance between the expected and the observed responses of text data. See Table 1 for snippets of answers and the respective similarity measures.

The first measure is $QSI = expected \# \ of \ clicks/observed \# \ of \ clicks$, and it ranges from 0 to 1. A score of 1 indicates (a) the student answered the items on the same order they were presented, *and* (b) no answer selection was changed. A score <1 indicates that the respondent answered at least one question out of order (e.g., answered a later question first and then returned to answer that question), or that, for at least one item, their selected answer was changed. The first property can be an indication of careless responding, especially if it happens often, while the second cannot. In fact, the second property could be an indication that the student is engaged in the survey to the point of weighing their options and possibly changing their minds later on.

QSI was affected more by changes to answer choices than by compliance with item order. Thus QSI can be interpreted as an "answer efficiency" measure, where the most efficient respondents select their answer and do not feel the need to change it later on in the survey.

Table 1 Snippets of the observed and expected order of example responses. In **bold**, responses that are out of order or changes in the selected answer. The last column presents percentile ranks for total response times

	Type	Sequence	QSI	NLLCS	% rank
Ex.1	Observed	c4,e1,**c6,a6,a2,e4**,c3,c2,o6,n4,o1,**o4,a3,a3**,...	0.85	0.85	48.8th
	Expected	c4,e1,c3,c6,a6,a2,e4,[o5],a3,o4,c2,o6,n4,o1,...			
Ex.2	Observed	a4,n6,**e1,e1**,a1,**n4,n4,n4**,a3,c5,**o6,o6,e5,e5**,...	0.73	1.00	31.7th
	Expected	a4,n6,e1,a1,n4,a3,c5,o6,e5,...			

The second similarity measure is NLLCS, a normalized value of the LLCS, that is $NLLCS = LLCS/total\ \#\ of\ items\ on\ the\ survey$. The length of the longest common sub-sequence is a measure of how close one's response sequence is to the expected sequence. Thus, it indicates how compliant one is with the item order. This normalized measure also varies within the [0,1] interval. A score of 1 indicates the person complied with the order of the items fully, while a score <1 indicates that they did not follow the order of the items for at least one of the items. Note that they may have also changed their answers to an item, but this does not affect the NLLCS. Thus NLLCS may be interpreted as a "compliance" measure.

Given the different characteristics between QSI and NLLCS, both measures were considered at first. However, the correlation between the two similarity measures was 0.79. With some evidence of multi-collinearity, the final person-explanatory model included only biological sex and NLLCS as predictors, which had a correlation of only −0.13. There was a total of 62 fixed effects. Note that the estimated item parameters have a different interpretation when the person-explanatory model is fit, but can be recovered by adding the average values of the predictors multiplied by the estimated fixed effects.

3.3 Item-Explanatory Model and Covariates

The item-explanatory model had the number of characters in the item statement ("Char. Count") and an indicator for "Reverse-Coded" items as fixed effects. The working speed parameter is a random effect centered around 0, and we estimate variance parameters for working speed τ and the error term ε.

3.4 Model Estimation Results

Fixed Effects. Fixed effects for the descriptive models' item parameters had a mean of 1 and standard deviation of 0.15. Due to space limitations, item parameter estimates are not reported here, but can be requested from the authors. The fixed effects for the person and item properties are presented on Table 2.

The person predictors are multiplied by a factor of −1 to conform to the model's parametrization and interpretation of τ_p as a person's working speed. The estimated effects were 0.144 for Males and −0.735 for NLLCS. Thus, if the student is Male, there is an increase in working speed; that is, Male students tend to work faster through the survey than their Female counterparts.

Additionally, there is a negative relationship between NLLCS and working speed. Thus low NLLCS scores are associated with an increase in working speed. Hence, the degree students *do not* comply with the item order are associated with working faster through the survey, after the person's intrinsic working speed has

Table 2 Estimated fixed effects for the explanatory models

Person-explanatory			
	Estimate	Std. error	Z value
Biological sex (male)	0.144	0.068	2.101
NLLCS	−0.735	0.366	−2.008
Item-explanatory			
	Estimate	Std. error	Z value
(Intercept)	0.672	0.057	11.732
Char. Count	0.010	0.001	7.355
Reverse-Coded	0.134	0.025	5.344

Table 3 Estimated standard deviations for descriptive-only, person-explanatory, and item-explanatory models

Parameter	Name	Descriptive	Person expl.	Item expl.
σ_ε	Residual	0.715	0.715	0.715
σ_τ	Working speed	0.485	0.476	0.485
σ_ζ	Item			0.101

been taken into account. Thus, NLLCS seems to indicate that students who are not complying with item order may be working more quickly, thus spending less time on the survey, likely due to a lack of engagement with the survey.

The estimated fixed effects for item properties in the item-explanatory model are 0.010 for "Char. Count", and 0.134 for "Reverse-coded" items. Note that the effect size for "Char. Count" is large due to its very small standard error. Thus, as expected, items with a larger number of characters require longer times to be answered. Interestingly, reverse-coded items seem to yield longer response time than regular items.

Random Effects. Estimated random effects are reported on Table 3. The standard deviation for working speed (i.e., between-person variability) was 0.485 for the descriptive-only model and the item-explanatory model, and 0.476 for the person-explanatory model. The residual standard deviation was about 0.715 for all models. The difference in estimated between-person variability between the descriptive and the explanatory models indicates that person properties accounted for some (small) portion of the variability in working speed. Finally, the between-item standard deviation was 0.101 for the item-explanatory model.

Model Comparison. Results are reported on Table 4. Given the descriptive-only and the person-explanatory models are nested, we perform a likelihood-ratio test (LRT). The LRT produces a p-value <0.01 in favor of the person-explanatory model. The cAIC is smaller for the person-explanatory model, while aBIC is smaller for the descriptive model. Note that the descriptive model is the model with the smaller number of parameters. Similarly, the descriptive-only and the item-explanatory models are compared using mAIC and aBIC statistics (Table 5). The comparisons

Table 4 Model comparison: LRT and fit indices cAIC and aBIC for the descriptive-only and the person-explanatory response time models

Model	# param.	cAIC	aBIC	*log-lik*	Deviance	χ^2	df	p-value
Descriptive	62	26,919.0	**27,863.7**	−13,644	27,288			
Person expl.	64	**26,918.8**	27,868.5	−13,639	27,278	9.664	2	0.008

Table 5 Model comparison: fit indices mAIC and aBIC for the descriptive-only and the item-explanatory response time models

Model	# param.	mAIC	aBIC
Descriptive	62	29,050.7	28,836.8
Item expl.	6	**28,967.0**	**28,471.7**

favor the item-explanatory model with both mAIC and aBIC. In this case, the item-explanatory model is the model with the smaller number of parameters.

4 Simulation

We perform a simulation study to evaluate (a) sample size and effect size requirements for parameter recovery under the true model, (b) model fit comparison between the explanatory and the descriptive models, when the person-explanatory or the item-explanatory model is the true model.

4.1 Simulation Design

The data generating processes are summarized on Table 6 and are described in detail in this section. We generate response time data while varying sample size $N = 200, 500, 1000$, and the number of items $M = 20, 40, 60$. Each simulation condition was replicated 100 times.

Person-Explanatory Model. When the person-explanatory model is the true model, we assume that a person's working speed is partly random, with a between-person error term, and partly predicted by two covariates. The first predictor, Z_1, is a continuous, Beta-distributed variable with values in [0, 1], and parameters $\alpha = 15$ and $\beta = 3$. The expected value of Z_1 is 0.83, and its standard deviation is 0.08. Z_1 was generated to replicate the behavior of a normalized LLCS variable, as described in the real data example. The second predictor, Z_2, is a categorical, Bernoulli-distributed variable of values 0 or 1 and with a probability of success $p = 1/2$. Z_2 was generated to mimic the "Biological Sex" variable, where 50% of the population is expected to be Female. The fixed effects for each covariate are $\eta_1 = -0.73$ and $\eta_2 = 0.14$. The other item effects are randomly generated from $N(1, 0.15)$. Finally,

Table 6 Data generating processes when the person-explanatory (on the left) or the item-explanatory model (on the right) is the true model

Person-explanatory model		*Item-explanatory model*	
Random effects		Random effects	
τ_p	$N(0, \sigma_\tau^2 = 0.5^2)$	τ_p	$N(0, \sigma_\tau^2 = 0.5^2)$
ε_{ip}	$N(0, \sigma_\epsilon^2 = 0.7^2)$	ε_{ip}	$N(0, \sigma_\epsilon^2 = 0.7^2)$
		ζ_i	$N(0, \sigma_\zeta^2 = 0.1^2)$
Fixed effects		Fixed effects	
η_1	-0.73	γ_1	0.01
η_2	0.14	γ_2	0.65
Observed variables		Observed variables	
Z_1	$Beta(15, 3)$	X_1	$N(30, 8.5^2)$
Z_2	$Bernoulli(0.5)$	X_2	$Bernoulli(0.5)$

the random effects are the between-person error, $\delta_p \sim N(0, \sigma_\tau^2 = 0.5^2)$, and the measurement error $\varepsilon_{ip} \sim N(0, \sigma_\varepsilon^2 = 0.7^2)$. A total of $M + 2$ fixed effects and two variances (one random effect) are estimated.

Item-Explanatory Model. We assume that the item parameters β_i' are predicted by two covariates. The first predictor, X_1, is a continuous variable generated from $N(30, 8.5^2)$, and the second predictor, X_2, is a Bernoulli-distributed variable with probability of success $p = 1/2$. The fixed effects related to each predictor are $\gamma_1 = 0.01$ and $\gamma_2 = 0.65$. As described in Equation 8, the item parameters are treated as a random effect. We generate the item error term as $\zeta_i \sim N(0, \sigma_\zeta^2 = 0.1^2)$. The person and error terms are generated the same as before. A total of three variances and two fixed effects are estimated for the item-explanatory model.

Parameter Recovery. Assuming either the person-explanatory or the item-explanatory model generates the data, we evaluate bias, and the root mean squared error (RMSE) of the variances, and the fixed effects associated with each true model.

Model Comparison. We evaluate model fit between the descriptive-only and the explanatory response time models using cAIC, mAIC, and aBIC.

4.2 Simulation Results

Random effects were recovered around the true value on average and revealed good parameter estimation precision across all simulation conditions. Just as expected, RMSE became smaller as sample size and test length increased. The fixed effects were mostly unbiased. However, they had a somewhat large RMSE for the person-explanatory model, which decreased as sample sizes increased (Tables 7 and 8).

Average rates for the difference in modified fit indices between the explanatory and the descriptive models are reported on Table 9 for when the true model is the

Table 7 Simulation: average bias and RMSE for standard deviation and covariates effects for the person-explanatory model

		σ_τ		σ_ε		η_1		η_2	
N	M	Bias	RMSE	Bias	RMSE	Bias	RMSE	Bias	RMSE
200	20	−0.0014	0.021	−0.0021	0.007	−0.0088	0.364	−0.0109	0.062
	40	−0.0018	0.021	0.0005	0.005	−0.0584	0.348	−0.0054	0.054
	60	−0.0020	0.021	−0.0005	0.003	−0.0916	0.360	0.0084	0.055
500	20	−0.0007	0.014	0.0002	0.003	−0.0211	0.213	0.0012	0.036
	40	0.0012	0.013	0.0001	0.003	0.0151	0.209	0.0045	0.033
	60	0.0015	0.013	0.0002	0.002	−0.0176	0.190	0.0032	0.036
1000	20	0.0002	0.010	0.0002	0.003	−0.0149	0.148	0.0022	0.029
	40	−0.0015	0.009	0.0001	0.002	−0.0034	0.152	0.0000	0.025
	60	0.0011	0.009	−0.0002	0.002	0.0031	0.147	−0.0037	0.026

Table 8 Simulation: average bias and RMSE for standard deviation and covariates effects for the item-explanatory model

		σ_ζ		σ_τ		σ_ε		γ_1		γ_2	
N	M	Bias	RMSE	Bias	RMSE	Bias	RMSE	Bias	RMSE	Bias	RMSE
200	20	−0.0060	0.018	0.0000	0.022	−0.0026	0.007	0.0000	0.001	−0.0111	0.047
	40	−0.0024	0.012	−0.0055	0.020	−0.0006	0.005	−0.0002	0.001	0.0047	0.029
	60	−0.0003	0.008	0.0032	0.017	−0.0007	0.003	0.0000	0.001	0.0050	0.023
500	20	0.0001	0.014	0.0026	0.014	−0.0009	0.004	0.0000	0.001	0.0017	0.044
	40	−0.0011	0.009	0.0010	0.015	0.0007	0.003	0.0000	0.001	−0.0012	0.027
	60	0.0013	0.008	0.0045	0.013	0.0006	0.003	0.0002	0.001	−0.0056	0.023
1000	20	−0.0009	0.015	−0.0037	0.010	0.0001	0.003	−0.0001	0.001	0.0091	0.038
	40	−0.0030	0.011	−0.0011	0.010	0.0003	0.002	0.0000	0.001	−0.0053	0.025
	60	−0.0007	0.007	−0.0003	0.011	0.0002	0.001	0.0001	0.001	−0.0062	0.022

Table 9 Simulation: average difference in modified AIC and BIC measures between the explanatory and the descriptive model, and the power of selecting the explanatory over the descriptive model

Descriptive vs. person-explanatory				
	$cAIC$		$aBIC$	
N	Diff.	Power	Diff.	Power
200	0.388	0.80	−1.850	0.32
500	1.090	0.96	4.091	0.68
1000	2.485	1.00	18.701	0.96
Descriptive vs. item-explanatory				
	$mAIC$		$aBIC$	
N	Diff.	Power	Diff.	Power
200	17.164	1.00	96.257	1.00
500	15.591	1.00	110.261	1.00
1000	15.511	1.00	121.964	1.00

person-explanatory model or the item-explanatory model. Due to space limitations, only results for $M = 20$ are shown. Preliminary results show that, on average, the mAIC and the cAIC favored the explanatory over the descriptive model. Power was high for both the person- and the item-explanatory model cases. The aBIC was a more conservative statistic than the cAIC, with low power for rates for small sample sizes ($N = 200$) but increasing with sample size. The cAIC increased in magnitude with increasing sample sizes, however the opposite trend was observed for the mAIC. This indicates that the mAIC may not be an appropriate measure for model comparison when the number of random effects differs between models.

5 Discussion

Understanding the sources of variability in response times is an essential step for differentiating between expected and aberrant response behavior. We propose an explanatory approach for response time modeling of psychological survey data, and demonstrate how one may use such a framework to gain insight into the relations between response times and person/item characteristics. Through a simulation study, we successfully recovered model parameters under varying sample size and test length conditions.

The person-explanatory model helps us explain the between-person variability, which was predicted by the random intercept after taking item effects into account. On the other hand, the item-explanatory model enabled us to explain item variability from item properties, and to obtain a simpler, more interpretable model than the descriptive one. In the real data analysis, the cAIC favored the person-explanatory model, but the aBIC favored the descriptive model. Given the simulation study results, where the aBIC had low power for small samples, the contradicting real data analysis results may be due to the small sample size ($N \approx 200$).

This study has some limitations. First, the descriptive model used in this study was a simplified version of the lognormal model (van der Linden, 2006), and it did not allow the items to have different variances. Our data suggests some items or groups of items could have different variability with respect to response times; thus, in the future, a model without such a constraint would be appropriate. Second, the similarity measure NLLCS is a proportion, which, due to the range restriction, may not be appropriate as a predictor in a linear regression model (Piepel, 2020). Therefore, alternative approaches should be considered. Third, in the simulation study comparing the descriptive and the item-explanatory models, the power of both mAIC and aBIC were equal to 1, thus a study of the false positive rates is required in the future. Lastly, the model comparison approach used in this study may be further developed to include more robust methods, such as a Bayesian approach.

As we have shown in this paper, both person and item properties may help explain variability in response times at the item level. Although not explored on this paper, an explanatory model including both item and person covariates in the model could reveal an even clearer picture and is the goal of future studies.

References

Bates, D., Mächler, M., Bolker, B., & Walker, S. (2015). Fitting linear mixed-effects models using **lme4**. *Journal of Statistical Software, 67*(1). https://doi.org/10.18637/jss.v067.i01

Cho, S.-J., & De Boeck, P. (2018). A note on N in Bayesian information criterion for item response models. *Applied Psychological Measurement, 42*(2), 169–172. https://doi.org/10.1177/0146621617726791

De Boeck, P., Bakker, M., Zwitser, R., Nivard, M., Hofman, A., Tuerlinckx, F., & Partchev, I. (2011). The estimation of item response models with the lmer function from the **lme4** package in *R. Journal of Statistical Software, 39*(12). https://doi.org/10.18637/jss.v039.i12

De Boeck, P., Cho, S.-J., & Wilson, M. (2016). Explanatory item response models. In *The Wiley handbook of cognition and assessment* (pp. 247–266). Wiley. https://doi.org/10.1002/9781118956588

Delattre, M., Lavielle, M., & Poursat, M.-A. (2014). A note on BIC in mixed-effects models. *Electronic Journal of Statistics, 8*(1), 456–475. https://doi.org/10.1214/14-EJS890

Hong, M., Rebouças, D. A., & Cheng, Y. (2021). Robust estimation for response time modeling. *Journal of Educational Measurement*. https://doi.org/10.1111/jedm.12286

Meade, A. W., & Craig, S. B. (2012). Identifying careless responses in survey data. *Psychological Methods, 17*(3), 437–455. https://doi.org/10.1037/a0028085

Piepel, G. F. (2020). Measuring component effects in constrained mixture experiments, 12.

R Core Team. (2020). R: A language and environment for statistical computing. *R Foundation for Statistical Computing.*

Säfken, B., Rügamer, D., Kneib, T., & Greven, S. (2018). Conditional model selection in mixed-effects models with cAIC4. *arXiv:1803.05664 [stat].*

Soto, C. J., & John, O. P. (2017). The next Big Five Inventory (BFI-2): Developing and assessing a hierarchical model with 15 facets to enhance bandwidth, fidelity, and predictive power. *Journal of Personality and Social Psychology, 113*(1), 117–143. https://doi.org/10.1037/pspp0000096

Vaida, F., & Blanchard, S. (2005). Conditional Akaike information for mixed-effects models. *Biometrika, 92*(2), 351–370.

van der Linden, W. J. (2006). A lognormal model for response times on test items. *Journal of Educational and Behavioral Statistics, 31*(2), 181–204. https://doi.org/10.3102/10769986031002181

Verbeke, G., & Molenberghs, G. (2001). *Linear mixed models for longitudinal data*. Springer.

Response Time Relationships Within Examinees: Implications for Item Response Time Models

Susan Embretson

1 Introduction

Due to the increased use of computerized testing, item response time (RT) data have become increasingly available. In conjunction with this increase, many item response theory models for using response times have been developed. The models vary in both primary purpose and underlying assumptions. For example, some models for response times provide person estimates that are presumed useful to directly or indirectly augment person estimates that are based on item accuracy (e.g., Roskam, 1997; Wang & Hanson, 2005). Other models use response time in mixture models to improving item parameter estimates by identifying subjects who are guessing (Meyer, 2010; Wise & DeMars, 2009; Molenaar & de Boeck, 2018).

As noted by van der Linden (2016), several item response models assume response time and response accuracy are highly dependent processes. However, the nature of this assumed relationship varies substantially between models; that is, greater accuracy may be associated with either increased (e.g., Roskam, 1997) or decreased response time (e.g., Thissen, 1983). Other models, such as hierarchical models (e.g., van der Linden & Fox, 2016), permit separate response time and accuracy estimates at the lower level, but allow for correlations of ability and response time speed at the higher level.

Although a wide variety of models and purposes exist, it is not clear to what extent response time patterns reflect the same qualities across different examinees. For example, some examinees may spend more time on relatively difficult items while others may spend less time on items that are difficult. In the current study,

S. Embretson (✉)
Georgia Institute of Technology, Atlanta, GA, USA
e-mail: susan.embretson@psych.gatech.edu

M. Wiberg et al. (eds.), *Quantitative Psychology*, Springer Proceedings in Mathematics & Statistics 353, https://doi.org/10.1007/978-3-030-74772-5_5

the relationship of item log response times to item differences in difficulty, mean item response times, test position and cognitive complexity was examined within subjects.

2 Method

2.1 Subjects

The examinees were 700 young adults at a military center. Examinees were administered several tests, including the one in the current study.

2.2 Test

The Form 1 of the *Spatial Learning Ability Test* (SLAT; Embretson, 1997) was administered by computer to all examinees. Both responses and response times on the 28 SLAT items were collected. Figure 1 shows an item from SLAT. Examinees are instructed to select the alternative that represents the stem when folded.

2.3 Variables Analyzed

Several variables were scored for each item and analyzed within subjects. These variables included mean item response time, IRT-calibrated item difficulty (β_i, Rasch model), item position on the test, item difficulty distance from examinees' estimated ability (i.e., $| \theta_j - \beta_i |$) and item cognitive complexity. Cognitive complexity was based on prior modeling of SLAT item difficulty to represent the complexity of folding the stem to the correct answer. On Fig. 1, folding the stem

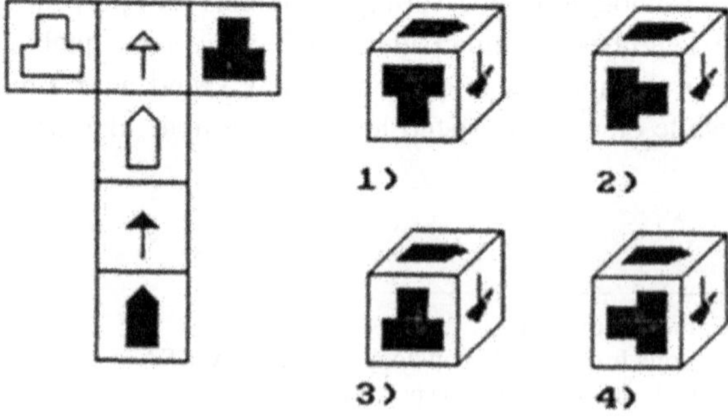

Fig. 1 An item from the Spatial Learning Ability Test

to the correct answer (#3) involves a rotation of the stem by 90 degrees and three surfaces carried, as the third side shown in the correct response is not attached to the other two sides in the stem.

3 Results

3.1 Between Person and Between Item Correlations

Initially, descriptive statistics on both between person differences (N = 700) and item differences (N = 28) were obtained. For persons, Table 1 shows that both trait levels and mean item response times (i.e., response time were log transformed to lnRT) varied. However, trait level was not correlated significantly with mean log response time. For items, Table 2 shows that item difficulty and response time also varied substantially. The inter-correlations of these variables as well as correlations with test position are also shown. Notice that at the item level, difficulty and response time have a moderately strong correlation. Test position, however, was negatively correlated with response time, indicating that less time is spent on items at the end of the test. Finally, cognitive complexity between items was analyzed by separately regressing item difficulty and mean item response time on the scored variables, degrees rotation and number of surfaces carried. A strong multiple correlation was found for item difficulty (R = .799). The item difficulty predicted from complexity had a moderate correlation (r = .495) with mean item lnRT as shown on Table 2.

Table 1 Descriptive statistics between persons

			Correlations	
Person variable	Mean	SD	Trait	RT
Trait level	.489	1.071	1.000	
Response time (ln)	3.175	.267	.038	1.000

Table 2 Descriptive statistics between items

			Correlations		
Item variable	Mean	SD	Diff.	RT	Position
Difficulty (Rasch β_i)	.000	.667	1.000		
Response time (ln)	3.014	.182	.691	1.000	
Test position	14.500	8.226	.029	−.483	1.000
Item complexity	.000	.508	.799	.495	.121

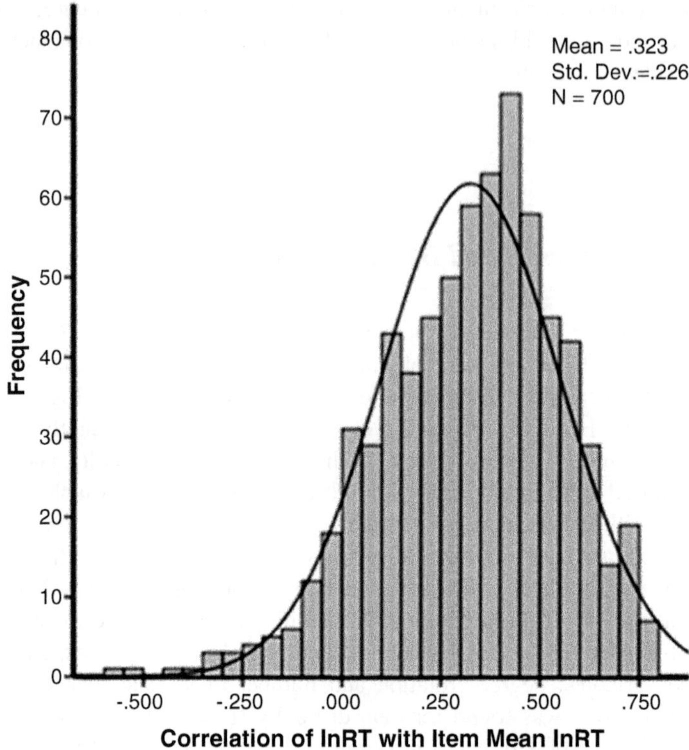

Fig. 2 Within person correlations of item response time with mean item response time

3.2 *Within Person Correlations*

Figure 2 presents the distribution of within person correlations with mean item response time. Although the mean correlation is positive (Mn = .323), substantial individual differences were found (SD = .226). The correlations ranged from −.587 to .799. Thus, the data show varying patterns of response times between persons.

Figure 3 presents the distribution of within person correlations of test position with mean item response time. Unlike the between item correlation of −.483 for mean item response time and test position, the within person correlation mean is nearly .000 (Mn = .120). Further, individual differences were found (SD = .247), with correlations ranging from −.870 to .708. Thus, examinees vary in whether they spend more or less time on items during testing.

Figure 4 presents the within person correlations of the item difficulty and mean item response time. While the mean correlation is positive (Mean = .240), individual differences were observed (SD = .238), with correlations ranging from −.547 to .764. A positive correlation indicates that an examinee spends more time on difficult items while a negative correlation implies less time. Again, this

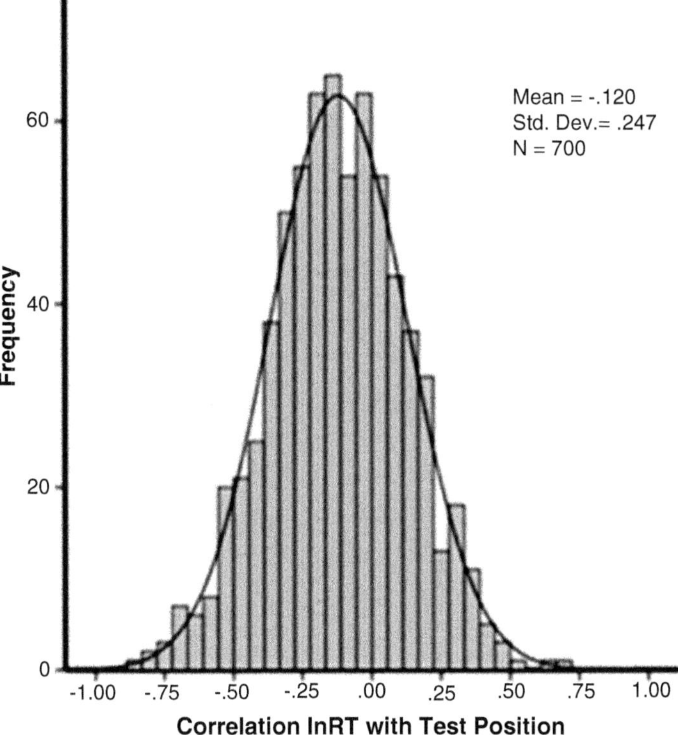

Fig. 3 Within person correlations of item response time with test position

distribution contrasts sharply with the strong positive correlation of item difficulty and mean response time found between items.

Figure 5 shows the within person correlations of relative item difficulty (i.e., absolute distance from their estimated trait level) and item response time. Although the mean correlation is negative (Mean = −.183), again substantial individual differences are observed (SD = .265), with a range from −.755 to .689. The negative correlations are found when an examinee spends more time on items near their trait level and less time on relatively or relatively hard items.

Finally, Fig. 6 presents the within person multiple correlations of the cognitive complexity variables with mean item response time. The multiple correlations range from .027 to .740, with a moderate mean (Mean = .350). The correlation must be positive but nonetheless individual differences are observed (SD = .132).

Between person correlations of the within person correlates of item response time are shown on Table 3. It can be seen, for example, that examinees whose response times are strongly related to mean item response time are also likely to spend more time on difficult items (r = .739) and somewhat more time on cognitively complex items (r = .230). Similarly, it can be seen that examinees with high trait levels are

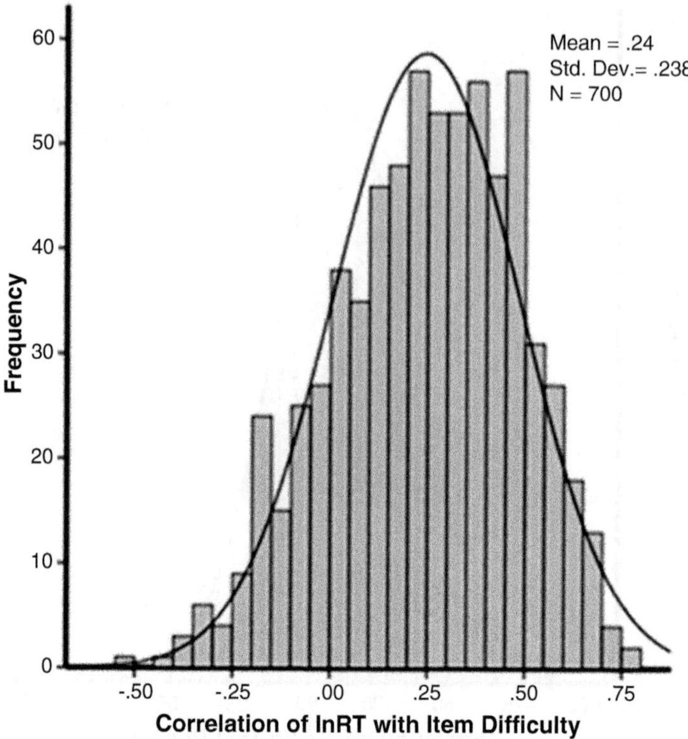

Fig. 4 Within person correlations of item response time with item difficulty

more likely to have positive correlations of their pattern of item response times with overall mean item response times, item difficulty and item cognitive complexity.

4 Discussion

The diversity of correlations examinees' pattern of item response times with the several variables in the current study do not provide widespread support for the assumptions of the various response time models that involve response times. That is, examinees vary widely in the correlates of their response times with variables such as mean item response time, item difficulty, test position, relative item difficulty and item cognitive complexity. Some examinees may have response time patterns that are consistent with a particular response time model, but others will not. Thus, a single response time model is not supported by the data in this study.

The results indicate significant strategy differences between examinees. Some examinees will devote more time to difficult items; others will devote less time. Some examinees devote less time to items near the end of the test, others devote

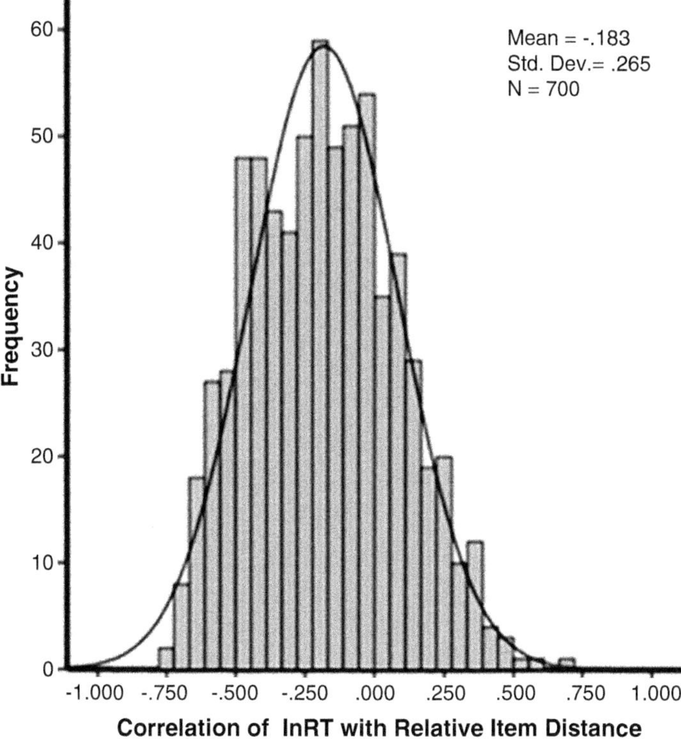

Fig. 5 Within person correlations of item response time with relative item difficulty distance

more time. Item cognitive complexity has little impact on item response time for some examinees; other examinees will devote more time to complex items.

The results obtained on the test used in the current study the Spatial Learning Ability Test may well generalize to many other tests. In fact, SLAT is a relatively homogeneous test, which is supported by internal consistency indices (i.e., Cronbach's alpha is .881). More heterogeneous tests may find even more diverse correlations of examinees' response times.

Given this diversity, mixture models could be important in identifying classes of examinees with varying strategies. Item parameter calibrations may vary by class as well as the validity of trait level interpretations. Thus, data relevant to the response processes aspect of validity or external relationships of trait levels aspect may vary by class.

Mixture models available for continuous variables are being developed and should be applied. Zopluoglu (2020) developed a finite mixture item response theory model for continuous measurement outcomes. This model could be applied in an exploratory mode to identify latent classes of examinees with varying item response strategies.

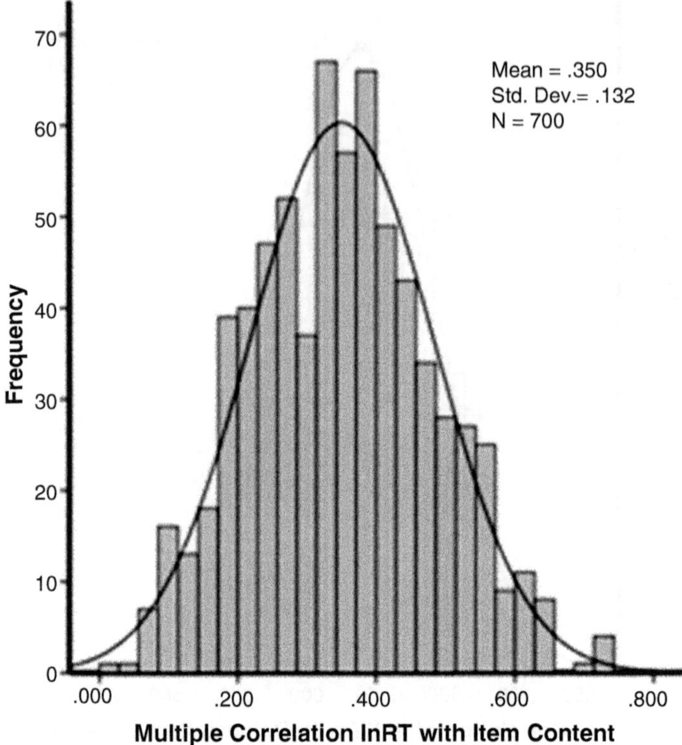

Fig. 6 Within person correlations of item response with cognitive complexity

Table 3 Between person correlations of within person relationships of item response times

	Overall test		Item response time correlations within persons			
	Trait level	Process time	MnlnRT	Diffic.	Distance	CogComp
Trait level	1.000	.038	.312	.406	−.556	.226
Processing time (mean lnRT)	.038	1.000	.118	.257	−.077	.188
Correlates of item lnRT within persons						
Mean lnRT	.312	.118	1.000	.739	−.387	.230
Item difficulty	.406	.257	.739	1.000	−.550	.453
Relative item difficulty distance	−.556	−.077	−.387	−.550	1.000	−.387
Item cognitive complexity (multiple R)	.226	.188	.230	.453	−.387	1.000

References

Embretson, S. E. (1997). The factorial validity of a cognitively designed test: The Spatial Learning Ability Test. *Educational and Psychological Measurement, 57*, 99–107.

Meyer, J. P. (2010). A mixture Rasch model with item response time components. *Applied Psychological Measurement, 34*(7), 521–538.

Molenaar, D., & de Boeck, P. (2018). Response mixture modeling: Accounting for heterogeneity of item characteristics across response times. *Psychometrika, 83*, 279–297.

Roskam, E. E. (1997). Models for speed and time-limit tests. In W. J. van der Linden & R. K. Hambleton (Eds.), *Handbook of modern item response theory* (pp. 187–208). Springer.

Thissen, D. (1983). Timed testing: An approach using item response theory. In D. J. Weiss (Ed.), *New horizons in testing: Latent trait test theory and computerized adaptive testing* (pp. 179–203). Academic.

Van der Linden, W. (2016). Lognormal response-time model. In W. van der Linden (Ed.), *Handbook of item response theory: Volume 1: Models* (pp. 261–300). Taylor & Francis Inc.

Van der Linden, W.J., & Fox, J.-P. (2016) Joint hierarchical modeling of responses and response times. In *Handbook of Modern Item Response Theory*, W.J van der Linden (Ed.), Vol 1, Chapter 29, Chapman and Hall/CRC Press.

Wang, T., & Hanson, B. A. (2005). Development and calibration of an item response model that incorporates response time. *Applied Psychological Measurement, 29*, 323–339.

Wise, S. L., & DeMars, C. E. (2009). An application of item-response time: The effort-moderated IRT model. *Journal of Educational Measurement, 43*, 19–38.

Zopluoglu, C. (2020). A finite mixture item response theory model for continuous measurement outcomes. *Educational and Psychological Measurement, 80*(2), 346–364.

Nonlinear Latent Effects in Diagnostic Classification Modeling Incorporating Response Times

Xin Qiao, Manqian Liao, and Hong Jiao

1 Introduction

The hierarchical modeling framework (van der Linden, 2007) has been widely used in the analysis of response and response time (RT) data. In this modeling framework, responses and RTs are modeled by separate measurement models at the first level; the correlational structures that capture the dependence between parameters from the item response model and the RT model are specified at the second level. To utilize RT in diagnostic classification modeling, Zhan et al. (2017) proposed the joint diagnostic classification model (DCM) of responses and RTs, where DCMs provide fine-grained diagnostic information on respondents' latent attributes.

Similar to the hierarchical modeling approach, a majority of studies assume linear relationship between RTs and person ability (e.g., Thissen, 1983). Recently, Molenaar et al. (2015) developed the bivariate generalized linear IRT modeling framework that allows both linear and nonlinear relations between responses and RTs, with the focus on applications in ability tests and personality tests. It is important to accommodate nonlinear relationships in the joint modeling of responses and RTs to further improve the measurement precision of latent ability. In diagnostic assessments, however, such nonlinear latent effects have not been investigated yet. Correctly modeling the potential nonlinear relationships between responses and RTs may improve the estimation of respondents' mastery status of the latent attributes.

X. Qiao (✉) · H. Jiao
University of Maryland, Pittsburgh, PA, USA
e-mail: xinqiao@umd.edu

M. Liao
Duolingo, Pittsburgh, PA, USA

M. Wiberg et al. (eds.), *Quantitative Psychology*, Springer Proceedings in Mathematics & Statistics 353, https://doi.org/10.1007/978-3-030-74772-5_6

Therefore, the current study aims to propose joint DCMs where both linear and nonlinear relationships between responses and RTs can be accommodated. Although the nonlinear relations can be diverse in real settings, the current study focuses on two common nonlinear latent effects (i.e., interaction and quadratic effects).

1.1 Nonlinear Joint Cognitive Diagnostic Modeling

In the present study, the deterministic input, noisy-and-gate (DINA; Junker & Sijtsma, 2001; Macready & Dayton, 1977) model is adopted as the measurement model for item responses. The lognormal model (van der Linden, 2006) is used as the measurement model for RTs. The two models are chosen due to their wide use in research. Then, DCMs incorporating RTs (i.e., JRT-DINA-linear, JRT-DINA-interaction, and JRT-DINA-quadratic) are proposed.

The JRT-DINA-Linear Model. At the first level, the dichotomous item response Y_{pi} is modeled using the DINA model with the logit scale parameterization (e.g., DeCarlo, 2011):

$$\text{logit}\left(P\left(Y_{pi}=1\right)\right)=\beta_i+\delta_i\prod_{k=1}^{K}\alpha_{pk}^{q_{ik}}, \tag{1}$$

where β_i and δ_i are item intercept and item interaction parameters, respectively; $\alpha_p = (\alpha_{p1}, \ldots, \alpha_{pK})^{'}$ denotes the attribute pattern for respondent p given all K attributes measured; $q_{ik} = 1$ indicates attribute k is required to correctly answer item i while $q_{ik} = 0$ otherwise. The higher-order latent structural model (de la Torre & Douglas, 2004) is further used to account for the correlation among latent attributes:

$$\text{logit}\left(P\left(\alpha_{pk}=1\right)\right)=\gamma_k\theta_p-\lambda_k, \tag{2}$$

where γ_k and λ_k are attribute-specific slope and difficulty parameters. log(T_{pi}) is modeled by an extension of the lognormal RT model (van der Linden, 2006) with the latent ability as predictor, which is written as:

$$\log\left(T_{pi}\right)=\zeta_i-\xi_p-\rho\theta_p+\varepsilon_{pi}, \tag{3}$$

where ξ_p can be interpreted as person speed due to idiosyncratic item-solving processes; ζ_i is interpreted as item intensity due to differences in item characteristics; ε_{pi} is the residual term and follows a normal distribution, ε_{pi}~$N(0, {\sigma_{\varepsilon i}}^2)$. The variation in log($T_{pi}$) is assumed to be partly due to the latent ability underlying the responses, θ_p (Thissen, 1983). At the second level, item parameters $\Psi_i = (\beta_i, \delta_i, \zeta_i)^{'}$ are assumed to follow a multivariate normal distribution. Person parameters $\Theta_p = (\theta_p, \xi_p)^{'}$ are assumed to be independently and normally distributed.

The JRT-DINA-Interaction Model. The formulation of the JRT-DINA-interaction model is the same as the JRT-DINA-linear model, except that the former accommodates the interaction between person speed and the latent ability in the RT measurement model:

$$\log\left(T_{pi}\right) = \zeta_i - \xi_p - \rho_1\theta_p - \rho_2\xi_p\theta_p + \varepsilon_{pi}, \tag{4}$$

where ρ_1 and ρ_2 capture the linear and interaction effects, respectively.

The JRT-DINA-Quadratic Model. The JRT-DINA-quadratic model accommodates a possible nonlinear relationship between response and response time by assuming a quadratic effect of the latent ability in the RT measurement model:

$$\log\left(T_{pi}\right) = \zeta_i - \xi_p - \rho_1\theta_p - \rho_2\theta_p^2 + \varepsilon_{pi}, \tag{5}$$

where ρ_1 and ρ_2 capture the linear and quadratic effects, respectively. When ρ_2 is set to be 0, the JRT-DINA-interaction and JRT-DINA-quadratic models reduce to the JRT-DINA-linear model. For all three models, we set $\mu_\theta = \mu_\tau = 0$ and ${\sigma_\theta}^2 = 1$ for scale identification purposes.

1.2 Bayesian Parameter Estimation

In the present study, JAGS (version 4.3.0; Plummer, 2015) was used to estimate the parameters using the full Bayesian approach with Markov chain Monte Carlo (MCMC) method. A Gibbs sampler (Gelfand & Smith, 1990) was implemented in JAGS.

The rest of the paper is organized as follows. First, we present a real data application of the proposed models. Then, a simulation study based on the real data application is conducted to evaluate the parameter recovery of the proposed models. In addition, the impact of ignoring possible nonlinear latent effects on the person parameter estimation, the attribute and pattern classification accuracy is evaluated in the simulation study. Lastly, the conclusions from the current study are summarized and future directions are discussed.

2 Method

2.1 Real Data Analysis

In this study, 10 dichotomously scored items from PISA 2012 mathematics assessment were used. Seven attributes were assessed: change and relationships (α_1), quantity (α_2), space and shape (α_3), uncertainty and data (α_4), occupational (α_5),

Table 1 Q matrix for PISA 2012 mathematics assessment items

Items	α_1	α_2	α_3	α_4	α_5	α_6	α_7
CM015Q01	0	1	0	0	1	0	0
CM015Q02D	1	0	0	0	1	0	0
CM015Q03D	1	0	0	0	1	0	0
CM020Q01	0	0	1	0	0	0	1
CM020Q02	0	0	1	0	0	0	1
CM020Q03	0	0	1	0	0	0	1
CM020Q04	0	0	1	0	0	0	1
CM038Q03T	0	0	0	1	0	1	0
CM038Q05	0	0	0	1	0	1	0
CM038Q06	0	0	0	1	0	1	0

societal (α_6), and scientific (α_7). The Q matrix is shown in Table 1. The natural logarithm of the RTs was calculated for the analysis. Zero RTs were treated as missing values which can easily be handled by our Bayesian estimation scheme. The final sample included 1582 respondents. No missing responses existed.

The JRT-DINA-linear, JRT-DINA-interaction, and JRT-DINA-quadratic models[1] were fitted to this dataset. The potential scale reduction factor (PSRF; Brooks & Gelman, 1998) lower than 1.1 was used as the convergence criterion. The Akaike information criterion (AIC; Akaike, 1974), the Bayesian information criterion (BIC; Schwarz, 1978), and the deviance information criterion (DIC; Spiegelhalter et al., 2002) were used for model selection. According to Congdon (2003), when used in the Bayesian MCMC estimation, the AIC, the BIC and the DIC model fit indices were specified as:

$$AIC = \overline{D} + p, \tag{6}$$

$$BIC = \overline{D} + p\,(\log N - 1) \tag{7}$$

$$DIC = \overline{D} + p_D, \tag{8}$$

where $\overline{D}$ denotes the posterior mean of the deviance; p denotes the number of parameters; N denotes the sample size; p_D is the effective number of parameters, which can be estimated by var(D)/2 (Gelman et al., 2014), that is, half of the posterior variance of the deviance. Smaller values of the AIC, the BIC and the DIC indicate better model fit.

A posterior predictive model check (PPMC; Gelman et al., 2014) was conducted to evaluate the absolute model-data fit. Posterior predictive probability (PPP) values near 0.5 indicate adequate model-data fit, while extreme PPP values (>.95 or <.05)

[1]For all three models, two Markov chains were used with 15,000 iterations per chain. The first 5000 iterations in each chain were discarded as burn-in and the thin interval was set as five.

indicate systematic differences between observed and predicted data. The current study followed Zhan et al. (2017) to evaluate the absolute model-data fit of RA and RT separately. The sum of the squared Pearson residuals for respondent p and item i (Yan et al., 2003) was used as the discrepancy measure for the RA model, which is written as:

$$D\left(Y_{pi};\boldsymbol{\alpha}_p,\beta_i,\delta_i\right)=\sum_{p=1}^{N}\sum_{i=1}^{I}\left(\frac{Y_{pi}-P\left(Y_{pi}=1\right)}{\sqrt{P\left(Y_{pi}=1\right)\left(1-P\left(Y_{pi}=1\right)\right)}}\right)^2, \tag{9}$$

where $P(Y_{pi}=1)$ has the same distribution as that in the Eq. 1. The sum of the standardized error function of $\log(T_{pi})$ for respondent p and item i (Marianti et al., 2014) was used as the discrepancy measure for the RT models. For the JRT-DINA-interaction model and the JRT-DINA-quadratic model, the discrepancy measures for the RT model are presented as:

$$D\left(\log T_{pi};\tau_p,\zeta_i,\varepsilon_i\right)=\sum_{p=1}^{N}\sum_{i=1}^{I}\left(\varepsilon_i\left(\log T_{pi}-\left(\zeta_i-\rho_1\tau_p-\rho_2\tau_p\theta_p\right)\right)\right)^2, \tag{10}$$

and

$$D\left(\log T_{pi};\tau_p,\zeta_i,\varepsilon_i\right)=\sum_{p=1}^{N}\sum_{i=1}^{I}\left(\varepsilon_i\left(\log T_{pi}-\left(\zeta_i-\rho_1\tau_p-\rho_2\theta_p^2\right)\right)\right)^2, \tag{11}$$

respectively. If ρ_2 reduces to zero, Eqs. 10 and 11 become the discrepancy measure for the RT model in the JRT-DINA-linear model.

2.2 *Simulation Study*

Data Generation and Analysis. The simulation study was based on real data analysis. Sample size and test length were fixed at 1000 respondents and 10 items, respectively. Q matrix was the same as shown in Table 1. Two data generating models were used: the JRT-DINA-quadratic and JRT-DINA-interaction models. Under each condition, the analysis models included the true data generating model and the JRT-DINA-linear model. True parameters were fixed as the same as those obtained from real data analysis. Thirty replications were conducted for each data generating model condition.

Outcome Measures. Model fit indices AIC, BIC, and DIC were examined in terms of how often they correctly identified the true data generating model. To evaluate parameter recovery, the bias and the mean root mean squared error (RMSE) were computed for person parameters. The correlation between estimated and true person parameter values were also calculated. The attribute correct classification accuracy (ACCR) and the pattern correct classification rate (PCCR) were computed to examine the classification accuracy of each attribute and each attribute profile.

3 Results

3.1 Real Data Analysis

According to Table 2, the JRT-DINA-linear model was favored by the AIC and the BIC, while the JRT-DINA-quadratic model was favored by the DIC. The PPMC procedure showed that all the three models had adequate model-data fit.

The posterior mean of the parameter estimates for ρ_1 were negative in all models (ranging from $-.172$ to -1.267), which indicates that respondents with higher ability spent more time on the items in general. In the JRT-DINA-interaction model, the posterior mean of ρ_2 was estimated to be $-.789$, which indicates that the relationship between ability and log RTs is positive for fast respondents but negative for slow respondents. In the JRT-DINA-quadratic model, the posterior mean of ρ_2 was estimated to be .172, which indicates that the relationship between latent ability and log RTs is negative for more proficient respondents but positive for less proficient respondents. The 95% credible intervals for the posterior means of ρ_1 and ρ_2 did not cover 0, which indicates that these parameter estimates were significantly different from 0.

Figure 1 further demonstrates the linear or nonlinear relationship between latent ability and log RTs based on the data analysis results. Three levels of person speed ξ were chosen: – 0.5, 0, and 0.5. Item intensity ζ was fixed at 4.473, which was mean of the posterior means of item intensity parameter estimates based on the JRT-DINA-quadratic model.

3.2 Simulation Study

Table 3 shows the frequencies that the AIC, BIC, and DIC identified each analysis model as the best fitting model under two data generating model conditions, respectively. When the JRT-DINA-interaction model was used as the data generating model, the AIC, BIC, and DIC all predominantly favored the JRT-DINA-interaction model over the JRT-DINA-linear model. When the JRT-DINA-quadratic model was used as the data generating model, the AIC and BIC tended to select the JRT-DINA-linear model, while the DIC tended to select the JRT-DINA-quadratic model. Therefore, it is suggested that the AIC and BIC should not the used for model comparison. In addition, the JRT-DINA-quadratic model should be preferred based on the DIC in the real data analysis.

Table 2 Model fit for PISA mathematics items

Model	Deviance	AIC	BIC	DIC	NP	pD	ppp_RA	ppp_RT
JRT-DINA-linear	36,937	**40,155**	**57,424**	46,861	3218	9925	0.580	0.590
JRT-DINA-interaction	36,963	40,182	57,457	49,435	3219	12,472	0.630	0.570
JRT-DINA-quadratic	37,021	40,240	57,515	**44,121**	3219	7099	0.570	0.542

Note. *Deviance* = posterior mean of the deviance; *AIC* = Akaike information criterion; *BIC* = Bayesian information criterion; *DIC* = deviance information criterion; *NP* = number of parameter; *pD* = effective parameter number; *ppp* = posterior predictive p-value; *RA* =item response accuracy; *RT* = item response time. Smallest fit values are bold face

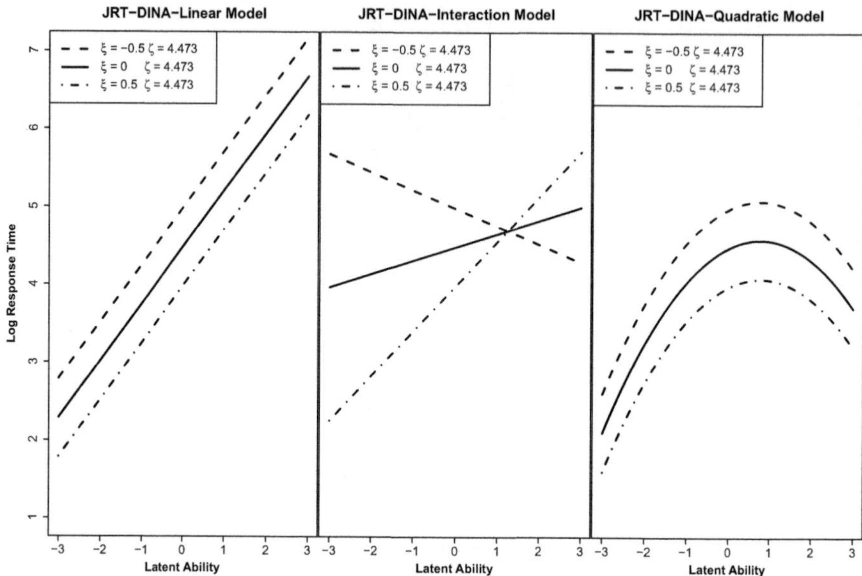

Fig. 1 Relations between latent ability and log response times (in seconds)

Table 3 Frequency of identifying each model as the best fitting model in simulation study

DGM	AM	AIC	BIC	DIC	NP	mean_pD
JDI	JDI	18	19	23	2055	5813
	JDL	12	11	7	2054	6367
JDQ	JDQ	1	2	25	2055	7310
	JDL	29	28	5	2054	10,211

Note. DGM = data generating model; *AM* = analysis model; *JDI* = JRT-DINA-interaction; *JRL* = JRT-DINA-linear; *JRQ* = JRT-DINA-quadratic; *Deviance* = posterior mean of the deviance; *AIC* = Akaike information criterion; *BIC* = Bayesian information criterion; *DIC* = deviance information criterion; *NP* = number of parameter; *pD* = effective parameter number

As shown in Table 4, the correlations between the true and estimated person parameter values obtained from the joint models with nonlinear latent effects were higher than the joint model with only a linear latent effect in both data generating model conditions. This indicates that ignoring nonlinear latent effects led to changes in the rank order of the respondents. Further, both the mean absolute biases and RMSEs of the person parameter estimates were inflated when nonlinear latent effects were neglected. This suggests that ignoring nonlinear latent effects led to larger estimation error in the latent ability parameters.

Table 5 presents the attribute and pattern correct classification rate in the simulation study. Pattern correct classification rate decreased when the analysis

Table 4 Summary of person parameter recovery in simulation study

Par.	DGM	AM	Cor.	Index	Min.	Mean	Max.	*SD*
θ	JDI	JDI	.811	Bias	.001	.403	2.852	.360
				RMSE	.054	.492	2.859	.327
		JDL	.788	Bias	.000	.433	2.787	.370
				RMSE	.031	.888	3.579	.653
	JDQ	JDQ	.903	Bias	.000	.307	1.528	.245
				RMSE	.074	.373	1.549	.223
		JDL	.877	Bias	.000	.846	3.945	.621
				RMSE	.058	.421	1.741	.245

Note. *Par.* = parameter; *DGM* = data generating model; *AM* = analysis model; *Cor.* = correlation; *JDI* = JRT-DINA-interaction; *JRL* = JRT-DINA-linear; *JRQ* = JRT-DINA-quadratic; *Min.* = minimum; *Max.* = maximum; *SD* = standard deviation; *RMSE* = root mean square error; *Bias* = absolute bias

Table 5 Attribute and pattern correct classification rate in simulation study

		ACCR							PCCR
DGM	AM	α_1	α_2	α_3	α_4	α_5	α_6	α_7	
JRI	JRI	.882	.717	.854	.868	.857	.878	.873	.438
	JRL	.883	.712	.851	.866	.853	.874	.870	.433
JRQ	JRQ	.811	.777	.905	.903	.893	.867	.881	.449
	JRL	.813	.766	.905	.902	.884	.864	.881	.443

Note. *DGM* = data generating model; *AM* = analysis model; *JDI* = JRT-DINA-interaction; *JRL* = JRT-DINA-linear; *JRQ* = JRT-DINA-quadratic; *ACCR* = attribute correct classification rate; *PCCR* = pattern correct classification rate

model was JRT-DINA-linear model in both data generating model conditions. In addition, attribute correct classification rates from the JRT-DINA-linear model was lower or equal to those from the JRT-DINA-interaction model or the JRT-DINA-quadratic model for all attributes except attribute 1. Therefore, ignoring nonlinear latent effects between response accuracy and RTs in the cognitive diagnostic context may lead to inaccurate classifications of the respondents.

4 Discussion

The current study proposed two joint DCMs with nonlinear latent effects between latent ability and RTs. Two findings from the real data analysis supported the nonlinear relationship between the responses and RTs: (1) the DIC model fit index favored the JRT-DINA-quadratic model; (2) the nonlinear latent effect parameters were significantly different from 0 in both models with nonlinear latent effects based on the 95% credible intervals of the posterior means. The follow-up simulation study mimicking the real data structure showed that the DIC generally supported the JRT-DINA models with nonlinear latent effects under all manipulated conditions. Given that Celeux et al. (2006) suggested that the DIC prefers models with nonlinear effects, future studies that generate data according to the linear model are needed to further validate the use of the DIC. In addition, ignoring nonlinear latent effects led to less accurate person parameter estimates and decrease of attribute correct classification rates and pattern correct classification rates.

In future studies, simulation studies may evaluate more factors. In addition, other nonlinear relations may be explored using different modeling techniques. Lastly, empirical datasets with more items and complete Q matrices should be used. Overall, this line of research is promising and more can be achieved in the future.

References

Akaike, H. (1974). A new look at the statistical model identification. *IEEE Transactions on Automatic Control, 19*(6), 716–723.

Brooks, S. P., & Gelman, A. (1998). General methods for monitoring convergence of iterative simulations. *Journal of Computational and Graphical Statistics, 7*, 434–455.

Celeux, G., Forbes, F., Robert, C. P., & Titterington, D. M. (2006). Deviance information criteria for missing data models. *Bayesian Analysis, 1*(4), 651–673.

Congdon, P. (2003). *Applied Bayesian modelling*. Wiley.

DeCarlo, L. T. (2011). On the analysis of fraction subtraction data: The DINA model, classification, latent class sizes, and the Q-matrix. *Applied Psychological Measurement, 35*, 8–26. https://doi.org/10.1177/0146621610377081

de la Torre, J., & Douglas, J. (2004). Higher-order latent trait models for cognitive diagnosis. *Psychometrika, 69*, 333–353. https://doi.org/10.1007/BF02295640

Gelfand, A. E., & Smith, A. F. M. (1990). Sampling-based approaches to calculating marginal densities. *Journal of the American Statistical Association, 85*, 398–409.

Gelman, A., Carlin, J. B., Stern, H. S., Dunson, D. B., Vehtari, A., & Rubin, D. B. (2014). *Bayesian data analysis*. CRC Press.

Junker, B. W., & Sijtsma, K. (2001). Cognitive assessment models with few assumptions, and connections with nonparametric item response theory. *Applied Psychological Measurement, 25*, 258–272. https://doi.org/10.1177/01466210122032064

Macready, G. B., & Dayton, C. M. (1977). The use of probabilistic models in the assessment of mastery. *Journal of Educational and Behavioral Statistics, 2*, 99–120. https://doi.org/10.2307/1164802

Marianti, S., Fox, J. P., Avetisyan, M., Veldkamp, B. P., & Tijmstra, J. (2014). Testing for aberrant behavior in response time modeling. *Journal of Educational and Behavioral Statistics, 39*(6), 426–451.

Molenaar, D., Tuerlinckx, F., & van der Maas, H. L. (2015). A bivariate generalized linear item response theory modeling framework to the analysis of responses and response times. *Multivariate Behavioral Research, 50*(1), 56–74.

Plummer, M. (2015). *JAGS version 4.0.0 user manual*. Lyon, France. Retrieved from https://sourceforge.net/projects/mcmc-jags/files/Manuals/4.x/

Schwarz, G. (1978). Estimating the dimension of a model. *The Annals of Statistics, 6*(2), 461–464.

Spiegelhalter, D. J., Best, N. G., Carlin, B. P., & Van Der Linde, A. (2002). Bayesian measures of model complexity and fit. *Journal of the Royal Statistical Society: Series B (Statistical Methodology), 64*(4), 583–639.

Thissen, D. (1983). Timed testing: An approach using item response theory. In D. J. Weiss (Ed.), *New horizons in testing: Latent trait test theory and computerized adaptive testing* (pp. 179–203). Academic.

van der Linden, W. J. (2006). A lognormal model for response times on test items. *Journal of Educational and Behavioral Statistics, 31*, 181–204. https://doi.org/10.3102/10769986031002181

van der Linden, W. J. (2007). A hierarchical framework for modeling speed and accuracy on test items. *Psychometrika, 72*, 287–308. https://doi.org/10.1007/s11336-006-1478-z

Yan, D., Mislevy, R. J., & Almond, R. G. (2003). *Design and analysis in a cognitive assessment* (ETS research report series, RR-03-32). ETS.

Zhan, P., Jiao, H., & Liao, D. (2017). Cognitive diagnosis modeling incorporating item response times. *British Journal of Mathematical and Statistical Psychology, 72*, 262–286. https://doi.org/10.1111/bmsp.12114

Sequential Monitoring of Aberrant Test-Taking Behaviors Based on Response Times

Suhwa Han and Hyeon-Ah Kang

1 Introduction

Identifying aberrant test-taking behaviors is essential to ensure valid inference on test outcomes. Traditional ways of detecting aberrant test-taking behaviors have been to investigate the agreement between the pattern of response scores within a person against a postulated measurement model, which are commonly referred to as person-fit methods. Recently, the increasing use of computers for testing has made response time (RT) data readily available, and various person-fit studies with respect to RTs were explored (e.g., Boughton, Smith & Ren, 2016; Marianti, Fox, Avetisyan, Veldkamp & Tijmstra, 2014; Meijer & Sotaridona, 2006; Sinharay, 2018, 2020; Toton & Maynes, 2019; van der Linden & Guo, 2008; van der Linden & van Krimpen-Stoop, 2003; Qian, Staniewska, Reckase & Woo, 2016). Although many person-fit studies have demonstrated the feasibility of using RTs for identifying aberrant test-taking behaviors, most of the existing methods utilize parameter estimates based on entire RT vectors of individuals, limiting their use to post-hoc analysis only. In this study, we suggest sequential procedures that monitor examinee RTs in real time and flag abnormalities as soon as they occur. Particularly, a cumulative sum (CUSUM) chart and a sequential generalized likelihood ratio (SGLRT) scheme are employed to allow for online detection. The suggested procedures can be applied to real-time detection of aberrancy for various types of assessments from traditional computer-based assessments to online testing and learning tools.

S. Han (✉) · H.-A. Kang
University of Texas at Austin, Austin, TX, USA
e-mail: suhwa@utexas.edu; hkang@austin.utexas.edu

M. Wiberg et al. (eds.), *Quantitative Psychology*, Springer Proceedings in Mathematics & Statistics 353, https://doi.org/10.1007/978-3-030-74772-5_7

2 Sequential Procedures for Detecting Aberrant Test-Taking Behaviors

To infer aberrant examinee behaviors, the current study considers RTs only. Hence, the log-normal response time model of van der Linden (2006) is used for the parametric evaluation throughout the study. The model assumes a normal density for the logarithm of the RTs:

$$\log T_i \sim N\left(\beta_i - \tau, \alpha_i^{-2}\right), \tag{1}$$

where T_i denotes the RT of an examinee for an item i; τ is a latent variable that indicates the working speed of the examinee; α_i is the time-discriminating parameter; β_i is the time intensity parameter.

2.1 *CUSUM-Based Approach*

The CUSUM procedure (Hawkins & Olwell, 1998; Page, 1954), which was originally developed for statistical quality control, is one of the most commonly used methods for tracking continuous, but possibly small, changes in the data. In this study, we suggest two CUSUM procedures based on (i) the observable RTs, and (ii) the estimable speed parameter.

Let T_i denote the response time of an examinee on item i. The first CUSUM procedure detects an unusual shift in the observed RTs by continuously accumulating the deviance between the observed RT and the expected RT under the in-control distribution:

$$W_i^T = \frac{\log T_i - E\left(\log T_i \mid \tau\right)}{\sqrt{\mathrm{Var}\left(\log T_i\right)}}. \tag{2}$$

Based on the monitoring statistic in (2), the upper and lower CUSUM are constructed as

$$C_i^+ = \max\left\{0, W_i + C_{i-1}^+ - d\right\}, \text{ and} \tag{3}$$

$$C_i^- = \min\left\{0, W_i + C_{i-1}^- + d\right\}, \tag{4}$$

where $C_0^+ = C_0^- = 0$ and d is the reference value. The reference value prevents CUSUM from being a mere accumulation of random errors in the data and thus needs to be carefully selected to optimize its performance. In the case of normally distributed data with a specified shift size to detect, it has been shown that the CUSUM statistic performs optimally when d is one half the magnitude between the target value and the out-of-control value that one wants to detect quickest (Lorden,

1971; Moustakides, 1986). When the CUSUM statistic exceeds a threshold, h, so called decision interval, the procedure signals a systematic change in the examinee's RTs, indicating a potential aberrant test-taking behavior. The decision interval is typically chosen such that the average number of observations evaluated until CUSUM signals out-of-control is minimized. The change point is estimated as the earliest time point at which $|C_i| > h$ (Siegmund & Venkatraman, 1995).

The second CUSUM procedure monitors change in the speed parameter estimates, $\hat{\tau}$, under the log-normal model. The monitoring statistic, W^t, sequentially tests the null hypothesis of no change in speed (i.e., $H_0 : \tau = E(\hat{\tau})$) via

$$W_i^t = \frac{\hat{\tau} - E(\hat{\tau})}{SE(\hat{\tau})}, \tag{5}$$

where $\hat{\tau}$ represents the most updated speed estimate. The W^t statistic is then plugged in the CUSUM equations presented in (3) and (4). The change point estimate is calculated in the same manner as in the first CUSUM procedure.

2.2 SGLRT-Based Approach

The optimality of CUSUM is grounded on the assumption that there is one specific size of a shift that CUSUM is to detect, meaning that the parameter after change is known. Such assumption is often not met when no prior information on the likely size of the shift is available. In this case, SGLRT procedure can be a viable alternative to CUSUM (Basseville & Nikiforov, 1993, p.14). As the name implies, SGLRT achieves online detection by sequentially conducting a generalized likelihood ratio test as the process moves along. The problem of the unknown post-change parameter is addressed by employing maximum likelihood (ML) estimates for the likelihood ratio test.

The new person-fit statistic based on SGLRT evaluates two likelihoods sequentially: the likelihood under the null hypothesis of no change (i.e., $H_0 : \tau = \tau_0$) against the alternative hypothesis of change (i.e., $H_1 : \tau = \tau_1$). Let τ_0 denote the hypothesized speed level under no aberrances. SGLRT then evaluates deviance in the likelihoods of τ sequentially across items:

$$s_k = \log \frac{f\left(\boldsymbol{t}_k \mid \hat{\tau}_k\right)}{f\left(\boldsymbol{t}_k \mid \hat{\tau}_0\right)} = \sum_{i=l}^{k} \log \frac{f\left(t_i \mid \hat{\tau}_k\right)}{f\left(t_i \mid \hat{\tau}_0\right)}, \tag{6}$$

where $\boldsymbol{t}_k$ refers to the vector of logarithms of RTs evaluated at evaluation point k. SGLRT statistic at each evaluation point contains most updated information on the degree of deviance between the two competing likelihoods. When the statistic exceeds its appropriate critical value, the procedure concludes there has been a change in the examinee's operating speed. As was done in the CUSUM-based approaches, the change point is determined as the earliest time point at which the statistic exceeds an appropriate threshold (Siegmund, 1985):

$$\hat{\upsilon} = \inf\left\{k : \max_{1\leq i\leq k} \log \frac{f\left(t_k \mid \hat{\tau}_k\right)}{f\left(t_k \mid \hat{\tau}_0\right)} > h\right\}. \tag{7}$$

2.3 *Moving Sample Strategy*

To allow for the real time detection of an abnormal shift in speed, the speed parameter has to be constantly updated to reflect a potential fluctuation in speed. A majority of existing applications of RT models, however, assumed that an examinee operates at a constant speed throughout the entire test. Particularly, when it comes to person-fit methods, calculating the fit statistic under the assumption of constant speed for all items can compromise detection power if an examinee indeed exhibited aberrant RTs. This consequence is unsurprising given that bias can be introduced in the speed parameter estimate from the contaminated observations. As a solution, we suggest a moving sample strategy that can avoid the parameter contamination, and yet, that can capture the changing speed estimate with increased sensitivity. The scope for the usual constant speed assumption is narrowed down from the entire test to each of the moving sample.

Figure 1 illustrates the possible sampling strategy under the scenario that abnormal upward shift in speed occurred toward the end of testing due to test speededness or loss of motivation. In this scenario, the expected speed (i.e., $E(\hat{\tau})$ in W^t and $\hat{\tau}_0$ in s_k) can be defined as the speed level that can be confidently said to be from the normal state. As the procedure seeks to detect changes in the later part of testing, we may employ a certain number of observations at the beginning of the test as a reference sample (marked as solid blocks in the figure) and use it throughout the sequential hypothesis testing. On the other hand, the most up-to-date speed level can be estimated based on a moving sample of a fixed size at each evaluation point as shown in the figure with blue diagonal patterns. As a result, the provisional speed estimate based on moving samples can reflect the most recent change because the sample constantly evolves by adding the most recent item into the sample and discarding the oldest one. The detection program can initiate the monitoring procedure as soon as it obtains the first moving sample.

3 Simulation Study

A Monte Carlo simulation study was conducted to investigate the performance of the proposed methods. The simulation study was designed to emulate a fixed-length large-scale educational testing situation where examinees tend to exhibit aberrant

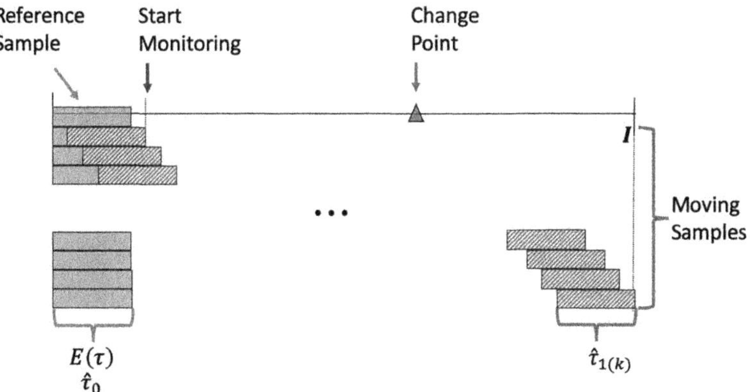

Fig. 1 A possible moving sampling strategy. The solid blocks represent a reference sample from which the benchmark speed estimates (i.e., $E(\hat{\tau})$ and $\hat{\tau}_0$) are calculated. The crosshatched blocks represent moving samples to reflect the most recent speed level

response behaviors toward the end of testing for reasons such as test speededness or loss of motivation. The focus of evaluation was on how accurately the proposed methods can identify individuals whose response times go through a systematic change and, if accurately identified, how promptly the change was signaled.

3.1 Data Generation and Simulation Design

Fictitious response time data for 1000 examinees were generated according to (1) for each replication. Examinees' true speed parameters, τ, were simulated to follow $N(0, 1)$ whereas the time discrimination parameters, α_i, were assumed to follow $N(2, 0.1^2)$. The true time intensity parameters, β_i, were generated from $N(0, 1)$ to place β_i and τ on the same scale.

To simulate aberrant response times, 10% of the examinee population (i.e., 100 examinees) was randomly selected to exhibit change in speed during the test. A change point was assumed to occur at the 16th item, and so the aberrant examinees' τ was increased by adding a constant (e.g., 0.5) at the 16th item. The study considered 3 factors: (i) test length, (ii) magnitude of change in τ (i.e., $\Delta\tau$ henceforth), and (iii) number of items in the reference/moving samples (sample size henceforth). Specifically, the simulation conditions were fully crossed by three different test lengths (30, 40, 50 items), four different $\Delta\tau$s (0.5, 0.75, 1, 1.25) and three different sample sizes (5, 10, 15 items), yielding a total of 36 conditions. In addition, different reference values, d, in the CUSUM procedures were tested to find out an optimal value that maximizes detection power given the nominal Type I error.

3.2 Evaluation

Calculation of the proposed statistics required known item parameter values. The study employed estimated item parameters to reflect real world settings where true parameters are unknown. Items were calibrated based on the Bayesian estimation procedure (Fox, Klein Entink, & Klotzke, 2017). Critical values for both the CUSUM procedures and the SGLRT procedure were empirically obtained by generating the null distributions through Monte Carlo simulation. The study defined Type I error as the proportion of incorrectly identified examinees out of all examinees. Therefore, the maximum statistic was taken within each examinee and used as a representative value to determine aberrancy. Power was defined accordingly as the proportion of examinees who were correctly identified as aberrant. By virtue of having sequential statistics, the procedures were evaluated on an additional criterion: average run length (ARL). Two types of ARL were considered. ARL_1, which is defined as the number of observations between the earliest possible detection point and the actual change point, was used to measure the promptness of detection. The shorter the ARL_1 is, the better the sequential procedure deems to work. ARL_0, on the other hand, refers to the number of observations taken from the onset of an evaluation until false detection. ARL_0 can be considered analogous to Type I error rates in classical hypothesis testing. One would like to see longer ARL_0 in the sense that the procedure was slow and conservative to make an errorneous signal. The performance of the proposed methods was also compared with another response-time-based person-fit statistic, namely χ_{pf} (Sinharay, 2018).

3.3 Results

Figure 2 presents power rates of the proposed statistics and χ_{pf} across the simulation conditions. Each subplot is conditioned on the $\Delta\tau$ size while the three test lengths were plotted on the X-axis. The four detection statistics and three sample sizes were represented as distinctive point and line types, respectively. The results suggest that the proposed statistics can achieve high power rates even with $\Delta\tau$ as small as 0.5 when the sample size is sufficiently large (i.e., 15 items). The impact of the sample size became smaller as the $\Delta\tau$ size increased. When $\Delta\tau$ was 1 or higher, the power rates approached 1 regardless of the sample size. Comparisons across the different detection methods revealed somewhat distinguishable performance from each procedure. Overall, among the sequential procedures, the CUSUM procedures, C^T and C^t, outperformed the s statistic while the two CUSUM procedures showed mixed results. For example, for $\Delta\tau = 0.5$, when the sample size was 5, C^t consistently outperformed C^T while this pattern was reversed when the sample size was 10. In all cases, the detection methods uniformly produced high power rates as the $\Delta\tau$ increased. χ_{pf} performed subpar under the current simulation settings,

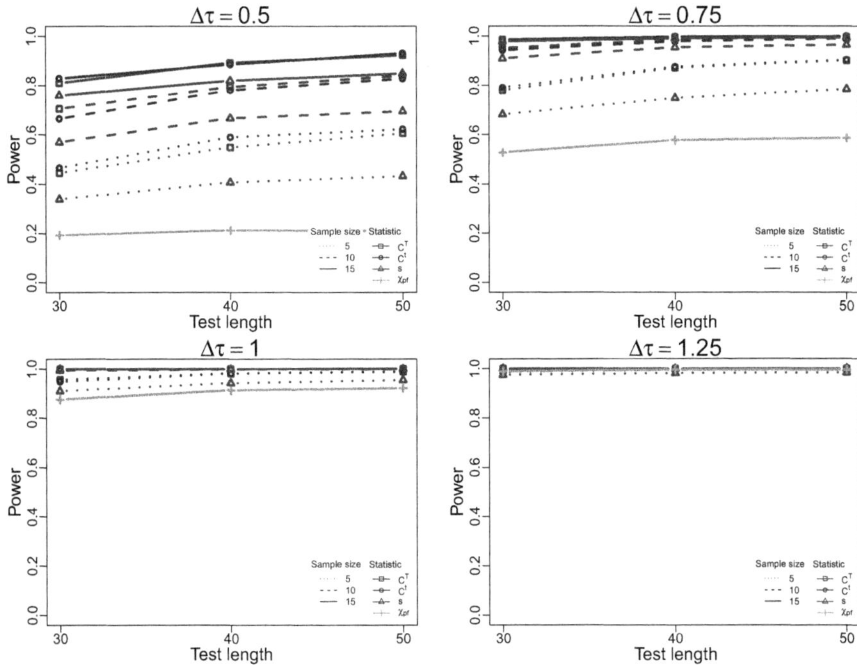

Fig. 2 Power rates across different $\Delta\tau$, test length and sample size conditions

particularly when $\Delta\tau$ was small. Longer tests led to slightly higher power rates when the test length increased from 30 items to 40 items, but the change afterwards was generally negligible.

Table 1 contains more detailed information on power, Type I error rates and ARL results across the statistics for the sample size of 15 condition. The results suggest that the sequential procedures were able to detect aberrant examinees with high power rates while maintaining Type I error rates near the nominal level. Although the results from the sample size of 5 and 10 conditions were omitted, we note that Type I error rates were all well controlled regardless of simulation conditions. χ_{pf} was found to be over conservative. The two CUSUM procedures had overall similar performance, as alluded to earlier. However, their ARL results differed as ARL_1 of C^t was relatively larger than that of C^T, indicating that the τ-based CUSUM detection was less prompt than its counterpart. In fact, it seems that the better ARL_1 in the RT-based CUSUM came at the expense of ARL_0. With much smaller ARL_0's than the other two methods, the RT-based CUSUM was quicker on average to produce an errorneous signal. The impact of $\Delta\tau$ can be clearly seen again in terms of ARL_1. As $\Delta\tau$ increased, ARL_1 became noticeably smaller, while the Type I error rates and ARL_0's remained in a comparable range.

Table 1 Power, Type I error and ARL for the proposed procedures for reference/moving sample size of 15 condition

Procedure	Statistic	$\Delta\tau$	Power	Type I error	ARL_1	ARL_0
CUSUM	C^T	0.5	0.810	0.050	6.675	10.041
		0.75	0.986	0.048	4.311	9.858
		1	1	0.051	2.788	9.836
		1.25	1	0.050	1.896	9.858
	C^t	0.5	0.829	0.050	9.526	12.170
		0.75	0.983	0.053	7.496	12.187
		1	1	0.050	5.972	12.212
		1.25	1	0.050	4.915	12.203
SGLRT	s	0.5	0.760	0.049	9.480	12.125
		0.75	0.979	0.049	7.378	12.068
		1	1	0.049	5.372	12.189
		1.25	1	0.049	4.296	12.108
Sinharay (2018)	χ_{pf}	0.5	0.195	0.032	NA	NA
		0.75	0.532	0.033	NA	NA
		1	0.876	0.035	NA	NA
		1.25	0.991	0.034	NA	NA

4 Application to Process Data

One potentially useful application of the proposed methods can be made with regard to innovative items. With the increasing emphasis on digital literacy skills, more and more computer-based testing programs started to incorporate innovative items that require a series of interactions with computers (e.g., clicking a button, dragging an object). All those user-computer interactions are recorded in log-file data, which are also known as process data. Process data provide interesting information about examinees' problem-solving behaviors by providing the type and sequence of entire actions that examinees took over the course of testing. More importantly, timing information is stored in the process data as computers automatically record each user action with its corresponding time stamp. By utilizing the timing information in the process data, we can deduce aberrant problem-solving behaviors.

4.1 Data

We analyzed process data from the Programme for the International Assessment of Adult Competencies (PIACC) 2012 survey. The PIACC survey measures a range of basic skills for adults including basic reading and numeracy competency. The survey also measures information technology skills of individuals through the problem solving in technology-rich environments (PSTRE) items. The PSTRE items require examinees to undertake a sequence of interactions with computer to access, retrieve, and save information for the successful completion of the requested task. Each user action was recorded with an appropriate label along with timestamp information. We extracted the RTs for each unique action and used them as the basis of our analysis. By treating the actions as if they are items, each unique action's time intensity parameter was calibrated according to the log-normal model. For the sequence of actions for each examinee, the CUSUM-based methods were applied to describe changes in examinee working speed. The moving sample strategy illustrated in Fig. 1 was applied. Specifically, for each individual, a sequence of actions for their first item was used as the reference sample, while the moving sample size was set to contain the same number of actions as in the reference sample. Critical values were calculated based on bootstrap simulations with the nominal level of 0.05.

4.2 Results

Figure 3 presents the charting statistics of the two CUSUM procedures for the PSTRE items from three different examinees in the PIACC 2012 survey. The subfigures on the left column plots the RT-based CUSUM statistics (i.e., C^T), and the column on the right presents plots of the τ-based CUSUM statistics (i.e., C^t) across the examinees' sequence of actions. The subfigures from each row correspond to a single examinee. Note that the two CUSUM statistics show opposite directions because of the inverse relationship between RT and speed.

The examinee on the first row represents a person whose action sequences follow the patterns expected from the parametric model. The CUSUM statistics of this examinee—both RT-based and τ-based—were maintained around zero. This may indicate that this person's response time patterns were normal throughout the testing. The examinees on the second and third row, on the other hand, exhibited response times that significantly deviate from the initial state. To be specific, the upper C^T statistics for Examinee 2184 showed a constantly increasing pattern, and this person ended up being flagged around the 50th action. In contrast, the lower C^T statistics of the examinee stayed near zero. This means that this person acted significantly slower than expected as he/she progressed through the exam. This pattern may signify a fatigue effect with slower reaction times. Interestingly, the examinee on the last row exhibited a completely opposite pattern. The examinee acted just as expected at the beginning of the test session, but acted faster and faster after half-way through the session. This pattern may be indicative of an inattentive test-taking behavior where in this context the examinee simply clicks around randomly without genuine problem solving.

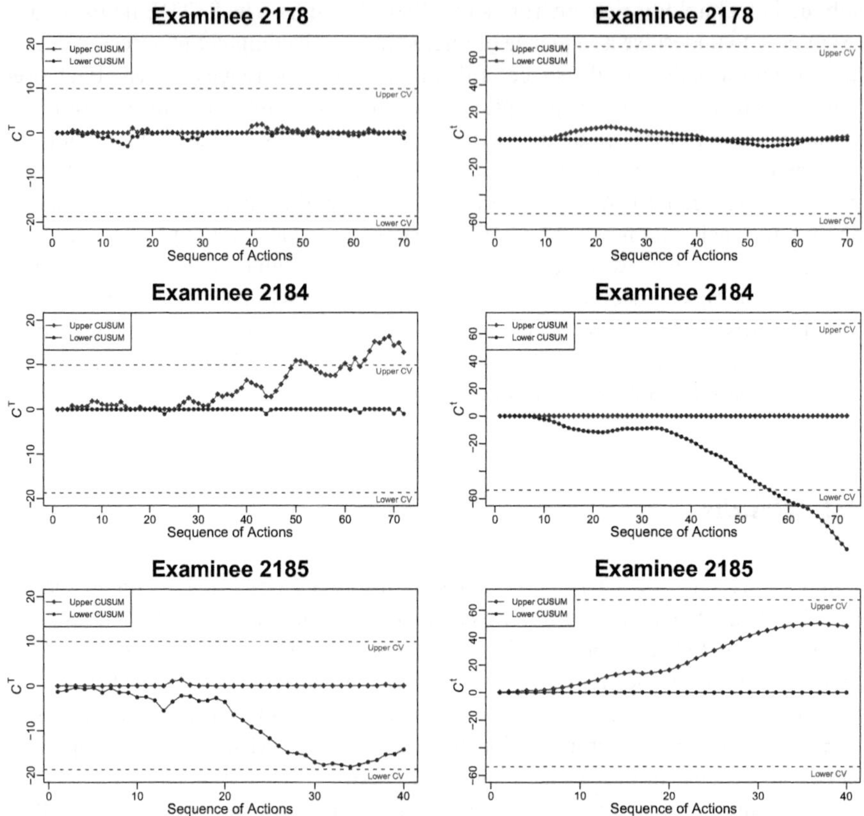

Fig. 3 CUSUM charts from PSTRE items in PIACC 2012 survey for three examinees

5 Discussion

Detecting abnormal test-taking behaviors is essential in psychological measurements to promote the validity of tests. As with the increasing use of RTs in psychometric research, RTs have been found to provide a valuable source of information in identifying aberrant behaviors, as they work as a proxy variable that manifests test-taking strategies. The current study presented sequential procedures that detect abnormalities in examinee RTs. The sequential procedures conduct continuous hypothesis testing where the degree of anomaly is evaluated each time the procedure receives a new observation. The simulation study results indicate promising outcomes: the proposed methods detected aberrant examinees with high detection power, even when the size of change in speed is quite small. The application to the real-world process data showed that the presented procedures can be useful in describing each individual's fluctuating RTs and speed in problem-solving items.

A few aspects of the study should be noted for discussion. As mentioned earlier, detection rates decreased as the reference/moving sample size decreased. This is an expected result because measurement error increases with a smaller sample size. When a larger τ change was imposed, however, the smallest sample condition (i.e., 5 items within the window) performed comparable to the larger sample conditions. Despite the seemingly obvious advantage of having a larger sample, caution should be exercised when determining the sample size. Although a larger sample size may be more appealing to obtain more precise estimates, a sample size that is too large will yield monotone speed estimates across items and be less sensitive for capturing ever-changing speed levels. In practice, an optimal sample size can be determined as the balanced point between the measurement error and the test length. For example, if we apply a reference/moving window size of 15 for a 20-item test, the detection power will drop simply because the procedure does not have enough evaluation points from which to accumulate evidence. We also note that our proposed methods can be more useful for detecting changes that continue for an extended duration because the methods are grounded on the principle of the accumulation of information. Plus, the fact that the suggested moving sample strategy relies on the reference sample at the beginning of testing makes our methods more suitable for behaviors from a continuing cause, such as speeded responses due to time limit or loss of motivation due to low stakes. However, our methods can still detect cases where an abnormal pattern appeared temporarily. In this case, the detection power may diminish because of small number of observations from the aberrant state. Nevertheless, if the magnitude of a change is sufficiently large despite the short duration, the procedures should be able to detect the change since the instance of the large and abrupt change is still well reflected in the maximum statistics within the person.

The paper concludes with implications and suggestions for future research. Indications based on RT only may not be sufficient. By incorporating another important source of information—response scores—into the procedure, examinee aberration may be detected with higher detection power and lower Type I error rates, promoting more confident decision. Another potential direction could be to extend our methods to multiple change point problems. It is entirely possible that examinees may change their working speed a few times during the test. Detecting multiple change points, if any, would allow for more fine-grained descriptions on examinee test-taking behaviors. With a recently opened era of online learning and testing, we believe that the suggested procedures can be highly relevant and timely. The fundamental ideas of the procedures—continuous testing and moving sample strategy—are flexible enough to be extended to other settings. For instance, in online learning settings where students learn a certain domain/skill through a sequence of tasks, the proposed methods can be used to detect dormant or haphazard actions and nudge the subjects on-site based on the detection results.

References

Basseville, M., & Nikiforov, I. V. (1993). *Detection of abrupt changes: Theory and application* (Vol. 104). Englewood Cliffs: Prentice Hall.

Boughton, K. A., Smith, J., & Ren, H. (2016). Using response time data to detect compromised items and/or people. *Handbook of quantitative methods for detecting cheating on tests* (pp. 177–192), Taylor & Francis.

Fox, J., Klein Entink, R., & Klotzke, K. (2017). *LNIRT: Lognormal response time item response theory models. R package version 0.2.0.*

Hawkins, D. M., & Olwell, D. H. (1998). *Statistics for engineering and physical science–cumulative sum charts and charting for quality improvement*. New York: Springer.

Lorden, G. (1971). Procedures for reacting to a change in distribution. *The Annals of Mathematical Statistics, 42*(6), 1897–1908.

Marianti, S., Fox, J.-P., Avetisyan, M., Veldkamp, B. P., & Tijmstra, J. (2014). Testing for aberrant behavior in response time modeling. *Journal of Educational and Behavioral Statistics, 39*(6), 426–451.

Meijer, R. R., & Sotaridona, L. (2006). Detection of advance item knowledge using response times in computer adaptive testing.

Moustakides, G. (1986). Optimal stopping times for detecting changes in distributions. *The Annals of Statistics, 14*(4), 1379–1387.

Page, E. S. (1954). Continuous inspection schemes. *Biometrika, 41*(1/2), 100–115.

Qian, H., Staniewska, D., Reckase, M., & Woo, A. (2016). Using response time to detect item preknowledge in computer-based licensure examinations. *Educational Measurement: Issues and Practice, 35*(1), 38–47.

Siegmund. (1985). *Sequential analysis: Tests and confidence intervals*. New York: Springer.

Siegmund, & Venkatraman, E. (1995). Using the generalized likelihood ratio statistic for sequential detection of a change-point. *The Annals of Statistics, 23*(1), 255–271.

Sinharay, S. (2018). A new person-fit statistic for the lognormal model for response times. *Journal of Educational Measurement, 55*(4), 457–476.

Sinharay, S. (2020). Detection of item preknowledge using response times. *Applied Psychological Measurement, 44*(5), 376–392.

Toton, S. L., & Maynes, D. D. (2019). Detecting examinees with pre-knowledge in experimental data using conditional scaling of response times. In *Frontiers in education* (Vol. 4, p. 49), Frontiers.

van der Linden, W. J. (2006). A lognormal model for response times on test items. *Journal of Educational and Behavioral Statistics, 31*(2), 181–204.

van der Linden, W. J., & Guo, F. (2008). Bayesian procedures for identifying aberrant response-time patterns in adaptive testing. *Psychometrika, 73*(3), 365–384.

van der Linden, W. J., & van Krimpen-Stoop, E. M. (2003). Using response times to detect aberrant responses in computerized adaptive testing. *Psychometrika, 68*(2), 251–265.

Estimating Approximate Number Sense (ANS) Acuity

Anne Thissen-Roe and Lewis Baker

1 Approximate Number Sense Acuity: Psychophysical Scaling Models as Item Response Models

The Approximate Number Sense (ANS) is a psychophysical construct thought to underlie quantity estimation, number processing, and the acquisition of number and math concepts during childhood (Feigenson, Dehaene & Spelke, 2004; Halberda & Feigenson, 2008). Humans (and some non-human animals) have numerosity-selective neurons that fire in response to specific quantities, and not in response to other quantities. This hard-wired brain response is approximate, with some activation for neighbor quantities and overlap between different neurons (Dietrich et al., 2016). The precision of the numerical representation increases through childhood and into adulthood, and differs between individuals of the same age (Halberda & Feigenson, 2008). ANS acuity can be measured through direct quantity estimation, or through the use of speeded quantitative comparison items. We will focus on the latter in this chapter.

As theories of ANS follow within the general psychophysical scaling tradition of Weber and Fechner (Odic, Im, Eisinger, Ly & Halberda, 2016), metrics of ANS acuity commonly include an "internal Weber fraction" w. This fraction is the minimum difference between two quantities at which the greater quantity can be reliably recognized by an individual, expressed as a fraction of the smaller quantity. The Weber fraction w of an individual relates to the ratio r of the quantities compared, the improper fraction of the larger over the smaller quantity, which yields 75% accurate performance by that individual (Hunt, 2007):

A. Thissen-Roe (✉) · L. Baker
pymetrics, inc., New York, NY, USA
e-mail: anne@pymetrics.com; lewis@pymetrics.com

M. Wiberg et al. (eds.), *Quantitative Psychology*, Springer Proceedings in Mathematics & Statistics 353, https://doi.org/10.1007/978-3-030-74772-5_8

$$w = r - 1 \quad . \tag{1}$$

Two competing mathematical models of internal sensory representations, including ANS, yield similar estimates of *w* via distinct forms of an equation predicting error rates from *w*, through least squares (Price, Palmer, Battista & Ansari, 2012) or by maximum likelihood estimation (Odic, Im, Eisinger, Ly & Halberda, 2016). Both models call for numerosity-sensitive neurons with overlapping tuning curves each responding to an approximate quantity, assuming that the tuning curves are Gaussian around the quantity of greatest sensitivity. The primary difference is in the spacing of the curves as the quantities to which they are sensitive increase, and the width of the tuning curves. The *Linear Spacing Model* calls for regularly spaced tuning curves as quantities increase, with increasingly wide tuning curves. Neurons in the Linear Spacing Model are sensitive to large quantities and are less particular about the quantities to which they respond than their counterparts that respond to small quantities. The *Logarithmic Spacing Model* calls for tuning curves of regular spacing and equal width on a log-transformed scale of quantity. As with the Linear Spacing Model, tuning curves for larger quantities are broader, specifically proportional to the quantities they register.

Prior research suggests that children gradually transition to a neural representation of numerosity consistent with the Linear Spacing Model as they learn to recognize and use symbolic numbers. By comparison, young children (and monkeys) tested with items that do not involve reading symbolic numbers produce data more consistent with the Logarithmic Spacing Model (Feigenson et al., 2004; Dehaene, 2007; Dietrich et al., 2016). An associated theory predicts that the same neural representation of the ANS is used in both symbolic and non-symbolic presentations in adults, albeit with an additional step wherein symbolic numbers are recognized and associated with their quantities, which impacts item response time. This theory predicts that regardless of item presentation, the Linear Spacing Model will fit adult response data better than the Logarithmic Spacing Model.

When a quantitative comparison item is presented, the two models imply mathematical functions of performance, or error rate, as a function of the internal Weber fraction *w* and the ratio of quantities *r*. Both functions take the familiar form of normal ogives in the inverse of *w*. Easier items have steeper slopes; all approach a limit of 50% correct performance (chance performance) as 1/*w* goes to 0, but the slope determines the critical location of 75% correct performance.

The Linear Spacing Model predicts:

$$P(correct) = \boldsymbol{\Phi}(\frac{1}{w} * \frac{(r-1)}{\sqrt{r^2+1}}) \tag{2}$$

and the Logarithmic Spacing Model predicts:

$$P(correct) = \boldsymbol{\Phi}(\frac{1}{w} * \frac{|\log r|}{\sqrt{2}}) \tag{3}$$

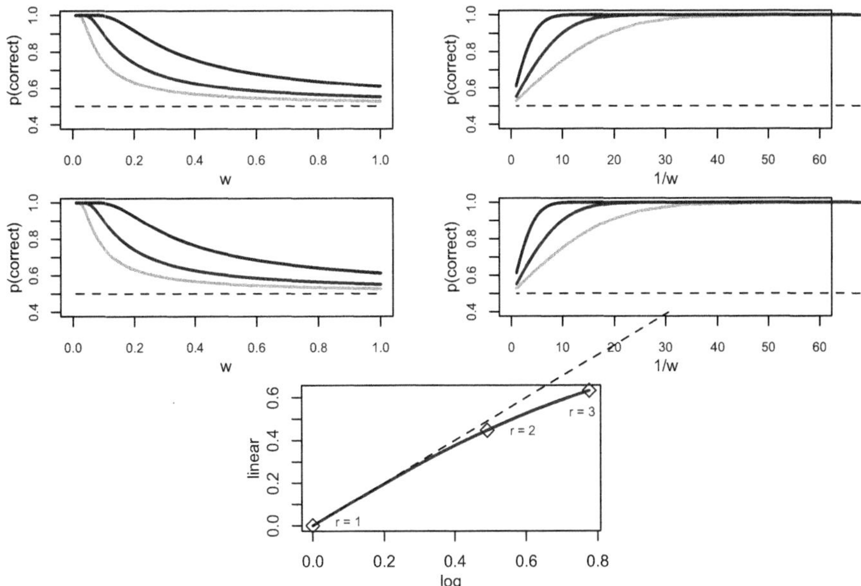

Fig. 1 Left side: Trace lines as a function of w. Upper panel: Trace lines of the Linear Spacing Model as a function of the internal Weber fraction w, at three ratios of numerosity: 1.1, 1.2, and 1.5 (left to right, and light to dark). Lower panel: Trace lines of the Logarithmic Spacing Model as a function of w; matching colors have matching ratios in all panels. **Right side: Trace lines as a function of 1/w.** Upper panel: Trace lines of the Linear Spacing Model as a function of 1/w. It is more apparent in this form that the trace lines are the upper halves of normal ogives. Lower panel: Trace lines of the Logarithmic Spacing Model as a function of the internal Weber fraction w. **Bottom center: Comparison of slope terms of the Linear and Logarithmic Spacing Models**

(Dietrich et al., 2016; Dehaene, 2007).[1]

This is not the usual form in which the error rate predictions are made in the ANS literature. However, presented in this form, it is readily apparent that the psychophysical scaling models make their predictions in the form of item characteristic curves, and w can be estimated using the latent trait methods common in item response theory. Trace lines for both models are presented in Fig. 1.

From the item response theory perspective, a few features are worth noting. First, the items have only a single parameter, r, which is an observed property of the item and does not require (or permit) calibration. Second, both models place persons and items on the same scale, by way of the relationship between r and w.

[1]Although Dietrich et al. (2016) give the logarithm in Equation 3 as base 2, w estimated using that base differ from the linear model by a constant scale factor. Dehaene (2007) does not specify a logarithm base, but his footnote 1 implies natural logarithm, which gives a much closer match to the linear model.

As has been noted before, the two models make quite similar predictions of behavior at the individual level. The trace lines shown in Fig. 1 are visually similar between the top and bottom panels. The Logarithmic Scaling Model gives slightly higher performance estimates, particularly for easy items. This difference has usually not been detectable in experimental contexts involving behavioral measures (Dietrich et al., 2016), but the fit of the two models can be compared in a sufficiently large sample.

In essence, w is a latent trait with two associated item models, which are uniquely grounded in psychophysical theory and modern neuroscience research. The theories and models are not limited to ANS, but past research shows them to be applicable. In the next section, using real-world data from two ANS scales, we compare and relate the parameters, fit and behavior of these models to "ordinary" IRT models.

2 An Application to Data: Magnitudes

Two scales designed to measure ANS exist within the pymetrics talent-matching platform. Each scale comprises 40 highly speeded quantitative comparison items of a single format. The items vary considerably in difficulty, where item difficulty is manipulated by the ratios of the paired quantities.

One scale, Fractions, measures ANS using symbolic stimuli: pairs of fractions, as its name suggests. A user is presented with two fractions side by side, and must choose the larger. The ratio of the two fractions is manipulated in order to increase or decrease difficulty. The left-right position of the correct option and known confounding variables, such as the presence of specific digits in the denominator, are counterbalanced.

The other scale, Dots, measures ANS using non-symbolic stimuli. Specifically, a pymetrics user is presented two side-by-side arrays of dots scattered on rectangular fields, and must select the array with proportionally more yellow dots in a mixture of yellow and blue. (The colors were selected such that recognizing them does not depend on color vision; the blue is substantially darker.) The numbers of blue and yellow dots are manipulated so as to contrive a range of ratios of proportions yellow, parallel to the difficulty manipulation in Fractions. Automatic item generation is used to produce item clones with the specified dot counts, with the variably-sized blue and yellow dots distributed in a unique, non-overlapping pattern for each user. As in Fractions, left-right position and some known confounds, such as the presence of subitizable dot counts, are counterbalanced. In both scales, items are presented very briefly and followed with a visual mask, in order to force users to estimate, rather than calculating or counting.

Dots and Fractions are always administered as a single application, called Magnitudes. See Baker and Thissen-Roe, this volume, for a more comprehensive discussion of the construct relationship between the symbolic and non-symbolic measures, their design, and their place in the larger pymetrics battery.

A sample was drawn of 38,435 users of the pymetrics platform, who had completed Magnitudes between November 2018 and August 2020, in the course of a job application or placement inquiry. A small number of users had incomplete records due to technical difficulties during completion. Of the sample drawn, 38,419 users had usable data for Dots, and 38,424 had usable data for Fractions. Over 89% of users selected English as their primary language, with the remaining selecting 25 other pymetrics localizations. The sample contained 14,605 men, 11,584 women, and 35 reporting as other, with 12,146 not disclosing.[2] Applicants disclosed their ethnicity as 12,537 White or European, 10,467 Asian, 660 Hispanic or Latino, 650 Black or African, and 2,099 as another race or ethnicity. The largest volume of applicants reported their citizenship as Australia (13,911), the United States (4,393) and the United Kingdom (1,932). As job applicants, all users were adults participating in the workforce.

2.1 Least Squares Estimation of ANS

In the present work, several methods were used to estimate the level of the underlying ANS construct in each of these individuals, separately within Dots and Fractions.

First, an individual's Weber fraction can be estimated using the least squares method of Price, Palmer, Battista and Ansari (2012). For w from 0 to 1 in steps of 0.01, the expected error rates at each ratio tested are calculated. For each individual and each potential w, the summed squared difference between observed and expected error is calculated, and the w with the least summed squared difference is selected for each individual.

This procedure has certain limitations. Most obviously, it introduces an absolute floor[3] beyond which poor performance cannot increase estimated w, because values of w above 1 are not considered. At the time Magnitudes was designed, values of w above 1 were not expected to appear in the user population; the extant literature formed the basis of the hypothesized population distribution. In actual practice, a floor effect was observed (see Fig. 2).

By a similar effect, a response pattern with perfect accuracy always results in the theoretically implausible estimate of w equal to zero. The maximum difficulty of the items presented constrains the next-lowest value of w which may be obtained through this method, with all items correct except for one. In our sample, we clearly see a gap between the perfect scores and the next-lowest scores.

[2]Pymetrics operates on voluntary data only, and as such demographic information is limited by applicant disclosure.

[3]This boundary might be considered a ceiling, as it is the *upper* limit of w; however, as high values of w go with poor performance, low ability, and low scores on traditional scales, we think of it as a performance floor.

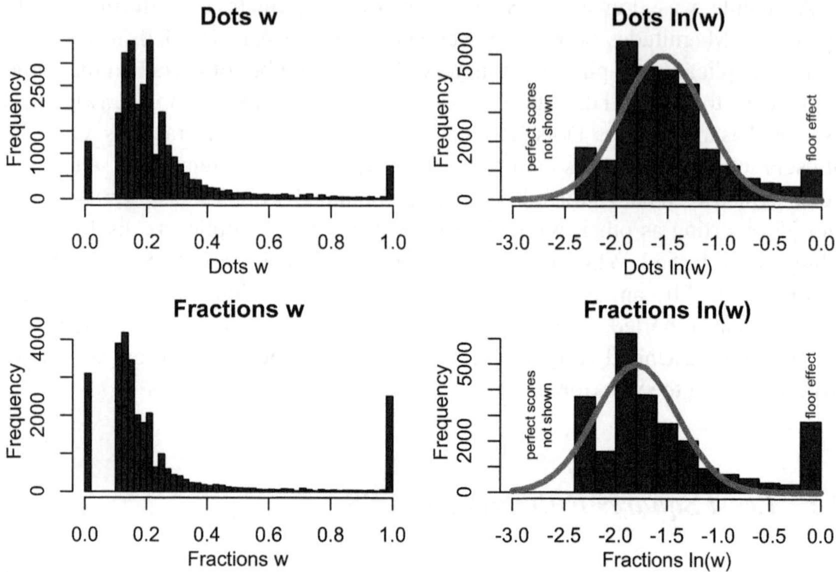

Fig. 2 Left side: Observed sample distributions of *w*, estimated by least squares. Upper panel: Dots. Note that aside from ceiling and floor effects, the distribution appears reasonably lognormal, with a long right tail and no negative values. Lower panel: Fractions. **Right side: Sample distributions under a logarithmic transform, with a normal distribution for comparison.** Upper panel: Dots. Note that perfect response patterns, assigned $w = 0$ by the scoring algorithm, are not shown in this panel. Lower panel: Fractions. Perfect response patterns are not shown

Despite these limitations, the least squares estimates provide usable individual scores, as well as certain useful information regarding the population distribution of ANS as an internal Weber fraction. Figure 2 shows the sample distributions of w, directly and under a logarithmic transform. The estimates of w appear to conform reasonably well to a lognormal distribution, a finding we use in our subsequent latent trait estimation.

2.2 *Latent Trait Estimation of ANS*

Latent trait estimation was used to produce estimates of w under both the Linear and Logarithmic Scaling Models, as well as several ordinary IRT models for comparison. Calibration of item and population parameters was accomplished using an algorithm similar to that described by Bock & Aitkin (1981), with fixed 41-point quadrature spanning $[-5, 5]$. For scoring of individuals, the Bayesian expectation a posteriori (EAP) method was used, again with fixed 41-point quadrature.[4]

Following from the finding of an approximately lognormal distribution of w in the previous section, a lognormal population prior was desirable for estimation of the Linear and Logarithmic Scaling Models, as was logarithmic spacing in the fixed quadrature. Accordingly, a normally distributed θ was defined such that

$$w = e^{\theta} \tag{4}$$

As noted, both the Linear Spacing Model and the Logarithmic Spacing Model call for only a single parameter, r, which is an observed property of the item and does not require (or permit) calibration. On the other hand, the mean and standard deviation of θ as it underlies w are latent parameters which need not be fixed for identification. In fact, the standard normal distribution often used as a prior for estimation of theta in IRT is likely inappropriate. Based on observations of the distribution of least-squares w and its logarithm, the distribution of θ is probably not centered at zero. Therefore, the parameters of the prior distribution, rather than the items, were calibrated.

An immediate advantage of latent trait estimation of w over least-squares estimation is the elimination of the structural floor effect. In cases of low performance, values of w above 1 may be obtained as scores, extending out to the point at which there are no longer sufficiently easy items to which to compare a user.

In addition, ordinary logistic IRT models were fit to the same data, using a fixed standard normal distribution as a prior. The models fit were the three-parameter logistic model (3PL), the two-parameter logistic model (2PL), a constrained version of the 3PL in which the lower asymptote was fixed to 0.5, and a further constrained 3PL in which the lower asymptote was fixed to 0.5 and the discrimination parameter was fixed to 1.

2.3 Results

Latent trait estimation permits evaluation of the fit of all six models to the available data, and comparison of models fit to the same dataset via the Bayesian Information Criterion (BIC). We chose the BIC over competing information criteria because it has a severe penalty imposed on less parsimonious models, a feature particularly important when working with large datasets. The BIC values obtained for all models are presented in Table 1.

[4]In anticipation of more involved future research, the authors implemented the calibration and scoring algorithm as a Java application, in lieu of using any of several publicly available estimation packages which would likely have sufficed for the current study.

Table 1 Bayesian Information Criterion (BIC) for All Latent Trait Models. The degrees of freedom are given as k

Model	k	Dots BIC	Fractions BIC
Linear Spacing Model	2	1,099,021.2	989,122.6
Logarithmic Spacing Model	2	1,103,894.7	998,994.4
Three-Parameter Logistic	120	987,110.0	878,570.2
Two-Parameter Logistic	80	988,630.6	879,157.4
3PL, fixed asymptote	80	986,781.8	877,991.9
3PL, location only	40	1,029,215.7	900,699.3

Several features are noteworthy. First, despite the superior theoretical grounding of the two psychophysical models, *all* of the IRT models fit better to both datasets. A likely partial explanation for this finding is that the IRT models all have more free parameters, and are capable of adapting more to the data. To the extent that this is the case, the IRT models may be useful in finding the causes of the misfit of the psychophysical models. This analysis is presented in the following section.

Second, between the two psychophysical models, the Linear Spacing Model gave a better fit to the data from both Fractions and Dots. This is consistent with the theory given in Dehaene (2007) that calls for a single underlying system that changes its nature with exposure to symbolic numerals. It is worth noting that we found only a modest correlation between w from the two scales (see Baker and Thissen-Roe, this volume), which is harder to explain under that theory.

From conversations between the authors and test-takers, we tested a variation of the psychophysical models for Dots that assumed a misinterpretation of the instructions. Although users are instructed to select the display with a greater proportion of yellow dots *relative to all dots in the display*, many users may have misinterpreted this to mean the greater proportion of yellow dots *relative to blue dots*. We find just that: a variation of the psychophysical models for Dots that used the ratio of yellow to blue rather than yellow to total fit considerably better, giving BIC values of 1,065,950.0 and 1,063,244.2 for the Linear and Logarithmic Spacing Models respectively. This suggests that many of our users are interpreting the instructions for Dots to ask for the higher odds of yellow, rather than the higher fraction of the total (and we ought to clarify our instructions); however, it is also notable that to the extent that the odds ratio is used, the Logarithmic Spacing Model fits better – even though all thirty-eight thousand users were adults in the workforce, applying to jobs that use symbolic numbers.

Third, among the IRT models, the same pattern of fit results was observed in both Dots and Fractions. In both cases, best fit was obtained with the constrained three-parameter logistic model in which the lower asymptote was fixed to 0.5, corresponding to a random draw between the two response options. Allowing the lower asymptote to vary did not improve model fit enough to compensate for the additional free parameters required. By contrast, the further-constrained model, in which item discrimination was fixed to unity, performed worst of the four on both datasets (though still better than the psychophysical models). It is apparent that some of the items on each scale are better measures of ANS than others; at least some of this may be attributable to previously known confounds that were counterbalanced rather than constrained.

Both the Linear Spacing Model and the Logarithmic Spacing Model place items and people on a common scale of ANS acuity and item difficulty, a relationship captured in the linear correspondence between w and r at the 75% performance level. This relationship mirrors the relationship in the logistic IRT models between an individual's latent trait standing θ and an item location parameter b. It follows that a mapping function that relates w to θ should match a mapping function between r and b, at least in the case of the most constrained IRT model. That is, given a function that predicts θ from w, one should be able to use the same function to predict b from $r - 1$, a useful feature should any new items be constructed!

As it turns out, the mapping occasionally holds but does not reliably do so; confounding item features and, potentially, alternate response strategies affect fitted b parameters, which then vary from their predicted values based on the r alone. In the cases of Dots and Fractions, the b parameters suggest that nearly all of the items are too easy for a majority of users, easier than expected given their ratios, although incorrect responses still occur. This effect is shown in Fig. 3.

3 Conclusion

We have shown here that psychophysical models based on Weber's law, applied to speeded quantitative comparison items as a measure of the Approximate Number Sense (ANS), imply item characteristic curves. The results indicate that ANS acuity can be estimated as a latent trait, with practical benefits relative to least squares estimation, such as an expanded range of measurement.

In our data, the Linear Spacing Model and Logarithmic Spacing Model did not fit as well as the more flexible, but less theoretically grounded, logistic models. There are variations on the psychophysical models that include terms for known confounds, such as dot size and sparsity (DeWind, Adams, Platt & Brannon, 2015). It is possible that a more complex and flexible model would enable the psychophysical models to fit as well as the logistic models.

We were also interested in the time it takes users to respond to each pair of quantities. In the course of the research described in this chapter, we did some initial exploration in the direction of fitting joint response time models, specifically using the hierarchical framework (van der Linden, 2006, 2007). However, diffusion models (Ratcliff, 1978; Ratcliff & Smith, 2008) were a better theoretical fit (Dehaene, 2007). For now, we leave response time modeling will to future studies.

Acknowledgments We would like to thank Frida Polli, founder of pymetrics. We would also like to thank Su Mei Lee for her work on the development of Magnitudes and the adaptation of the least-squares scoring algorithm, and Fedor Garin and Zachary Smith for leading the front-end design of the Magnitudes app. Finally, we would like to thank David Thissen and Dylan Molenaar for helpful comments on earlier drafts.

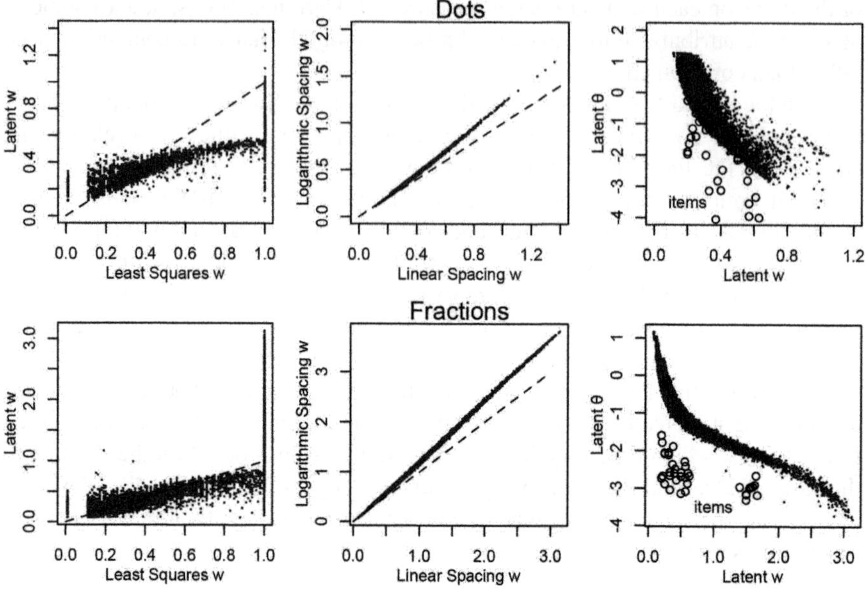

Fig. 3 Left panels: Latent trait estimation of w improves on least squares estimation by permitting measurement below the "floor" of $w = 1$. Latent w has a long right tail, particularly for Fractions (lower panel). **Center panels:** Estimates based on the Linear Spacing Model and Logarithmic Spacing Model are nearly perfectly correlated, but do not scale the same. The Logarithmic Spacing Model predicts higher performance on the easy items; one might say it is less forgiving of mistakes. **Right panels:** The relationship between θ and w is strong, particularly for Fractions, and monotonic but not linear. One would expect that if one plotted $r - 1$ against the location parameter for each item, it would fall along the line; instead, these items (open circles) fall below the line, indicating that they are probably easier than the psychophysical models predict

References

Bock, R. D., & Aitkin, M. (1981). Marginal maximum likelihood estimation of item parameters: Application of an EM algorithm. *Psychometrika, 46*, 443–459.

Dehaene, S. (2007). Symbols and quantities in parietal cortex: Elements of a mathematical theory of number representation and manipulation. In P. Haggard & Y. Rossetti (Eds.), *Attention and performance xxii sensorimotor foundations of higher cognition* (pp. 527–574). Cambridge: Harvard University Press.

DeWind, N. K., Adams, G. K., Platt, M. L., & Brannon, E. M. (2015). Modeling the approximate number system to quantify the contribution of visual stimulus features. *Cognition, 142*, 247–265.

Dietrich, J. F., Huber, S., Klein, E., Willmes, K., Pixner, S., & Moeller, K. (2016). A systematic investigation of accuracy and response time based measures used to index ans acuity. *PLoS ONE, 11*, 1–45.

Feigenson, L., Dehaene, S., & Spelke, E. (2004). Core systems of number. *TRENDS in Cognitive Science, 8*, 307–314.

Halberda, J., & Feigenson, L. (2008). Developmental change in the acuity of the 'number sense': The approximate number system in 3-, 4-, 5-, and 6-year-olds and adults. *Developmental Psychology, 44*, 1457–1465.

Hunt, E. (2007). *The mathematics of behavior*. New York, NY: Cambridge University Press.

Odic, D., Im, H. Y., Eisinger, R., Ly, R., & Halberda, J. (2016). Psimle: A maximum-likelihood estimation approach to estimating psychophysical scaling and variability more reliably, efficiently, and flexibly. *Behavioral Research Methods, 48*, 445–462.

Price, G. R., Palmer, D., Battista, C., & Ansari, D. (2012). Nonsymbolic numerical magnitude comparison: Reliability and validity of different task variants and outcome measures, and their relationship to arithmetic achievement in adults. *Acta Psychologica, 140*, 50–57.

Ratcliff, R. (1978). A theory of memory retrieval. *Psychological Review, 85*, 59–108.

Ratcliff, R., & Smith, P. L. (2008). A comparison of sequential sampling models for two-choice reaction time. *Psychological Review, 111*, 333–367.

van der Linden, W. J. (2006). A lognormal model for response times on test items. *Journal of Educational and Behavioral Statistics, 31*, 181–204.

van der Linden, W. J. (2007). A hierarchical framework for modeling speed and accuracy on test items. *Psychometrika, 77*, 287–308.

Differences in Symbolic and Non-symbolic Measures of Approximate Number Sense

Lewis Baker and Anne Thissen-Roe

1 Introduction

Researchers have shown increasing interest in the human capacity to represent numbers and numerical information. In particular, research has focused on how adults, children, and even some animals appear to efficiently represent the relative numerosity of objects. The early developmental onset of relative numerosity is apparent to any adult who has unevenly divided sweets between two children: even relatively small inequalities are detected rapidly (and with vigor). Two decades of research have theorized an innate cognitive process that represents large numerosities (Xu & Spelke, 2000; Xu et al., 2005; Dehaene, 2011), with later theories further hypothesizing an approximate number sense or system (ANS) that innately and automatically represents the approximate, relative cardinality of sets of objects (Halberda & Feigenson, 2008). The existence of the ANS is supported by neurological evidence suggesting a double dissociation between verbal knowledge and intuitive understanding of quantitative values from specific brain damage (Dehaene & Cohen, 1997). Moreover, evidence that nonverbal infants and animals can also estimate quantities suggests an innate, biologically based predicate for arithmetic representation (Dehaene et al., 1998). Such a specialized process has led to expansive research on the ANS and its potential for exposing a new understanding of mathematical cognition.

Numerical representation attributed to the ANS has demonstrated stable individual differences across a predictable developmental trajectory, which, importantly, appears to be predictive of future mathematics ability. Infants as young as six months can reliably identify differences in magnitude of two groups of objects

L. Baker (✉) · A. Thissen-Roe
pymetrics, inc., New York, NY, USA
e-mail: lewis@pymetrics.com; anne@pymetrics.com

M. Wiberg et al. (eds.), *Quantitative Psychology*, Springer Proceedings in Mathematics & Statistics 353, https://doi.org/10.1007/978-3-030-74772-5_9

at a ratio 1:2, refining to a 2:3 ratio by nine months of age (Lipton & Spelke, 2003). Acuity with judgements of relative magnitude rapidly increase throughout development, until reaching stability in early adulthood, where adults can reliably judge a magnitude difference between 9:10 to 10:11 (Pica et al., 2004; Halberda & Feigenson, 2008). An increasingly refined sense of quantity and ability to compare quantities correlates with elementary school children's acquisition of arithmetic facts, as well as adult mathematics achievement (Fazio et al., 2016; Halberda et al., 2008). Further research indicates that precision with ANS tasks at age 3–4 can predict mathematics performance two and half years later ($R^2 = 0.352$, $N = 13$), but not performance in verbal reasoning (Mazzocco et al., 2011). For this reason, ANS measures are increasing popular measures of math aptitude (Bonny & Lourenco, 2013).

ANS acuity is often measured through speeded judgments of relative magnitude. Participants in such tasks view two sets of objects and select which set contains more items. This can be done using non-symbolic items, where users compare sets of colored dots or familiar objects, or using symbolic items such as Arabic numerals or fractions. In either method, the items must not require multiple steps or formal operations, and must be amenable to rapid presentation and response. Many researchers prefer non-symbolic measures of ANS acuity because of their broad application to very young children, adults without formal education, or non-human animals. Meanwhile, symbolic measures of ANS acuity have an advantage of face validity, as they require a level of mathematics expertise, and may therefore be more closely related to math achievement. However, these two measures are not always comparable. Fazio and colleagues (2014) found that both symbolic and non-symbolic measures correlate with math achievement in fifth graders, although the relationship was much stronger for symbolic numbers. On the other hand, Sasanguie and colleagues (2013) found no significant relationships between symbolic and non-symbolic measures, while also finding that symbolic measures had a greater correlation with performance on a curriculum-based math assessment. Other work validates that non-symbolic magnitude comparison can predict math ability in children; however, they fail to find predictive validity in adults (Inglis et al., 2011). Other evidence supports a causal relationship between training children in non-symbolic estimation and symbolic math performance, using a related non-symbolic ANS task based on summing approximate magnitudes (Park & Brannon, 2013).

In summary, the exact relationship between symbolic and non-symbolic measures of ANS acuity is very much unknown, as is their respective contribution to mathematics ability. To assist the academic study of these different procedures, we leveraged a dataset of over twenty-two thousand responses to ANS acuity measures taken from a subset of an online job assessment. The assessment included measures of symbolic ANS (comparing fractions) and non-symbolic ANS (comparing dot patterns), alongside three other measures of numerical reasoning, spatial reasoning and working memory. With this data, we attempt to answer two questions. First, how closely related are symbolic and non-symbolic measures of the approximate number sense? And second, how are the two ANS methods related to other measures of mathematics ability?

2 Method

The current study analysed data completed by job applicants through the pymetrics platform. Pymetrics is a job matching platform that uses behavioral data and machine learning methods to recommend applicants to roles where they best fit (see www.pymetrics.ai). Here we analyse the results from four tests that comprise a broader suite of 16 tests in the pymetrics battery. Each test is described in depth below.

Participants were 27,720 job applicants to 18 distinct positions at 5 client companies over the time period from November 2018 to June 2020. Participants with missing data from any of the four tests outlined below were removed from analysis. Also, only participants who played on the desktop computer app were included (mobile apps are also available). This left 22,187 applicants for analysis. The sample contained 8579 men, 7638 women and 14 reporting as other, with 5879 not disclosing.[1] Applicants disclosed their ethnicity as 7851 White or European, 6415 Asian, 367 Hispanic or Latino, 366 Black or African, and 1334 as another race or ethnicity. Data was collected from a global sample of applicants, with 87.1% reporting English as their primary language (the remaining users reported a mix of 22 other languages covered by pymetrics). Participants hailed from six continents, with the largest volume of applicants from Australia (8469), the United States (1687) and the United Kingdom (1486). The entire 16-test battery took a median of 36 min to complete. This study compares performance on 4 of these tests, outlined below.

3 Measurements

ANS Acuity: Magnitudes. *Magnitudes* measures a participant's discrimination of relative magnitude. It was developed as a replication of Fazio et al. (2014), with a user interface compatible with web and mobile apps. Magnitudes has both non-symbolic and symbolic subtests, named *Dots* and *Fractions*, respectively. Subtest order was standardized for all participants, with Dots always coming before Fractions. Figure 1a–b illustrates the test flow for both subtests.

Each subtest contained 40 trials consisting of two side-by-side displays. In the non-symbolic subtest, Dots, displays contained a mix of blue and yellow dots of different sizes and randomized location. The object of the test was for users to select which display contained a larger proportion of yellow dots. The displays were uniquely generated images built from an algorithm that ensured non-overlapping dots. The true ratio difference in magnitude ranged from 1.19 to 2.67 across all

[1]Pymetrics operates on voluntary data only, and as such demographic information is limited by applicant disclosure.

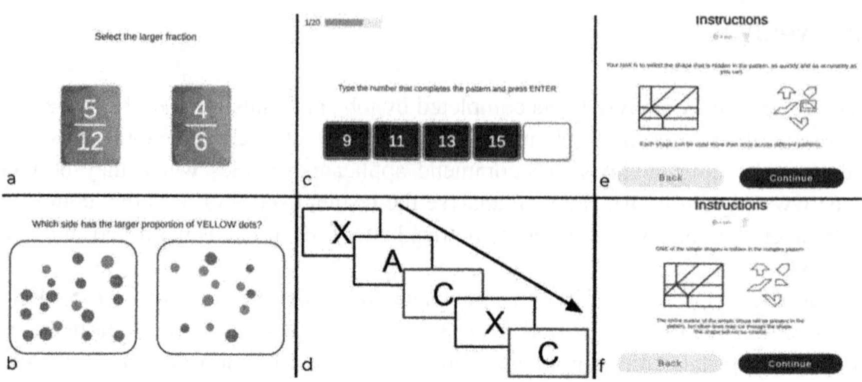

Fig. 1 Test Battery. All images are single displays from the pymetrics game battery except (**d**), which is a composite diagram of five sample displays. (**a**) Fractions. Users select the larger fraction ($\frac{5}{12} < \frac{4}{6}$, a ratio difference of 1.6 : 1). (**b**) Dots. Users select the display with proportionally more yellow dots ($\frac{4}{18} < \frac{7}{13}$, a ratio difference of 2.42 : 1). (**c**) Sequences. Users type the number that completes the pattern ($x_{i-1} + 2 = 17$). (**d**) Letters. Users respond when a display repeats from n − 2 displays previous (in pink). (**e–f**) Shapes. Users identify which simple shape (right) can be found in the complex shape (left); pink highlights for illustration only

trials. Trials were randomly counterbalanced by target location so that the target was equally likely to appear on either side. The total pixel coverage of all dots were set so that both sides always had equal colored area. Likewise, the side with the largest surface area of yellow color was counterbalanced so as not to be predictive of target side. Participants were given two practice trials with feedback. After that, participants were instructed that they would complete 40 trials without stopping, and to respond as quickly and as accurately as possible. Upon starting the test, participants had a 5000 ms response window for each trial. Stimuli were displayed for only 1500 ms to discourage counting. The next trial began 500 ms following a response or timeout. The boundary around the selected display would change colors to indicate a registered response, but did not provide feedback for response accuracy. Trials were randomized for each participant.

The symbolic subtest, Fractions, was similar to Dots with some notable exceptions. Fractions trials presented two whole number fractions. Participants were instructed to select the fraction that was greater in magnitude. Unlike Dots, Fractions displays would be visible for the entire 5000 ms response window, as pilot testing indicated that 1500 ms was too brief for reliable responding. As with Dots, Fractions trials were counterbalanced for target side, but also for a variety of potential heuristics that a savvy user might use rather than estimating relative magnitudes, following the supplemental documents provided in Fazio et al. (2016). For example, trials were counterbalanced so users could not guess the larger fraction simply by selecting the fraction greater than $\frac{1}{2}$.

Three key metrics were obtained for both Dots and Fractions. Accuracy was measured as the overall proportion of correct answers. Response time (RT) was measured as the time (ms) required to complete correct trials. A third metric, w, is the subject of Thissen-Roe and Baker, this volume. Briefly, w is the internal Weber fraction, the estimated threshold of the Just Noticeable Difference of presented items. The coefficient w can be calculated by least squares or latent trait methods using its predicted relationship to correct response:

$$P(correct) = \Phi(\frac{1}{w} * \frac{(r-1)}{\sqrt{r^2+1}}) \tag{1}$$

wherein r is the ratio of the two presented quantities (e.g., the fractions). In this chapter, we use least squares estimation, which is the summed square of observed performance minus expected performance, where formula (1) is the expected performance, minimized across several groups of similarly difficult items, binned by the four quartiles of r.

Research supports that w is a reliable, robust psychophysical measure of the sensitivity of ANS acuity (Price et al., 2012). As w was highly correlated with accuracy in this study ($r_{Dots:w,acc} = -0.945$, $r_{Fractions:w,acc} = -0.946$), all analyses were conducted using only w.

Symbolic Pattern Completion: Sequences. Sequences is a symbolic pattern completion task, a measure of numerical reasoning ability, and is modeled after Thurstone's Number Series Test (Thurstone, 1938). Sequence completion ability is a robust component of quantitative reasoning subscales of general intelligence (Carroll et al., 1993) and is correlated with academic achievement and mathematical aptitude (Mayer et al., 1984).

In Sequences, participants view sequences of numbers with one item omitted, as shown in Fig. 1c. Participants were instructed to fill in the missing number that fit the pattern. Omitted numbers could appear in any location in the sequence. Patterns were generated so that trials included the a variety of arithmetic operations, including addition by a constant, multiplication and exponentiation. Participants had 30 s to complete each of the 20 patterns. The metrics from Sequences were overall accuracy and average response time for correct trials.

Spatial Reasoning: Shapes Shapes assesses spatial reasoning ability. It is modeled after Thurstone's Gottschaldt Figures test (Thurstone, 1938), and is correlated with mathematics achievement (Tosto et al., 2014). In this test, a number of simple shapes are presented, along with one complex pattern (Fig. 1e–f). The task is to identify which of the simple shapes is embedded in the complex pattern. Participants had 45 s to complete each of the 14 trials. The metrics from Shapes were overall accuracy and average response time for correct trials.

Working Memory: Letters Letters is an adaptation of Kirchner's n-back test, designed to assesses working memory ability (Kirchner, 1958). Working memory is correlated with general mental ability (GMA) and academic achievement, including mathematical problem solving ability (Friso-Van den Bos et al., 2013). Here it is included as a predictor of math ability that is not domain-specific to numerical cognition. In Letters, users view a sequence of individually displayed letters (Fig. 1d). The user must respond whether the letter currently seen is the same as a letter seen two presentations previous. For example, in the sequence [L, L, T, R, T, T], the user would respond to the fifth letter, since it appears two steps after another "T", but they would not respond to the sixth letter, since two steps previous was the letter "R". Each letter appears for 1 s followed by a 200 ms ISI and 1 s fixation cross. Sequences of letters are algorithmically generated so that there are always 10 targets within a 40 letter stream. The primary metrics of Letters were hit and false alarm rates and their corresponding response times.

4 Results

4.1 Symbolic vs Non-symbolic ANS

The first comparison of interest is the similarity of the non-symbolic measure of the approximate number system, Dots, and the symbolic measure, Fractions. The two Weber fractions, w, were modestly correlated ($r = 0.32$, $t_{22185} = 50.658$, $p < 10^{-16}$), as were their response times ($r = 0.40$, $t_{22185} = 65.199$, $p < 10^{-16}$).

The mean w for Fractions ($\mu = 0.269, median = 0.170, \sigma = 0.273$) was greater than the mean w for Dots ($\mu = 0.257, median = 0.210, \sigma = 0.189$). A Kolmogorov-Smirnov test indicated that the distributions significantly deviated to a modest extent ($D = 0.170$, $p < 10^{-16}$).

A speed-accuracy trade-off was observed for Dots ($r_{w,rt} = -0.186$), indicating that slower participants had more refined estimates of magnitude in visual comparisons. However, this trade-off did not exist for Fractions ($r_{w,rt} = 0.084$). The differences in these correlations were moderate and significant using Steiger's correlation comparison formulation ($r_{diff} = -0.27$, $z_{diff} = -28.69$, $p < 10^{-11}$) (Steiger, 1980).

These results indicate a modest relationship between symbolic and non-symbolic measures of the ANS. The most noticeable difference is that participants demonstrate a higher mean w but lower median w for Fractions versus Dots. The distribution of w from Fractions has a longer and heavier right tail than Dots, with more users having w greater than 1. There are a few potential reasons for this: Fractions is more difficult (as interpreted from higher response times), and the additional effort may lead to participants giving up. Fractions also relies on learned skills, which may lead to relatively worse responding for participants with less confidence in mathematics.

In a different effect, we see that users with slower average response times have a finer w for Dots, but not for Fractions. This is a curious effect that warrants further study in a more controlled setting. It may be that slower users for Dots are simply fast counters. However, as the Dots displays vanish after 1.5 s, this strategy would rely heavily on visual working memory capacity. Another possibility is that the underlying neurocognitive process of Dots is substantively different than that of Fractions. Dots may be more akin to the random walk-type evidence accumulation based on the pooling of estimates from multiple neurons, as described by Dehaene (2007). Longer viewing might improve estimates. Meanwhile, symbolic ANS measures like Fractions are theorized to have sequential process components, such that merely looking at the item longer may not result in greater certainty as to the answer without relying on elaborative thinking. This possibility could be tested by fitting a diffusion model (Ratcliff & Smith, 2008) to data from both scales. We leave this to future research.

4.2 *Relationship of ANS to Other Measures of Math Ability*

The second comparison of interest is the similarity of ANS measures to other indicators of math performance. Table 1 shows the correlation matrix of all measures of interest.

Sequences. Numerical reasoning as measured by Sequences was significantly correlated with both Dots w ($r = -0.304$, $t_{22185} = -47.53$, $p < 10^{-16}$) and Fractions w ($r = -0.445$, $t_{22185} = -74.01$, $p < 10^{-16}$). Furthermore, Sequences was significantly more correlated with Fractions than with Dots ($r_{diff} = 0.141$, $z_{diff} = 17.33$, $p < 10^{-16}$).

Shapes. Spatial reasoning as measured by Shapes accuracy was significantly correlated with both Dots w ($r = 0.258$, $t_{22185} = -39.77$, $p < 10^{-16}$) and Fractions w ($r = 0.300$, $t_{22185} = -46.84$, $p < 10^{-16}$), although both correlations were less than when comparing ANS measures to numerical reasoning. There was a significant difference between the correlation of ANS domains and Shapes ($r_{diff} = 0.042$, $z_{diff} = 4.800$, $p < 10^{-6}$), although this difference was trivially small.

Letters. Both Fractions and Dots were only marginally correlated with the working memory task, Letters. Higher hit rates were associated with smaller w ($r_{Frac} = -0.148$, $r_{Dots} = -0.122$, $t_{22185} < -18.16$, $p < 10^{-16}$). Conversely, higher false alarm rates were associated with larger w ($r_{Frac} = 0.216$, $r_{Dots} = 0.215$, $t_{22185} > 31.99$, $p < 10^{-16}$). However, there were no practical differences between either ANS subtest and working memory ($z_{diffhitrate} = 2.79$, $p = 0.005$, $z_{diffFArate} = 0.111$, $p = 0.914$).

Altogether, we see modest evidence that both ANS tasks predict numerical and spatial reasoning ability, with the symbolic measure, Fractions, being more strongly correlated with numerical reasoning, and only slightly more correlated with spatial reasoning. Meanwhile, we see only minor relationships between measures of working memory, without differentiation by ANS subtests. This supports a theory of ANS as a domain-specific mathematical construct, with convergent validity between two domain-relevant measures and far less with a related by domain-agnostic construct.

Table 1 Correlation matrix for all experimental measures. *ACC* proportionate accuracy, *FA* false alarm rate, *Hit* hit rate, *RT* response time (ms), *w* estimated Weber fraction

	Dots RT	Dots w	Frac RT	Frac w	Letters FA RT	Letters FAs	Letters Hit RT	Letters Hits	Seq Acc	Seq RT	Shapes Acc	Shapes RT
Dots RT	1											
Dots w	−0.186	1										
Frac RT	0.401	−0.029	1									
Frac w	0.024	0.322	0.084	1								
Letters FA RT	0.072	−0.067	0.066	−0.059	1							
Letters FAs	−0.065	0.210	−0.007	0.213	−0.133	1						
Letters Hit RT	0.132	−0.068	0.133	−0.074	0.216	−0.181	1					
Letters Hits	−0.062	−0.121	−0.070	−0.148	0.118	0.028	0.061	1				
Seq Acc	0.015	−0.304	−0.095	−0.445	0.047	−0.215	0.076	0.184	1			
Seq RT	0.172	0.106	0.337	0.266	0.032	0.091	0.048	−0.132	−0.285	1		
Shapes Acc	0.020	−0.258	−0.029	−0.300	0.048	−0.223	0.098	0.159	0.388	−0.157	1	
Shapes RT	0.218	−0.139	0.217	−0.085	0.049	−0.114	0.104	−0.018	0.138	0.155	0.175	1

5 Discussion

Through collection of a large amount of behavioral data on five separate measures relating to math achievement, we find that symbolic and non-symbolic measures of the approximate number sense are moderately correlated, but distinct. We report that the symbolic task was significantly more correlated with a simple numerical reasoning measure than the non-symbolic task. There are significant relationships between both ANS measures and spatial reasoning and working memory, with no practical distinction between symbolic and non-symbolic ANS variants. This agrees with previous research comparing symbolic and non-symbolic tasks and math achievement, which found that symbolic measures better predicted school math achievement, and through meta-analysis found a similar correlation symbolic and non-symbolic magnitude comparison accuracy ($r \sim 0.31$).

The primary contribution of this report is to provide substantial data to support existing theories of the approximate number sense. However, it should be noted that what these analyses provide in volume may also be detracted in control. The pymetrics battery is offered to job applicants to complete in their own time. Although participants are given instructions to complete the battery in a distraction-free setting, they may still complete in the coffee shops and bus stations of the real world, adding more noise than a laboratory. Likewise, many of the test featured here are substantially shorter than their laboratory counterparts. This is a necessary compromise to remove some burden from job applicants; however, laboratory experiments with 10, if not 100 times the trials are likely to find more subtle effects than those presented here. In exchange, the current study offers a view of tens of thousands of participants from a broader range of demographics than typically available to college campuses. We hope that this information may be useful for further understanding the cognitive substrates of mathematical cognition.

Acknowledgments We would like to thank Frida Polli, founder of pymetrics. We would also like to thank Su Mei Lee, Janelle Szary, Eugenia Fernandez and Nicholas DeVeau for their work on the development and testing of Magnitudes, Shapes, and Sequences; and Fedor Garin and Zachary Smith who led front-end design of the tests.

References

Bonny, J. W., & Lourenco, S. F. (2013). The approximate number system and its relation to early math achievement: Evidence from the preschool years. *Journal of Experimental Child Psychology, 114*(3), 375–388.

Carroll, J. B., et al. (1993). *Human cognitive abilities: A survey of factor-analytic studies.* Cambridge University Press.

Dehaene, S. (2007). Symbols and quantities in parietal cortex: Elements of a mathematical theory of number representation and manipulation. In P. Haggard & Y. Rossetti (Eds.), *Attention and performance XXII sensorimotor foundations of higher cognition.* Cambridge: Harvard University Press.

Dehaene, S. (2011). *The number sense: How the mind creates mathematics*. OUP.
Dehaene, S., & Cohen, L. (1997). Cerebral pathways for calculation: Double dissociation between rote verbal and quantitative knowledge of arithmetic. *Cortex, 33*(2), 219–250.
Dehaene, S., Dehaene-Lambertz, G., & Cohen, L. (1998). Abstract representations of numbers in the animal and human brain. *Trends in Neurosciences, 21*(8), 355–361.
Fazio, L. K., Bailey, D. H., Thompson, C. A., & Siegler, R. S. (2014). Relations of different types of numerical magnitude representations to each other and to mathematics achievement. *Journal of Experimental Child Psychology, 123*, 53–72.
Fazio, L. K., DeWolf, M., & Siegler, R. S. (2016). Strategy use and strategy choice in fraction magnitude comparison. *Journal of Experimental Psychology: Learning, Memory, and Cognition, 42*(1), 1.
Friso-Van den Bos, I., Van der Ven, S. H., Kroesbergen, E. H., & Van Luit, J. E. (2013). Working memory and mathematics in primary school children: A meta-analysis. *Educational Research Review, 10*, 29–44.
Halberda, J., & Feigenson, L. (2008). Developmental change in the acuity of the" number sense": The approximate number system in 3-, 4-, 5-, and 6-year-olds and adults. *Developmental Psychology, 44*(5), 1457.
Halberda, J., Mazzocco, M. M., & Feigenson, L. (2008). Individual differences in non-verbal number acuity correlate with maths achievement. *Nature, 455*(7213), 665–668.
Inglis, M., Attridge, N., Batchelor, S., & Gilmore, C. (2011). Non-verbal number acuity correlates with symbolic mathematics achievement: But only in children. *Psychonomic Bulletin & Review, 18*(6), 1222–1229.
Kirchner, W. K. (1958). Age differences in short-term retention of rapidly changing information. *Journal of Experimental Psychology, 55*(4), 352.
Lipton, J. S., & Spelke, E. S. (2003). Origins of number sense: Large-number discrimination in human infants. *Psychological Science, 14*(5), 396–401.
Mayer, R. E., Larkin, J. H., & Kadane, J. B. (1984). A cognitive analysis of mathematical problem-solving ability. In R. J. Sternberg (Ed.), *Advances in the Psychology of Human Intelligence* (Vol. 2, pp. 231–273). Hoillsdale, NJ: Erlbaum.
Mazzocco, M. M., Feigenson, L., & Halberda, J. (2011). Preschoolers' precision of the approximate number system predicts later school mathematics performance. *PLoS One, 6*(9), e23749.
Park, J., & Brannon, E. M. (2013). Training the approximate number system improves math proficiency. *Psychological Science, 24*(10), 2013–2019.
Pica, P., Lemer, C., Izard, V., & Dehaene, S. (2004). Exact and approximate arithmetic in an amazonian indigene group. *Science, 306*(5695), 499–503.
Price, G. R., Palmer, D., Battista, C., & Ansari, D. (2012). Nonsymbolic numerical magnitude comparison: Reliability and validity of different task variants and outcome measures, and their relationship to arithmetic achievement in adults. *Acta Psychologica, 140*(1), 50–57.
Ratcliff, R., & Smith, P. L. (2008). A comparison of sequential sampling models for two-choice reaction time. *Psychological Review, 111*, 333–367.
Sasanguie, D., Göobel, S. M., Moll, K., Smets, K., & Reynvoet, B. (2013). Approximate number sense, symbolic number processing, or number–space mappings: What underlies mathematics achievement? *Journal of Experimental Child Psychology, 114*(3), 418–431.
Steiger, J. H. (1980). Tests for comparing elements of a correlation matrix. *Psychological Bulletin, 87*(2), 245.
Thurstone, L. L. (1938). *Primary mental abilities* (Vol. 119). Chicago: University of Chicago Press.
Tosto, M. G., Hanscombe, K. B., Haworth, C. M., Davis, O. S., Petrill, S. A., Dale, P. S., Malykh, S., Plomin, R., & Kovas, Y. (2014). Why do spatial abilities predict mathematical performance? *Developmental Science, 17*(3), 462–470.
Xu, F., & Spelke, E. S. (2000). Large number discrimination in 6-month-old infants. *Cognition, 74*(1), B1–B11.
Xu, F., Spelke, E. S., & Goddard, S. (2005). Number sense in human infants. *Developmental Science, 8*(1):88–101.

Formulas of Multilevel Reliabilities for Tests with Ordered Categorical Responses

Zhenqiu (Laura) Lu, Minju Hong, and Seohyun Kim

1 Introduction

Reliability is a measure of overall internal consistency of a test. It has been widely used in statistical, psychological, educational, social and behavioral research when data are collected by responding to items in a test or a questionnaire (Bollen, 1989; Finney & DiStefano, 2006). A high value of reliability indicates the measure provides similar, reliable, and stable results under consistent conditions. There are many approaches that have been proposed to estimate reliabilities. Among them, the classical test theory (CTT) approach has been widely used, and the Cronbach alpha is the most popular reliability. But it only measures the lower bound on the consistency of a test (Green et al., 1977; Novick & Lewis, 1967; Sijtsma, 2009). Another approach using structural equation modeling (SEM) has been proposed to obtain more accurate reliabilities (Bentler, 2009; Bollen, 1989; Green & Yang, 2009; Miller, 1995; Raykov, 1997; Raykov & Shrout, 2002). But these methods focus on addressing continuous outcomes.

For tests with ordered categorical responses, Green and Yang (2009) proposed a nonlinear reliability coefficient within an SEM framework, and the nonlinear reliability has been found to be more accurate than the linear reliability that treats categorical scores as continuous. But they only considered the items with the same number of categories. Kim, Lu and Cohen (2020) extended their research to broader situations and proposed a general formula for reliabilities. But these formulas are only for single level data structure. And their research did not consider the composite

Z. Lu (✉) · M. Hong
University of Georgia, Athens, GA, USA
e-mail: zlu@uga.edu

S. Kim
University of Virginia, Charlottesville, VA, USA

M. Wiberg et al. (eds.), *Quantitative Psychology*, Springer Proceedings in Mathematics & Statistics 353, https://doi.org/10.1007/978-3-030-74772-5_10

reliability or the coefficient Omega (McDonald, 1985) and the maximal reliability H of weighted sum (Bentler, 2007) for tests with categorical responses. So far, there has been no research on this topic.

In order to fill the gap, the current study reviewed various approaches to reliabilities, extended single level reliabilities to multilevel reliabilities, and provided closed-form formulas for multilevel nonlinear SEM reliabilities for tests with ordered categorical responses via a multilevel confirmatory factor analysis (MCFA) approach. Multilevel alpha was also considered.

2 Reliabilities

2.1 CTT Approach

Suppose there are J items in a test. In classical test theory (CTT), an observed score X_j on item j ($j = 1, \ldots, J$) is composed of two uncorrelated components, a latent true score or trait, T_j, and an error score, ϵ_j, with mean of 0:

$$X_j = T_j + \epsilon_j$$

Let X, T and ϵ be the sum of observed scores, of true scores, and of error scores, respectively, across J items. Then

$$X = X_1 + X_2 + \cdots + X_J = \sum_{j=1}^{J} X_j,$$

and $T = \sum_{j=1}^{J} T_j, \epsilon = \sum_{j=1}^{J} \epsilon_j$, so we have $X = T + \epsilon$.

We want to make sure how much of variance of observed score is due to the latent true score versus the error. One measure is to use reliability. The reliability coefficient of a test is defined as the ratio of the true variance to the total variance, which is the sum of the true variance and the error variance. Mathematically, it is

$$\rho = \frac{\sigma_T^2}{\sigma_x^2},$$

where σ_T^2 is the variance of T, and σ_x^2 is the variance of X (Lord & Novick, 1968). The reliability quantifies the proportion or ratio. It is an estimation of how much random error might be in the scores around the true score.

Cronbach Alpha Under CTT, there are many ways to estimate reliability: test-retest, alternative forms, split-half, Spearman-Brown prophecy formula, and the Cronbach alpha (or coefficient Alpha). Among them, the Cronbach alpha (Cronbach, 1951) is the most commonly used. The Cronbach alpha is defined as

$$\alpha = \frac{J^2 \overline{\sigma}_{xx'}}{{\sigma_x}^2}$$

where J is the total number of items, ${\sigma_x}^2$ is the variance of observed scores of the test X, and $\overline{\sigma}_{xx'}$ is the mean of off-diagonal covariance between two parallel tests X and X'. Specifically, the alpha can be calculated as

$$\alpha = \frac{J^2 * \frac{\sum_i \sum_{j,i<j} \sigma_{x_i,x_j}}{\frac{J(J-1)}{2}}}{{\sigma_x}^2}$$

where $\sum_i \sum_{j,i<j} \sigma_{\varepsilon_i,\varepsilon_j}$ is the sum of lower (or upper) off-diagonal covariance between items i and j.

2.2 CFA Approach

However, the Cronbach alpha is only a lower bound on the internal consistency of the test (Green et al., 1977; Novick & Lewis, 1967; Sijtsma, 2009). To get a better estimate, another approach to reliability is the structural equation modeling (SEM) approach. Specifically, this approach uses confirmatory factor analysis (CFA) to estimate reliability. Tests are assumed to have underlying factorial structure (factors, e.g., reading ability, math ability, or personality).

$$X_j^* = \lambda_{1j}\eta_1 + \lambda_{2j}\eta_2 + \cdots + \lambda_{Mj}\eta_M + e_j,$$

where X_j^* is a continuous score for item j, M is the number of latent factors, η_m $(1 \leq m \leq M)$ are latent factors weighted by corresponding factor loadings λ_m, and e_j is a measurement error term. We assume errors are independent and have variance $\sigma^2_{\varepsilon_j}$ for item j.

Suppose there are J items in the test and X^* and T are the sum of observed scores and of true scores, respectively. Then $X^* = \sum_{j=1}^{J} X_j^*$ and $T = \sum_{j=1}^{J} \sum_{m=1}^{M} \lambda_{mj}\eta_m$. Because item scores are presented by a confirmatory factor analysis model, the linear reliability ρ_{lin} is calculated as the ratio of true sum score variance to observed sum score variance where the true score variance is estimated using the CFA model above.

$$\rho_{lin} = \frac{\sigma_T^2}{\sigma_{X^*}^2} = \frac{Var\left(\sum_{j=1}^{J} \sum_{m=1}^{M} \lambda_{mj}\eta_m\right)}{Var\left(\sum_{j=1}^{J} X_j^*\right)}.$$

Here ρ_{lin} measures the linear proportion of observed sum score variance that is attributed to the latent factors, $\eta_1, \eta_2, \ldots, \eta_M$ (Bollen, 1989).

Composite Reliability/Coefficient Omega ω

If item scores have only one factor, then $M = 1$ and the reliability above becomes

$$\rho_{lin} = \frac{\sigma_T^2}{\sigma_{X^*}^2} = \frac{Var\left(\sum_{j=1}^{J} \lambda_j \eta\right)}{Var\left(\sum_{j=1}^{J} X_j^*\right)}.$$

And if we assume that latent factor have unit variance $Var(\eta) = 1$, then the reliability ρ_{lin} is referred to as composite reliability or coefficient omega ω (McDonald, 1985)

$$\omega = \frac{\left(\sum \lambda_{x_j}\right)^2}{\left(\sum \lambda_{x_j}\right)^2 + \sum \sigma_{\varepsilon_j}^2}$$

where $\sum \lambda_{x_j}$ is a sum of the factor loading of item *j*, and $\sum \sigma_{\varepsilon_j}^2$ is a sum of all error variances.

Maximal Reliability *H* for Weighted Sum

Composite reliability represents the relation between a scale's underlying latent factor and its unit-weighted composite, but a scale's unit-weighted composite may not optimally reflect its underlying latent construct. The true score variance estimated in factor analysis allows for heterogeneous indicator weights, so it is reasonable to allow heterogeneous weights when creating a scale's composite score.

$$X = w_1 X_1 + w_2 X_2 + \cdots + w_J X_J = \sum_{j=1}^{J} w_j X_j$$

One approach to comparing true score variance for one common factor to the variance of a unit-weighted scale is presented as maximal reliability *H* (e.g., Bentler, 2007). When the weight vector

$$W = \left(\lambda' \psi^{-1} \lambda\right)^{-1/2} \psi^{-1} \lambda,$$

where λ is the factor loading matrix and ψ is the residue variance matrix, then the maximal reliability is given by

$$\rho_{w\prime x(\max)} = \frac{\lambda' \psi^{-1} \lambda}{\lambda' \psi^{-1} \lambda + 1}$$

By assuming that the variance of each item is 1, the standardized version of maximal reliability for a single common factor model can be expressed as follows (e.g., Hancock & Mueller, 2001; Geldhof et al., 2014).

$$H = \frac{\sum \frac{\lambda_{x_j}^2}{\sigma_{\varepsilon_j}^2}}{1 + \sum \frac{\lambda_{x_j}^2}{\sigma_{\varepsilon_j}^2}} = \frac{\sum \frac{\lambda_{x_j}^2}{1-\lambda_{x_j}^2}}{1 + \sum \frac{\lambda_{x_j}^2}{1-\lambda_{x_j}^2}} = \frac{1}{1 + \frac{1}{\sum \frac{\lambda_{x_j}^2}{1-\lambda_{x_j}^2}}}$$

where $\lambda_{x_j}^2$ is the squared standardized factor loading of item j, and $\sigma_{\varepsilon_j}^2$ is the error variance of item j.

3 Multilevel Reliabilities

The data collected from social and educational areas often have multilevel structure. In these cases, multilevel reliabilities for multilevel structure were proposed.

3.1 Multilevel Confirmatory Factor Analysis (MCFA)

Muthén (2011) defined a multilevel confirmatory factor analysis (MCFA) by assuming a one-factor model holds for both the between and the within components. The observed value of the p-dimensional variable y_{gi} is partitioned into three components:

$$y_{gi} = V + y_{Bg} + y_{wgi}$$

where y_{gi} is the observed value of individual i in group g, V is a grand mean, y_{Bg} is the between-group part of the observed value, and y_{wgi} is the within-group part of the observed value. The multilevel CFA specifies a model at between-group level and within-group level separately. Suppose there are h factors between groups and m factors within groups, the between-group level CFA model is

$$y_{Bg} = \Lambda_{Bg}\eta_{Bg} + \varepsilon_{Bg}$$

where Λ_{Bg} is a $(p \times h)$ matrix of factor loadings with elements λ_{Bg}'s, η_{Bg} is a h-dimensional vector of factor scores with the assumption of $\eta_{Bg} \sim MN(0_h, \Psi_{h \times h})$, and ε_{Bg} is a p-dimensional vector of errors with the assumption of $\varepsilon_i \sim MN(0_p, \Phi_{p \times p})$. And the within-group CFA model level is defined as

$$y_{wgi} = \Lambda_{wg}\eta_{wgi} + \varepsilon_{wgi}$$

where Λ_{wg} is a $(p \times m)$ matrix of factor loadings with elements λ_{wg}'s, η_{wgi} is a m-dimensional vector of factor scores with the assumption of

η_{wgi}~$MN(0_m, \Psi_{m \times m})$, and ε_{wgi} is a p-dimensional vector of errors with the assumption of ε_i~$MN(0_p, \Phi_{p \times p})$.

If there is only one factor either between-group or within-group, then the variance of the observed variable y, $\sigma^2_{y_{gi}}$, is decomposed (Muthén, 2011) as

$$\sigma^2_{y_{gi}} = \lambda^2_{Bg}\sigma^2_{\eta Bg} + \sigma^2_{\varepsilon Bg} + \lambda^2_{wg}\sigma^2_{\eta wgi} + \sigma^2_{\varepsilon wgi}$$

$$= \sigma^2_{BF} + \sigma^2_{BE} + \sigma^2_{WF} + \sigma^2_{WE}$$

where λ_{Bg} is between-group factor loadings, $\sigma^2_{\eta Bg}$ is the variances of between-group factor scores, $\sigma^2_{\varepsilon Bg}$ is the variances of between-group errors, λ_{wg} is within-group factor loadings, $\sigma^2_{\eta wg}$ is the variances of within-group factor scores, and $\sigma^2_{\varepsilon wg}$ is the variances of within-group errors, ${\sigma_{BF}}^2$ is a between-level factor score variance, ${\sigma_{BE}}^2$ is a between-level error variance, ${\sigma_{WF}}^2$ is a within-level factor score variance, and ${\sigma_{WE}}^2$ is an within-level error variance.

3.2 *Multilevel Reliabilities*

Applying MCFA to reliability calculation, p dimensions become J items, and we assume there is only one factor either between-group or within-group.

Multilevel Alpha The multilevel alpha is calculated as

$$\text{within} - \text{group level } \alpha = \frac{J^2 * \overline{\sigma}_{wgi,wgj}}{\sigma^2_{wg}}$$

$$\text{between} - \text{group level } \alpha = \frac{J^2 * \overline{\sigma}_{Bgi,Bgj}}{\sigma^2_{Bg}}$$

where J is the number of items, $\overline{\sigma}_{wgi,wgj}$ is the average of the within-group covariance between items i and j. σ^2_{wg} is the variance of the within-group part of observed value, $\overline{\sigma}_{Bgi,Bgj}$ is the mean of the between-group covariance between items i and j, and σ^2_{Bg} is the variance of the between-group part of observed value.

Multilevel Omega And multilevel omega is obtained as

$$\text{within} - \text{group level } \omega = \frac{\left(\sum \lambda_{wg_j}\right)^2}{\left(\sum \lambda_{wg_j}\right)^2 + \sum \sigma^2_{\varepsilon wg_j}}$$

$$\text{between} - \text{group level } \omega = \frac{\left(\sum \lambda_{Bg_j}\right)^2}{\left(\sum \lambda_{Bg_j}\right)^2 + \sum \sigma^2_{\varepsilon Bg_j}}$$

where $\sum \lambda_{wgj}$ is a sum of within-group level squared factor loading of item j, and $\sum \sigma^2_{\varepsilon \text{wgi}}$ is a sum of within-group level error variances, $\sum \lambda_{Bgj}$ is a sum of within-group level squared factor loading of item i, and $\sum \sigma^2_{\varepsilon Bgj}$ is a sum of within-group level error variances.

Multilevel *H* Maximal H is calculated by

$$\text{within} - \text{group level } H = \frac{1}{1 + \frac{1}{\sum \frac{\lambda^2_{wg_j}}{1-\lambda^2_{wg_j}}}}$$

$$\text{between} - \text{group level } H = \frac{1}{1 + \frac{1}{\sum \frac{\lambda^2_{Bg_j}}{1-\lambda^2_{Bg_j}}}}$$

where λ^2_{wgj} is the squared standardized within-group factor loading of item j, λ^2_{Bgj} is the squared standardized between-group factor loading of item j.

4 Multilevel Reliability for Categories Responses

It is very common in social and behavioral sciences that items have ordered categories. When the observed data are ordinal categorical, fitting linear SEM models using the linear estimation method is not desirable because it violates the assumption and provides inflated chi-square estimates and attenuated factor loadings (Bollen, 1989). To address this problem, we consider the observed categorical scores ($\mathrm{X_j}$) are from underlying continuous variables $\left(\mathrm{X_j^*}\right)$ and the nonlinear relationship between $\mathrm{X_j}$ and $\mathrm{X_j^*}$ is

$$X_j = \begin{cases} C_j - 1, & if \quad X_j^* \geq v_{C_j-1} \\ \vdots & \vdots \\ 1, & if \quad v_1 \leq X_j^* < v_2 \\ 0, & if \quad X_j^* < v_1. \end{cases}$$

where C_j is the number of categories for X_j, and the ν_i $(i = 1, 2, \ldots, C_j - 1)$ are the category thresholds. If X_j^* is less then ν_1, $\mathrm{X_j}$ is equal to 0, for $\upsilon_1 \leq \mathrm{X_j^*} < \upsilon_2$, $\mathrm{X_j}$ is equal to 1, and if $\mathrm{X_j^*}$ is above ν_{C_j-1}, $\mathrm{X_j}$ is equal to $\mathrm{C_j} - 1$. If the structure of the test is well-specified, this approach can estimate reliability more accurately than the linear SEM approach.

Multilevel Alpha for Tests with Categorical Responses Single level alpha for categorical responses can be calculated by using polychoric correlations if we assume the variance of each item is 1. Reliability calculated from parallel measures. For multilevel alpha, both within- and between-group levels reliabilities are calculated.

Multilevel Composite Reliability for Tests with Categorical Responses Single level composite reliabilities have been proposed by Kim, Lu and Cohen (2020) to investigated reliability with items having the same or different numbers of ordered categories. For multilevel composite reliabilities, the same formula can be applied at both within- and between-group levels. Multilevel Omega for tests with categorical responses is a simplified version for one factor models.

Multilevel Maximal Reliability for Tests with Categorical Responses There has been no research on this topic done before. In this article, we derived the numerical formula as follows. Suppose X and $\tilde{X}$ are two parallel tests, which are two weighted sums, $X = \sum_{j=1}^{J} w_j X_j$ and $\tilde{X} = \sum_{j'=1}^{J} w_{j'} \tilde{X}_{j'}$. To estimate the reliability for the nonlinear measurement model, the correlation between X and $\tilde{X}$is used, which is

$$\rho_{X\tilde{X}} = \frac{Cov\left(X, \tilde{X}\right)}{\sqrt{\mathrm{var}(X)\mathrm{var}\left(\tilde{X}\right)}}.$$

The numerator for weighted sums is

$$Cov\left(X, \tilde{X}\right) = Cov\left(\sum_{j=1}^{J} w_j X_j, \sum_{j'=1}^{J} w_{j'} \tilde{X}_{j'}\right) = \sum_{j=1}^{J}\sum_{j'=1}^{J} w_j w_{j'} Cov\left(X_j, \tilde{X}_{j'}\right),$$

in which

$$Cov\left(X_j, \tilde{X}_{j'}\right) = E\left(X_j \tilde{X}_{j'}\right) - E\left(X_j\right) E\left(\tilde{X}_{j'}\right)$$

$$= \left(\sum_{k=1}^{C_j-1} \sum_{l=1}^{C_{j'}-1} \Phi_2 \left(\nu_{jk}, h_{j_l'}; \rho_M \right) - (C_{j'} - 1) \sum_{k=1}^{C_j-1} \Phi_1 \left(\nu_{jk} \right) - (C_j - 1) \right.$$

$$\left. \times \sum_{l=1}^{C_{j'}-1} \Phi_1 \left(h_{j_l'} \right) + (C_j - 1) (C_{j'} - 1) \right)$$

$$- \left(- \sum_{k=1}^{C_j-1} \Phi_1 \left(\nu_{jk} \right) + (C_j - 1) \right) \left(- \sum_{k=1}^{C_{j'}-1} \Phi_1 \left(h_{j_l'} \right) + (C_{j'} - 1) \right)$$

$$= \sum_{k=1}^{C_j-1} \sum_{l=1}^{C_{j'}-1} \Phi_2 \left(\nu_{jk}, h_{j_l'}; \rho_M \right) - \sum_{k=1}^{C_j-1} \Phi_1 \left(\nu_{jk} \right) \sum_{l=1}^{C_{j'}-1} \Phi_1 \left(h_{j_l'} \right)$$

and

$$\rho_M = \sum_{m=1}^{M} \sum_{m'=1}^{M} \lambda_{mj} \lambda_{m'j'} \rho_{\eta_m \eta_{m'}}$$

The denominator is

$$Var(X) = Var \left(\sum_{j=1}^{J} w_j X_j \right) = \sum_{j=1}^{J} \sum_{j'=1}^{J} w_j w_{j'} Cov \left(X_j, X_{j'} \right)$$

$$= \sum_{j=1}^{J} \sum_{j'=1}^{J} w_j w_{j'} \left(\sum_{k=1}^{C_j-1} \sum_{l=1}^{C_{j'}-1} \Phi_2 \left(\nu_{jk}, h_{j_l'}; \rho_{X_j^* X_{j'}^*} \right) \right.$$

$$\left. - \sum_{k=1}^{C_j-1} \Phi_1 \left(\nu_{jk} \right) \sum_{l=1}^{C_{j'}-1} \Phi_1 \left(h_{j_l'} \right) \right)$$

Therefore the reliability is calculated from parallel measures of ordered categories responses

$$\rho_{Cat} = \frac{\sum_{j=1}^{J} \sum_{j'=1}^{J} w_j w_{j'} \left[\sum_{k=1}^{C_j-1} \sum_{l=1}^{C_{j'}-1} \Phi_2 \left(\nu_{jk}, h_{j_l'}; \rho_M \right) - \sum_{k=1}^{C_j-1} \Phi_1 \left(\nu_{jk} \right) \sum_{l=1}^{C_{j'}-1} \Phi_1 \left(h_{j_l'} \right) \right]}{\sum_{j=1}^{J} \sum_{j'=1}^{J} w_j w_{j'} \left[\sum_{k=1}^{C_j-1} \sum_{l=1}^{C_{j'}-1} \Phi_2 \left(\nu_{jk}, h_{j_l'}; \rho_{X_j^* X_{j'}^*} \right) - \sum_{k=1}^{C_j-1} \Phi_1 \left(\nu_{jk} \right) \sum_{l=1}^{C_{j'}-1} \Phi_1 \left(h_{j_l'} \right) \right]}$$

For one factor models, the formula above can be greatly simplified. The multilevel maximal reliability of weighted sum will apply the formula at both within-group and between-group levels.

5 Conclusions

This study proposed a confirmatory factor analysis approach to multilevel reliability for tests with ordered categories item responses. It extended single level reliabilities to multilevel reliabilities, and provided closed–form formulas for calculating various types of multilevel nonlinear reliabilities, including the composite reliability, the coefficient Omega, and the maximal reliability.

References

Bentler, P. M. (2007). Covariance structure models for maximal reliability of unit-weighted composites. In *Handbook of latent variable and related models* (pp. 1–19). North-Holland.

Bentler, P. M. (2009). Alpha, dimension-free, and model-based internal consistency reliability. *Psychometrika, 74*(1), 137–143.

Bollen, K. A. (1989). *Structural equations with latent variables*. Wiley.

Cronbach, L. J. (1951). *Coefficient alpha and the internal structure of tests. psychometrika, 16*(3), 297–334.

Finney, S. J., & DiStefano, C. (2006). Non-normal and categorical data in structural equation modeling. In G. R. Hancock & R. O. Mueller (Eds.), *Structural equation modeling: A second course* (pp. 269–314). Information Age.

Geldhof, G. J., Preacher, K. J., & Zyphur, M. J. (2014). Reliability estimation in a multilevel confirmatory factor analysis framework. *Psychological Methods, 19*(1), 72–91.

Green, S. B., Lissitz, R. W., & Mulaik, S. A. (1977). Limitations of coefficient alpha as an index of test unidimensionality. *Educational and Psychological Measurement, 37*(4), 827–838.

Green, S. B., & Yang, Y. (2009). Reliability of summed item scores using structural equation modeling: An alternative to coefficient alpha. *Psychometrika, 74*(1), 155–167.

Hancock, G. R., & Mueller, R. O. (2001). Rethinking construct reliability within latent variable systems. In R. Cudeck, S. du Toit, & D. Sörbom (Eds.), *Structural equation modeling: Present and future – A festschrift in honor of Karl Jöreskog* (pp. 195–216). Scientific Software International.

Kim, S., Lu, Z., & Cohen, A. S. (2020). Reliability for tests with items having different numbers of ordered categories. *Applied psychological measurement, 44*(2), 137–149.

Lord, F. M., & Novick, R. (1968). Statistical theories of mental test scores. Reading MA: Addison-Wesley.

McDonald, R. P. (1985). *Factor analysis and related methods*. Erlbaum.

Miller, M. B. (1995). Coefficient alpha: A basic introduction from the perspectives of classical test theory and structural equation modeling. *Structural Equation Modeling, 2*(3), 255–273.

Muthén, B. O. (2011). Mean and covariance structure analysis of hierarchical data. UCLA: Department of Statistics, UCLA. Retrieved from https://escholarship.org/uc/item/1vp6w4sr.

Novick, M., & Lewis, C. (1967). Coefficient alpha and the reliability of composite measurements. *Psychometrika, 32*(1), 1–13.

Raykov, T. (1997). Estimation of composite reliability for congeneric measures. *Applied Psychological Measurement, 21*(2), 173–184.

Raykov, T., & Shrout, P. E. (2002). Reliability of scales with general structure: Point and interval estimation using a structural equation modeling approach. *Structural Equation Modeling, 9*(2), 195–212.

Sijtsma, K. (2009). On the use, the misuse, and the very limited usefulness of Cronbach's alpha. *Psychometrika, 74*(1), 107–120.

Polytomous IRT Models Versus IRTree Models for Scoring Non-cognitive Latent Traits

Francisca Calderón and Jorge González

1 Introduction

Non-cognitive latent traits are unobservable variables related to personality characteristics defined as patterns of thoughts, feelings, and behaviours (Borghans et al., 2008). Examples of non-cognitive assessments are personality tests, opinion surveys, and satisfaction questionnaires, among others.

Non-cognitive assessments are distinguished from the cognitive evaluations in that for the former there is not a correct or incorrect response option. Rather, these instruments collect information mostly using Likert type items of ordinal categorical response (e.g., "Strongly Disagree", "Disagree", "Agree", "Strongly Agree") yielding score data defined on a polytomous scale. Thus, respondents know or probably have an insight about which option is "most appropriate" to answer, depending on the context that the non-cognitive instrument is applied.

Item response theory (IRT, Lord, 1980), is a useful framework to measure latent traits from the answers to measurement instruments. An IRT model specifies the relation between the observable variables (i.e., item responses on a test) and non-observable ones (i.e., latent trait). The mathematical model describes the conditional probabilities of responses given one or more latent variables. When items are scored in more than two categories, polytomous IRT models such as the Graded Response Model (GRM, Samejima, 1969) and the Generalized Partial Credit Model (GPCM, Muraki, 1992) have been usually used to measure the latent trait of interest.

F. Calderón (✉) · J. González
Departamento de Estadística, Pontificia Universidad Católica de Chile, Santiago, Chile

Laboratorio Interdiciplinario de Estadística Social, LIES, Facultad de Matemáticas, Pontificia Universidad Católica de Chile, Santiago, Chile
e-mail: flcalderon@mat.uc.cl; jorge.gonzalez@mat.uc.cl

M. Wiberg et al. (eds.), *Quantitative Psychology*, Springer Proceedings in Mathematics & Statistics 353, https://doi.org/10.1007/978-3-030-74772-5_11

The statistical modeling of polytomous score data in non-cognitive assessments is challenging because respondents can use different strategies or show different tendencies to choose categories independently of the item content, leading to response styles in their answers. Ignoring response styles can result in biased latent trait estimates, which invalidate inferences on an individual's construct of interest being measured.

Under the IRT framework, IRTree models (Böckenholt, 2012; De Boeck & Partchev, 2012; Jeon & De Boeck, 2016) have been used to analyze polytomous items taking into account response styles. IRTree models are appealing because of their unique ability to decompose Likert-type scale item responses into a series of binary pseudo-item responses represented in a tree structure specified for the response categories (Jeon & De Boeck, 2019). This decomposition allows to model not only the main trait of interest being measured, but also additional traits representing response style in answers. Thus, IRTree models can be considered as part of the tool kit of models for modeling polytomous items response data.

The aim of this paper is to compare the performance of some traditional polytomous IRT models with the more recently introduced IRTree models in the modeling of self-report non-cognitive latent traits. Such comparison is motivated by the fact that IRTree models allow to account for extreme response style (ERS) effects in attitudinal measurements, while at the same time provide estimates of the target trait. Thus, two specific goals of this research are; (i) to detect the presence of ERS in self-report questionnaires measuring non-cognitive traits, and (ii) to compare the target trait estimations produced by both the traditional IRT and the IRTree approaches.

The paper is organized as follows. Two traditional polytomous IRT models, the GRM and the GPCM are first described in Sect. 2. Next, a brief account on IRTree is presented in Sect. 3. An application to compare the performance of both the traditional polytomous IRT and the IRTree models is illustrated in Sect. 4. The paper ends with conclusions and discussion in Sect. 5.

2 Traditional Polytomous IRT Models

In this section we briefly revise the basics of two traditional polytomous IRT models that have been used to model non-cognitive latent traits.

2.1 The Graded Response Model

The GRM (Samejima, 1969) has been used to model ordered polytomous categories, to evaluate students' performance on items with partial credit, and for analysing Likert-type agreement scales predominantly used in attitude or opinion surveys (Kuhlmann et al., 2017; Weng & Cheng, 2000).

In a first step, the GRM describes the probability that an answer is at or above a particular ordered category given the latent trait of interest θ. Secondly, the actual probability of responding on a particular category is computed by subtracting adjacent probabilities estimated in the first step.

Let X_{ij} be a random variable representing an answer of individual j to item i taking values $k = 0, \ldots, m_i$. The probability of answering item i at or above category k can be written as

$$P_{ik}^{*} = \frac{\exp^{a_i(\theta - b_{ik})}}{1 + \exp^{a_i(\theta - b_{ik})}}, \tag{1}$$

where, a_i is an item discrimination parameter, b_{ik} is the category location parameter, and P_{ik}^{*} is known as the cumulative probability curve.

By definition, the probability of responding at or above the lowest category is $P_{i0}^{*}(\theta) = 1$ whereas the probability of responding above the highest category is $P_{im_i}^{*}(\theta) = 0, \forall\theta$. For others values of k, the probabilities $P_{ik}^{*}(\theta)$ are computed by specific dichotomizations. For instance, for an item with five categories ($m_i = 4$), the first dichotomization refers to category 0 versus 1–4, the second to 0–1 versus 2–4, and so on until the latest dichotomization 0–3 versus 4.

By computing the difference between adjacent cumulative probabilities, the probability of responding on a particular category k is obtained as

$$P_{ik} = Pr\{X_i = k|\theta\} = P_{ik}^{*} - P_{i(k+1)}^{*}. \tag{2}$$

It is important to note that under this model, the cumulative probability curves are parallel because only one a_i is estimated for each item. Hence, the slope (a_i) is shared among $m_i - 1$ category response curves. The threshold (location) parameters represent the value on the θ-scale when the probability of responding at or above the particular category is equal to 0.5.

2.2 *The Generalized Partial Credit Model*

The GPCM (Muraki, 1992) is an extension of the Partial Credit Model (PCM; Masters, 1982) which relaxes the restriction of all items having the same discrimination parameter. The GPCM was developed in a parallel way to developments of the PCM by using the two-parameter logistic (2PL) model instead of the Rasch model (Dodd et al., 1995) and is based on the assumption that the probability of choosing the $k-$th category over the first category is governed by a dichotomous response model.

The probability of an answer in category k of item i is modeled as

$$P_{ik}(\theta) = \frac{\exp^{\sum_{v=1}^{k} Z_{iv}(\theta)}}{\sum_{c=1}^{k} \exp^{\sum_{v=1}^{c} Z_{iv}(\theta)}}, \tag{3}$$

with

$$Z_{ik}(\theta) = a_i(\theta - b_{ik}) = a_i(\theta - b_i + d_k), \tag{4}$$

where a_i and b_{ik} are defined as before. Note that for this model, item-category parameters, b_{ik}, correspond to the points on the θ scale at which the curves of $P_{ik-1}(\theta)$ and $P_{ik}(\theta)$ are intersected. Also, they decompose into two parameters; b_i being the item-location parameter and d_k is the category-location parameter. To avoid indeterminacies, the following location constraint is typically imposed (Muraki & Muraki, 2016):

$$\sum_{k=1}^{m_i-1} d_k = 0 \tag{5}$$

An important assumption in these models relates to the unidimensionallity of the latent trait θ. Also, local independence is required. More details on traditional IRT models for polytomous items can be found in Nering and Ostini (2011).

3 Non Traditional Polytomous IRT Models

In this section we describe IRTree models, which can be considered a less traditional family of IRT models used for modeling polytomous score data.

3.1 IRTree Models

In comparison with the traditional polytomous IRT models described in the previous section that measure only a unidimensional trait, Item response-Tree (IRTree) models (Böckenholt, 2012; De Boeck & Partchev, 2012; Jeon & De Boeck, 2016) make use of multiple latent traits to explain the responses to polytomous items. As it will be explained below, a key distinguishing feature is that polytomous items are recoded into binary pseudo-items so that the model can be estimated as a multidimensional IRT model for binary items.

IRTree models can describe a postulated internal decision process with a tree structure, which is composed of sub-trees, nodes and branches (Jeon & De Boeck, 2016). The categorical responses can thus be interpreted as a sequential process of going through the tree to its end nodes. The probability of answering in a category

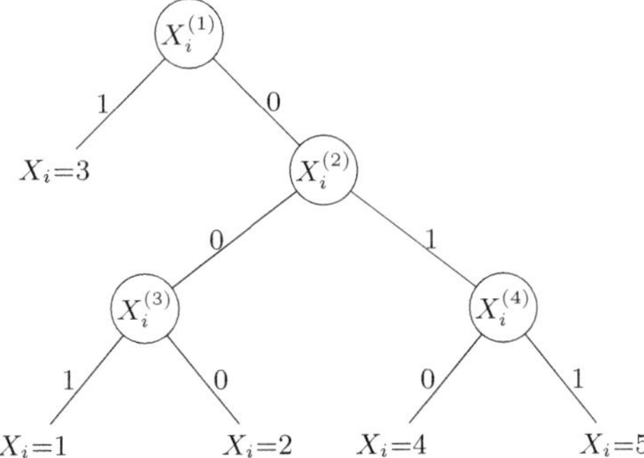

Fig. 1 Tree structure for a nested scale with 4 response categories plus one middle category

is thus obtained as the product of the probabilities at each node which are modeled using traditional binary IRT models, such as the 1PL or 2PL models.

As an example, consider the tree structure for a 5-point Likert scale (1: Strongly disagree, 2: Disagree, 3: Neutral, 4: Agree and 5: Strongly agree) shown in Fig. 1. Branch values are assigned according to research interests and postulated theories. In Fig. 1, the first node has a value of 1 related to category 3 and a value of 0 related to all other categories. This value assignment indicates that the first node is modeling the propensity to answer in the middle category. The second node has a value of 1 related to agreement categories and a value of 0 related to disagreement categories. Then, the second node is modeling the propensity to agree. Additionally, the third and four nodes have a value of 1 related to extreme negative and extreme positive categories, respectively, and a value of 0 related to the other categories. Therefore, these nodes are modeling the propensity of responding in the extreme categories. This is an example of what is called a nested response tree structure. Linear structures can also be considered in which case one branch from each internal node leads directly to an end node (a response category). Examples of other type of tree structures can be found in Jeon and De Boeck (2016) and Böckenholt (2012).

As mentioned before, IRTree models need the polytomous items to be recoded into several dichotomous pseudo-items. The recodification is made using the so-called mapping matrix's, denoted here as $\mathbf{M}^*$ and whose entries are defined by

$$m^*_{cn} = \begin{cases} 1 & \text{if } n\text{-th node is modeling the propensity to answer in category } c \\ \text{NA} & \text{when there is no connection between category } c \text{ and node } n \\ 0 & \text{otherwise} \end{cases}$$

For a test instrument composed of I polytomous items, a total of $I \times N$ dichotomous pseudo-items need to be generated. For the five categories item example, there will be $N = 4$ pseudo items, one for each node in the tree representation. The mapping matrix in this case reads as

$$
\mathbf{M}^* := \begin{array}{c} X_i = c \\ 1 \\ 2 \\ 3 \\ 4 \\ 5 \end{array} \begin{array}{c} \begin{array}{cccc} X_i^{(1)} & X_i^{(2)} & X_i^{(3)} & X_i^{(4)} \end{array} \\ \left[\begin{array}{cccc} 0 & 0 & 1 & \text{NA} \\ 0 & 0 & 0 & \text{NA} \\ 1 & \text{NA} & \text{NA} & \text{NA} \\ 0 & 1 & \text{NA} & 0 \\ 0 & 1 & \text{NA} & 1 \end{array} \right] \end{array},
$$

The values in the first column of $\mathbf{M}^*$ indicates that the first node is modeling the propensity to answer in the middle category. For this reason, a 1 is assigned for the third row and 0 for the others. Entries in the second column are 1 for agreement categories ($c = 4, 5$) and 0 for disagreement categories ($c = 1, 2$). Additionally, because there is no connection between category 3 and the second node (see Fig. 1) an entry "NA" is used for the middle category. The third and four nodes have a value of 1 related to extreme negative ($c = 1$) and extreme positive ($c = 5$) categories, respectively, and a value of 0 related to the other categories involved. Note that for the third and fourth nodes, the middle category is again not related and, consequently, the third and fourth column have also the value "NA" for $c = 3$.

In order to obtain an explicit expression for the probability of answering in a category, we define two additional matrices (**M** and **T**) with entries

$$
m_{cn} = \begin{cases} 0 & \text{if } m^*_{cn} \text{ is 0 or NA} \\ 1 & \text{if } m^*_{cn} \text{ is equal to 1} \end{cases},
$$

and

$$
t_{cn} = \begin{cases} 1 & \text{if the } n\text{-th node is related to category } c \\ 0 & \text{if the } n\text{-th node is not related to category } c \end{cases},
$$

respectively. For the example item, these matrices are

$$
\mathbf{M} := \begin{array}{c} X_i = c \\ 1 \\ 2 \\ 3 \\ 4 \\ 5 \end{array} \begin{array}{c} \begin{array}{cccc} X_i^{(1)} & X_i^{(2)} & X_i^{(3)} & X_i^{(4)} \end{array} \\ \left[\begin{array}{cccc} 0 & 0 & 1 & 0 \\ 0 & 0 & 0 & 0 \\ 1 & 0 & 0 & 0 \\ 0 & 1 & 0 & 0 \\ 0 & 1 & 0 & 1 \end{array} \right] \end{array},
$$

and

$$\mathbf{T} := \begin{bmatrix} 1\,1\,1\,0 \\ 1\,1\,1\,0 \\ 1\,0\,0\,0 \\ 1\,1\,0\,1 \\ 1\,1\,0\,1 \end{bmatrix}.$$

If the probability at each node is modeled using a 2PL model, namely

$$P(X_i^{(n)} = m_{cn}|\theta^{(n)}) = \frac{\exp[m_{cn}\alpha_i^{(n)}(\theta^{(n)} + \beta_i^{(n)})]}{1 + \exp[\alpha_i^{(n)}(\theta^{(n)} + \beta_i^{(n)})]}, \tag{6}$$

for all $i \in \{1, \ldots, I\}$ and $m_{cn} \in \{0, 1\}$, then the polytomous probability can be written as

$$\begin{aligned} P(X_i = c|\theta) &= P(X_i^{(1)} = m_{c1}, X_i^{(2)} = m_{c2}, ..., X_i^{(N)} = m_{cN}|\theta^{(1)}, \theta^{(2)}, ..., \theta^{(N)}) \\ &= \prod_{n=1}^{N} P(X_i^{(n)} = m_{cn}|\theta_p^{(n)})^{t_{cn}}. \end{aligned} \tag{7}$$

For the example item, the probability of responding in category c of item i can then be expressed as

$$\begin{aligned} P(X_i = c|\theta) = P(X_i^{(1)} &= m_{c1}|\theta^{(1)})^{t_{c1}} \\ \times P(X_i^{(2)} &= m_{c2}|X_i^{(1)}, \theta^{(2)})^{t_{c2}} \\ \times P(X_i^{(3)} &= m_{c3}|X_i^{(1)}, X_i^{(2)}, \theta^{(3)})^{t_{c3}} \\ \times P(X_i^{(4)} &= m_{c4}|X_i^{(1)}, X_i^{(2)}, \theta^{(4)})^{t_{c4}} \end{aligned} \tag{8}$$

Note that the latest probability term in Eq. (8) does not contain $X_i^{(3)}$ in the conditional term. This is due to the tree specification, namely, the node outcomes, conditional on the earlier decisions and the latent variables involved, are independent of each other.

Other variants of the model consider only one latent trait for all nodes leading to specify an unidimensional model; node-specific item parameters or shared across nodes; and explanatory variables at the individual and item level. A detailed description of these and other variants of IRTree models can be found in Jeon and De Boeck (2016).

4 Application

In Chile, the Agency of Quality of Education[1] is the governmental organization responsible for measuring cognitive and non-cognitive aspects in the educational system. Currently, together with the "Education Quality Measurement System" test (*Sistema de Medición de la Calidad de Educación*, SIMCE, by their initials in spanish) (Agencia de Calidad de la Educación, 2015), Chilean students, teachers and parents, express their perceptions and attitudes towards different non-academic aspects, through the Quality and Education Context (QEC) questionnaires (Agencia de Calidad de la Educación, 2017). These questionnaires collect information used to build personal and social development indicators (IDPS, for their initials in spanish). The IDPS are indexes that provide information related to the personal and social development of the students of an educational institution, complementary to the results of the cognitive test and the achievement of the Learning Standards. The QEC are administered annually on a census application and are composed of Likert-type items.

4.1 Data

For the illustration we consider the QEC questionnaire applied to students which include a series of questions that seek to collect their perceptions and attitudes on Academic self-esteem and Motivation, School Climate, Participation and Civic education, and Healthy lifestyle.

The QEC student questionnaire is composed of 210 items and each student has around 50 min to answer it. In this application we are focus only on one IDPS, the School Climate, and more specifically, on items related with Safe-Environment. The analyzed data set contained answers to six items measuring the degree to which 4th grade students agree with several affirmative sentences about their teachers. Table 1 shows the items analyzed, each having a response scale with four categories: 1 strongly disagree; 2 disagree; 3 agree; 4 strongly agree.

Table 1 shows the response category distribution for each item. It can be seen that the largest proportion of students choose the strongly agree category, which would indicate most of the students have a "good" perception of their teacher related to safe-environment. However, such observed frequency could be due to response styles in their answers. To investigate it, we compare the performance between traditional IRT models and the IRTree approach that accounts for response styles.

[1] www.agenciaeducacion.cl

Table 1 Six safe-environment items analyzed from student QEC 2017 and the response proportion in each category

Item	Do your teachers teach the following to your course?	SD	D	A	SA
1	My teachers teach us what to do if a classmate hits us	10.23	6.73	24.61	54.63
2	My teachers teach us what to do if a classmate hits another classmate	8.33	6.89	25.79	54.90
3	My teachers teach us what to do if a classmate takes the materials from us	8.76	9.21	27.96	49.66
4	My teachers teach us what to do when a classmate is very upset	6.37	5.12	22.73	61.46
5	My teachers teach us that stealing is wrong	4.92	2.39	13.38	75.42
6	My teachers teach us that it is wrong to hit classmates	3.53	2.26	13.5	76.39

SD strongly disagree, *D* disagree, *A* agree, *SA* strongly agree

4.2 Analyses

Two traditional polytomous IRT models and two IRTree models were fitted to the data. Model fit was assessed using the Akaike information criterion (AIC; Akaike, 1974), and the Bayesian information criterion (BIC; Schwarz, 1978). The reliability of the scale was evaluated using Cronbach's alpha (Cronbach, 1951). The dimensionality of the safe-environment construct was assessed using methods based on eigenvalues. All the analyses were conducted using the Flexmirt (Cai, 2012), and R (R Core Team, 2020) software.

4.3 Results

The Cronbach's alpha coefficient was 0, 83 for the sample in study ($N = 1000$). The eigenvalues analysis and a scree-plot (not shown) suggested that the items could be adequately represented by a single dimension (Cattell, 1966; Joreskog, 2007), and consequently a unidimensional polytomous IRT model can be fitted.

Table 2 shows model fit indices for the GRM, GPCM, and two IRTree models. IRTree model 1 refers to a tree structure similar to the one shown in Fig. 1 but with no middle category in their options. Consequently, a three-dimensional model was fitted, considering a 2PL model in each node. IRTree model 2 refers to the same tree structure as model 1 but considering node 2 and node 3 specification as the same latent trait. In other words, both nodes represent the extreme response style, no matter whether it is positive or negative. The IRTree model 1 shows the best fitting, followed by IRTree model 2, the GRM and GPCM, respectively. These results indicate that possible response styles are better accounted by the IRTree models (Plieninger, 2020).

For the comparison of estimated latent traits, the perception that students have towards a safe environment was the main trait of interest to be evaluated. This trait

Table 2 Model selection

Type	Model	Npars	Log-likehood	AIC	BIC
Polytomous	GPCM	24	−4540.97	9129.94	9247.72
Polytomous	GRM	24	−4468.68	8985.37	9103.16
IRTree	model 1 (3−dim)	36	−4200.44	8476.88	8663.37
IRTree	model 2 (2−dim)	24	−4247.99	8545.98	8668.68

was assumed to be modelled by the first node in the two IRTree models (model 1 and model 2), whereas the other two nodes accounted for extreme response styles. The estimated traits using the four IRT models correlated high (over 0.9) as shown in Table 3. The correlations between the target trait with both the extreme negative response style (ENRS) and the extreme positive response style (EPRS) in IRTree model 1 were −0.761 and 0.627, respectively. The large correlations would indicate that the extreme response latent variables are not enough separated from the main trait; which in turn would be indicative of possible bias in the measuring of the target trait (e.g., Plieninger, 2017). The correlation between the target trait (θ_1) and the ERS (θ_2) in the IRTree model 2 was 0.490. This lower correlation indicates that the ERS component is not severely picking up on trait information as it was the case for IRTree model 1. Thus, although model 2 does not fit better than model 1, it allows the interpretation of the results in a less ambiguous way.

The pattern of estimated traits by each IRT model plotted against the observed sum scores is shown in Fig. 2. It can be seen that these patterns are very similar for the GRM and GPCM estimates, and that there are no much differences between the estimated traits for the IRTree models and those by the traditional IRT models. This means that latent trait estimates by IRTree models can be used as a reliable alternative to traditional polytomous IRT models.

5 Conclusions and Discussion

Two traditional polytomous IRT models and two IRTree models were compared in terms of model fit and the estimation of non-cognitive latent traits. The IRTree models had a better fit than traditional polytomous IRT models, and the estimated traits of interest produced by these non traditional polytomous IRT models were highly correlated and aligned to the ones obtained using the GRM and the GPCM.

Given that the preliminary inspection of the analysed data showed that a large proportion of students chose the extreme positive category, suggesting possible response styles present in the data sample, the fact that the two IRTree models fitted better than traditional IRT model is reassuring. Although IRTree model 1 had the best fit, the model tree specification (negative/positive ERS) does not yield independent components and thus it captures part of the target trait. This is not the case for the IRTree model 2 which allows to separate the target trait and the response style component in a better way.

Table 3 Correlations among estimated traits

Model	GRM	GPCM	IRTree 1(θ_1)	IRTree 1(θ_2)	IRTree 1 (θ_3)	IRTree 2(θ_1)	IRTree 2(θ_2)
GRM	1						
GPCM	0.991	1					
IRTree 1(θ_1)	0.907	0.923	1				
IRTree 1(θ_2)	−0.513	−0.551	−0.761	1			
IRTree 1(θ_3)	0.846	0.832	0.627	−0.042	1		
IRTree 2(θ_1)	0.875	0.889	0.995	−0.761	0.627	1	
IRTree 2(θ_2)	0.740	0.737	0.524	0.106	0.962	0.490	1

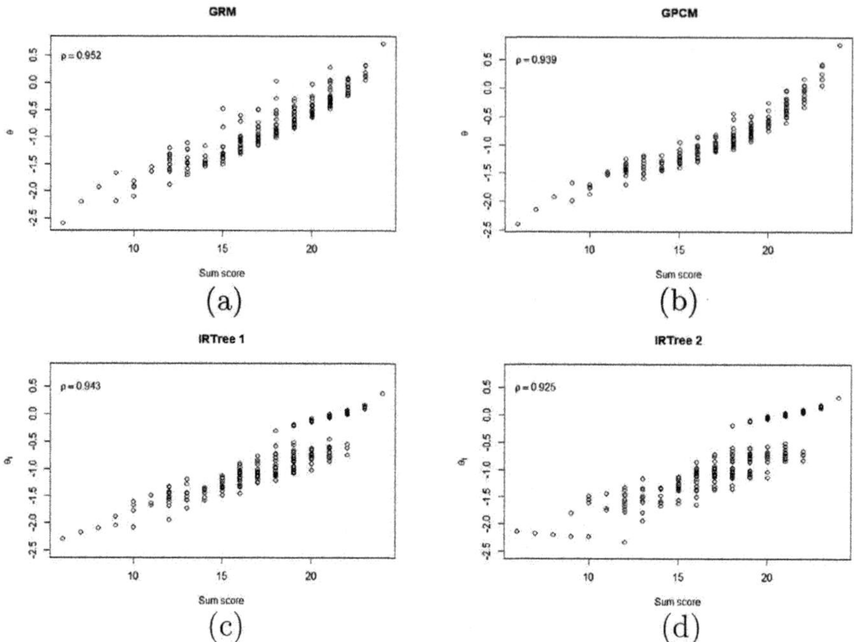

Fig. 2 Correlation between latent trait estimates and the sum score. (**a**) GRM (uni-dimensional). (**b**) GPCM (uni-dimensional). (**c**) IRTree model 1 (three-dimensional). (**d**) IRTree model 2 (two-dimensional)

Finally, the highly correlated and aligned results with the traditional polytomous IRT models for the estimates of the measured trait of interest (safe-environment) allow us to conclude that the IRTree model can be safely used to estimate traits of interest while at the same time account for response styles.

Acknowledgments Francisca Calderón was funded by the National Agency for Research and Development (ANID)/Scholarship Program/Doctorado Nacional/2017 – 21171096. Jorge González was partially funded by the FONDECYT grant 1201129.

References

Agencia de Calidad de la Educación. (2015). Informe técnico simce 2015. Accessed 3 July 2020. http://archivos.agenciaeducacion.cl/Informe_Tecnico_SIMCE_2015_Final.pdf

Agencia de Calidad de la Educación. (2017). Informe técnico 2017. indicadores de desarrollo personal y social (idps) medidos a través de cuestionarios. Accessed 3 July 2020. http://archivos.agenciaeducacion.cl/Informe_tecnico_IDPS_2017.pdf

Akaike, M. (1974). A new look at the statistical model identification. *IEEE Transactions on Automatic Control, 19*, 716–723.

Borghans, L., Duckworth, A. L., Heckman, J. J., & ter Weel, B. (2008). The economics and psychology of personality traits. Working Paper 13810, National Bureau of Economic Research.

Böckenholt, U. (2012). Modeling multiple response processes in judgment and choice. *Psychological Methods, 17*(4), 665–678.

Cai, L. (2012). *flexmirt: Flexible multilevel item factor analysis and test scoring [computer software]*. Seattle, WA: Vector Psychometric Group, LLC.

Cattell, R. B. (1966). The scree test for the number of factors. *Multivariate Behavioral Research, 1*(2), 245–276. PMID: 26828106.

Cronbach, L. (1951). Coefficient alpha and internal structure of tests. *Psychometrika, 16*(3), 297–334.

De Boeck, P., & Partchev, I. (2012). Irtrees:tree-based item response models of the glmm family. *Journal of Statistical Software, 48*(1), 1–28.

Dodd, B. G., Ayala, R. D., & Koch, W. R. (1995). Computerized adaptive testing with polytomous items. *Applied Psychological Measurement, 19*(1), 5–22.

Jeon, M., & De Boeck, P. (2016). A generalized item response tree model for psychological assessments. *Behavior Research Methods, 48*(3), 1070–1085.

Jeon, M., & De Boeck, P. (2019). Evaluation on types of invariance in studying extreme response bias with an irtree approach. *British Journal of Mathematical and Statistical Psychology, 72*(3), 517–537.

Joreskog, K. G. (2007). Factor analysis and its extensions. In R. Cudeck & R. C. MacCallum (Eds.), *Factor analysis at 100: Historical developments and future directions* (pp. 47–77). Lawrence Erlbaum Associates Publishers.

Kuhlmann, T., Dantlgraber, M., & Reips, U.-D. (2017). Investigating measurement equivalence of visual analogue scales and likert-type scales in internet-based personality questionnaires. *Behavior Research Methods, 49*(6), 2173–2181.

Lord, F. (1980). *Applications of item response theory to practical testing problems*. Hillsdale, NJ: Lawrence Erlbaum Associates.

Masters, G. (1982). A rasch model for partial credit scoring. *Psychometrika, 47*, 149–174.

Muraki, E. (1992). A generalized partial credit model: Application of an EM algorithm. *ETS Research Report Series, 1992*(1), i–30.

Muraki, E., & Muraki, M. (2016). Generalized partial credit model. In W. J. van der Linden (Ed.), *Handbook of item response theory. Three volume set* (Vol. 1, pp. 127–137). Boca Raton, FL: Chapman and Hall/CRC.

Nering, M. L., & Ostini, R. (2011). *Handbook of polytomous item response theory models*. Taylor and Francis.

Plieninger, H. (2017). Mountain or molehill? A simulation study on the impact of response styles. *Educational and Psychological Measurement, 77*(1), 32–53.

Plieninger, H. (2020). Developing and applying ir-tree models: Guidelines, caveats, and an extension to multiple groups. *Organizational Research Methods, 24*(3), 654–670. http://dx.doi.org/10.1177/1094428120911096

R Core Team. (2020). *R: A language and environment for statistical computing*. Vienna: R Foundation for Statistical Computing.

Samejima, F. (1969). *Estimation of latent ability using a response pattern of graded scores*. Psychometrika Monograph Supplement.

Schwarz, G. (1978). Estimating the dimension of a model. *The Annals of Statistics, 6*, 461–464.

Weng, L.-J., & Cheng, C.-P. (2000). Effects of response order on likert-type scales. *Educational and Psychological Measurement, 60*(6), 908–924.

[illegible] (2007). [illegible] and psychology of [illegible] (Working Paper [illegible]). National Bureau of Economic Research.

[illegible]

[illegible] Seattle, WA: [illegible]

[illegible]

[illegible] Psychometrika, [illegible]

[illegible]

[illegible] A cognitive model for [illegible] (1984). [illegible]

[illegible]

[illegible]

[illegible] Psychometrika Monograph [illegible]

[illegible] and Psychological Measurement [illegible]

On the Coefficient Alpha in High-Dimensions

Kentaro Hayashi, Ke-Hai Yuan, and Regan Sato

1 Introduction

The coefficient alpha (Cronbach, 1951) remains very important as a measure of reliability in the social sciences. Whenever a new questionnaire is developed by psychologists, the coefficient alpha is consistently reported to demonstrate that the measure has good reliability. Moreover, the coefficient alpha itself remains an active research area in psychometrics (e.g., Yuan & Bentler, 2002; Zhang & Yuan, 2016).

It is well known that, under certain conditions, the coefficient alpha increases as the number of items increase. The fact has been noted via the Spearman-Brown formula (Brown, 1910; Spearman, 1910). This implies that as the number of items goes to infinity, the coefficient alpha eventually approaches 1. Therefore, the issue of reliability is closely associated with that of dimensionality of the manifest variables.

Regarding high dimensionality, there is another interesting phenomenon. It has been known that the results from factor analysis (FA; e.g., Lawley & Maxwell, 1971) approach those from principal component analysis (PCA; e.g., Jolliffe, 2002) as the number of variables increase (Guttman, 1956).

In this work, we show that the coefficient alpha approaching 1 is related to the increased closeness between FA and PCA in high dimensions. Here, the closeness between FA and PCA includes the closeness with respect to both their loadings and factor score (principal component). More specifically, we show that as the dimension increases the phenomenon of the coefficient alpha approaching 1 is related to four different phenomena: (1) the closeness between FA and PCA

K. Hayashi (✉) · R. Sato
University of Hawaii, Honolulu, HI, USA
e-mail: hayashik@hawaii.edu; regans@hawaii.edu

K.-H. Yuan
University of Notre Dame, Notre Dame, IN, USA
e-mail: kyuan@nd.edu

M. Wiberg et al. (eds.), *Quantitative Psychology*, Springer Proceedings in Mathematics & Statistics 353, https://doi.org/10.1007/978-3-030-74772-5_12

loadings, (2) the inverse of the covariance matrix of the manifest variables becoming a diagonal matrix, assuming a FA model in the population, (3) the communalities between FA and PCA approaching each other, and (4) the factor score and the principal component agreeing with each other.

2 Definitions and Assumptions

Suppose that there exists a p-dimensional vector of random variables, $\boldsymbol{x} = (x_1, \ldots, x_p)^T$, measuring the same construct. Denote the covariance matrix and the correlation matrix of $\boldsymbol{x}$ as $\boldsymbol{\Sigma}$ and $\mathbf{P}$, respectively. Then the coefficient alpha is defined as:

$$\alpha(\boldsymbol{\Sigma}) = \frac{p}{p-1}\left(1 - \frac{tr(\boldsymbol{\Sigma})}{\mathbf{1}_p^T\boldsymbol{\Sigma}\mathbf{1}_p}\right).$$

When the x_j's are all standardized, the alpha coefficient is defined as:

$$\alpha(\mathbf{P}) = \frac{p}{p-1}\left(1 - \frac{tr(\mathbf{P})}{\mathbf{1}_p^T\mathbf{P}\mathbf{1}_p}\right) = \frac{p\overline{\rho}}{1 + (p-1)\overline{\rho}},$$

where $\overline{\rho} = (\mathbf{1}_p{}^{\mathbf{T}}\mathbf{P}\mathbf{1}_p - p)/p^*$ is the average of the $p^* = p(p-1)$ correlation coefficients between the distinct pairs of the items in $\boldsymbol{x}$ (Hayashi & Kamata, 2005).

***Assumption* 1** We assume a one-factor model holds and all the factor loadings are positive. Also, all the elements of eigenvector corresponding to the largest eigenvalue of the covariance matrix have a positive sign.

This assumption is necessary for the alpha coefficient to be justified. We can make the sign of factor loadings always positive by reversing the items if necessary.

Let the one-factor model be $\boldsymbol{x} = \boldsymbol{\mu} + \boldsymbol{\lambda}f + \varepsilon$, where $\boldsymbol{\mu} = E(\boldsymbol{x})$ is a $p \times 1$ vector of intercepts, $\boldsymbol{\lambda}$ is a $p \times 1$ vector of factor loadings, f is a (scalar) latent variable, and ε is a $p \times 1$ vector of random errors. We assume that the mean and the variance of the factor and the errors are $E(f) = 0$, $\text{Var}(f) = 1$, $E(\boldsymbol{\varepsilon}) = \mathbf{0}$, and $\text{Cov}(\boldsymbol{\varepsilon}) = \boldsymbol{\Psi}$, where $\boldsymbol{\Psi}$ is a diagonal matrix with positive elements (i.e., the errors are uncorrelated with each other), respectively. Also, we assume that the factor and the errors are uncorrelated (i.e., $\text{Cov}(f, \boldsymbol{\varepsilon}) = \mathbf{0}$). Then, the covariance matrix of $\boldsymbol{x}$ is expressed as $\boldsymbol{\Sigma} = \boldsymbol{\lambda}\boldsymbol{\lambda}^T + \boldsymbol{\Psi}$. Here, $\boldsymbol{\lambda}$ is defined as $\boldsymbol{\lambda} = \omega^{1/2}\boldsymbol{\lambda}_+$, where $\boldsymbol{\lambda}_+$ is the standardized (i.e., $||\boldsymbol{\lambda}_+||_2 = 1$) eigenvector corresponding to the single nonzero eigenvalue ω of $\boldsymbol{\Sigma} - \boldsymbol{\Psi}$ (i.e., $\omega = \text{ev}_1(\boldsymbol{\Sigma} - \boldsymbol{\Psi})$).

Likewise, express the principal component analysis (PCA) loadings as $\boldsymbol{\lambda}^* = {\omega_1}^{1/2}{\boldsymbol{\lambda}_1}^*$, where ${\boldsymbol{\lambda}_1}^*$ (p x 1) is the standardized (i.e., $||{\boldsymbol{\lambda}_1}^*||_2 = 1$) eigenvector corresponding to the largest eigenvalue ω_1 of $\boldsymbol{\Sigma}$ (i.e., $\omega_1 = \text{ev}_1(\boldsymbol{\Sigma})$). Then, the first principal component (PC) is obtained as $f^* = \boldsymbol{\lambda}^{*T}(\boldsymbol{x} - \boldsymbol{\mu})$. Because $\boldsymbol{\Sigma} = \sum_{i=1}^{p} \omega_i \boldsymbol{\lambda}_i^* \boldsymbol{\lambda}_i^{*T}$, where ω_i is the i-th largest eigenvalue of $\boldsymbol{\Sigma}$ and $\boldsymbol{\lambda}_i^*$ is the corresponding standardized eigenvector, we can also express $\boldsymbol{\Sigma}$ as $\boldsymbol{\Sigma} = \boldsymbol{\lambda}^* \boldsymbol{\lambda}^{*T} + \boldsymbol{\Psi}^*$, where $\boldsymbol{\Psi}^* = \sum_{i=2}^{p} \omega_i \boldsymbol{\lambda}_i^* \boldsymbol{\lambda}_i^{*T}$ is not a diagonal matrix, in general, unlike the FA model.

Denote the i-th element of $\boldsymbol{\lambda}$ and $\boldsymbol{\lambda}^*$ as λ_i andλ_i^*, respectively. Then the i-th communalities based on a one-factor FA model and the corresponding PCA are λ_i^2 and λ_i^{*2}, respectively. That is, for a one-factor model, the i-th communalities for the FA and the PCA reduce to the squared i-th loading for the FA and the PCA, respectively. Also, denote the i-th diagonal element of $\boldsymbol{\Sigma}$ as σ_{ii}, and the supremum and the infimum of σ_{ii}, $i = 1, \ldots, p$, as $\sigma_{\sup}$ and $\sigma_{\inf}$ (i.e., $\sigma_{\sup} = \sup_{i \geq 1}(\sigma_{ii})$ and $\sigma_{\inf} = \inf_{i \geq 1}(\sigma_{ii})$), respectively. Likewise, we write the i-th diagonal element of $\boldsymbol{\Psi}$ as ψ_{ii}, and denote the supremum and the infimum of ψ_{ii} as $\psi_{\sup} = \sup_{i \geq 1}(\psi_{ii})$ and $\psi_{\inf} = \inf_{i \geq 1}(\psi_{ii})$, respectively.

***Assumption* 2** The supremum of the diagonal elements of $\boldsymbol{\Sigma}$ is finite (i.e., $\sigma_{\sup} < \infty$) and the infimum of the unique variances is bounded away from zero ($0 < \psi_{\inf}$). Then obviously, $0 < \psi_{\inf} \leq \psi_{ii} \leq \psi_{\sup} \leq \Sigma_{\sup} < \infty$.

The direct consequence of *Assumption* 2 is that not only the diagonal elements of $\boldsymbol{\Psi}$ are bounded above and also bounded away from zero, but the inverse $\boldsymbol{\Psi}^{-1}$ are also bounded above and bounded away from zero. That is, $0 < {\psi_{\sup}}^{-1} \leq {\psi_{ii}}^{-1} \leq {\psi_{\inf}}^{-1} < \infty$. Because $0 < \psi_{\inf} \leq \sigma_{\inf}$, $\sigma_{\inf}$ is also bounded away from zero.

With more latent variables, Schneeweiss and Mathes (1995) and Schneeweiss (1997) suggested to use non-centered canonical correlations to measure the closeness between the loadings of PCA and FA. Now, with a single factor, the non-centered squared canonical correlation between FA loadings and PCA loadings for the one-factor model is defined as:

$$\rho^2(\boldsymbol{\lambda}, \boldsymbol{\lambda}^*) = \left(\boldsymbol{\lambda}^T\boldsymbol{\lambda}\right)^{-1}\left(\boldsymbol{\lambda}^T\boldsymbol{\lambda}^*\right)\left(\boldsymbol{\lambda}^{*T}\boldsymbol{\lambda}^*\right)^{-1}\left(\boldsymbol{\lambda}^{*T}\boldsymbol{\lambda}\right)$$

$$= \frac{\left(\boldsymbol{\lambda}^T\boldsymbol{\lambda}^*\right)^2}{\|\boldsymbol{\lambda}\|_2^2\|\boldsymbol{\lambda}^*\|_2^2} = \left\{Corr\left(\boldsymbol{\lambda}, \boldsymbol{\lambda}^*\right)\right\}^2.$$

That is, for a one-factor model, the squared canonical correlation reduces to the squared correlation.

Now, express $\boldsymbol{\Sigma}$ as $\boldsymbol{\Sigma} = \boldsymbol{\Delta}\mathbf{P}\boldsymbol{\Delta}$, where $\boldsymbol{\Delta} = \text{diag}({\sigma_{ii}}^{1/2})$ is the diagonal matrix whose diagonal elements are standard deviations. Then, we can express $\boldsymbol{\Sigma} = \boldsymbol{\lambda}\boldsymbol{\lambda}^T + \boldsymbol{\Psi}$ as $\boldsymbol{\Sigma} = \boldsymbol{\Delta}\mathbf{P}\boldsymbol{\Delta} = \boldsymbol{\Delta}(\boldsymbol{l}\boldsymbol{l}^T + \boldsymbol{U})\boldsymbol{\Delta}$, where $\mathbf{P} = (\rho_{ij}) = \boldsymbol{l}\boldsymbol{l}^T + \boldsymbol{U}$

is the covariance (correlation) matrix of the standardized variables $\mathbf{\Delta}^{-1}\boldsymbol{x}$ with the standardized FA loading vector $\boldsymbol{l} = (l_i)$ and the standardized (diagonal) error variance matrix $\boldsymbol{U} = \text{diag}(u_{ii})$. Because the diagonal elements of $\mathbf{P}$ are all 1's, the diagonal elements of $\boldsymbol{U}$ are functions of $\boldsymbol{l}$, that is, $\boldsymbol{U} = \boldsymbol{I}_p - \text{diag}(\boldsymbol{l}\boldsymbol{l}^T)$ with $u_{ii} = 1 - l_i^2$. Therefore, $\sigma_{ii} = \lambda_i^2 + \psi_{ii} = (\sigma_{ii})(l_i^2 + u_{ii}) = (\sigma_{ii})\{l_i^2 + (1 - l_i^2)\}$, and $\psi_{ii} = (\sigma_{ii})(1 - l_i^2)$.

***Assumption* 3** Let $c > 0$ be a small positive constant. Then, under *Assumption* 2, $0 < c \le l_i^2 < 1$.

Recall that $\overline{\rho}$ be the average correlation. Then, we can show that $0 < c \le l_i^2 < 1$ implies $c \le \overline{\rho} < 1$. Because l_i's take the same positive sign (due to *Assumption* 1), $c \le l_i^2$ implies $c^{1/2} \le l_i$. Thus, $c \le \rho_{ij} = l_i l_j$. Also, due to *Assumption* 2, $\psi_{\inf} \le \psi_{ii} = (\sigma_{ii})(1 - l_i^2)$, so that $l_i^2 \le 1 - \psi_{\inf}\sigma_{ii}{}^{-1} < 1$ and $l_i < 1$. Thus, $\rho_{ij} = l_i l_j < 1$. Combining both, we have $c \le \rho_{ij} < 1$. Because $\overline{\rho}$ is the average of $p(p-1)/2$ distinct ρ_{ij}'s, $\overline{\rho}$ has the same lower and upper bounds as those for ρ_{ij}'s. Thus, $c \le \overline{\rho} < 1$ follows.

Because $\psi_{ii} = (\sigma_{ii})(1 - l_i^2) \le \psi_{\sup}$, we can show that $l_i^2 \ge 1 - \psi_{\sup}(\sigma_{ii})^{-1} \ge 1 - \psi_{\sup}(\sigma_{\inf})^{-1}$. If $1 - \psi_{\sup}(\sigma_{\inf})^{-1} > 0$, that is, if $\sigma_{\inf} > \psi_{\sup}$, then $0 < c^* < l_i^2$, where $c^* = 1 - \psi_{\sup}(\sigma_{\inf})^{-1}$. However, in general, may not exist such a positive constant c^*.

3 Theorem

Now, we state our main theorem connecting the coefficient alpha and the closeness between FA and PCA in high dimensions.

***Theorem* 1**

(1) (FA loadings and PCA loadings) The squared non-centered correlation between FA loadings and PCA loadings approaches 1 (i.e., $\rho^2(\lambda, \lambda^*) = \{\text{Corr}(\boldsymbol{\lambda}, \boldsymbol{\lambda}^*)\}^2 \to 1$) if and only if the coefficient alpha approaches 1 (i.e., $\alpha(\mathbf{\Sigma}) \to 1$).
(2) (Precision matrix) The precision matrix (i.e., the inverse of the covariance matrix $\mathbf{\Sigma}$) approaches the inverse of the diagonal matrix of unique variances (i.e., $\mathbf{\Sigma}^{-1} - \mathbf{\Psi}^{-1} \to \mathbf{0}$) if and only if the coefficient alpha approaches 1 (i.e., $\alpha(\mathbf{\Sigma}) \to 1$).
(3) (Communality) The difference between the i-th communalities based on FA and PCA approaches zero for almost all i as the number of observed variables increases (i.e., $\lambda_i^2 - \lambda_i^{*2} \to 0$ as $p \to \infty$) if and only if the coefficient alpha approaches 1 (i.e., $\alpha(\mathbf{\Sigma}) \to 1$).
(4) (Factor score and principal component) The factor score and the principal component agree with each other (i.e., $\{\text{Corr}(f, f^*)\}^2 \to 1$) if and only if the coefficient alpha approaches 1 (i.e., $\alpha(\mathbf{\Sigma}) \to 1$).

4 Preliminary Results

In this section, we present *lemmas* that are needed to prove *Theorem* 1.

***Lemma* 1** $\alpha(\mathbf{\Sigma}) \to 1$ as $p \to \infty$ if and only if $\alpha(\mathbf{P}) \to 1$ as $p \to \infty$.

Proof As before, $\mathbf{\Sigma} = \mathbf{\Delta P \Delta}$, where $\mathbf{\Delta}$ is the diagonal matrix whose elements are standard deviations. Due to *Assumption* 2, $\mathbf{P} = \mathbf{\Delta}^{-1}\mathbf{\Sigma}\mathbf{\Delta}^{-1}$. Thus, $\mathbf{0} < \sigma_{\inf}\mathbf{P} \leq \mathbf{\Sigma} \leq \sigma_{\sup}\mathbf{P} < \infty$ and $\mathbf{0} < \sigma_{\sup}^{-1}\,\mathbf{\Sigma} \leq \mathbf{P} \leq \sigma_{\inf}^{-1}\,\mathbf{\Sigma} < \infty$.

(<=) Taking the trace on each term of the inequality $\sigma_{\inf}\mathbf{P} \leq \mathbf{\Sigma} \leq \sigma_{\sup}\mathbf{P}$ yields $(\sigma_{\inf})tr(\mathbf{P}) \leq tr(\mathbf{\Sigma}) \leq (\sigma_{\sup})tr(\mathbf{P})$. Because $\sigma_{\inf}{}^{1/2}\boldsymbol{I}_p \leq \mathbf{\Delta} \leq \sigma_{\sup}{}^{1/2}\boldsymbol{I}_p$, it follows that $(\sigma_{\inf})(\mathbf{1}_{\mathrm{p}}{}^T\mathbf{P}\mathbf{1}_{\mathrm{p}}) \leq \mathbf{1}_p{}^T\mathbf{\Sigma}\mathbf{1}_p = \mathbf{1}_p{}^T\mathbf{\Delta P \Delta}\mathbf{1}_p \leq (\sigma_{\sup})(\mathbf{1}_p{}^T\mathbf{P}\mathbf{1}_p)$. Thus,

$$\begin{aligned}\alpha\,(\mathbf{\Sigma}) \quad &= \{p/\,(p-1)\}\left\{1 - tr(\mathbf{\Sigma})\,/\,\left(\mathbf{1}_p{}^T\mathbf{\Sigma}\mathbf{1}_p\right)\right\}\\ &\geq \{p/\,(p-1)\}\left\{1 - \left(\sigma_{\sup}\right) tr(\mathbf{P})\,/\,\left(\left(\sigma_{\inf}\right)\mathbf{1}_p{}^T\mathbf{P}\mathbf{1}_p\right)\right\}\\ &= \{p/\,(p-1)\}\left\{1 - \left(\sigma_{\sup}/\sigma_{\inf}\right) tr(\mathbf{P})\,/\,\left(\mathbf{1}_p{}^T\mathbf{P}\mathbf{1}_p\right)\right\}\\ &\geq 1 - \left(\Sigma_{\sup}/\sigma_{\inf}\right) tr(\mathbf{P})\,/\,\left(\mathbf{1}_p{}^T\mathbf{P}\mathbf{1}_p\right).\end{aligned}$$

Now, $p/(p\text{-}1)\ p \to 1$ as $p \to \infty$, and $\alpha(\mathbf{P}) = \{p/(p\text{-}1)\}\{1 - tr(\mathbf{P})/(\mathbf{1}_p{}^T\mathbf{P}\mathbf{1}_p)\} \to 1$ implies $tr(\mathbf{P})/(\mathbf{1}_p{}^T\mathbf{P}\mathbf{1}_p) \to 0$. Because $\sigma_{\sup}$ is bounded and $\sigma_{\inf}$ is bounded away from zero, $(\sigma_{\sup}/\sigma_{\inf})$ is also bounded and bounded away from zero. Thus, $tr(\mathbf{P})/(\mathbf{1}_p{}^T\mathbf{P}\mathbf{1}_p) \to 0$ implies $(\sigma_{\sup}/\sigma_{\inf})tr(\mathbf{P})/(\mathbf{1}_p{}^T\mathbf{P}\mathbf{1}_p) \to 0$, and $\alpha(\mathbf{\Sigma}) \to 1$ follows.

(=>) Taking the trace on each term of the inequality $\sigma_{\sup}^{-1}\mathbf{\Sigma} \leq \mathbf{P} \leq \sigma_{\inf}^{-1}\mathbf{\Sigma}$ yields $(\sigma_{\sup}^{-1})tr(\mathbf{\Sigma}) \leq tr(\mathbf{P}) \leq (\sigma_{\inf}^{-1})tr(\mathbf{\Sigma})$. Because $\sigma_{\sup}{}^{-1/2}\boldsymbol{I}_p \leq \mathbf{\Delta}^{-1} \leq \sigma_{\inf}{}^{-1/2}\,\boldsymbol{I}_p$, it follows that $(\sigma_{\sup}^{-1})(\mathbf{1}_p{}^T\mathbf{\Sigma}\mathbf{1}_p) \leq \mathbf{1}_p{}^T\mathbf{P}\mathbf{1}_p = \mathbf{1}_p{}^T\mathbf{\Delta}^{-1}\mathbf{\Sigma}\mathbf{\Delta}^{-1}\mathbf{1}_p \leq (\sigma_{\inf}^{-1})(\mathbf{1}_p{}^T\mathbf{\Sigma}\mathbf{1}_p)$. Thus,

$$\begin{aligned}\alpha\,(\mathbf{P}) \quad &= \{p/\,(p-1)\}\left\{1 - tr\,(\mathbf{P})\,/\,\left(\mathbf{1}_p{}^T\mathbf{P}\mathbf{1}_p\right)\right\}\\ &\geq \{p/\,(p-1)\}\left\{1 - \left(\sigma_{\inf}^{-1}\right) tr(\mathbf{\Sigma})\,/\,\left(\left(\sigma_{\sup}^{-1}\right)\mathbf{1}_p{}^T\mathbf{\Sigma}\mathbf{1}_p\right)\right\}\\ &= \{p/\,(p-1)\}\left\{1 - \left(\sigma_{\sup}/\sigma_{\inf}\right) tr(\mathbf{\Sigma})\,/\,\left(\mathbf{1}_p{}^T\mathbf{\Sigma}\mathbf{1}_p\right)\right\}\\ &\geq 1 - \left(\Sigma_{\sup}/\sigma_{\inf}\right) tr(\mathbf{\Sigma})\,/\,\left(\mathbf{1}_p{}^T\mathbf{\Sigma}\mathbf{1}_p\right).\end{aligned}$$

As before, because $(\sigma_{\sup}/\sigma_{\inf})$ is bounded and bounded away from zero, $tr(\mathbf{\Sigma})/(\mathbf{1}_p{}^T\mathbf{\Sigma}\mathbf{1}_p) \to 0$ implies $(\sigma_{\sup}/\sigma_{\inf})tr(\mathbf{\Sigma})/(\mathbf{1}_p{}^T\mathbf{\Sigma}\mathbf{1}_p) \to 0$. Thus $\alpha(\mathbf{P}) \to 1$ follows.

***Lemma* 2** Under *Assumption* 3, $\alpha\,(\mathbf{P}) \to 1$ if and only if $p \to \infty$.

Proof (<=) With *Assumption* 3 that $0 < c \leq \overline{\rho} < 1$, it follows from $\alpha(\mathbf{P}) = \overline{\rho}\{p^{-1} + \overline{\rho}(1-p^{-1})\}^{-1} = \{1 + p^{-1}(\overline{\rho}^{-1} - 1)\}^{-1}$ that $\alpha(\mathbf{P}) \to 1$ as $p \to \infty$ (i.e., as $p^{-1} \to 0$).

(=>) $\alpha(\mathbf{P}) = \{1 + p^{-1}(\overline{\rho}^{-1} - 1)\}^{-1} \to 1$ is equivalent to $p^{-1}(\overline{\rho}^{-1} - 1) \to 0$. This happens either when $\overline{\rho} \to 1$ or when $p \to \infty$. By *Assumption* 3 (i.e., $\overline{\rho} < 1$), $p \to \infty$ follows.

The following results are also needed for the proof of *Theorem* 1. Only the result of Bentler and Kano (1990) was for a single factor, as other results have been stated in the context of multi-factor model. Their proof and conditions for one-factor model were much simpler.

***Lemma* 3** (Bentler & Kano, 1990; Schneeweiss & Mathes, 1995; Schneeweiss, 1997; Krijnen, 2006b): If $\boldsymbol{\lambda}^T\boldsymbol{\Psi}^{-1}\boldsymbol{\lambda} \to \infty$, then $\rho^2(\boldsymbol{\lambda}, \boldsymbol{\lambda}^*) \to 1$.

***Lemma* 4**

(1) (Krijnen, 2006a, *Theorem* 3): $\boldsymbol{\lambda}^T\boldsymbol{\Psi}^{-1}\boldsymbol{\lambda} \to \infty$ implies $p \to \infty$.
(2) With *Assumption* 3, the converse of (1) also holds. That is, $p \to \infty$ implies $\boldsymbol{\lambda}^T\boldsymbol{\Psi}^{-1}\boldsymbol{\lambda} \to \infty$.
(3) (Krijnen, 2006a, *Theorem* 2): Let σ^{ii} be the (i, i) element of $\boldsymbol{\Sigma}^{-1}$. Then, $\psi_{ii}\sigma^{ii} \to 1$ for almost all i implies $p \to \infty$.

Notes: (i) For a m-factor model, *Lemma* 4 (1) states that "$\boldsymbol{\Lambda}^T\boldsymbol{\Psi}^{-1}\boldsymbol{\Lambda} \to \infty$ then $m/p \to 0$ as $p \to \infty$."

(ii) "For almost all i" means that "the limit holds almost everywhere on the set of positive integers except possibly on a subset of measure zero" (Krijnen, 2006a, p. 195).

***Proof* of (2)**

With *Assumption* 2, "$p \to \infty$ implies $\boldsymbol{\lambda}^T\boldsymbol{\Psi}^{-1}\boldsymbol{\lambda} \to \infty$" is equivalent to "$p \to \infty$ implies $\boldsymbol{\lambda}^T\boldsymbol{\lambda} \to \infty$," which is further equivalent to "$\boldsymbol{\lambda}^T\boldsymbol{\lambda} < \infty$ implies $p < \infty$." Now, by *Assumption* 3,

$$\begin{aligned}
\infty > \boldsymbol{\lambda}^T\boldsymbol{\lambda} &= tr\left(\boldsymbol{\lambda}\boldsymbol{\lambda}^T\right) = tr(\boldsymbol{\Sigma} - \boldsymbol{\Psi}) = tr\{\boldsymbol{\Delta}\,(\mathbf{P} - U)\,\boldsymbol{\Delta}\} \\
&\geq (\Sigma_{\text{inf}})\,tr(\mathbf{P} - U) = (\Sigma_{\text{inf}})\,tr\left(\boldsymbol{l}\boldsymbol{l}^T\right) = (\Sigma_{\text{inf}})\,tr\left(\boldsymbol{l}^T\boldsymbol{l}\right) = (\Sigma_{\text{inf}})\,\left(\textstyle\sum_{i=1}^{p} l_i^2\right) \\
&\geq (\Sigma_{\text{inf}})\,(c)(p)
\end{aligned}$$

with a small positive constant c. Thus, $p < \infty$ follows.

The Woodbury formula (See e.g., Harville, 1997, Chap. 16) is given by:

$$\boldsymbol{\Sigma}^{-1} = \boldsymbol{\Psi}^{-1} - \boldsymbol{\Psi}^{-1}\boldsymbol{\lambda}\left(1 + \boldsymbol{\lambda}^T\boldsymbol{\Psi}^{-1}\boldsymbol{\lambda}\right)^{-1}\boldsymbol{\lambda}^T\boldsymbol{\Psi}^{-1}.$$

***Lemma* 5** (1) (Hayashi, Yuan, & Jiang, 2019): If $\boldsymbol{\lambda}^T\boldsymbol{\Psi}^{-1}\boldsymbol{\lambda} \to \infty$, then $\boldsymbol{\Sigma}^{-1} - \boldsymbol{\Psi}^{-1} \to \mathbf{0}$.

(2) If $\boldsymbol{\Sigma}^{-1} - \boldsymbol{\Psi}^{-1} \to \mathbf{0}$, then $\boldsymbol{\lambda}^T\boldsymbol{\Psi}^{-1}\boldsymbol{\lambda} \to \infty$.

***Proof* of (2)** $\boldsymbol{\Sigma}^{-1} - \boldsymbol{\Psi}^{-1} \to \mathbf{0}$ implies $\sigma^{ii} - \psi_{ii}{}^{-1} \to 0$ for almost all i, which can also be expressed as $\psi_{ii}\sigma^{ii} \to 1$ for almost all i. Then, by *Lemma* 4 (3), $\psi_{ii}\sigma^{ii} \to 1$ for almost all i implies $p \to \infty$. Finally, by *Lemma* 4 (2), $p \to \infty$ implies $\boldsymbol{\lambda}^T\boldsymbol{\Psi}^{-1}\boldsymbol{\lambda} \to \infty$.

***Lemma* 6** (Bentler & Kano, 1990): If $\boldsymbol{\lambda}^T\boldsymbol{\Psi}^{-1}\boldsymbol{\lambda} \to \infty$ as $p \to \infty$, then the squared correlation between the PC f^* and the factor f converges to 1, i.e., $\{\mathrm{Corr}(f, f^*)\}^2 \to 1$.

***Lemma* 7** (Bentler and Kano, 1990): (1) For a one-factor model, the PCA loading vector can be expressed as a linear combination of the FA loading vector, as follows:

$$\boldsymbol{\lambda}^* = \boldsymbol{c}\,(\boldsymbol{\lambda}, \boldsymbol{\Psi}, \omega_1)\,\boldsymbol{\lambda},$$

where

$$c\,(\boldsymbol{\lambda}, \boldsymbol{\Psi}, \omega_1) = \frac{\omega_1^{1/2}\left(\omega_1 \boldsymbol{I}_p - \boldsymbol{\Psi}\right)^{-1}}{\sqrt{\boldsymbol{\lambda}^T\left(\omega_1 \boldsymbol{I}_p - \boldsymbol{\Psi}\right)^{-2}\boldsymbol{\lambda}}} = \frac{\omega_1^{1/2}\left(\boldsymbol{I}_p - \omega_1^{-1}\boldsymbol{\Psi}\right)^{-1}}{\sqrt{\boldsymbol{\lambda}^T\left(\boldsymbol{I}_p - \omega_1^{-1}\boldsymbol{\Psi}\right)^{-2}\boldsymbol{\lambda}}} \tag{1}$$

with ω_1 being the largest eigenvalue of $\boldsymbol{\Sigma}$.

(2) If $\boldsymbol{\lambda}^T\boldsymbol{\Psi}^{-1}\boldsymbol{\lambda} \to \infty$ as $p \to \infty$, then $\boldsymbol{\lambda}^* - \boldsymbol{\lambda} \to \boldsymbol{0}$. That is, $\boldsymbol{c}(\boldsymbol{\lambda},\boldsymbol{\Psi},\omega_1) \to \boldsymbol{I}_p$.

5 *Proof* of *Theorem* 1

Due to *Lemma* 1, our proofs can apply to either $\alpha\,(\boldsymbol{\Sigma})$ or $\alpha\,(\mathbf{P})$.

***Proof* of Part 1**

(<=) By *Lemma* 2, $\alpha\,(\mathbf{P}) \to 1$ implies $p \to \infty$. Due to *Lemma* 4 (2), $p \to \infty$ implies $\boldsymbol{\lambda}^T\boldsymbol{\Psi}^{-1}\boldsymbol{\lambda} \to \infty$. Finally, by *Lemma* 3, $\boldsymbol{\lambda}^T\boldsymbol{\Psi}^{-1}\boldsymbol{\lambda} \to \infty$ results in $\rho^2(\boldsymbol{\lambda}, \boldsymbol{\lambda}^*) \to 1$.

(=>) $\rho^2(\boldsymbol{\lambda}, \boldsymbol{\lambda}^*) \to 1$ implies $\boldsymbol{\lambda}^* - c\boldsymbol{\lambda} \to \boldsymbol{0}$ for some non-zero constant c (due to the Cauchy-Schwarz inequality). By *Lemma* 7 (1), $\boldsymbol{\lambda}^* = \boldsymbol{c}(\boldsymbol{\lambda},\boldsymbol{\Psi},\omega_1)\boldsymbol{\lambda}$, where $\boldsymbol{c}(\boldsymbol{\lambda},\boldsymbol{\Psi},\omega_1)$ is given as in Eq. (1). The only way that the vector $\boldsymbol{c}(\boldsymbol{\lambda},\boldsymbol{\Psi},\omega_1)$ behaves as if it were a scalar is when the numerator converges to a constant times the identity matrix. That is, ${\omega_1}^{-1}\boldsymbol{\Psi} \to \boldsymbol{0}$. This implies $\omega_1 \to \infty$. Because $\sigma_{\sup} < \infty$ due to *Assumption* 2, the unbounded largest eigenvalue of $\boldsymbol{\Sigma}$ (i.e., $\omega_1 = \mathrm{ev}_1(\boldsymbol{\Sigma}) \to \infty$) implies $p \to \infty$. Thus, by *Lemma* 2, $p \to \infty$ implies $\alpha(\mathbf{P}) \to 1$.

***Proof* of Part 2**

(<=) As in the necessity proof of part 1, $\alpha(\mathbf{P}) \to 1$ implies $\boldsymbol{\lambda}^T\boldsymbol{\Psi}^{-1}\boldsymbol{\lambda} \to \infty$. By *Lemma* 5 (1), $\boldsymbol{\lambda}^T\boldsymbol{\Psi}^{-1}\boldsymbol{\lambda} \to \infty$ results in $\boldsymbol{\Sigma}^{-1} - \boldsymbol{\Psi}^{-1} \to \boldsymbol{0}$.

(=>) By *Lemma* 5 (2), $\boldsymbol{\Sigma}^{-1} - \boldsymbol{\Psi}^{-1} \to \boldsymbol{0}$ implies $\boldsymbol{\lambda}^T\boldsymbol{\Psi}^{-1}\boldsymbol{\lambda} \to \infty$. By *Lemma* 4 (1), $\boldsymbol{\lambda}^T\boldsymbol{\Psi}^{-1}\boldsymbol{\lambda} \to \infty$ implies $p \to \infty$. Finally, by *Lemma* 2, $p \to \infty$ results in $\alpha(\boldsymbol{P}) \to 1$.

***Proof* of Part 3**

(<=) By *Lemma* 2, $\alpha\,(\mathbf{P}) \to 1$ implies $p \to \infty$. Also, as in the necessity proof of part 1, $\alpha(\mathbf{P}) \to 1$ implies $\boldsymbol{\lambda}^T\boldsymbol{\Psi}^{-1}\boldsymbol{\lambda} \to \infty$. Now, by *Lemma* 7 (2), $\boldsymbol{\lambda}^T\boldsymbol{\Psi}^{-1}\boldsymbol{\lambda} \to \infty$ as $p \to \infty$ implies. $\boldsymbol{\lambda}^* - \boldsymbol{\lambda} \to \boldsymbol{0}$. Thus, ${\lambda_i}^{*2} - {\lambda_i}^2 \to 0$ for almost all i.

(=>) If ${\lambda_i}^{*2} - {\lambda_i}^2 = ({\lambda_i}^* - \lambda_i)({\lambda_i}^* + \lambda_i) \to 0$ for almost all i, the i-th FA loading and the i-th PCA loading converge to each other for almost all i, except for a possible difference of the sign. (Due to *Assumption* 1, λ_i^* and λ_i have the same positive sign.) This implies $\rho^2(\boldsymbol{\lambda}, \boldsymbol{\lambda}^*) \to 1$. Thus, applying the sufficiency proof for part 1, $\alpha(\mathbf{P}) \to 1$ follows.

***Proof* of Part 4**

(<=) Due to the necessity proof of part 1, α $(\mathbf{P}) \to 1$ implies $\boldsymbol{\lambda}^T \boldsymbol{\Psi}^{-1} \boldsymbol{\lambda} \to \infty$ as well as $p \to \infty$. Thus, by *Lemma* 6, $\{\mathrm{Corr}(f, f^*)\}^2 \to 1$ follows.

(=>) Noting $f^* = \boldsymbol{\lambda}_1^{*T}(\boldsymbol{x} - \boldsymbol{\mu})$ and $\mathrm{Var}(f) = 1$,

$$
\begin{aligned}
\{\mathrm{Corr}\,(f, f^*)\}^2 &= \{\mathrm{Cov}\,(f, f^*)\}^2 / \{\mathrm{Var}(f)\mathrm{Var}\,(f^*)\} \\
&= \left(\boldsymbol{\lambda}^T\boldsymbol{\lambda}_1^*\right)^2 / \left(\boldsymbol{\lambda}_1^{*T}\boldsymbol{\Sigma}\boldsymbol{\lambda}_1^*\right) \\
&= \left\{\boldsymbol{\lambda}_1^{*T}\left(\boldsymbol{\lambda}\boldsymbol{\lambda}^T\right)\boldsymbol{\lambda}_1^*\right\} / \left(\boldsymbol{\lambda}_1^{*T}\boldsymbol{\Sigma}\boldsymbol{\lambda}_1^*\right) \\
&= \left\{\boldsymbol{\lambda}_1^{*T}\left(\boldsymbol{\Sigma} - \Psi\right)\boldsymbol{\lambda}_1^*\right\} / \left(\boldsymbol{\lambda}_1^{*T}\boldsymbol{\Sigma}\boldsymbol{\lambda}_1^*\right) \\
&= 1 - \left\{\boldsymbol{\lambda}_1^{*T}\Psi\boldsymbol{\lambda}_1^*\right\} / \left(\boldsymbol{\lambda}_1^{*T}\boldsymbol{\Sigma}\boldsymbol{\lambda}_1^*\right) \\
&\le 1 - \psi_{\inf}/\omega_1^*.
\end{aligned}
$$

Because $\{\mathrm{Corr}(f, f^*)\}^2 \to 1$, $\omega_1^* \to \infty$. Because $\sigma_{\sup} < \infty$ due to *Assumption* 2, $\omega_1^* \to \infty$ implies $p \to \infty$. Finally, due to *Lemma* 2, $p \to \infty$ implies α $(\mathbf{P}) \to 1$.

6 Illustration with Simulated Data

We illustrate Theorem 1 with some simulated data sets. The design of the simulation is as follows: The sample size (n) is 400 and the numbers of items (p) are 6, 12, 24, 48, and 96. For $p = 6$, the population factor loadings (as a column vector) are $\boldsymbol{\lambda}_6 = (0.8, 0.7, 0.6, 0.8, 0.65, 0.5)^T$. For $p = 12$, 24, 48, and 96, the population factor loadings are $\boldsymbol{\lambda}_{12} = \mathbf{1}_2 \otimes \boldsymbol{\lambda}_6$, $\boldsymbol{\lambda}_{24} = \mathbf{1}_4 \otimes \boldsymbol{\lambda}_6$, $\boldsymbol{\lambda}_{48} = \mathbf{1}_8 \otimes \boldsymbol{\lambda}_6$, and $\boldsymbol{\lambda}_{96} = \mathbf{1}_{16} \otimes \boldsymbol{\lambda}_6$, respectively, where $\mathbf{1}_k$ is the k-dimensional column vector whose elements are all 1's, and $\otimes$ is the Kronecker product. Based on the population factor loadings, the population correlation matrices ($\mathbf{P}$) were created. Data were simulated from multivariate normal distributions with population mean vectors **0's** and covariance matrices $\mathbf{P}$ (i.e., covariances = correlations). Twenty data sets were generated for each value of p. For each data set, the following values were computed: (1) the coefficient alpha, (2) the Fisher-z transformed (square root of the) squared correlation between FA loadings and PCA loadings (see e.g., Fisher, 1915), (3) the ratio of the average absolute off-diagonal element to the average diagonal element of the precision matrix (i.e., the inverse of the sample correlation matrix), (4) the average absolute difference between communalities based on FA and PCA, and (5) the Fisher-z transformed correlation between the Bartlett factor scores and the PCs. We employed the Fisher-z transformation because the correlation values were very close to 1 even when the number of variables (p) were small. Furthermore, we will use regression analysis to investigate how much (additional) variance of outcome variables (i.e., (2) through (5) above) is explained by the number of variables (p)

and the coefficient alpha if the coefficient alpha is included as the second predictor, when the number of variables (p) is the only initial predictor. The sample size for the regression analysis is equal to 100, which are the number of replications (20) times the number of different values of p (5).

The results are shown in Tables 1 and 2. According to the results, as p increases, the value of the coefficient alpha also increases (from 0.834 when $p = 6$ to 0.988 when $p = 96$). In relation to *Theorem* 1, the results shown in Tables 1 and 2 have the following pattern.

(1) FA and PCA loadings: As the value of the coefficient alpha increases, the Fisher-z transformed correlation between FA and PCA loadings also increases (from z = 3.52 when alpha = 0.843 to z = 4.02 when alpha = 0.988), indicating the greater closeness between FA and PCA loadings. This illustrates part 1 of *Theorem* 1. When the number of items (p) was the only predictor, only 21.8% of the variance for the Fisher-z transformed correlation between FA and PCA loadings was explained (i.e., $R^2 = .218$). However, when coefficient alpha is added as the second predictor, the corresponding R^2 increased to 50.0%, an increment of 28.2%.
(2) Precision matrix: As the value of the coefficient alpha increased, the ratio of the average absolute value of off-diagonal elements to the average diagonal element of the inversed sample correlation matrix decreased (from 0.164 when alpha = 0.843 to 0.046 when alpha = 0.988), indicating that the inversed sample correlation matrix approached a diagonal matrix. This illustrates part 2 of *Theorem* 1. When the number of items (p) was the only predictor, only 43.2% of the variance for the ratio of the average absolute value of off-diagonal elements to the average diagonal element was explained. However, when adding coefficient alpha as the second predictor, R^2 increased to 97.0%, resulting in an increment of 53.8%.
(3) Communality: As the value of coefficient alpha increases, the average absolute value of the difference between communalities based on FA and those based on PCA decreased (from 0.0790 when alpha = 0.843 to 0.0276 when alpha = 0.988). This illustrates part 3 of *Theorem* 1. When the number of items (p) is the only predictor, only 39.3% of the variance for the average absolute value of the differences in communalities was explained. However, when coefficient alpha is added as the second predictor, R^2 increased to 86.0%, resulting in an increment of 46.7%.
(4) Factor score and principal component: As the value of the coefficient alpha increases, the Fisher-z transformed correlation between the Bartlett factor scores and the PCs increases (from z = 2.79 when alpha = 0.843 to z = 4.28 when alpha = 0.988). This illustrates part 4 of Theorem 1. When the number of items (p) was the only predictor, 84.1% of variance for the Fisher-z transformed correlation between the factor scores and the PCs was already explained. However, when adding coefficient alpha as the second predictor, the R^2 becomes even higher at 97.9%, resulting in an increment of 13.8%.

Table 1 The sample means across 20 replications for five measures

			Inverse Corr.	Difference	
# of items (p)	Alpha	Z (closeness)	Ratio off/diag	Communality	Z (scores)
6	0.8343	3.5225	0.16399	0.07895	2.7891
12	0.9067	3.8453	0.08582	0.05043	3.1911
24	0.9519	3.9518	0.05495	0.03397	3.5554
48	0.9759	3.9781	0.04553	0.02842	3.9356
96	0.9877	4.0225	0.04551	0.02759	4.2830

Note. Z (Closeness) = Fisher-z transformed (square-root of) squared correlation between FA and PCA loadings; Inverse Corr. Ratio off/diag = ratio of average absolute off-diagonal element to average diagonal element of the precision (inverse correlation) matrix; Difference Communality = average absolute difference between communalities based on FA and PCA; Z (Scores) = Fisher-z transformed correlation between factor scores and PCs, all averaged over 20 replications

Table 2 R-Squares with predictor p alone and by adding alpha

	Dependent variables			
		Inverse Corr.	Difference	
Predictor(s)	Z (closeness)	Ratio off/diag	Communality	Z (scores)
# of items (p) only	0.218	0.432	0.393	0.841
# of items (p) and alpha	0.500	0.970	0.860	0.979

Note. Z (Closeness) = Fisher-z transformed (square-root of) squared correlation between FA and PCA loadings; Inverse Corr. Ratio off/diag = ratio of average absolute off-diagonal element to average diagonal element of the precision (inverse correlation) matrix; Difference Communality = average absolute difference between communalities based on FA and PCA; Z (Scores) = Fisher-z transformed correlation between factor scores and PCs

7 Discussion

We showed that the phenomenon of the coefficient alpha approaching 1 is related to the increased closeness between FA and PCA. The relationship implies that when the value of coefficient alpha is close to 1, we can confidently use PCA in place of FA and trust that the results are almost the same whether we use FA or PCA. A practical implication for this work is that we can use the value of coefficient alpha as an index for the degree of closeness between FA and PCA. It is easier for applied researchers to compute the coefficient alpha with popular statistical software such as SPSS than computing the squared correlation between FA loadings and PCA loadings. If the results are similar whether we use either FA or PCA, then we recommend that applied researchers should use PCA rather than FA. This is because PCA is straight-forward to compute and it only involves eigenvalue-eigenvector decomposition. Also, unlike FA, PCA never encounters difficulties such as non-convergence and improper solutions (also called the Heywood cases). In addition, the solution for PCA does not require or depend on any iterative numerical algorithms such as the quasi-Newton's methods, except for the numerical computations of standard linear algebra. These problems might become a concern for FA if the number of items becomes very large. We demonstrated that if there is a relatively large number of items and the value of coefficient alpha is also very high, then the results will be very close between FA and PCA. In the numerical illustration of Sect. 6, we demonstrated that the number of items and the coefficient alpha together can predict the degree of closeness between FA and PCA substantially better than the number of items alone.

In our study, we focused on the relationship of coefficient alpha and FA/PCA with high dimensional data. Theoretically, we focused on the case where the number of items go to infinity. On the other hand, in the numerical illustration, we demonstrated that the high level of agreement between FA and PCA as measured by the squared correlation can occur with only about 100 items. That is, the high level of agreement between FA and PCA seems to occur with much smaller number of items than researchers such as in machine learning defined as high dimensions, in which the number of variables often far exceed the number of subjects. For the closeness between FA and PCA without reference to high dimensions, refer to e.g., Bentler and de Leeuw (2011). There are also numerous research on factor scores (in)determinacy, which is beyond the scope of our work. For the topic, refer to e.g., Bentler and Yuan (1997).

The coefficient alpha is not the only measure for reliability. As a matter of fact, there is a connection between the coefficient omega (cf., McDonald, 1985) and FA, as well as between the coefficient theta (Armor, 1974) and PCA. The coefficient omega is defined as

$$\omega\left(\boldsymbol{\lambda},\boldsymbol{\Psi}\right)=\frac{\left(\mathbf{1}_p^T\boldsymbol{\lambda}\right)^2}{\left(\mathbf{1}_p^T\boldsymbol{\lambda}\right)^2+tr(\boldsymbol{\Psi})}.$$

Here, if $(\mathbf{1}^T\boldsymbol{\lambda})^2/tr(\boldsymbol{\Psi})\to\infty$, then $\omega(\boldsymbol{\lambda},\boldsymbol{\Psi})\to 1$. Due to the Cauchy-Schwarz inequality, $(\mathbf{1}^T\boldsymbol{\lambda})^2\le(p)(\boldsymbol{\lambda}^T\boldsymbol{\lambda})$. Also, $(\mathbf{1}^T\boldsymbol{\lambda})^2/tr(\boldsymbol{\Psi})\le\{(p)(\boldsymbol{\lambda}^T\boldsymbol{\lambda})\}\{(\psi_{\text{inf}}^{-1})(p^{-1})\}=(\boldsymbol{\lambda}^T\boldsymbol{\lambda})(\psi_{\text{inf}}^{-1})$, where ψ_{inf}^{-1} is bounded and bounded away from zero due to *Assumption* 2. Thus, $(\mathbf{1}^T\boldsymbol{\lambda})^2/tr(\boldsymbol{\Psi})\to\infty$ implies $\boldsymbol{\lambda}^T\boldsymbol{\Psi}^{-1}\boldsymbol{\lambda}\to\infty$ (again due to *Assumption* 2). That is, $(\mathbf{1}^T\boldsymbol{\lambda})^2/tr(\boldsymbol{\Psi})\to\infty$ implies both $\omega(\boldsymbol{\lambda},\boldsymbol{\Psi})\to 1$ and $\boldsymbol{\lambda}^T\boldsymbol{\Psi}^{-1}\boldsymbol{\lambda}\to\infty$.

Thus, if the ratio of the square of sum of FA loadings to the sum of unique variances goes to infinity, i.e., $(\mathbf{1}^T\boldsymbol{\lambda})^2/tr(\boldsymbol{\Psi})\to\infty$, then

(1) the coefficient omega approaches 1, i.e., $\omega(\boldsymbol{\lambda},\boldsymbol{\Psi})\to 1$;
(2) the coefficient alpha approaches 1, i.e., $\alpha(\boldsymbol{\Sigma})\to 1$ (due to *Lemma* 4 (1) and *Lemma* 2);
(3) the squared non-centered correlation between FA loadings and PCA loadings approaches 1, i.e., $\rho^2(\boldsymbol{\lambda},\boldsymbol{\lambda}^*)\to 1$ (due to *Lemma* 3);
(4) the precision matrix approaches the inverse of the diagonal matrix of unique variances, i.e.,
$\boldsymbol{\Sigma}^{-1}-\boldsymbol{\Psi}^{-1}\to\mathbf{0}$ (due to *Lemma* 5 (1));

(5) the difference between the i-th communalities based on FA and PCA approaches zero for almost all i as the number of observed variables increases, i.e., $\lambda_i^2 - \lambda_i^{*2} \to 0$ as $p \to \infty$ (due to *Lemma* 7 (2));
(6) The factor score and the PC agree with each other, i.e., $\{\mathrm{Corr}(f, f^*)\}^2 \to 1$ (due to *Lemma* 6).

The coefficient theta (Armor, 1974) is defined as $\theta(\mathbf{P}) = \{p/(p-1)\}(1-1/\omega_1(\mathbf{P}))$, where $\omega_1(\mathbf{P})$ is the largest eigenvalue of the correlation matrix $\mathbf{P}$. Obviously, if $\omega_1(\mathbf{P}) \to \infty$ (as $p \to \infty$), then $\theta(\mathbf{P}) \to 1$. Due to *Assumption* 2, σ_{sup} and σ_{inf} are bounded and bounded away from zero. Thus, $\omega_1(\mathbf{P}) \to \infty$ (as $p \to \infty$) if and only if the largest eigenvalue ω_1 of $\mathbf{\Sigma}$ goes to infinity, i.e., $\omega_1(\mathbf{\Sigma}) \to \infty$ (as $p \to \infty$). Here, due to the boundedness of the supremum of the diagonal elements (i.e., $\sigma_{\text{sup}} < \infty$) of the covariance matrix $\mathbf{\Sigma}$, $\omega_1(\mathbf{P}) \to \infty$ or $\omega_1(\mathbf{\Sigma}) \to \infty$ implies $p \to \infty$. Also, due to *Lemma* 4 (2), $p \to \infty$ implies to $\boldsymbol{\lambda}^T \mathbf{\Psi}^{-1} \boldsymbol{\lambda} \to \infty$. Thus, if the largest eigenvalue of either the correlation matrix or the covariance matrix goes to infinity, i.e., either $\omega_1(\mathbf{\Sigma}) \to \infty$ or $\omega_1(\mathbf{P}) \to \infty$, then the coefficient theta approaches 1, i.e., $\theta(\mathbf{P}) \to 1$, and the results (2) through (6) above also hold.

One limitation for our work is that when the number of items is very large, it may be hard for a one-factor model to hold in practice. However, we conjecture that our results can be extended to a multi-factor case. It is noteworthy to mention that besides Bentler and Kano (1990), all the results on the closeness between FA and PCA were proved under a multi-factor case. For a multi-factor model, we may be able to employ, for example, Krijnen (2004) Corollary 2*a* in place of our *Lemma* 6. We showed that the coefficient alpha approaches 1 even if limited number of items that are nearly uncorrelated with each other are added, as long as the mean correlation is bounded away from zero. Therefore, as long as the multi-factor model includes a general factor, it is likely that our results still hold for a multi-factor case.

Acknowledgments We are thankful to Dr. Jorge Andres Gonzalez Burgos for his valuable comments on an earlier version of the article. This work was supported by Grant 31971029 from the Natural Science Foundation of China.

References

Armor, D. J. (1974). Theta reliability and factor scaling. In H. L. Costner (Ed.), *Sociological methodology 1973–1974*. Jossey-bass. https://doi.org/10.1007/BF00151900

Bentler, P.M., & Kano, Y. (1990). On the equivalence of factors and components. *Multivariate Behavioral Research, 25*, 67–74. https://doi.org/10.1207/s15327906mbr2501_8

Bentler, P. M., & de Leeuw, J. (2011). Factor analysis via component analysis. *Psychometrika, 76*, 461–470. https://doi.org/10.1007/s11336-011-9217-5

Bentler, P. M., & Yuan, K.-H. (1997). Optimal conditionally unbiased equivariant factor score estimators. In M. Berkane (Ed.), *Latent variable modeling with applications to causality* (pp. 259–281). Springer.

Brown, W. (1910). Some experimental results in the correlation of mental ability. *British Journal of Psychology, 3*, 271–295.

Cronbach, L. I. (1951). Coefficient alpha and the internal structure of tests. *Psychometrika, 16*, 297–334. https://doi.org/10.1007/BF02310555

Fisher, R. A. (1915). Frequency distribution of the values of the correlation coefficient in samples of an indefinitely large population. *Biometrika, 10*, 507–521. http://doi:10.2307/2331838

Guttman, L. (1956). Best possible systematic estimates of communalities. *Psychometrika, 21*, 273–285. https://doi.org/10.1007/BF02289137

Harville, D. A. (1997). *Matrix algebra from a statistician's perspective*. Springer.

Hayashi, K., & Kamata, A. (2005). A note on the estimator of the alpha coefficient for standardized variables under normality. *Psychometrika, 70*, 579–586. https://doi.org/10.1007/s11336-001-0888-1

Hayashi, K., Yuan, K.-H., & Jiang, G. (2019). On extended Guttman condition in high dimensional factor analysis. In M. Wiberg, S. Culpepper, R. Janssen, J. Gonzalez, & D. Molenaar (Eds.), *Quantitative psychology: The 83-rd annual meeting of the psychometric society, new York City, 2018* (pp. 221–228). Springer.

Jolliffe, I. T. (2002). *Principal component analysis* (2nd ed.). Springer.

Krijnen, W. P. (2004). Convergence in mean square of factor predictors. *British Journal of Mathematical and Statistical Psychology, 57*, 311–326. https://doi.org/10.1348/000711004230714O

Krijnen, W. P. (2006a). Convergence of estimates of unique variances in factor analysis, based on the inverse sample covariance matrix. *Psychometrika, 71*, 193–199. https://doi.org/10.1007/s11336-000-1142-9

Krijnen, W. P. (2006b). Necessary conditions for mean square convergence of the best linear factor predictor. *Psychometrika, 71*, 593–599.

Lawley, D. N., & Maxwell, A. E. (1971). *Factor analysis as a statistical method* (2nd ed.). American Elsevier.

McDonald, R. P. (1985). *Factor analysis and related methods*. Erlbaum.

Schneeweiss, H. (1997). Factors and principal components in the near spherical case. *Multivariate Behavioral Research, 32*, 375–401. https://doi.org/10.1207/s15327906mbr3204_4

Schneeweiss, H., & Mathes, H. (1995). Factor analysis and principal components. *Journal of Multivariate Analysis, 55*, 105–124. https://doi.org/10.1006/jmva.1995.1069

Spearman, C. C. (1910). Correlation calculated from faulty data. *British Journal of Psychology, 3*, 271–295. https://doi.org/10.1111/j.2044-8295.1910.tb00206.x

Yuan, K.-H., & Bentler, P. M. (2002). On robustness of the normal-theory based asymptotic distributions of three reliability coefficient estimates. *Psychometrika, 67*, 251–259. https://doi.org/10.1007/BF02294845

Zhang, Z., & Yuan, K.-H. (2016). Robust coefficients alpha and omega and confidence intervals with outlying observations and missing data: Methods and software. *Educational and Psychological Measurement, 76*, 387–411. https://doi.org/10.1177/0013164415594658

IRT Analysis of Dimensional Structure and Item Wording Effects

Ki Cole, Ronna Turner, and Sohee Kim

1 Introduction

The Perceived Stress Scale (PSS; Cohen & Williamson, 1988) is a widely used measure of self-report of perceived stress. Principal components factor analysis often results in a two-factor solution composed of either positively or negatively directed items (Lee, 2012). Cohen and Williamson (1988) stated that the distinction between factors was irrelevant for purposes of measuring perceived stress. In addition to the overall directional meaning of an item, the orientation may also have an influence on how an item operates. When a negatively worded item stem contains a contraction, such as "not" or "no," or a negative prefix, such as "un-," or "non-," the term or prefix indicates a change in the orientation of the meaning (Swain et al., 2008). Other times, the meaning of the item can be changed by using terms of opposite meaning, such as "happy" and "sad".

The purpose of this study was to investigate the potential effects item direction and orientation on model fit, item parameters, and respondent scores by comparing the calibrations of various multidimensional structures using the multidimensional graded response IRT model.

K. Cole (✉) · S. Kim
Oklahoma State University, Stillwater, OK, USA
e-mail: ki.cole@okstate.edu

R. Turner
University of Arkansas, Fayetteville, AR, USA

M. Wiberg et al. (eds.), *Quantitative Psychology*, Springer Proceedings in Mathematics & Statistics 353, https://doi.org/10.1007/978-3-030-74772-5_13

1.1 Item Wording: Directionality and Orientation

When assessing some psychological constructs, survey instruments composed of items are used to measure the underlying latent trait. The wording of items used in the survey are a key component for the instrument's sound psychometric properties, including reliability, validity, item functioning, and information. Studies have extensively investigated the effects of wording direction – whether positive or negative (Benson & Hocevar, 1985; DiStefano & Motl, 2009; Ebesutani et al., 2012; Gitchel et al., 2011; Magazine et al., 1996; Matlock et al., 2016; Michaelides et al., 2016; Mook et al., 1991; Motl & DiStefano, 2002; Tomás & Oliver, 1999; Weems et al., 2003; Weijters & Baumgartner, 2012). Theoretically, if a respondent answers strongly agree to a positively directed item, "I am happy," the respondent would answer at the exact opposite end of a Likert-type response scale, strongly disagree, to a negatively directed item "I am sad," assuming happy and sad are viewed as exact opposite feelings. Having a mixture of positive and negative items within a scale is most often used and supported by many psychometric studies (Baumgartner & Steenkamp, 2001; Couch & Keniston, 1960; Gu et al., 2015; Michaelides et al., 2016; Weijters & Baumgartner, 2012; Wong et al., 2003); this design is intended to diminish response bias due to non-construct related factors, such as item directionality. Others favor a scale of only positively worded items due to the problematic issues that negative items may cause (Matlock et al., 2016; Wong et al., 2003).

An additional component of the wording effect not included in the aforementioned studies was the orientation of the item. Swain et al. (2008) further characterized negative items as having a negative context due to the negative meaning of the root-terminology, e.g., sad as opposed to happy in the previous example, or due to negatively orienting the item using the words "not" or "no" or the prefix "un-" or "non". Swain et al.(2008) focused primarily on the orientation of NW items; Weijters and Baumgartner (2012) also included the orientation of positive items when reviewing studies of direction and orientation. Table 1 presents four closely related items intended to measure the same construct in order to distinguish among the four wording types.

1.2 Multidimensional Structure

Dimensionality of a dataset refers to the number of factors or constructs a dataset is intended to measure. Sometimes the dimensions are based on content-specific

Table 1 Four items to illustrate direction and wording/orientation effects

	Worded	Oriented
Positive	I am happy. (PW)	I am not sad. (PO)
Negative	I am sad. (NW)	I am not happy. (NO)

stimuli, and others for some non-content-specific stimulus, e.g., item directionality (Gu et al., 2015; Michaelides et al., 2016; Wang et al., 2015; Xin & Chi, 2010).

Many times, item directionality will affect the outcome of exploratory factor analysis resulting in two factors according to direction. Cohen and Williamson (1988) supported the use of a single-level, unidimensional analysis even when items loaded in this way. Hence, many apply unidimensional analysis when studying wording effects. Others indicate that directionality and wording effects should be taken into account (Michaelides et al., 2016; Wang et al., 2015; Xin & Chi, 2010).

Multidimensional structures may be more appropriate for modeling survey data, considering whether to take into account construct related components or to control for non-construct related effects. A first-order multidimensional model includes more than one factor. A simple structure multidimensional arrangement is one in which each item is associated with only one factor, and factors may be correlated or uncorrelated.

A traditional bifactor model is one in which subsets of items are associated with a single specific factor, and all items are associated with a general factor. A reduced bifactor model is one in which all items are associated with a general factor but only some items are associated with a specific factor. Because the general factor is modeled to account for what all items have in common and the specific factors account for what is distinct within subgroups of factors, the general factor and specific factors are often assumed to be uncorrelated.

Almost all research studies that compare psychometric properties of various model structures include the unidimensional model and traditional bifactor models (Gignac, 2006; Gu et al., 2015; Michaelides et al., 2016; Reise et al., 2007; Wang et al., 2015; Xin & Chi, 2010) and a simple-structure multidimensional model (with the exception of Gu et al. (2015)). In most cases, the traditional bifactor model consistently provided the best model-fit statistics. However, none distinguish between items with different orientations. Wang et al. (2015), in conclusion, recognized that some negative items were based on wording or orientation, but they do not make the distinction in the analyses. Of those that only accounted for positive or negatively directed items, Xin and Chi (2010) supported a model that accounted only for negative items, while Michaelides et al. (2016) favored a model that accounted only for positive items.

1.3 Graded Response IRT Model

Item response theory (IRT) is a modern approach to analyze item response data. Several IRT models exist for polytomous data – the graded response (GR), generalized partial credit (GPC), and nominal response (NR). These differ in the assumptions of the data, whether responses are truly ordinal, and in the number of characteristics hypothesized about each item. Polytomous IRT models are used to estimate item and category characteristics, such as item slope and category intercepts, or as traditional IRT parameters discrimination and category location. Item discrimination is a measure of how well an item distinguishes among respondents with similar construct scores. Category location provides an indication of which category a respondent with a specific construct score is likely to choose. Because parameter estimates are compared across various models and for pairs of items, the slope and intercepts are used in this study in order to utilize the standard errors of the estimates. The GR model (Samejima, 1969) is specifically for ordinal data and is used in this study. This model is considered an extension of the dichotomous two-parameter logistic (2PL) IRT model; furthermore, the multidimensional GR (MGR) model is an extension of the multidimensional 2PL model. For the MGR model, an underlying latent construct score and each item's discrimination is assumed to be unique across each dimension, while the category location parameters are consistent across dimensions for each item.

1.4 Summary

Previous research has investigated the effects of item directionality on the dimensional structure of psychological and personality instruments. None (to our knowledge) have also included the confounding effects of direction and orientation on the dimensional structures of survey instruments. The research questions of this study are,

1. What multidimensional structure(s) best model item response data to items that have a mixture of positively and negatively directed items confounded with wording and orientation characteristics?
2. What are the effects of modeling direction and orientation wording characteristics on item parameter estimates?
3. What are the effects of modeling direction and orientation wording characteristics on ability parameter estimates?

2 Method

2.1 Instrument

Perceived Stress Scale (PSS; Cohen & Williamson, 1988) contains ten items, a combination of positively and negatively worded and oriented items. A corresponding item was written in the opposite direction for each of the selected items for a total of 20 items; participants responded to the full set of 20 items. Of those, two were positively oriented (PO), eight were positively worded (PW), seven items were negatively oriented (NO), and three items were negatively worded (NW). Of the ten pairs of items, seven have a NO item matched with a PW item; one pair matches a NW item with a PW item; two pairs match a NW item with a PO item. Item stems are provided in Table 2.

Table 2 Descriptive statistics of responses

	Negative item			Positive item			Item pair response	
		M	*SD*		*M*	*SD*	Agree[a]	Disagree[b]
1	Been upset because of something that happened unexpectedly	2.85	0.87	Remained calm when something happened unexpectedly.	2.35	0.85	73.7%	26.3%
2	Felt you were unable to control the important things in your life.	2.75	1.05	Felt you were able to control the important things in your life.	2.31	0.91	68.0%	32.0%
3	Felt nervous and "stressed."	3.38	1.01	Not felt nervous and "stressed."	2.89	1.03	86.4%	13.6%
4	Felt unsure about your ability to handle your personal problems.	2.45	0.97	Felt confident about your ability to handle your personal problems.	2.11	0.92	59.0%	41.0%
5	Felt that things were not going your way.	2.68	0.89	Felt that things were going your way.	2.45	0.90	60.3%	39.7%
6	Found that you could not cope with all the things you had to do.	2.40	1.02	Found that you were able to cope with all the things you had to do.	2.27	0.88	62.2%	37.8%
7	Been unable to control irritations in your life.	2.80	0.98	Been able to control irritations in your life.	2.41	0.89	59.6%	40.4%
8	Felt that you were not on top of things.	2.71	0.94	Felt that you were on top of things.	2.45	0.89	57.8%	42.2%
9	Been angered because of things that were outside of your control.	2.84	0.93	Have not gotten angry at things that were outside your control.	2.71	0.97	71.5%	28.5%
10	Felt difficulties were piling up so high that you could not overcome then.	2.42	1.06	Felt that you could successfully confront difficulties as they occurred.	2.25	0.86	62.5%	37.5%

Note. Response options were 1 = *Never*, 2 = *Almost Never*, 3 = *Sometimes*, 4 = *Fairly Often*, 5 = *Very Often*. Responses to positive were items were reverse coded so that to any item, a higher value (maximum of 5) corresponds to a higher level of perceived stress and a lower value (minimum of 1) corresponds to a lower level of perceived stress
[a]Responses "Agree" if the response to each item is within ± 1 of each other
[b]Responses "Disagree" if the response to each item with more than ±1 of each other

2.2 Participants

Complete item responses were collected from 3176 participants after observations were removed for missing data and/or patterns of acquiescence or inattention. The sample was primarily female (N = 2010, 63.3%); 19.4% (N = 617) were male, and 17.3% (N = 549) did not indicate a self-selected gender. A majority of the sample was White (N = 2476, 78.0%); 4.9% (N = 155) self-identified as Black/African American, and 4.7% (N = 148) identified themselves as Hispanic. The sample was diverse in their age; 34.3% (N = 1089) were between 18 and 29 years old, 22.6% (N = 718) were between 30 and 39 years old, 15.0% (N = 477) were between 40 and 49 years old, and 18.4% (N = 583) were 50 or older.

2.3 Analysis

The (multidimensional) graded response IRT model was used to calibrate the dataset under various dimensional structures. One unidimensional and ten different multidimensional structures were used. Models to compare were:

1. Unidimensional (ignoring directionality and orientation effects)
2. Multidimensional, correlated traits, with two direction-specific dimensions: positive and negative (ignoring orientation effects)
3. Multidimensional, correlated traits, with two orientation-specific dimensions: wording and orientation (ignoring directional effects)
4. Multidimensional, correlated traits, with four dimensions: positive wording, positive orientation, negative wording, and negative orientation
5. Bifactor with one general factor and two direction-specific factors: positive and negative (ignoring orientation effects)
6. Bifactor with one general factor and one direction-specific factor: positive
7. Bifactor with one general factor and one direction-specific factor: negative
8. Bifactor with one general factor and two orientation-specific factors: wording and orientation (ignoring directional effects)
9. Bifactor with one general factor and one orientation-specific factor: wording (items that do not use the word "not" or prefix "un-")
10. Bifactor with one general factor and one orientation-specific factor: orientation (items that do use the word "not" or prefix "un-")
11. Bifactor with one general factor and four specific factors: positive wording, positive orientation, negative wording, and negative orientation

Data calibrations were performed using the 'mirt' package (Chalmers, 2014) in the R software (R Core Team, 2014) to conduct confirmatory, full-information (maximum likelihood) multidimensional item response theory analyses. The graded response model was used, with the quasi-Monte Carlo EM estimation procedure; this method was chosen for its stability for models with three or more factors. To fit the bifactor models, both the 'bfactor()' and 'mirt()' functions were used so that comparisons to the non-bifactor multidimensional models could be made without bias. Results were nearly equivalent, and the results section includes the output from the data fit with the 'bfactor()' model.

Analyses were as follows. The model-data fit statistics were compared across the eleven different structures to determine which models had a better data-model fit. Item parameter estimates for items were compared across the top model-fit structures in order to determine the modeling effects of each structure on parameter estimates. Comparisons were made using correlations and repeated measures analysis. The item parameter estimates for item pairs having different direction and orientations were compared using t-tests in order to investigate item wording and orientation effects within top model-fit structures. Estimated trait scores across the different structures were compared to traditional sum scores. Comparisons were made using correlations and repeated-measures analysis.

3 Results

3.1 Descriptive Statistics

Descriptive statistics of responses within categories for items and across pairs of positively and negatively worded items are reported in Table 2. Overall, negative items tended to have a higher mean response, indicating a higher level of perceived stress, than the positive item pair.

Response agreement was investigated, such that having an ‘Agree’ in responses for a pair of items is defined as having a same response value or having an adjacent response value for the two items. (Positive items were reverse coded such that for all items a response of 1 corresponds to little to no perceived stress and 5 corresponds to a very high perceived stress.) One item pair (items 1 and 11) had a negatively worded item paired with a positively worded items. Seventy four percent of responses were in agreement for this pair. Two item pairs were a negatively worded item paired with a positively oriented item (item 3 and 13 and items 9 and 19). On average, 86.4% and 71.5% of respondents had agreement on items 3 and 13 and items 9 and 19, respectively. Seven item pairs were a negatively oriented item paired with a positively worded item (items 2 and 12, 4 and 14, 5 and 15, 6 and 16, 7 and 17, 8 and 18, and 9 and 19). On average, these items tended to have lower agreement of responses.

3.2 Model Fit

According to all the fit statistics reported in Table 3, the bifactor models with two or four specific dimensions (M5, M8, and M11) and the four-dimensional model (M4) had the smallest model fit index values. Furthermore, the bifactor model with two specific factors had a better fit than the bifactor model with four factors or the multidimensional model. In the subsequent results, we will consider and compare estimates from both bifactor models with two specific factors, either direction-specific factors (M5) or orientation-specific (M8) factors, the bifactor model with four specific factors (M11), and the multidimensional model with four dimensions (M4).

3.3 Item Parameter Estimates

Seven sets of estimated item discrimination parameters were compared: that of the UD model, between the item and the general factor for each bifactor model, between the item and the specific factor for each bifactor model, and between the item and the unique factor for the multidimensional model.

The unidimensional model discrimination estimate was strongly and positively correlated with the discrimination from the multidimensional model ($r_{U,\,MD} = 0.95$) and the general factor of each of the bifactor models ($0.93 < r < 0.96$). The unidimensional model discrimination estimate was moderately correlated with the specific factor from the BFWO model ($r_{U,\,BFWO\_S} = 0.745$), but had a low correlation with the specific factor from the other bifactor models ($|r| < 0.16$). A similar pattern happened for the multidimensional model discrimination estimate with the general factors of the bifactor models ($0.92 < r < 0.99$), specific factor of the BFWO model ($r_{MD,\,BFWO\_S} = 0.531$), and specific factors of other bifactor models ($|r| < 0.25$).

The discrimination estimate on the general factors from each of the bifactor models were highly correlated ($r > 0.95$). The item discrimination parameters on each item related to the specific factors had a lower correlations ($r_{BFPN\_S,\,BFWO\_S} = -0.158$, $r_{BFPN\_G,\,BFPNWO\_G} = 0.731$, $r_{BFWO\_G,\,BFWO\_G} = 0.016$). Within a single bifactor model, the general and specific factors had a very low correlation within the BFPN model ($r = 0.010$) and

Table 3 Fit statistics of seven model structures using the GR model (N = 3176)

Model	Loglik	GoF	AIC	AICC	BIC	SABIC
1. UD	−69408.4	87794.7	139016.8	139023.3	139623.1	139305.4
2. MD PN	−68749.0	86469.8	137699.9	137706.6	138312.3	137991.4
3. MD WO	−69261.5	87501.5	138725.1	138731.8	139337.5	139016.6
4. MD NPWO	−68536.1	86036.4	137284.2	137291.6	137927.0	137590.2
5. BF PN	−68466.5	85910.8	137172.9	137182.4	137900.5	137519.2
6. BF P	−68680.0	86337.9	137580.0	137587.9	138246.9	137897.4
7. BF N	−68686.4	86350.7	137592.8	137600.8	138259.8	137910.2
8. BF WO	−68447.3	85872.6	137134.7	137144.2	137862.3	137481.0
9. BF W	−68678.3	86334.6	137578.6	137586.8	138251.7	137899.0
10. BF O	−69085.1	87148.0	138388.1	138395.9	139049.0	138702.7
11. BF NPWO	−68578.2	86134.3	137396.4	137405.9	138124.0	137742.7

UD Unidimensional, *MD* Multidimensional [first order, correlated dimensions], *BF* Bifactor, *P* Positive, *N* Negative, *W* Wording, *O* Orientation

the BFPNWO model ($r = 0.159$); however, the general and specific factors within the BFWO model had a moderate correlation ($r = 0.562$).

Table 4 reports the mean and standard deviation ($M(SD)$) of the discrimination estimate and standard errors within subsets of items based on direction and orientation. The averages of the estimated discrimination within subsets of items for the unidimensional model, multidimensional model, and the general factor of the bifactor models were very similar. A repeated measures analysis was used to test the significant differences in the item discrimination estimate across these five models. A Greenhouse-Geisser (GG) adjustment was used due to the violation of sphericity. The results indicated significant differences ($p < .05$). Post hoc analysis with a Bonferroni adjustment indicated that the estimated discrimination from the unidimensional model was significantly smaller than the estimated discrimination from the multidimensional model and from the general factor from the BFWO model (bifactor model with two orientation-specific factors). The estimated discrimination from the multidimensional model was significantly greater than that on the unidimensional model and the general factor from the BFWO. No other models had significantly different estimates.

The differences in standard errors were also evaluated using repeated measures analysis. A GG adjustment was used, and the results were statistically significant ($p < .05$). The standard errors of the unidimensional estimate and the multidimensional estimate were significantly lower than the standard error on the general factor of the BFWO and BFNPWO models.

By design, pairs of items existed such that one item was positively worded and one item was negatively worded. Furthermore, within 9 of the 10 pairs of items, one item was worded without using the negative "not" or prefix "un-" in the item stem and one item was worded using the negative "not" or prefix "un-". Here, paired-samples t-tests were used to compare the estimated item discrimination within pairs of items based on item direction or orientation within each of the five models. Item pairs worded in the positive or negative direction did not have significantly different estimated discriminations for any of the models. Items that were worded without the use of "not" or "un-"tended to be more discriminating than those without. This difference was significant ($p < .003$) only for the BFNP model.

3.4 Trait Score Estimates

A traditional sum score was calculated for the original first 10 items, as directed for scoring the PSS. This was compared to the estimated trait scores from the various model The sum score had strong positive correlation with the UD IRT score and with the estimated score on the general factor from the bifactor models ($r > .95$). The UD score was most correlated with the trait estimate on the general factor from each of the bifactor models ($r > .95$). The scores on the general factors from each bifactor model were also highly correlated ($r > 0.970$). Within each bifactor model, the trait scores on the general and specific factors had low correlations ($|r| < 0.235$).

Table 4 Descriptive statistics (M(SD)) of estimated item slope/discrimination parameter and standard errors within sets of items based on direction and orientation across models

	Factor	Item Set	Count	M1: UD		M4: MDPNWO		M5: BFNP		M8: BFWO		M11: BFNPWO	
Estimate	General	NO	7	2.025	(0.553)	2.159	(0.619)	2.214	(0.651)	2.084	(0.595)	2.255	(0.673)
		NW	3	1.535	(0.170)	2.014	(0.316)	1.831	(0.201)	1.916	(0.259)	1.860	(0.137)
		PO	2	1.257	(0.378)	1.601	(0.568)	1.151	(0.379)	1.417	(0.424)	1.281	(0.407)
		PW	8	2.116	(0.364)	2.290	(0.445)	2.066	(0.418)	2.178	(0.414)	2.079	(0.402)
		Total	20	1.911	(0.496)	2.134	(0.514)	1.991	(0.556)	2.028	(0.545)	2.029	(0.493)
	Specific[a]	NO	7					0.170	(0.251)	0.719	(0.262)	0.320	(0.526)
		NW	3					1.265	(0.819)	−0.721	(0.071)	1.033	(0.561)
		PO	2					0.510	(0.005)	−0.436	(0.021)	0.701	(0.055)
		PW	8					1.126	(0.283)	0.874	(0.236)	1.091	(0.260)
		Total	20					0.751	(0.593)	0.774	(0.524)	0.449	(0.666)
Standard Errors	General	NO	7	0.062	(0.011)	0.049	(0.018)	0.072	(0.016)	0.068	(0.015)	0.084	(0.030)
		NW	3	0.050	(0.003)	0.052	(0.009)	0.090	(0.051)	0.070	(0.010)	0.082	(0.035)
		PO	2	0.046	(0.006)	0.050	(0.011)	0.046	(0.005)	0.053	(0.009)	0.054	(0.008)
		PW	8	0.065	(0.009)	0.066	(0.012)	0.070	(0.013)	0.071	(0.013)	0.070	(0.012)
		Total	20	0.060	(0.011)	0.056	(0.015)	0.071	(0.023)	0.068	(0.013)	0.075	(0.024)
	Specific[a]	NO	7					0.066	(0.009)	0.068	(0.012)	0.106	(0.036)
		NW	3					0.130	(0.102)	0.067	(0.004)	0.118	(0.077)
		PO	2					0.048	(0.001)	0.063	(0.003)	0.114	(0.014)
		PW	8					0.066	(0.009)	0.062	(0.006)	0.066	(0.008)
		Total	20					0.072	(0.016)	0.068	(0.015)	0.084	(0.030)

UD Unidimensional, *BFPN* bifactor model with two direction-specific factors, *BFWO* bifactor model with two orientation-specific factors, *BFPNWO* bifactor model with four direction-specific factors, *NO* negatively oriented, *NW* negatively worded, *PO* positively oriented, *PW* positively oriented

[a]Bifactor models had two or four specific dimensions. Regardless of the number of specific dimensions, the descriptive statistics are reported within subsets of NO, NW, PO, and PW items

The correlations between the four MD trait scores and the general dimension score of the bifactor models were moderate to high. The correlation between the general dimension score of the bifactor models had the highest correlation with the estimated trait score on the negatively oriented dimension ($r > 0.92$), and it had the lowest correlation with the estimated trait score on the positively oriented dimension ($0.56 < r < 0.66$).

4 Discussion

The results of this study have implications to survey writers, administrators, and scorers. Previous recommendations are inconsistent on creating instruments with a mixture of positively and negative directed items or with items uniformly written in a single direction. Results of this study recommend a combination of negatively oriented and positively worded items. When items are written in the reverse, or negated, direction, items tend to be more discriminating when direction is indicated with the use of a contraction or negative prefix. However, items written with a positive direction should not use contractions or negating prefixes, but instead use positive terms and expressions. When scoring, if a single construct score is desired, a unidimensional or BF model is preferred. If a distinction is desired across the construct measured by different item types (direction and orientation), the MD model with four dimensions is preferred.

Limitations of this study include the unbalanced number of items worded or oriented in a specific direction and that only a single construct was being measured. In the future, including a balanced number of the four item types is recommended, along with evaluations with other instruments measuring negative constructs, positive constructs, and neutral constructs.

References

Baumgartner, H., & Steenkamp, E. (2001). Response styles in marketing research: A cross-national investigation. *Journal of Marketing Research, 38*(2), 143–156.

Benson, J., & Hocevar, D. (1985). The impact of item phrasing on the validity of attitude scales for elementary school children. *Journal of Educational Measurement, 22*(3), 231–240.

Chalmers, P. (2014). Mirt: A multidimensional item response theory package for the R environment. *Journal of Statistical Software, 48*(6), 1–29.

Cohen, S., & Williamson, G. M. (1988). Perceived stress in a probability sample of the United States. In S. Spacapan & S. Oskamp (Eds.), *The social psychology of health* (pp. 31–67). Sage.

Couch, A., & Keniston, K. (1960). Yeasayers and naysayers: Agreeing response set as a personality variable. *Journal of Abnormal and Social Psychology, 60*(2), 151–174.

DiStefano, C., & Motl, R. W. (2009). Personality correlates of method effects due to negatively worded items on the Rosenberg Self-Esteem scale. *Personality and Individual Differences, 46*(3), 309–313.

Ebesutani, C., Drescher, C. F., Reise, S. P., Heiden, L., Hight, T. L., Damon, J. D., & Young, J. (2012). The Loneliness Questionnaire – Short Version: An evaluation of reverse-worded and non-reverse-worded items via item response theory. *Journal of Personality Assessment, 94*(4), 427–437.

Gignac, G. (2006). A confirmatory examination of the factor structure of the multidimensional aptitude battery: Contrasting oblique, higher order, and nested factor models. *Educational and Psychological Measurement, 66*(1), 136–145.

Gitchel, D., Roessler, R. T., & Turner, R. C. (2011). Gender differential item functioning according to item wording on the Perceived Stress Scale for adults with Multiple Sclerosis. *Rehabilitation Counseling Bulletin, 55*(1), 20–28.

Gu, H., Wen, Z., & Fan, X. (2015). The impact of wording effect on reliability and validity of the Core Self-Evaluation Scale (CSES): A bi-factor perspective. *Personality and Individual Differences, 83*, 142–147.

Lee, E. (2012). Review of the psychometric evidence of the Perceived Stress Scale. *Asian Nursing Research, 6*, 121–127.

Magazine, S. L., Williams, L. J., & Williams, M. L. (1996). A confirmatory factor analysis examination of reverse coding effects in Meyer and Allen's Affective and Continuance Commitment Scales. *Educational and Psychological Measurement, 56*(2), 241–250.

Matlock, K., Turner, R., & Gitchel, D. (2016). A study of reverse-worded matched item pairs using the generalized partial credit and nominal response models. *Educational and Psychological Measurement, 78*(1), 103–127.

Michaelides, M. P., Koutsogiorgi, C., & Panayiotou, G. (2016). Method effects on an adaptation of the Rosenberg self-esteem scale in Greek and the role of personality traits. *Journal of Personality Assessment, 98*(2), 178–188.

Mook, J., Kleijn, W. C., & van der Ploeg, H. M. (1991). Symptom positively and negatively worded items in two popular self-report inventories of anxiety and depression. *Psychological Reports, 69*, 551–560.

Motl, R. W., & DiStefano, C. (2002). Longitudinal invariance of self-esteem and method effects associated with negatively worded items. *Structural Equation Modeling, 9*(4), 562–578.

R Core Team. (2014). *R: A language and environment for statistical computing*. R Foundation for Statistical Computer. Retrieved from http://www.R-project.org

Reise, S., Morizot, J., & Hays, R. (2007). The role of the bifactor model in resolving dimensionality issues in health outcomes measures. *Quality of Life Research, 16*, 19–31.

Samejima, F. (1969). Estimation of latent ability using a response pattern of graded scores. In *Psychometrika* (Monograph supplement no. 17).

Swain, S. D., Weathers, D., & Niedrich, R. W. (2008). Assessing three sources of misresponse to reversed Likert items. *Journal of Marketing Research, 45*(1), 116–131.

Tomás, J. M., & Oliver, A. (1999). Rosenberg's self-esteem scale: Two factors or method effects. *Structural Equation Modeling, 6*, 84–98.

Wang, W., Chen, H., & Jin, K. (2015). Item response theory models for wording effects in mixed-format scales. *Educational and Psychological Measurement, 75*(1), 157–178.

Weems, G. H., Onwuegbuzie, A. J., Schreiber, J. B., & Eggers, S. J. (2003). Characteristics of respondents who respond differently to positively and negatively worded items on rating scales. *Assessment and Evaluation in Higher Education, 28*(6), 587–607.

Weijters, B., & Baumgartner, H. (2012). Response to reversed and negated items in surveys: A review. *Journal of Marketing Research, 49*(5), 737–747.

Wong, N., Rindfleisch, A., & Burroughs, J. E. (2003). Do reverse-worded items confound measures in cross-cultural consumer research? The case of the material values scale. *Journal of Consumer Research, 30*, 72–91.

Xin, Z., & Chi, L. (2010). Wording effect leads to a controversy over the construct of the Social Dominance Orientation Scale. *The Journal of Psychology, 144*(5), 473–488.

Item Level Measurement of Extreme Response Style

Tongtong Zou and Daniel M. Bolt

1 Introduction

Response styles reflect individual variability in the use of rating scales that are exhibited by respondents when answering survey questions (Bolt, Lu, & Kim, 2014). Among the various forms of response style heterogeneity that have been documented, extreme response style (ERS), which is defined as a content-irrelevant propensity to overselect the endpoints of a rating scale, is commonly observed on self-report rating scale instruments.

In the area of item response theory, one approach to the measurement of ERS uses a multidimensional nominal response model (MNRM) as an extension of the traditional nominal response model (NRM; Bock, 1972, 1997) to incorporate ERS as a continuous latent trait (Bolt & Johnson, 2009). Falk and Cai (2016) further revised this model by adding item discrimination parameters to the response style trait. As a result, under the Falk and Cai model items may show greater or lesser sensitivities to a response style such as ERS.

The probability that respondent j selects category k from $k = 1, \ldots,$ K categories of item i under the influence of $m = 1, \ldots,$ M latent traits (including both substantive and response styles traits) is modeled in a "divide by total" fashion, with each item category having a unique intercept parameter c_{ik} and a slope parameter s_{ikm} for each trait dimension m. Each item also has a unique discrimination parameter for each dimension $a_{i,m}$ that applies across all categories. The general structure of the Falk and Cai model is thus given by:

T. Zou (✉) · D. M. Bolt
University of Wisconsin-Madison, Madison, WI, USA
e-mail: tzou9@wisc.edu

M. Wiberg et al. (eds.), *Quantitative Psychology*, Springer Proceedings in Mathematics & Statistics 353, https://doi.org/10.1007/978-3-030-74772-5_14

$$P(U_{ij}=k \mid \theta_1, \theta_2, \ldots, \theta_M) = \frac{exp(a_{i1}\, s_{ik1}\, \theta_{j1} + \ldots + a_{iM}\, s_{ikM}\, \theta_{jM} + c_{ik})}{\sum_{h=1}^{K} exp(a_{i1}\, s_{ih1}\, \theta_{j1} + \ldots + a_{iM}\, s_{ihM}\, \theta_{jM} + c_{ih})}$$

where some of the $\theta_1, \theta_2, \ldots, \theta_M$ traits reflect intended-to-be-measured content traits, and others are response style traits. An assumption underlying Falk and Cai's model is that the same level of item discrimination on response style traits applies for all respondents regardless of their content trait levels. Such an assumption might be called into question by tree-based models of response style, where the ERS trait is portrayed as being invoked only at a later node in the tree-based sequential response process. Such an occurrence should make the equal discrimination assumption questionable as the same item should be less informative regarding ERS for a respondent unlikely to reach such nodes. It thus might be speculated that an item shows more discriminating power on ERS for a respondent whose content trait level is expected to lead to a response away from the midpoint on a given item.

The present paper explores the possibility of such systematic variation of ERS discrimination through the use of an anchoring vignette design. The appeal of a vignette design is that it allows exploration of response style discrimination without the need to attend to the unknown respondent content trait level. Specifically, we can apply a psychometric model similar to the Falk and Cai model that only attends to response style traits when fitting the empirical vignette response data. As the vignettes are designed with known and varying expected responses, they provide a convenient way of testing our hypothesis that items expected to produce responses toward the middle of the rating scale should show reduced ERS discrimination. We consider extensions of this model for self-report items in discussion.

1.1 Anchoring Vignettes

Anchoring vignettes are hypothetical scenarios rated by respondents that use the same rating scale as for self-report items. The scenarios are designed so as to elicit the same subjective response across respondents, implying that the same rating should ideally be given by each respondent. For a given rating scale, vignettes often target a particular response option on the scale, so that systematic departures from the expected response can be clearly recognized. Responses to a set of anchoring vignettes are theorized to reflect respondents' personalized tendencies to over-/under-select certain rating scale options. Unlike self-report ratings, vignette responses have the benefit of not being influenced by an underlying content trait that varies across respondents.

The current study uses data from 30 vignettes from the cross-national study on conscientiousness by Mõttus et al. (2012). In their survey questionnaire, 6 different self-report rating scales are distinguished by the usage of different labels for the end points, with each scale having 5 score categories. Correspondingly, a total of $5 \times 6 = 30$ anchoring vignettes are used, resulting in five vignettes per self-report item. For vignettes based on the same rating scale, each of the five vignettes is targeted toward a different rating scale category, what we refer to as the expected response level for the vignette. As a result, each vignette can be defined by levels on two factors, the type of rating scale and the expected response level.

Below are a few examples of vignettes from the Mottus et al. questionnaire that were used in the present study. Among them, vignettes 1 and 2 have the same rating scale (in this case associated with a self-report item on accountability), whereas vignette 3 illustrates a different rating scale type (in this case associated with a self-report item on capability). Despite applying the same rating scale, vignettes 1 and 2 are distinguished by the level of expected response. For the first vignette, Kevin seems to be more reliable compared to Dick, thus the expected response level for vignette 2 is higher than for vignette 1. The example vignettes are as follows:

Please rate the persons described in the short text below:

1	[Kevin] often stays at work after office-hours to recheck the finished documents. During his ten-year employment history he has never missed a day at work or been late in finishing an assignment
	Dutiful, Scrupulous _ _ _ _ _ Unreliable, Undependable
2	Generally [Dick's] friends trust him, but sometimes they have been really annoyed by him. For example, [Dick] does not always return the things he has borrowed on time and sometimes he completely forgets about his promises
	Dutiful, Scrupulous _ _ _ _ _ Unreliable, Undependable
3	[Mary] runs a company she founded on her own, raises three children and takes care of her household. In addition, she is active in sports and in community life. Despite her wide range of activities, she has time for her parents and to go hiking with friends
	Capable, efficient, competent_ _ _ _ _ Inept, unprepared

1.2 Item Response Model for Anchoring Vignette Data

Based on the assumption that the anchoring vignettes invoke the same subjective responses across respondents, we apply a special case of Falk and Cai's model where self-report content trait(s) are omitted and only the ERS trait is present with its accompanying item discrimination parameter. The probability for respondent j to select category k from the $k = 1, \dots, K$ categories of item i under the influence of an ERS latent trait is thus modeled as:

$$P(U_{ij} = k \mid \theta_{ERS}) = \frac{exp(a_{ERS,i}\, s_{ik}\, \theta_{ERS} + c_{ik})}{\sum_{h=1}^{5} exp(a_{ERS,i}\, s_{ih}\, \theta_{ERS} + c_{ih})}$$

where s_{ik} denote specified category slope parameters, $a_{ERS,i}$ denotes an item's discrimination parameter related to the ERS trait, c_{ik} denote item category intercepts, and θ_{ERS} is the ERS trait. To define the trait as an ERS trait, we constrain s_{ik} to $\{1, -0.67, -0.67, -0.67, 1\}$ for all items i.

2 Methods

For the present paper we use only the response data of the 30 vignette items (not the self-report rating items) collected for a total of 2965 participants from the Mottus et al. nationwide conscientiousness study. There are five potential response categories for each vignette, coded 1 to 5. As mentioned above, these 30 vignettes can be grouped according to: (1) the level of the expected response (five levels corresponding to rating categories from 1 to 5); (2) the type of rating scale (6 rating scale types varied according to the rating scale used for self-report items).

Our methodological study consists of two parts. In the first part, we carry out a unidimensional IRT analysis on the response data using the mirt routine (Chalmers et al., 2018) in R. In this analysis, we fit the ERS model as shown above. We then examine the resulting item discrimination estimates by rating scale type and expected response level, with an expectation of reduced discrimination for items that target the middle of the rating scale (i.e., expected response level = 3). A two-way ANOVA using the two factors of level and rating scale type is carried out for validation of the ERS discrimination patterns.

In the second part of the analysis, three additional constrained models are fit along with the model described above to further examine our hypothesis. The three constrained models are defined as follows:

(1) A restricted model where ERS discrimination varies only according to rating scale type, where $t = 1, 2, \ldots, 6$ denotes the type of scale:

$$P(U_{ij} = k \mid \theta_{ERS}) = \frac{exp(a_{ERS,t(i)}\, s_k\, \theta_{ERS} + c_{ik})}{\sum_{h=1}^{5} exp(a_{ERS,t(i)}\, s_h\, \theta_{ERS} + c_{ih})}$$

(2) A restricted model where ERS discrimination varies only according to expected response level, where $l = 1, 2, \ldots, 5$ denotes the expected level of vignette response:

$$P(U_{ij} = k \mid \theta_{ERS}) = \frac{exp(a_{ERS,l(i)}\, s_k\, \theta_{ERS} + c_{ik})}{\sum_{h=1}^{5} exp(a_{ERS,l(i)}\, s_h\, \theta_{ERS} + c_{ih})}$$

(3) A restricted model where ERS discrimination varies systematically with respect to both rating scale type and level factors with additive effects for each factor. For simplicity, we use $n = t \times l$ to index the scale and level of each vignette:

$$P(U_{n(i)j} = k \mid \theta_{ERS}) = \frac{exp(a_{ERS,t(i)}\, a_{ERS,l(i)}\, s_k\, \theta_{ERS} + c_{ik})}{\sum_{h=1}^{5} exp(a_{ERS,t(i)}\, a_{ERS,l(i)}\, s_h\, \theta_{ERS} + c_{ih})}$$

All four models (the original unrestricted model and the three restricted models) were estimated using Markov chain Monte Carlo methods in WINBUGS 1.4. Prior distributions are specified as N(0,1) for both a_{ERS} and θ_{ERS}. The initial values for all parameters are generated randomly by the program. A Gibbs sampling procedure is used to sample from the joint posterior density of the model parameters. To define parameter estimates, the number of burn-in iterations is set to 4000 with an additional 1000 iterations used for the final estimation of a_{ERS}. The Deviance Information Criterion (DIC) for each model was used for model comparison. Meanwhile, the same two-way ANOVA analysis was also applied to the ERS discrimination parameter estimates of the baseline model from the MCMC procedure for comparison to the results from the mirt routine. The results are then interpreted.

3 Results

3.1 IRT Analysis

The estimates of the item discrimination parameter a_{ERS} for all vignette items are plotted in Fig. 1 for the six scale types by the five expected response levels. A common pattern emerges across scale types in that the middle-level vignettes (those expected to yield a response of “3”) have lower ERS discrimination than vignettes with expected response levels away from “3”. Further, the ANOVA results in Table 1 show that the level factor is significant ($p < 0.001$), which indicates that there exists a relationship between an item’s ERS discrimination and the expected response level.

3.2 Model Comparison Analysis

The item discrimination estimates a_{ERS} under the baseline model are again plotted in Fig. 2 across different vignette levels for each of the six vignette rating scale types. As for the mirt analysis, it can be seen that the discrimination increased as the

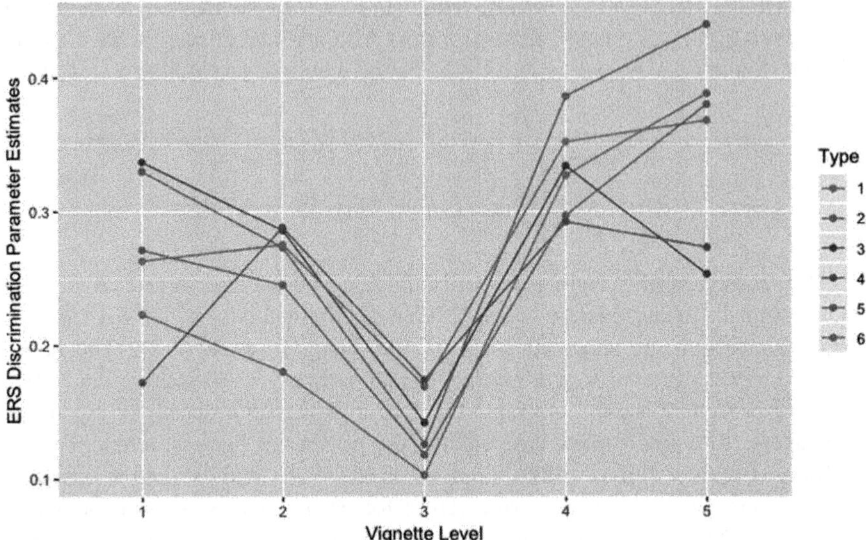

Fig. 1 Estimates of a_{ERS} across vignette levels by scale type, mirt analysis

Table 1 ANOVA results of MIRT a_{ERS} estimates

	Df	Sum Sq	Mean Sq	F-value	p-value
Type	5	0.02	0.00	1.51	0.23
Level	4	0.17	0.04	17.68	0.00
Error	20	0.05	0.00		
Total	29	0.24			

vignette level moves away from the middle category, suggesting that the influence of ERS is greater when the expected response level is away from the center of the rating scale.

A two-way ANOVA was likewise applied to ERS item discrimination estimates for the baseline model including factors for the rating scale type and level. The results in Table 2 show that the level effect is again significant at $p < 0.001$, results in line with those of the mirt analysis.

For the restricted Model 2 where item discrimination varies across the vignette expected response levels, the estimates of $a_{ERS,l(i)}$ ($l = 1, 2, \ldots, 5$) along with their standard errors are shown in Table 3. It can be seen that the ERS discrimination indicated by the absolute value of $a_{ERS,l(i)}$ deceases when moving away from the two ends towards the middle category, which is the result also observed in the baseline model.

The values of the Deviance Information Criterion (DIC) for the four models are presented in Table 4 below. It can be seen that the model in which ERS discrimination differs only according to level (Model 3) fits better than the restricted version where ERS discrimination differs only according to scale type (Model 2).

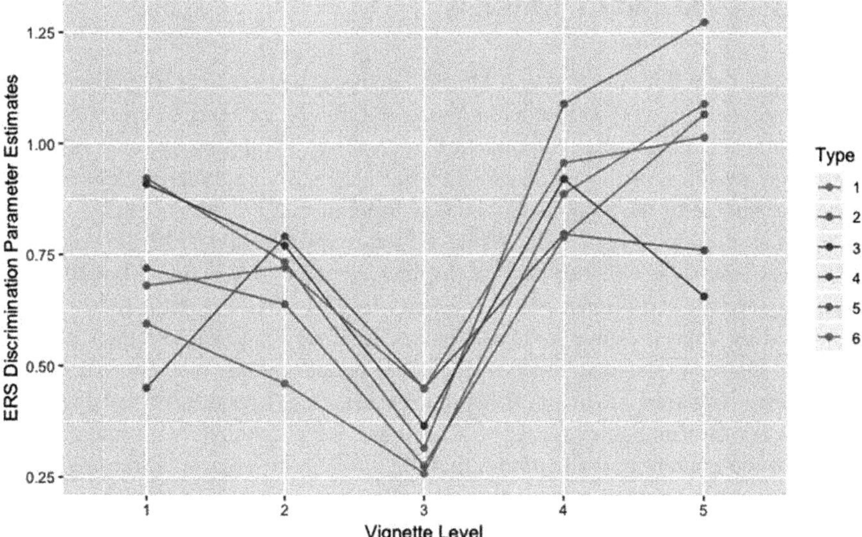

Fig. 2 Estimates of a_{ERS} across vignette levels by scale type, MCMC analysis

Table 2 ANOVA results of MCMC a_{ERS} estimates

	Df	Sum Sq	Mean Sq	F value	Pr(>F)
Type	5	0.16	0.03	1.49	0.23
Level	4	1.42	0.35	16.35	0.00
Error	20	0.43	0.02		
Total	29	2.01			

Table 3 $a_{ERS,l(i)}$ estimates of Restricted Model 2 from MCMC analysis

	Mean	Std.	MC error	Start	Sample
$a_{ERS,1}$	0.68	0.01	0.00	4000	1001
$a_{ERS,2}$	0.67	0.01	0.00	4000	1001
$a_{ERS,3}$	0.37	0.01	0.00	4000	1001
$a_{ERS,4}$	0.88	0.02	0.00	4000	1001
$a_{ERS,5}$	0.93	0.02	0.00	4000	1001

Table 4 DIC values for four models

Model	*D*	*Dhat*	*pD*	DIC
Restricted Model 1	149,158.0	146,505.0	2653.1	151,811.0
Restricted Model 2	148,645.0	146,002.0	2642.6	151,287.0
Restricted Model 3	148,514.0	145,715.0	2799.8	151,314.0
Baseline Model	148,270.0	145,607.0	2663.1	150,934.0

Model 4, where there is an interaction between both level and rating scale type (the baseline model), appears to fit best. Therefore, it would appear that while only level shows a systematic effect, there is likely also some interaction between level and rating scale type.

4 Discussion and Conclusions

The results from both the mirt and MCMC analyses suggests that ERS discrimination is reduced for vignette items targeting the middle categories of the response scale, which indicates that respondent tendencies in exhibiting extreme response style may be more readily invoked when the item pushes subject responses away from the middle of the response scale. One limitation of the current study is that it is based strictly on vignette data. While vignettes have the appeal of allowing us to study response style behavior without the interference of a respondent-level content trait, the vignette conditions are less relevant to real-world measurement than a self-report rating scale instrument. Thus a natural next step is to explore the results of this study in relation to data involving actual self-report items. When both ERS trait and content traits are involved, we might nevertheless hypothesize that the same item's ERS discrimination power will be lower for individuals with intermediate levels of the content trait (assuming that places them on average at the middle of the rating scale) than for individuals with higher or lower levels of the content trait (assuming that places them on average away from the middle of the response scale). To that end, it may be useful to develop a psychometric model that allows ERS discrimination to vary in relation to a respondent's content trait for self-report items.

There are some other limitations to the current analysis. Our ANOVA analyses are applied to discrimination estimates rather than the parameters themselves. Although the sample sizes are large, estimation error still likely has an effect. In addition, while the vignettes were designed to be manipulated with respect to two primary factors, it is possible that there are other aspects of the vignettes associated the level factor that contribute to the effects found and attributed to the expected response level. Clearly the ability to replicate these findings with other instruments (including self-report rating scale instruments) are needed.

Despite these limitations to the current study, it appears there is likely value in applying the current paradigm toward more formal comparisons of tree-based versus MIRT-based modeling of response style. The current results would appear consistent with a tree-based representation of response process in which respondents first decide whether to select the middle category, and only at a later stage (if the middle category is NOT chosen) decide to select an extreme response. There is likely value in exploring further the degree to which tree-based response style models can be made manifest in the discrimination parameter estimate variability seen in this study. Such an evaluation may be best performed through simulation studies, or alternatively through the type of real data studies presented by Böckenholt (2017). While this comparison can be examined with real or simulated vignette data, it will again find its greatest meaning when applied to self-report data.

References

Bock, R. D. (1972). Estimating item parameters and latent ability when responses are scored in two or more nominal categories. *Psychometrika, 37*, 29–51.

Bock, R. D. (1997). The nominal categories model. In W. J. van der Linden & R. K. Hambleton (Eds.), *Handbook of modern item response theory* (pp. 33–49). New York: Springer.

Bolt, D. M., & Johnson, T. R. (2009). Addressing score bias and DIF due to individual differences in response style. *Applied Psychological Measurement, 33*, 335–352.

Bolt, D. M., Lu, Y., & Kim, J. S. (2014). Measurement and control of response styles using anchoring vignettes: A model-based approach. *Psychological Methods, 19(4)*, 528–541.

Böckenholt, U. (2017). Measuring response styles in Likert items. *Psychological Methods, 22(1)*, 69–83.

Chalmers, R. P., Pritikin, J., Robitzsch, A., Zoltak, M., Kim, K., Falk, C. F. et al. (2018). Mirt: Multidimensional item response theory. *R package* version 1.27.1.

Falk, C. F., & Cai, L. (2016). A flexible full-information approach to the modeling of response styles. *Psychological Methods, 21*, 328–347.

Mõttus, R., Allik, J., Realo, A., Pullman, H., Rossier, J., Zecca, J., Tseung, C. N. (2012). Comparability of self-reported conscientiousness across 20 countries. *European Journal of Personality, 26*, 307–317.

On the Marginal Effect Under Partitioned Populations: Definition and Interpretation

Eduardo Alarcón-Bustamante, Ernesto San Martín, and Jorge González

1 Introduction

In social sciences and other fields, the impact that an exogenous explanatory random variable, X, (e.g., the score of a selection test) has on the outcome random variable, Y, (e.g., the grade point average, GPA) is usually measured through the marginal effect (see Geiser & Studley, 2002; DEMRE, 2016; Manzi et al., 2008; Grassau, 1956). The marginal effect quantifies the changes in the conditional expectation with respect to changes in the values of X: if changes in X produces large (small) changes in Y, then the effect of X will be high (low) on Y.

In predictive validity studies involving university selection tests, one of the main goals is to characterise the marginal effect taking into account that the population of interest is partitioned in groups or clusters (universities, countries, sex, among others). In this context, the conditional expectation of the GPA is conditioned not only on the test score, but also on a random variable, Z, characterising the groups. The most common approach is to use a multiple linear regression model with

E. Alarcón-Bustamante (✉) · J. González
Faculty of Mathematics, Department of Statistics, Pontificia Universidad Católica de Chile, Santiago, Chile

Interdisciplinary Laboratory of Social Statistics, Santiago, Chile
e-mail: esalarcon@mat.uc.cl; jorge.gonzalez@mat.uc.cl

E. San Martín
Faculty of Mathematics, Department of Statistics, Pontificia Universidad Católica de Chile, Santiago, Chile

Interdisciplinary Laboratory of Social Statistics, Santiago, Chile

The Economics School of Louvain, Université Catholique de Louvain, Ottignies-Louvain-la-Neuve, Belgium
e-mail: esanmart@mat.uc.cl

M. Wiberg et al. (eds.), *Quantitative Psychology*, Springer Proceedings in Mathematics & Statistics 353, https://doi.org/10.1007/978-3-030-74772-5_15

interaction terms between the test score and the group variable Z. By taking the difference between the marginal effect of a group of interest and one of reference, researchers compare the impact of the test scores on the GPA between groups. As a matter of fact, the effect that X has on the group z with respect to the reference, z', corresponds to the "interaction effect", which is quantified by the corresponding interaction regression coefficient (see Cameron & Trivedi, 2005; Cornelissen, 2005; Powers & Xie, 1999; Norton et al., 2004; Ai & Norton, 2003; Long & Mustillo, 2018).

Formally, researchers are learning about the marginal effect of X on Y in a partitioned population by using the regression $\mathbb{E}(Y|X, Z)$, typically a linear one with some interaction terms. Thus, the analysis is separately made for each group while the interest is to report and draw conclusions based on a global analysis. As an example, in Miller and Frech (2000) a regression analysis is used to determine the effect of each explanatory variables on life expectancy measures and infant mortality for 21 OECD countries. Among the explanatory variables, the authors consider pharmaceutical consumption indexes, per capita income and other lifestyle factors such as tobacco use, alcohol consumption and richness of diet. Their study focuses on both a global analysis, reporting the effects of the explanatory variables on the outcomes, and an analysis by group, reporting the marginal effect of some explanatory variables for four countries (France, Italy, US and Ireland). In this paper, we will show that this type of analysis needs to be carefully improved. The motivation being that a trend can appear when different groups are analysed separately, and possibly disappear when they are combined. This phenomenon is related to the Simpson's Paradox (see Simpson, 1951; Blyth, 1972).

As a matter of fact, we combine the groups through the Law of Total Probability, which lead to define $\mathbb{E}(Y|X)$ as a mixture of the corresponding conditional expectations for each group with mixing weights depending on each group. Thus, we compute the marginal effect of X on Y by using $\mathbb{E}(Y|X)$, instead of $\mathbb{E}(Y|X, Z)$. We define this marginal effect as the *Global Marginal Effect*, which is interpreted as the total marginal effect for partitioned populations. Although from this result it might be intuitive that the global marginal effect is obtained as a convex combination of the marginal effects for each group, we show that an additional term that depends on the predictive outcomes Y's by X's is also included in the definition.

The rest of the paper is organised as follows. In Sect. 2 the concept of *Global Marginal Effect* is formally defined and its properties are discussed. A detailed analysis of the function that characterise the Global Marginal Effect is also presented in this section. An illustration showing the use of the global marginal effect in a real data set is presented in Sect. 3. The paper ends in Sect. 4 drawing conclusions and with a discussion.

2 Global Marginal Effect

2.1 Definition of the Global Marginal Effect

Let us consider a population that is partitioned in groups or clusters and for which score data (X, Y) are observed. Let Z be a categorical random variable such that $Z = z$ if the statistical unit belongs to the group z for $z \in \{0, \dots, G\}$. Thus, each member of the population is characterised by a triple (Y, X, Z). By applying the Law of Total Probability, the conditional expectation, $\mathbb{E}(Y|X)$, for the full population is obtained as

$$\mathbb{E}(Y|X) = \sum_z \mathbb{E}(Y|X, Z = z)\mathbb{P}(Z = z|X). \tag{1}$$

Equation (1) provides a global and unique conditional expectation function for the population, which contains the information of all the groups. In particular, this function could be characterised as a global model composed by different regression models (one for each group). The component models are those that relate the scores variables for each group, and a model for the categorical variable Z. The *Global Marginal Effect* is accordingly obtained by taking the derivative with respect to X in Equation (1), namely

$$\frac{d\mathbb{E}(Y|X)}{dX} = \tag{2}$$

$$\sum_z \frac{d\mathbb{E}(Y|X,Z=z)}{dX}\mathbb{P}(Z=z|X) + \sum_z \mathbb{E}(Y|X, Z = z)\frac{d\mathbb{P}(Z=z|X)}{dX}.$$

From (2), it can be seen that the Global Marginal Effect is not only the weighted average of the marginal effects in $Z = z$, but it also depends on the marginal effects observed through the categorical regression, $\mathbb{P}(Z = z|X)$. In particular, it follows that if $Z \perp\!\!\!\perp X$, Equation (2) reduces to

$$\frac{d\mathbb{E}(Y|X)}{dX} = \sum_z \left[\frac{d\mathbb{E}(Y|X, Z = z)}{dX}\right]\mathbb{P}(Z = z).$$

Thus, the marginal effect in partitioned populations is a weighted average of the marginal effects in $Z = z$, if belonging to the group Z does not depend on X.

For the case when $Z \not\perp\!\!\!\perp X$, and taking into account that $\sum_z P(Z = z \mid X) = 1$, the Global Marginal Effect in Equation (2) can be rewritten as follows:

$$\frac{d\mathbb{E}(Y|X)}{dX} = \sum_z \frac{d\mathbb{E}(Y|X, Z = z)}{dX}\mathbb{P}(Z = z|X) +$$

$$+ \sum_{z \neq z'} [\mathbb{E}(Y|X, Z = z) - \mathbb{E}(Y|X, Z = z')]\frac{d\mathbb{P}(Z = z|X)}{dX}; \tag{3}$$

here z' is the label of a reference group. It can be verified that the Global Marginal Effect is invariant under the chosen reference group; for a proof, see Appendix A.1.

Equation (3) corresponds to the sum of two functions, namely

$$a(X) = \sum_{z} \frac{d\mathbb{E}(Y|X, Z = z)}{dX} \mathbb{P}(Z = z|X), \text{ and}$$

$$b(X) = \sum_{z \neq z'} [\mathbb{E}(Y|X, Z = z) - \mathbb{E}(Y|X, Z = z')] \frac{d\mathbb{P}(Z = z|X)}{dX},$$

where $a(X)$ is a convex combination of the marginal effects in each group with weights being a function of X. Then, $a(X)$ will vary according to the variations of the weights as a function of X. The term $b(X)$ is the sum of the differences of the predicted Y, multiplied by the marginal effect of X on Z.

In the next section, both functions $a(X)$ and $b(X)$ are analysed when the population is assumed to be partitioned in three groups. A linear and a multinomial logistic regression model are considered for $\mathbb{E}(Y|X, Z = z)$ and $\mathbb{P}(Z = z|X)$, respectively.

2.2 Interpretation of the Global Marginal Effect

Let us consider three groups, (i.e., $z \in \{0, 1, 2\}$). By using the invariant property of the global marginal effect, without loss of generality we take $z' = 0$ as the reference group, then

$$\frac{d\mathbb{E}(Y|X)}{dX} = \sum_{z=0}^{2} \frac{d\mathbb{E}(Y|X, Z = z)}{dX} p_z(X) + \\ + \sum_{z=1}^{2} [\mathbb{E}(Y|X, Z = z) - \mathbb{E}(Y|X, Z = 0)] \frac{dp_z(X)}{dX},$$

where $p_z(X) = \mathbb{P}(Z = z|X)$. If a linear function for $\mathbb{E}(Y|X, Z = z)$ is considered (i.e., $\mathbb{E}(Y|X, Z = z) = \delta_z + \gamma_z X$), the marginal effect is a constant function of X, namely γ_z. On the other hand, if a multinomial logistic function $F(u_z) = \exp\{u_z\}/(1 + \sum_{j=1}^{2} \exp\{u_j\})$, $u_z = \alpha_z + \beta_z X$ and $z \in \{1, 2\}$, is used for the prediction function, $p_z(X)$, the marginal effect of X on Z is given by

$$\frac{dp_z(X)}{dX} = \begin{cases} p_z(X) \left(\beta_z - \sum_{j=1}^{2} \beta_j p_j(X) \right) & \text{if } z \in \{1, 2\} \\ - \sum_{z=1}^{2} p_z(X) \left(\beta_z - \sum_{j=1}^{2} \beta_j p_j(X) \right) & \text{if } z = 0 \end{cases}$$

(See Wooldridge, 2010; Greene, 2003). This marginal effect inform us about the change in predicted probabilities due to the changes in X (Wulff, 2014).

Analysis of $a(X)$ Note that:

$$a(X) = \sum_{z=0}^{2} \gamma_z p_z(X),$$

which corresponds to a mixture of γ_z's with mixing weights defined by $p_0(X)$, $p_1(X)$, and $p_2(X)$.

For ease of exposition, let us consider the following particular case as an example

$$\mathbb{E}(Y|X, Z = 1) \geq \mathbb{E}(Y|X, Z = 0); \quad \text{and} \quad \mathbb{E}(Y|X, Z = 2) \geq \mathbb{E}(Y|X, Z = 0),$$

and $\gamma_0 > \gamma_2 > \gamma_1$. The group 0 has the lowest predicted Y for all the values of X, but its marginal effect, γ_0, is higher than both γ_1 and γ_2. Hence, its "importance" in $a(X)$ will depends on how $p_0(X)$ varies with respect to X. This case is graphically illustrated in Fig. 1. From the right-side panel in Fig. 1, it can be seen that $p_0(X)$ is a decreasing function of X (i.e., for higher values of X, a lower probability of belonging to the group 0 is found), then for lower values of X, $a(X)$ is influenced by $\gamma_0 p_0(X)$. In this sense, $a(X)$ can be interpreted as a trade-off among the marginal effects of the groups: as a function of X, it depends not only on the highest value γ_z for a specific group z, but also on the size of such a group.

Analysis of $b(X)$ In our example,

$$b(X) = \sum_{z=1}^{2} [(\delta_z - \delta_0) + (\gamma_z - \gamma_0)X] \left(p_z(X)[\beta_z(1 - p_z(X)) - \beta_j p_j(X)]\right),$$

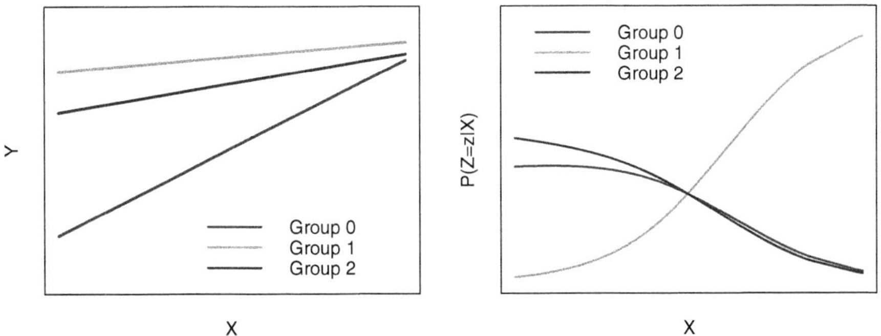

Fig. 1 Example situation. The left-side panel shows $\mathbb{E}(Y|X, Z = z) = \delta_z + \gamma_z X$. The right-side panel shows $p_z(X) = F(u_z)$ for $z \in \{1, 2\}$, and $p_0(X) = 1 - \sum_{z=1}^{2} p_z(X)$

with $j \neq z$. Let us analyse the first component of $b(X)$, namely

$$b_1(X) = [(\delta_1 - \delta_0) + (\gamma_1 - \gamma_0)X]\,(p_1(X)[\beta_1(1 - p_1(X)) - \beta_2 p_2(X)])\,.$$

When

$$\mathbb{E}(Y|X, Z = 1) \geq \mathbb{E}(Y|X, Z = 0),$$

$b_1(X)$ will increase (or decrease) according to

$$p_1(X)[\beta_1(1 - p_1(X)) - \beta_2 p_2(X)],$$

which can be written as

$$p_1(X)[\beta_1 p_0(X) - (\beta_2 - \beta_1)p_2(X)]. \tag{4}$$

Note that Equation (4) depends not only on the probability of belonging to the group 1, but also on the probability of belonging to the group 0 and 2. In this context, if x_1^* is the inflection point of $p_1(X)$, which is a monotonic increasing function of X, then for all $x > x_1^*$

$$\mathbb{P}(Z = 1|X = x) > \mathbb{P}(Z \neq 1|X = x).$$

Thus, for all $x > x_1^*$, $b_1(X)$ is influenced by $\mathbb{P}(Z = 1|X = x)$. In contrast, for all $x < x_1^*$, $b_1(X)$ is influenced by $\mathbb{P}(Z \neq 1|X = x)$. For the other groups, the function $b(X)$ can be analysed analogously.

Collecting all the components of $b(X)$ and after some algebra, it can be shown that

$$b(X) = \sum_{z=1}^{2} \beta_z p_z(X)[f_z(X)p_0(X) + (f_z(X) - f_j(X))p_j(X)], \tag{5}$$

where $z \neq j$, and $f_z(X) = \mathbb{E}(Y|X, Z = z) - \mathbb{E}(Y|X, Z = 0)$. Then, $b(X)$ is a function that depends not only on the differences between the predictions of Y with respect to a reference group, but also on the probability of being in the groups which in turn change across X.

In summary, the Global Marginal Effect is not only a weighted average of the marginal effects in each group, but it also considers a term accounting for the differences between the predicted outcome weighted by the marginal effect of the probability of belonging to the group z. Moreover, it is not a fixed value as it changes as a function of X. In other words, the Global Marginal Effect does not reduce to a slope, but it also considers the relevance of the predicted outcomes.

3 Application

The university admission system in Chile includes two mandatory selection tests (Mathematics and Language and Communication) and two elective ones (Sciences and History, Geography and Social Sciences). Other selection factors, namely, the Ranking and High school GPA are also considered in the selection process. A score, in the 150–850 scale, is assigned to each selection factor, which are weighted to obtain a unique application score.

To illustrate the interpretation of the Global Marginal Effect, we analyse the effect of the Mathematics selection test score, X, over the GPA[1] in the first year, Y, of selected students in the Faculty of Biological Sciences of a Chilean university. We analyse the three undergraduate programs offered by this Faculty: Marine Biology, Biochemistry, and Biology. The last enrolled student in each program scored 631, 631, and 623 in the Mathematics test, respectively.

To estimate the Global Marginal Effect in Equation (1), the same functions described in Sect. 2.2 (i.e., a linear function $\mathbb{E}(Y|X, Z = z) = \delta_z + \gamma_z X$, and a multinomial logistic model for $p_z(X)$) were considered. By using the invariant property of the global marginal effect, the chosen reference group was the Marine Biology program.

3.1 Results

To have a general picture on how the Global Marginal Effect varies in terms of test scores, study programs, and the proportion of students in each program, we used the functions $a(X)$ and $b(X)$ described in the preceding section. Figure 2 shows a graphical representation of both functions which will be analysed together with the information provided in Table 1 that include the estimation of the marginal effects and the proportion of students in each program.

From Table 1, it can be seen that the Marine Biology program has the largest marginal effect and the lowest proportion of enrolled students. In contrast, the smallest marginal effect is found for the group of students enrolled in the Biochemistry program. The central-top panel in Fig. 2 shows the probability of belonging to each program as a function of the Mathematics test score. From the figure, it can be seen that higher score values are associated with higher probabilities of being in the Biochemistry program (i.e., $p_1(X)$ is an increasing function of X). In contrast, $p_0(X)$ (the probability of being in the Marine Biology program), is a decreasing function for all the range of scores. Regarding the Biology program group, it can be seen that up to a score 619 (approx.), $p_2(X)$ is an increasing function of X that decreases for higher score values. In summary, low scores in the Mathematics test

[1]The scale score for the GPA is 1.0–7.0. The minimum score to pass a course is 4.0.

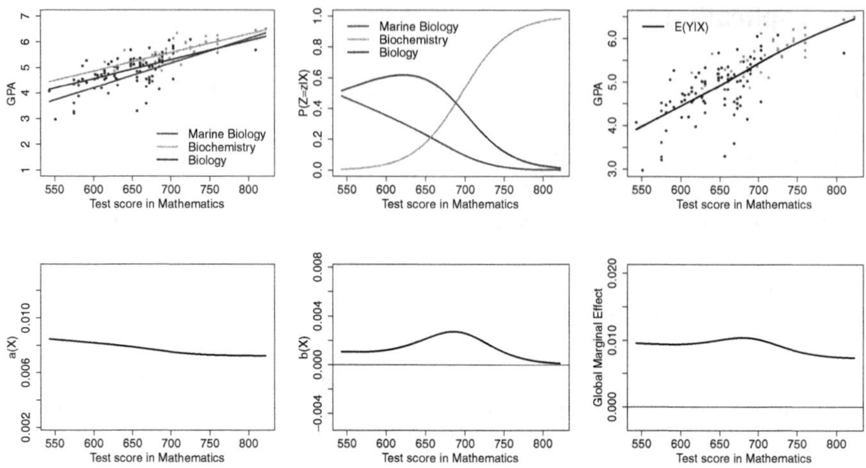

Fig. 2 Functions involved in the Global Marginal Effect

Table 1 γ_z and the empirical proportion of students in undergraduate programs in the faculty of Biological Sciences

z	Program	Prop	γ_z
0	Marine Biology	0.20	0.0096
1	Biochemistry	0.33	0.0072
2	Biology	0.47	0.0074

are associated with a higher probability to find students in the Marine Biology or Biology Programs than students in Biochemistry. Likewise, higher scores in the Mathematics test are associated with a higher probability to find students in the Biochemistry than students from Marine Biology or Biology programs.

The preceding analysis is useful to inspect more deeply how the two functions $a(X)$ and $b(X)$ looks like. As a matter of fact, $a(X) = \gamma_0 p_0(X) + \gamma_1 p_1(X) + \gamma_2 p_2(X)$ and thus, both γ_0 and γ_2 have larger weights for lower values of X, while γ_1 has a larger weight for higher values of X. Considering that $\gamma_0 > \gamma_2 > \gamma_1$, it follows that $a(X)$ is a decreasing function of X as it can be seen in the left-bottom panel of Fig. 2.

Let us analyse $b(X)$ by taking into account Equation (5), which can be rewritten as follows:

$$\begin{aligned} b(X) &= p_0(X)(\beta_1 p_1(X) f_1(X) + \beta_2 p_2(X) f_2(X)) \\ &\quad + (\beta_1 - \beta_2)(f_1(X) - f_2(X)) p_1(X) p_2(X). \end{aligned}$$

Because for low scores in the Mathematics test, $p_1(X) \to 0$, then

$$b(X) \to \beta_2 p_0(X) p_2(X) f_2(X).$$

On the other hand, for higher values of X, $p_0(X) \to 0$, $p_2(X) \to 0$, then

$$b(X) \to 0.$$

Moreover, as it is seen from the top-left panel of Fig. 2, the score range $619 < x < 703$ contains most of the students from all the programs, and thus $b(X)$ is influenced by $p_0(X)$, $p_1(X)$, and $p_2(X)$, which is reflected in the central-bottom panel of Fig. 2.

The Global Marginal Effect, reported in the right-bottom panel of Fig. 2, is the effect that the Mathematics test score has in students of the Faculty of Biology. For the analysed data, it turns to be positive for the whole range of test scores. For lower score values, there is a larger proportion of students belonging to a program where the marginal effect of Mathematics test score is high. In contrast, for higher scores, a larger proportion of students will be found for a program where the marginal effect is low. Note that the concavity of the curve in central range of scores is due to the fact that of both $f_1(X) > 0$ and $f_2(X) > 0$ (see the top-left panel in Fig. 2).

4 Conclusions and Discussion

We have introduced the concept of Global Marginal Effect which is obtained by computing the marginal effect of X on Y by decomposing $\mathbb{E}(Y|X)$ with respect to Z through the Law of Total Probability. The Global Marginal Effect is useful when the main interest is to learn about the effect of X on Y in a partitioned population.

By means of a physiognomy of the studied population based on Fig. 2, we have proposed a new way to analyse and interpret a marginal effect for the case of partitioned populations. Such interpretation shows the effect of X by considering other characteristics of the population (differences in predicted outcomes and the size of each group) which are accordingly defined as a non-constant function of X. Note that, although the physiognomy of the studied population considered a particular reference group, the derived result related to the invariant property of the global marginal effect with respect to the chosen reference group ensures that the type of interpretation proposed generalises no matter the group chosen as reference.

The studied scenario makes sense if both X and Y are fully observed. In the selection context, however, there is a partial observability of the outcome, whereas the explanatory random variable is fully observed (e.g., the GPA in the university is observed in selected students only, whereas the test scores are observed for all the applicants). Thus, a relevant future work is to combine the results of this paper and the ideas in Alarcón-Bustamante, San Martín and González (2020) in order to have a whole overview of the effect that a selection test score has over the GPA in the higher education system.

Acknowledgments Eduardo Alarcón-Bustamante was funded by the National Agency for Research and Development (ANID)/Scholarship Program/Doctorado Nacional/2018-21181007. Ernesto San Martín was partially funded by the FONDECYT grant 1181261. Jorge González was partially funded by the FONDECYT grant 1201129.

A.1 Invariant Property of the Global Marginal Effect

Proof The global marginal effect in Equation (2) is a function that depends on both X and Z, namely $g(X, Z)$. Let z' be any chosen reference group. Noting that $p_{z'}(X) = 1 - \sum_{z \neq z'} p_z(X)$, where $p_z(X) = \mathbb{P}(Z = z|X)$ we have

$$g(X, Z = z') = \frac{d\mathbb{E}(Y|X, Z = z')}{dX} + \sum_{z \neq z'} \left[\frac{d\mathbb{E}(Y|X, Z = z)}{dX} - \frac{d\mathbb{E}(Y|X, Z = z')}{dX} \right] p_z(X)$$
$$+ \sum_{z \neq z'} \left[E(Y|X, Z = z) - \mathbb{E}(Y|X, Z = z') \right] \frac{dp_z(X)}{dX}$$

Now, suppose that another reference group, z'' ($z' \neq z''$), is chosen. Then,

$$g(X, Z = z'') = \frac{d\mathbb{E}(Y|X, Z = z'')}{dX} + \sum_{z \neq z''} \left[\frac{d\mathbb{E}(Y|X, Z = z)}{dX} - \frac{d\mathbb{E}(Y|X, Z = z'')}{dX} \right] p_z(X)$$
$$+ \sum_{z \neq z''} \left[E(Y|X, Z = z) - \mathbb{E}(Y|X, Z = z'') \right] \frac{dp_z(X)}{dX}$$

By subtracting both functions we obtain

$$g(X, Z = z') - g(X, Z = z'') = \left[\frac{d\mathbb{E}(Y|X, Z = z'')}{dX} - \frac{d\mathbb{E}(Y|X, Z = z')}{dX} \right] \left[\sum_z p_z(X) - 1 \right]$$
$$+ \left[E(Y|X, Z = z'') - \mathbb{E}(Y|X, Z = z') \right] \frac{d\left[\sum_z p_z(X) \right]}{dX}$$

Finally, because $\sum_z p_z(X) = 1$, hence

$$\left[\sum_z p_z(X) - 1 \right] = 0 \quad ; \quad \frac{d\left[\sum_z p_z(X) \right]}{dX} = 0$$

This fact implies that

$$g(X, Z = z') - g(X, Z = z'') = 0,$$

and therefore $g(X, Z = z') = g(X, Z = z'')$, for all $z' \neq z''$. □

Remark 1 *Analogously, it can be proven that $g(X, Z)$ is invariant under the chosen reference group when $Z \perp\!\!\!\perp X$.*

References

Ai, C., & Norton, E. C. (2003). Interaction terms in logit and probit models. *Economic Letters, 80*, 123–129.

Alarcón-Bustamante, E., San Martín, E., & González, J. (2020). Predictive validity under partial observability. In M. Wiberg, D. Molenaar, J. González, U. Böckenholt, & J.-S. Kim (Eds.), *Quantitative psychology* (pp. 135–145). Cham: Springer International Publishing.

Blyth, C. (1972). On Simpson's paradox and the sure-thing principle. *Journal of the American Statistical Association, 67*(338), 364–366.

Cameron, A., & Trivedi, P. (2005). *Microeconometrics. Methods and applications*. New York: Cambridge University Press.

Cornelissen, T. (2005). *Standard errors of marginal effects in the heteroskedastic probit model.* (Discussion paper)

DEMRE. (2016). *Prueba de selección universitaria* (Technical Report). Universidad de Chile.

Geiser, S., & Studley, R. (2002). UC and the SAT: Predictive validity and differential impact of the SAT I and SAT II at the University of California. *Educational Assessment, 8*(1), 1–26.

Grassau, E. (1956). Análisis estadístico de las pruebas de bachillerato. *Anales de la Universidad de Chile, 102*, 77–93.

Greene, W. H. (2003). *Econometric analysis* (5 Ed.). Upper Saddle River, NJ: Prentice Hall.

Long, J. S., & Mustillo, S. A. (2018). Using predictions and marginal effects to compare groups in regression models for binary outcomes. *Sociological Methods & Research*, 1–37. https://doi.org/10.1177/0049124118799374

Manzi, J., Bravo, D., del Pino, G., Donoso, G., Martínez, M., & Pizarro, R. (2008). *Estudio de la validez predictiva de los factores de selección a las universidades del consejo de rectores, admisiones 2003 al 2006*. Comité Técnico Asesor, Honorable Consejo de Rectores de las Universidades Chilenas.

Miller, R., & Frech, H. (2000). Is there a link between pharmaceutical consumption and improved health in OECD countries? *Pharmacoeconomics, 18*(1), 33–45.

Norton, E. C., Wang, H., & Ai, C. (2004). Computing interaction effects and standrard errors in logit and probit models. *The Stata Journal, 4*(2), 154–167.

Powers, D. A., & Xie, Y. (1999). *Statistical methods for categorical data analysis*. Academic Press, Inc.

Simpson, E. (1951). The interpretation of interaction in contingency tables. *Journal of the Royal Statistical Society, Series B, 13*(2), 238–241.

Wooldridge, J. M. (2010). *Econometric analysis of cross section and panel data* (2 Ed.). Cambridge, MA: The MIT Press.

Wulff, J. N. (2014). Interpreting results from the multinomial logit model: Demonstrated by foreign market entry. *Organizational Research Methods, 18*(2), 1–26.

References

Range-Preserving Confidence Intervals and Significance Tests for Scalability Coefficients in Mokken Scale Analysis

Letty Koopman, Bonne J. H. Zijlstra, and L. Andries van der Ark

1 Introduction

Mokken scale analysis is a popular scaling method used in questionnaires and is based on nonparametric item response theory models (see, e.g., Mokken, 1971; Sijtsma & Molenaar, 2002; Sijtsma & Van der Ark, 2017, for an elaborate introduction). The most popular aspect of Mokken scale analysis is scalability coefficients, which can be used to construct questionnaires from a larger set of items or to evaluate questionnaires that have a fixed set of items (Sijtsma & Van der Ark, 2017). Let I denote the total number of items, indexed by i or j ($i, j = 1, 2, \ldots, I$). There are three types of scalability coefficients: item-pair scalability coefficient H_{ij} is a normed correlation between items i and j, item scalability coefficient H_i is a normed item–rest correlation that can be considered a discrimination index, and total-scale coefficient H is the weighted sum of the H_is across all items, for which higher values indicate a more accurate ordering of respondents (e.g., Sijtsma & Molenaar, 2016, p. 309). The standard errors of the three types of scalability coefficients were derived using the delta method as $SE_{H_{ij}}$, SE_{H_i} and SE_H, respectively (Kuijpers et al., 2013). Snijders (2001) generalized the coefficients to two-level scalability coefficients for multi-rater data, in which multiple raters score the subjects of interest. Two-level scalability coefficients consist of within-rater and between-rater coefficients, which provide information on the scalability on the respondent- and the group-level, respectively (see also, Koopman et al., 2020). Within-rater coefficients have a similar interpretation to Mokken's coefficients.

A Mokken scale is defined as a set of items for which

L. Koopman (✉) · B. J. H. Zijlstra · L. A. van der Ark
Research Institute of Child Development and Education, University of Amsterdam, Amsterdam, The Netherlands
e-mail: V.E.C.Koopman@UvA.nl

M. Wiberg et al. (eds.), *Quantitative Psychology*, Springer Proceedings in Mathematics & Statistics 353, https://doi.org/10.1007/978-3-030-74772-5_16

$$\begin{aligned} H_{ij} &> 0 \quad \text{for all item-pairs } (i, j), \\ H_i &\geq c > 0 \quad \text{for all items } i, \end{aligned} \tag{1}$$

where c is some positive lower bound for which $c = 0.3$ is often used (Mokken, 1971, p. 184). All scalability coefficients can take values from $-\infty$ to 1. If the items are statistically independent, the scalability coefficients equal 0; if the items are perfectly correlated, the scalability coefficients equal 1. The strength of a scale can be interpreted as follows:

$$\begin{aligned} 0.3 \leq H &< 0.4 : \text{ weak scale}, \\ 0.4 \leq H &< 0.5 : \text{ medium scale}, \\ 0.5 \leq H &: \text{ strong scale}. \end{aligned} \tag{2}$$

For more information on suggested thresholds for two-level scalability coefficients, see Snijders (2001). The actual minimum of scalability coefficients depends on the marginal frequencies (Sijtsma & Molenaar, 2002, p. 59). Away from the boundary, the sampling distribution of scalability coefficients is approximately normal (Koopman et al., 2020; Mokken, 1971, pp. 166–167), but if a coefficient is close to the boundary or the SE is large, the sampling distribution is skewed to the left.

The point estimates of a scalability coefficient and its SE in sample data can be combined by a normal approximation Wald-based confidence interval or significance test (Koopman et al., 2020; Kuijpers et al., 2013). Two-sided confidence intervals are useful to determine the strength of total-scale coefficient H with confidence (Eq. 2), whereas one-sided significance tests are useful to test the two criteria of a Mokken scale (Eq. 1; Koopman et al., 2021). If the sampling distribution of the scalability coefficients is skewed, Wald-based confidence intervals and significance tests may be biased. This can result in deteriorated coverage of the confidence interval, inclusion of values larger than 1 in the confidence interval, and inflated Type I error rates of the significance tests. In this chapter, we propose a range-preserving confidence interval and significance test using a logarithmic transformation that can be applied to all scalability coefficients, both in nonclustered data (i.e., obtained by a simple random sampling design) and clustered data (i.e., obtained by a cluster sampling design). We compare the performance of the Wald-based and range-preserving methods in terms of coverage and Type I error rate using simulated data. Applications of the range-preserving methods in software are demonstrated.

2 Sampling Distribution of Scalability Coefficients

The sampling distribution of both Mokken's and Snijders' scalability coefficients are asymptotically normal (Mokken, 1971, pp. 166–167; Koopman et al., 2020,

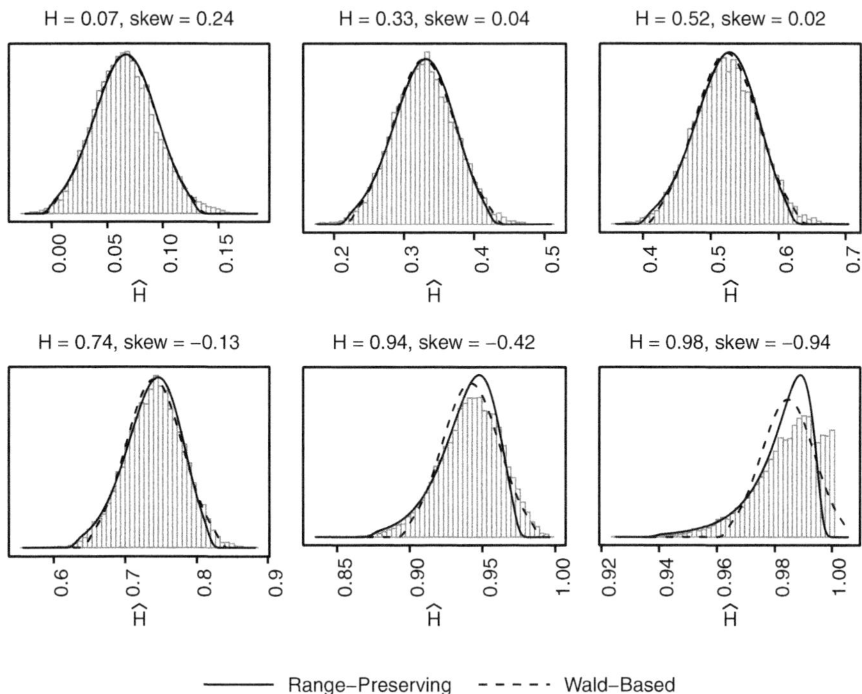

Fig. 1 Six empirical distributions of total-scale coefficient H, with Wald-based (dashed line) and range-preserving (solid line) approximations of the sampling distribution based on the average $\widehat{H}$ and $SE^2_{\widehat{H}}$ across the datasets. The distribution is based on 10,000 simulated datasets with 10 dichotomous items and 100 respondents

respectively). Therefore, it is common practice to use normal-theory approaches to confidence interval estimation and significance testing. Let $\widehat{H}$ denote the point estimate of H with standard error $SE_{\widehat{H}}$. Figure 1 shows six histograms of the empirical sampling distribution of $\widehat{H}$ for a range of population values for H, created with 10,000 simulated datasets using 100 respondents and 10 dichotomous items. For H away from the boundary of 1, the distribution is approximately normal (as is expected according to asymptotic theory), but as H comes closer to the boundary, the distribution becomes increasingly skewed. For skewed sampling distributions, normal-theory approaches may be biased, in which case, range-preserving approaches are desirable because they only take values on the possible range of the coefficient and tend to be more accurate and reliable (Efron & Tibshirani, 1993, Section 13.7).

Confidence interval and significance tests can be applied to the scalability coefficients by using point estimates of the item-pair coefficients $\widehat{H}_{ij}$, item coefficients $\widehat{H}_i$, and total-scale coefficient $\widehat{H}$, along with $SE_{\widehat{H}_{ij}}$, $SE_{\widehat{H}_i}$, and $SE_{\widehat{H}}$, respectively. Two-sided confidence intervals of H are appropriate to estimate whether a scale is weak, medium, or strong (Eq. 2). One-sided significance tests (or one-sided confidence intervals) are appropriate to evaluate the two criteria of a Mokken scale (Eq. 1; Koopman et al., 2021). For the first criterion, the null hypothesis is $H_{ij} = 0$ and the alternative hypothesis is $H_{ij} > 0$ for each item pair (i, j). For the second criterion, the null hypothesis is $H_i = c$ and the alternative hypothesis is $H_i > c$ for each item i.

2.1 *Wald-Based Methods*

Wald-based methods assume a normal sampling distribution. A two-sided confidence interval contains two confidence limits. Let $z_{\alpha/2}$ denote the z score pertaining to significance level $\alpha/2$. Then, the two-sided $(1-\alpha)\times 100\%$ Wald-based confidence interval (denoted CI) is computed as

$$\text{CI} = \widehat{H} \pm z_{\alpha/2} \times SE_{\widehat{H}}. \tag{3}$$

Consider a two-sided 95% CI, $z_{\alpha/2} \approx 1.96$. Note that the upper confidence limit may exceed the boundary of 1, which is the maximum value of H. One-sided CIs also exist and can be constructed by replacing $z_{\alpha/2}$ in Eq. 3 with z_α and by selecting the confidence limit of interest, which is the lower limit for H_{ij} and H_i. For a one-sided 95% CI $z_\alpha \approx 1.645$.

The Wald-based significance test is a z test to standardize the difference between $\widehat{H}$ and the value of H under the null-hypothesis to a z score. For example, using the null hypothesis $H = c$, z is computed as

$$z = \frac{\widehat{H} - c}{SE_{\widehat{H}}}. \tag{4}$$

The corresponding one-sided p value can be found in the standard normal z table.

A problem with the Wald-based method is that the sampling distribution is skewed for very high values of H or SE, in which case the results cannot be trusted.

2.2 *Range-Preserving Methods*

A confidence interval is range-preserving if its values are in the possible range of the parameter of interest. We propose a strategy to compute a range-preserving interval and to apply a similar strategy to compute a z score, which we collectively refer to as range-preserving methods. Range-preserving methods also apply asymptotic normal theory, but rather than using the original estimate $\widehat{H}$, which is bounded by 1, confidence interval and z scores are computed using a transformation of $\widehat{H}$ and its SE.

Let $g(\widehat{H})$ denote the transformation of $\widehat{H}$, and let $\log(x)$ denote the natural logarithm of x. Then

$$g(\widehat{H}) = -\log(1 - \widehat{H}). \tag{5}$$

The range for the transformed scalability coefficient is the real space $(-\infty, \infty)$. Let $g^{-1}(\widehat{H})$ denote inverse of $g(\widehat{H})$, and let $\exp(x)$ denote the exponential of x. It follows that

$$g^{-1}(g(\widehat{H})) = 1 - \exp(-g(\widehat{H})) = \widehat{H}. \tag{6}$$

Let $g'(\widehat{H})$ denote the first derivative of $g(\widehat{H})$ with respect to $\widehat{H}$. By the chain rule (Stewart, 2008, p. 197),

$$g'(\widehat{H}) = \frac{d}{d\widehat{H}}\, g(\widehat{H}) = \frac{1}{1 - \widehat{H}}. \tag{7}$$

Using the delta method (Agresti, 2012, pp. 577–594), the SE of $g(\widehat{H})$, $SE_{g(\widehat{H})}$, is then approximated as

$$\begin{aligned} SE_{g(\widehat{H})} &\approx \sqrt{[g'(\widehat{H})]^2 SE^2_{\widehat{H}}} \\ &= SE_{\widehat{H}}/(1 - \widehat{H}). \end{aligned} \tag{8}$$

To obtain the range-preserving confidence interval (denoted CI*), we first construct a Wald-based confidence interval using the result of Eqs. 5 and 8,

$$\begin{aligned} \mathrm{CI}_{g(\widehat{H})} &= g(\widehat{H}) \pm z_{\alpha/2} \times SE_{g(\widehat{H})} \\ &= -\log(1 - \widehat{H}) \pm z_{\alpha/2} \times SE_{\widehat{H}}/(1 - \widehat{H}). \end{aligned} \tag{9}$$

Then, this interval is transformed back to the original scale of H, which reflects the range-preserving confidence interval:

$$\begin{aligned} \mathrm{CI}^* &= 1 - \exp(-CI_{g(\widehat{H})}) \\ &= 1 - \exp(\log(1 - \widehat{H}) \pm z_{\alpha/2} \times SE_{\widehat{H}}/(1 - \widehat{H})). \end{aligned} \tag{10}$$

The range-preserving z score (denoted z^*) is computed by transforming both $\widehat{H}$ and c,

$$z^* = \frac{g(\widehat{H}) - g(c)}{SE_{g(\widehat{H})}}. \tag{11}$$

If $\widehat{H} = 1$, then the SE is estimated as $SE_{\widehat{H}} = 0$, resulting in $g(\widehat{H}) = \infty$ and an undefined $SE_{g(\widehat{H})}$, z, and z^*. In that case, we define CI* as [1, 1] and evaluate z and z^* as significant.

Similarly, confidence intervals and z scores can be computed for item pairs as CI_{ij} and z_{ij}, and for items as CI_i and z_i (superscript * is added for range-preserving confidence intervals and z scores), by replacing $\widehat{H}$ and $SE_{\widehat{H}}$ in Eqs. 3, 4, 10, and 11 with $\widehat{H}_{ij}$ and $SE_{\widehat{H}_{ij}}$ or with $\widehat{H}_i$ and $SE_{\widehat{H}_i}$ respectively.

Multivariate Case. The range-preserving transformation is easily generalized to the multivariate case, which is useful to, for example, construct a variance–covariance matrix for a set of transformed item-pair or item coefficients. Let $\mathbf{H} = [H_{(1)}, H_{(2)}, \ldots, H_{(k)}, \ldots, H_{(K)}]^T$ denote a transposed vector containing K scalability coefficients $H_{(k)}$, $(k = 1, 2, \ldots, K)$. The transformation of $\mathbf{H}$ is

$$g(\mathbf{H}) = [g(H_{(1)}), g(H_{(2)}), \ldots, g(H_{(k)}), \ldots, g(H_{(K)})]^T. \tag{12}$$

Let $\mathbf{G} = \frac{\partial g(\mathbf{H})}{\partial \mathbf{H}^T}$ be the Jacobian of $g(\mathbf{H})$, that is, the matrix of first-order partial derivatives with respect to $\mathbf{H}$. Let $\bigoplus$ indicate the direct sum. For $g(\mathbf{H})$,

$$\mathbf{G} = \bigoplus_{k=1}^{K} 1/(1 - H_{(k)}). \tag{13}$$

$\mathbf{G}$ is a diagonal matrix with the first derivative of $g(H_{(k)})$ (Eq. 7) on the kth diagonal element and zero on the off-diagonal elements. Let $\mathbf{V_H}$ denote the variance–covariance of $\mathbf{H}$, $V_{(k)}$ the variance of $H_{(k)}$, and $V_{(k,l)}$ the covariance between $H_{(k)}$ and $H_{(l)}$. Applying the multivariate delta method, the variance–covariance matrix of $g(\mathbf{H})$, $\mathbf{V}_{g(\mathbf{H})}$, is approximated by

$$\mathbf{V}_{g(\mathbf{H})} \approx \mathbf{G}\mathbf{V_H}\mathbf{G} \tag{14}$$

$\mathbf{V}_{g(\mathbf{H})}$ is a diagonal matrix for which the kth diagonal element equals $V_k/(1 - H_k)^2$ and the off-diagonal element (k, l) equals $V(k, l)/[(1 - H_{(k)})(1 - H_{(l)})]$. In data samples, $\mathbf{H}$ and $\mathbf{V_H}$ in Eqs. 12 to 14 are replaced by their estimates $\widehat{\mathbf{H}}$ and $\mathbf{V}_{\widehat{\mathbf{H}}}$, respectively, to get estimates $g(\widehat{\mathbf{H}})$ and $\mathbf{V}_{g(\widehat{\mathbf{H}})}$.

2.3 Approximating the Sampling Distribution

In Fig. 1, the Wald-based and range-preserving approximations of the distribution are plotted over the distributions. This visualization shows that when H does not approach the boundary of 1, the approximated distributions are similar (upper panels), but close to the boundary the range-preserving approximation (solid line) approaches the distribution more accurately than the Wald-based approximation (dashed line), especially in the left tail (lower panels). Note that the left tail is of interest because the one-sided significance tests evaluate whether H_{ij} or H_i is significantly larger than some hypothesized value. Hence, the left tail is compared to the hypothesized value.

3 Simulation Study

We performed a small-scale simulation study to investigate the coverage of the two-sided confidence interval and Type I error rate of the one-sided significance test for the Wald-based and range-preserving methods.

Method. We simulated data for 10 dichotomous items using a two-parameter logistic model (Birnbaum, 1968, p. 458). The difficulty parameter was fixed to equidistant values between -1 and 1 across the items. We included the following independent variables:

Item discrimination: The magnitude of the total-scale scalability coefficient was manipulated by increasing a_i in the two-parameter logistic model. The higher the discrimination, the better the item can distinguish between respondents, which results in higher scalability of the item, and thus the total scale. There were six levels in which a_i varied across items at equidistant values between 0 and 1: between 0.8 and 2, between 1 and 4, between 2 and 8, between 10 and 25, or between 25 and 75, resulting in $H = 0.07$ (unscalable), 0.33 (weak), 0.52 (strong), 0.74 (very strong), 0.94 (extremely strong), and 0.98 (near unity), respectively.

Sample size: The sample size N was 100, 500, or 1,000. Although 100 respondents is not considered sufficient for a Mokken scale analysis (Straat, Van der Ark & Sijtsma, 2014), the difference between the methods is expected to be more distinct.

Method: The Wald-based and range-preserving methods were used to compute the dependent variables.

We evaluated the following dependent variables, for which the population value H was determined by using the mean of $\widehat{H}$ across all replications within a condition, assuming it was unbiased.

Coverage: The coverage of the two-sided 95% confidence interval was determined to be the proportion of times H was included in the 95% CI or CI*. Its value should be close to 0.95.

Type I error rate: The Type I error rate of the one-sided significance test was determined as the proportion of times the p value of z or z^* was below significance level 0.05. Its value should be close to the significance level. Statistics z and z^* were computed by replacing c by H in Eqs. 4 and 11.

Method was a within-subject variable, whereas item discrimination and sample size were between-subject variables. There were $4 \times 3 = 12$ conditions and for each condition 10,000 datasets were simulated. Data were simulated

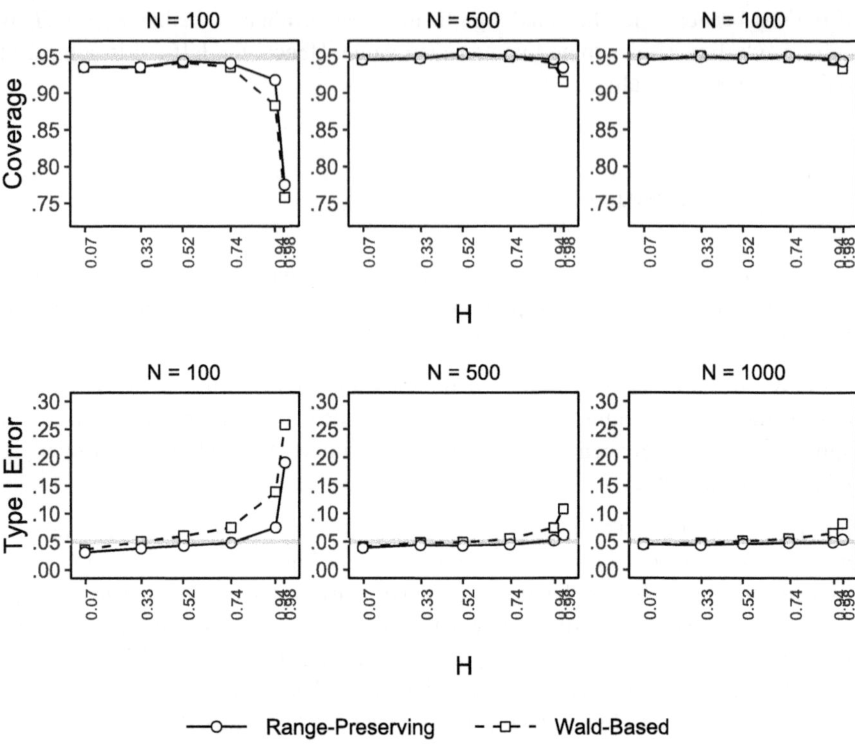

Fig. 2 Coverage rates of the two-sided confidence interval (top panels) and Type I error rates of the one-sided significance test (bottom panels) for the Wald-based (dashed line) and range-preserving (solid line) method. The row panels represent the sample size N. Each panel displays the population values H on the horizontal axis

in R (R Development Core Team, 2017) using the function `simdata()` from package `mirt` (Chalmers et al., 2012).[1]

Results. Figure 2 shows the coverage rates of CI and CI* and the Type I error rates of z and z^* for all conditions. CI* outperformed CI in all conditions—more substantially for conditions where H approached its upper boundary of 1. Overall, the coverage rates were poorer in the conditions with 100 respondents compared to the conditions with more respondents, especially for the highest two H conditions. In general, for the two highest H conditions, the average undercoverage of CI was divided in 9.2% on the left side and 1.2% on the right side, indicating that the CI had mainly undercoverage in the left tail of the distribution, whereas the right tail was overcovered. The undercoverage of CI* was divided more symmetrically, with 5.3% on the left tail and 3.6% on the right tail. When looking only at the 500 and 1,000 respondents conditions, the undercoverage of CI was 5.5% in the left tail and

[1]Syntax files are available to download from the Open Science Framework: https://osf.io/5m827/.

1.2% in the right tail, compared to 2.8% in both tails for CI*. This indicates that the tails of the sampling distribution are better approximated using the range-preserving method compared to the Wald-based method.

The Type I error rate of z^* was close to that of z in most conditions, but for conditions in which $H \geq 0.74$, z^* outperformed z. For 100 respondents, the Type I error rate of both z and z^* was below the nominal value for the lowest H condition, but improved with increased sample size.

Note that for the condition with 100 respondents and $H = 0.98$, in approximately 10% of the replications $\widehat{H}$ was (very close to) 1 (i.e., $\widehat{H} > 0.999$) and $SE_{\widehat{H}}$ was estimated (very close to) 0 (i.e., the mean of $SE_{\widehat{H}} = 0.0002$, compared to a mean of 0.0086 for $\widehat{H} < 0.999$). Regardless of the method, this estimation issue made it problematic to construct accurate intervals or to perform accurate tests, resulting in deteriorated coverage and Type I error rates for both methods.

4 Implementation in Software

The range-preserving methods are implemented in R (R Development Core Team, 2017) in the package `mokken` (Van der Ark, 2007, 2012). Here we give an overview of how to get CI* and z^* for Mokken's scalability coefficients in nonclustered and clustered data and for Snijders' two-level scalability coefficients in multi-rater data, using scores of 639 students nested in 30 schools on 7 items measuring their well-being with teachers. The first column in the dataset contains a grouping variable, which we will ignore for nonclustered computations but which we use for clustered data. Throughout we will use the significance level $\alpha = 0.05$ and a null hypothesis for coefficients $c = 0.3$. Wald-based results can be obtained by replacing `"RP"` by `"WB"` in the R code. Let `R>` denote the R prompt. The R script and output are available to download from the Open Science Framework: https://osf.io/5m827/.

```
R> # Preliminary code:
R> # Load package, get data
R> # Set significance level and value c
R> library(mokken)
R> data(SWMD)
R> X <- SWMD[, -1] # item scores SWMD
R> groups <- SWMD[, 1] # grouping variable
R> alpha <- .05 # Significance level
R> c <- .3 # Null hypothesis value
R> ## Mokken's scalability coefficients in nonclustered data:
R> # Point estimates, standard errors,
R> # and two-sided range-preserving confidence intervals
R> coefH(X, ci = 1 - alpha, type.ci = "RP")
R> # Range-preserving z-scores using null hypothesis c
R> coefZ(X, lowerbound = c, type.z = "RP")
R> ## Mokken's scalability coefficients in clustered data:
R> # Point estimates, standard errors,
R> # and two-sided range-preserving confidence intervals
```

```
R> coefH(X, ci = 1 - alpha, type.ci = "RP", level.two.var
             = groups)
R> # Range-preserving z-scores using null hypothesis c
R> coefZ(X, lowerbound = c, type.z = "RP", level.two.var
             = groups)
R> ## Snijders' two-level scalability coefficients:
R> # Point estimates, standard errors,
R> # and two-sided range-preserving confidence intervals
R> MLcoefH(SWMD, ci = 1 - alpha, type.ci = "RP")
R> # Range-preserving z-scores using null hypothesis c
R> MLcoefZ(SWMD, lowerbound = c, type.z = "RP")
```

5 Discussion

We proposed a method to compute range-preserving confidence intervals and significance tests, which we implemented in the R package mokken. Simulation results showed that for H not close to 1, Wald-based and range-preserving methods are very similar and both are useful. However, for very strong scales ($H > 0.7$), the range-preserving methods return more accurate results and are preferred over the Wald-based method, especially for the left tail of the sampling distribution (which is used in the one-sided significance tests). The results were poorer for only 100 respondents, confirming that larger samples are desirable (Straat et al., 2014). Note that we only investigated range-preserving methods for scalability coefficients in nonclustered data. Whether the results are similar in clustered data and for two-level scalability coefficients is a topic for further research.

In our method, we used $(-\infty, 1]$ as the range for H. However, the actual minimum of scalability coefficients depends on the marginal frequencies (Sijtsma & Molenaar, 2002, p. 59). This minimum has the undesirable property that it must be estimated and thus varies across finite samples. We explored an alternative and more complex logistic transformation that takes the estimated minimum into account. The results were very similar to the results obtained using the logarithmic transformation presented in this chapter, so we did not investigate this method any further.

A limitation of the logarithmic transformation is that the value 1 can not be included in the interval (although values very close to 1 can), as this value corresponds to ∞ on the transformed scale. However, 1 is a possible value for scalability coefficients, both in the population and in data samples. Alternative transformations that can include 1 may approximate the sampling distribution more closely. However, this will not solve the deteriorated coverage and Type I error rates for very high H entirely because there remain samples where the SE can not be estimated because $\widehat{H} = 1$.

References

Agresti, A. (2012). *Categorical data analysis* (3rd ed.). Wiley.

Birnbaum, A. (1968). Some latent trait models and their use in inferring an examinee's ability. In F. M. Lord & M. R. Novick *Statistical theories of mental test scores* (pp. 395–479). Addison-Wesley.

Chalmers, R. P., et al. (2012). mirt: A multidimensional item response theory package for the R environment. *Journal of Statistical Software, 48*(6), 1–29.

Efron, B., & Tibshirani, R. J. (1993). *An introduction to the bootstrap* (1st ed.). Chapman & Hall.

Koopman, L., Zijlstra, B. J. H., & Van der Ark, L. A. (2020). Standard errors of two-level scalability coefficients. *British Journal of Mathematical and Statistical Psychology, 73*(2), 213–236. https://doi.org/10.1111/bmsp.12174

Koopman, L., Zijlstra, B. J. H., & Van der Ark, L. A. (2021). *A two-step test-guided Mokken scale analysis, for nonclustered and clustered data*. Quality of Life Research. Advance online publication. https://doi.org/10.1007/s11136-021-02840-2

Kuijpers, R. E., Van der Ark, L. A., & Croon, M. A. (2013). Standard errors and confidence intervals for scalability coefficients in Mokken scale analysis using marginal models. *Sociological Methodology, 43*(1), 42–69. https://doi.org/10.1177/0081175013481958

Mokken, R. J. (1971). *A theory and procedure of scale analysis*. Mouton.

R Development Core Team. (2017). *R: A language and environment for statistical computing* [Computer software] R Foundation for Statistical Computing. http://www.R-project.org/

Sijtsma, K., & Molenaar, I. W. (2002). *Introduction to nonparametric item response theory*. Sage. https://doi.org/10.1007/s11136-007-9281-6

Sijtsma, K., & Molenaar, I. W. (2016). Mokken models. In W. J. van der Linden (Ed.), *Handbook of item response theory. volume 1: Models* (pp. 303–321). CRC Press.

Sijtsma, K., & Van der Ark, L. A. (2017). A tutorial on how to do a Mokken scale analysis on your test and questionnaire data. *British Journal of Mathematical and Statistical Psychology, 70*(1), 137–158. https://doi.org/10.1111/bmsp.12078

Snijders, T. A. B. (2001). Two-level non-parametric scaling for dichotomous data. In A. Boomsma, M. A. J. van Duijn, & T. A. B. Snijders (Eds.), *Essays on item response theory* (pp. 319–338). Springer. https://doi.org/10.1007/978-1-4613-0169-1_17

Stewart, J. (2008). *Calculus: Early transcendentals* (6th ed.). Thompson Brooks/Cole.

Straat, J. H., Van der Ark, L. A., & Sijtsma, K. (2014). Minimum sample size requirements for Mokken scale analysis. *Educational and Psychological Measurement, 74*(5), 809–822. https://doi.org/10.1177/0013164414529793

Van der Ark, L. A. (2007). Mokken scale analysis in R. *Journal of Statistical Software, 20*(11), 1–19. https://doi.org/10.18637/jss.v020.i11

Van der Ark, L. A. (2012). New developments in Mokken scale analysis in R. *Journal of Statistical Software, 48*(5), 1–27. https://doi.org/10.18637/jss.v048.i05

References

[illegible]

Equating Nonequivalent Groups Using Propensity Scores: Model Misspecification and Sensitivity Analysis

Gabriel Wallin and Marie Wiberg

1 Introduction

Test score equating comprises statistical models and methods to make test scores from different test forms comparable (Kolen & Brennan, 2014; González & Wiberg, 2017). Equating is therefore an essential part for an educational testing program to ensure fairness. The statistical parameter of interest is a function that maps the scores from one test form (e.g. the most recent administration of the test) to another test form. The test forms to be equated will in the following be referred to as the new test form X and the old test form Y. How this function is calculated depends to a great extent on the data collection design that has been adopted. Generally, testing programs employ either common test-takers or common items. The former refers to the underlying assumption that test-takers from different administrations are only randomly different from each other in terms of the latent trait the test is constructed to measure. The observed test score differences between the test groups would thus solely be due to differences in difficulty level between the test forms. Equating methods that utilize common items on the other hand uses a set of items common for both the new and old test form to adjust not only for difficulty differences but also for ability differences between the test groups. The underlying assumption is thus that the groups of test-takers are drawn from different populations. These common items are often referred to as anchor items, and the data collection design as nonequivalent groups with anchor test (NEAT) design (von Davier et al., 2004). There are however testing programs that face nonequivalent

G. Wallin (✉)
CNRS, Laboratoire J.A. Dieudonné, team Maasai, Université Côte d'Azur, Inria, Nice, France
e-mail: gabriel.wallin@inria.fr

M. Wiberg
Department of Statistics, USBE, Umeå University, Umeå, Västerbottens Län, Sweden

M. Wiberg et al. (eds.), *Quantitative Psychology*, Springer Proceedings
in Mathematics & Statistics 353, https://doi.org/10.1007/978-3-030-74772-5_17

groups but lack common items, for example the Invalsi test (Invalsi, 2013) and the Armed Services Vocational Aptitude Battery (Quenette et al., 2006). To falsely assume that the test groups are samples from the same population, i.e. not adjusting for ability differences, will yield a biased estimate of the equating function that for example can lead to unfair admission decisions to university programs. One way of controlling for ability imbalance between the test groups when there are no anchor items is to use background information about the test-takers. This is known as the nonequivalent groups with covariates (NEC) design (Wiberg & Bränberg, 2015).

Background information, that from now on will be referred to as covariates, has been used to equate test forms before. Kolen (1990), Cook et al. (1990) and Wright and Dorans (1993) used it as a tool to balance the test groups, Liou et al. (2001) used covariates instead of anchor items, Bränberg and Wiberg (2011) developed a linear equating method using covariates and Hsu et al. (2002) incorporated covariates into item response theory (IRT) true-score equating. To use covariates within a propensity score has also been investigated in previous equating research, and was first proposed by Livingston et al. (1990). Among the more recent studies, Moses et al. (2010) incorporated two anchor test scores within a propensity score, Powers (2010) used them for chained equating (CE) frequency estimation, IRT true-score and observed-score equating, Longford (2015) used propensity scores to for matching and Haberman (2015) used them to transform nonequivalent groups to pseudo-equivalent groups.

This study builds on the study of Wallin and Wiberg (2019), where propensity scores for the first time were introduced within the kernel equating (von Davier et al., 2004) framework. Both post-stratification equating (PSE) and CE were considered, and the underlying assumptions for using propensity scores were for the first time formalized. In their study, they did however assume that the functional form of the propensity score was known. Since this is never the case in practical applications, this study investigates how sensitive the equated scores are for misspecification of the propensity score estimation model. Specifically, three different kinds misspecification are considered: Misspecification of the link function, misspecification by leaving out a covariate and by missing a second-order moment, respectively. The intention is to quantify how severe each of the misspecifications are in terms of bias of the equated scores and the precision of the equating function estimate. This follows the study by Waernbaum (2012) were propensity score model misspecification were analyzed for the estimation of causal treatment effects. The same model misspecifications as in this paper were considered, but a different, scalar, parameter was evaluated.

The rest of the paper is structured as follows. In Sect. 2, the kernel equating framework is briefly described. In Sect. 3, propensity scores for equating are introduced, and in Sect. 4 a simulation study is presented. The paper is concluded with a discussion of the results.

2 Kernel Equating

Test scores from the new test form X are denoted by X and test scores from the old test form Y are denoted by Y. For this study, test-takers given test form X are thought of as a random sample from population P and test-takers given test form Y as a random sample from population Q. As test-takers are randomly sampled from their respective populations, X and Y are treated as random variables with sample spaces $\mathcal{X}$ and $\mathcal{Y}$. Their respective realizations are denoted x_j, $j = 1, \ldots, J$, and y_k, $k = 1, \ldots K$, where number-correct scoring is assumed throughout the paper. The equating function $\varphi(x)$ is a mapping from $\mathcal{X}$ to $\mathcal{Y}$, but not all such functions are equating functions, see Kolen and Brennan (2014) for a list of requirements. The most commonly used equating function is the equipercentile function (Braun & Holland, 1982), defined as

$$\varphi(x) = G_Y^{-1}(F_X(x)), \tag{1}$$

where G_Y and F_X denote the cumulative distribution functions (CDFs) of test score Y and X.

Kernel equating is a semi-parametric method to estimate the equating function $\varphi(x)$, using both kernel smoothing techniques of the score distributions and maximum likelihood estimation of the score probabilities. To define the kernel equating estimator, let μ_X denote the mean of X, σ_X^2 denote the variance of X, let V be a continuous random variable with $\mathbb{E}(V) = 0$ and $\mathbb{V}(V) = \sigma_V^2$, and $a_X^2 = \sigma_X^2/(\sigma_X^2 + \sigma_V^2 h_X^2)$, where $h_X > 0$ is a smoothing parameter. Now a continuous version of the test score variable X is introduced as

$$X(h_X) = a_X(X + h_X V) + (1 - a_X)\mu_X.$$

The random variable $X(h_X)$ has the same mean and variance as X, and a corresponding continuous score variable is introduced for Y as well. The estimated CDF of $X(h_X)$ equals

$$F_{h_X}(x) = P(X(h_X) \leq x) = \sum_j \hat{r}_j K(\hat{R}_{jX}(x)) \tag{2}$$

for which $r_j = P(X = x_j)$ is the jth X score probability, usually estimated using a log-linear model, $R_{jX}(x) = (x - \hat{a}_X x_j - (1 - \hat{a}_X)\hat{\mu}_X)/\hat{a}_X h_X$, and K is the kernel function defined by the probability distribution of V. The most common distributional choice of V is the Gaussian distribution, and such assumption will be made in this study as well, meaning that K will equal the standard Gaussian CDF.

With corresponding definitions for $G_{h_Y} = P(Y(h_Y) \leq y)$, the estimated kernel equating function equals

$$\varphi(x; \hat{\mathbf{r}}, \hat{\mathbf{s}}) = \hat{G}_{h_Y}^{-1}(\hat{F}_{h_X}(x)),$$

with $\hat{\mathbf{r}} = (\hat{r}_1, \hat{r}_2, \ldots, \hat{r}_J)^\top$ and $\hat{\mathbf{s}} = (\hat{s}_1, \hat{s}_2, \ldots, \hat{s}_K)^\top$.

3 Propensity Scores

This paper considers the NEC design (Wiberg & Bränberg, 2015), where the population P sample has received test form X, the population Q sample has received test form Y, and the test-takers in both samples have an associated covariate vector $\mathbf{D} = (D_1, \ldots, D_m)$ recorded. In the NEC design, these covariates serve the purpose of controlling for ability imbalance between the test groups. The aim is to control for all covariates that affect the relationship between (X, Y) and the test form assignment mechanism. This test form assigment is denoted by $Z = 1$ if test form X is administered to a randomly selected test-taker, and $Z = 0$ if test form Y is administered.

The variables Z, $\mathbf{D}$ and (X, Y) are depicted in Fig. 1. The covariate vector $\mathbf{D}$ confounds the relationship between test form assignment and test score, which motivates the goal to control for such disturbance. It should be pointed out that in reality, the true confounder of the Z-(X, Y) relationship is the latent ability. By successfully controlling for ability, it would only be the difficulty differences between the test forms that would cause observed differences in the distributions of X and Y. The covariates in the NEC design thus play the role of a proxy for ability. Although rarely pointed out, the same underlying assumption is made when using anchor items A: replace $\mathbf{D}$ with A in Fig. 1 and it will illustrate the NEAT design. Anchor items are therefore, just as covariates, used as a proxy for ability. However, since anchor items are constructed as mini-versions of the full test forms, there is often a good reason to treat them as an ability proxy. It is reasonable to believe that if $\mathbf{D}$ is going to be an equally good ability proxy as the anchor items, it needs to include several covariates that all relate to the latent construct that the test is constructed to measure.

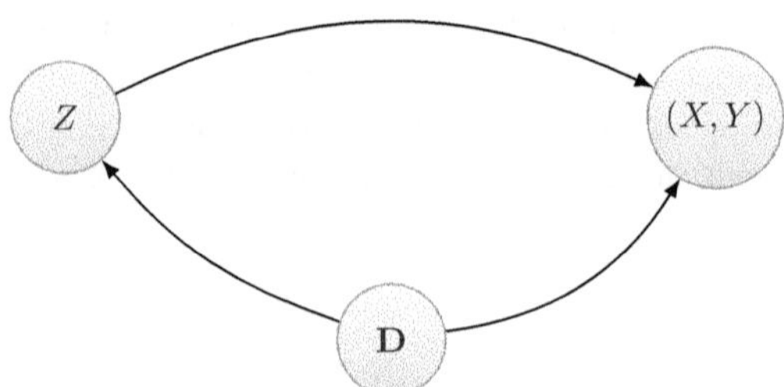

Fig. 1 The nonequivalent groups with covariates design

A practical problem arises when using more than just a few covariates since the number of empty cells in the data matrix quickly proliferates. To be able to use all available information, some dimension-reducing function of the covariate vector is needed. This study considers the use of propensity scores to tackle the dimensionality problem. The propensity score is a scalar function of the covariate vector and is defined as $e(\mathbf{D}) = P(Z = 1|\mathbf{D})$. It is a balancing score, meaning that if $\mathbf{D}$ contains all confounders of the relationship between Z and (X, Y), it is sufficient to control for $e(\mathbf{D})$ to achieve covariate balance between the test groups. Since it actually is the latent ability we wish to control for, the positive effect of balancing the groups on the covariates fully depends on the quality of $\mathbf{D}$ as a proxy for ability. We again emphasize that this however is no different from the underlying assumption behind using an anchor test.

Since the propensity score is unknown, it has to be estimated. The most common estimation method, and the one employed in this study, is logistic regression. After retrieving the estimated propensity score for each test-taker, it is subdivided into strata based on the percentiles, following the proposition by Rosenbaum and Rubin (1984). All test-takers within a stratum are considered equivalent in terms of the latent trait, and the method proposed thus creates strata for where the assumption underlying the common test-taker approach holds.

4 Simulation Study

4.1 Equating Estimators

The simulation study considers both PSE- and CE-based estimators using propensity scores, as they were derived and presented in Wallin and Wiberg (2019). To define the PSE-based estimator, consider the score probabilities

$$\begin{aligned} r_{Pj} &= P(X = x_j|P), \\ r_{Qj} &= P(X = x_j|Q), \\ s_{Pk} &= P(Y = y_k|P), \\ s_{Qk} &= P(Y = y_k|Q), \end{aligned} \tag{3}$$

where the notation P, Q and T refer to the underlying population for which the terms are calculated on. The term T denotes the target population that the equating function is defined on. For PSE, $T = w_P P + w_Q Q$ where w_P and w_Q denote weights that often are set to respect the relative sample sizes, and such that $0 \leq w_P, w_Q \leq 1$, $w_P + w_Q = 1$. Following from this definition of the target population, the test score probabilities for the target population can be calculated as

$$r_j = P(X = x_j|T) = w_P r_{Pj} + w_Q r_{Qj} \tag{4}$$

and

$$s_k = P(Y = y_k|T) = w_P s_{Pk} + w_Q s_{Qk}, \tag{5}$$

As can be seen in Equations 4 and 5, there is a missing data structure by design since the terms r_{Qj} and s_{Pk} cannot be directly estimated from the data. However, if the propensity score is a proper ability proxy, it will be able to unbiasedly estimate the quantities $w_Q r_{Qj}$ and $w_P s_{Pk}$. See Wallin and Wiberg (2019) for the details. The score probability vectors $\mathbf{r}$ and $\mathbf{s}$ can thus be estimated, which leads to the PSE estimator

$$\varphi(x; \hat{\mathbf{r}}, \hat{\mathbf{s}})_{PSE} = \hat{G}_{h_Y}^{-1}(\hat{F}_{h_X}(x)), \tag{6}$$

To define the CE estimator, consider the score CDFs

$$\begin{aligned} F_{H_P}(x) &= P(X(h_X) \leq x|P), \\ G_{H_Q}(y) &= P(Y(h_Y) \leq y|Q), \\ H_{h_{eX}}(e(\mathbf{d})) &= P(e(\mathbf{D}) \leq e(\mathbf{d})|P). \\ H_{h_{eY}}(e(\mathbf{d})) &= P(e(\mathbf{D}) \leq e(\mathbf{d})|Q), \end{aligned} \tag{7}$$

Now gather the score probabilities in (3) in the vectors $\mathbf{r}_P = (r_{P1}, \ldots, r_{PJ})^\top$ and $\mathbf{s}_Q = (s_{Q1}, \ldots, s_{QK})^\top$. Further let $\mathbf{t}_P = (t_{P1}, \ldots, t_{PJ})^\top$ and $\mathbf{t}_Q = (t_{Q1}, \ldots, t_{QK})^\top$, where $t_{Pj} = P(e(\mathbf{D}) = e(\mathbf{d})|P)$ and $t_{Qk} = P(e(\mathbf{D}) = e(\mathbf{d})|Q)$. Note that the score CDFs in (7) together with $\mathbf{r}_P$, $\mathbf{s}_Q$, $\mathbf{t}_P$ and $\mathbf{t}_Q$ all are possible to estimate from data. For the CE estimator, the underlying assumption instead is that there is a functional link between the X scores and the propensity scores in population P, and a functional link between the propensity scores and the Y scores in population Q. To get the explicit assumptions, we refer to Wallin and Wiberg (2019).

By linking the CDFs in (7) together in a chain, the CE estimator is retrieved:

$$\varphi(x; \hat{\mathbf{r}}_P, \hat{\mathbf{t}}_P, \hat{\mathbf{t}}_Q, \hat{\mathbf{s}}_Q)_{CE} = \hat{G}_{h_Q}^{-1}(\hat{H}_{h_{eY}}(\hat{H}_{h_{eX}}^{-1}(\hat{F}_{h_P}(x)))), \tag{8}$$

4.2 Simulation Design

To evaluate how sensitive the equated scores are to propensity score model misspecification, the finite sample properties of the PSE and CE estimators in Equations 6 and 8 are evaluated in a simulation study where misspecification is introduced. The results are based on 10,000 simulated test-takers and 1,000 iterations.

The data generating process (DGP) follows Wallin and Wiberg (2019) and is as follows:

1. Draw the covariates $D_1, D_2 \sim \text{Uniform}(1, 5)$.
2. Draw a sequence of 10,000 Bernoulli trials to generate the treatment variable $Z \sim \text{Bernoulli}(e(\mathbf{D}))$, where

$$e(\mathbf{D}) = (1 + \exp(-0.36 + 1.25D_1 + 1.25D_2 - 0.35D_1^2 - 0.35D_2^2))^{-1}. \quad (9)$$

   This creates test groups of about the same size.
3. The test scores on test form X for all test-takers were calculated as

$$X = -6 + 4D_1 + 5D_2 + \epsilon_X$$

   and the test scores on test form Y for all test-takers were calculated as

$$Y = -9 + 3D_1 + 6D_2 + \epsilon_Y,$$

   where $\epsilon_X \sim \mathcal{N}(2, 1.5)$ and $\epsilon_Y \sim \mathcal{N}(0, 1)$. The covariate distributions thus differ between the test groups, and the ϵ terms represent difference in difficulty between the test forms. Since only integer scores are considered, X and Y were rounded to the nearest integer, and the upper limit we set equal to a test score of 40.
4. Calculate the observed score for each test-taker as

$$U = ZX + (1 - Z)Y.$$

5. Estimate the propensity score $e(\mathbf{D})$ in Equation 9 using logistic regression. Next, subdivide the estimated propensity score into 20 categories based on the percentiles. This number was set to achieve covariate balance between the test groups as measured by the Absolute Standardized Mean Difference (Austin, 2008). For each iteration and both equating estimators, there will be three estimated propensity scores for each test-taker: one with a misspecified link function (probit link instead of logit link), one that leaves out D_2 and one that leaves out the second-order terms.

With the DGP described above, each test-taker had a potential test score on both test forms (the test score he/she would have got if taken test form X/Y), an observed test score indicating which administration was actually assigned to the test-taker, a measurement on both covariates and three estimated propensity scores. We furthermore created two alternative versions of the covariates by subdividing them into five equally spaced groups, in the same spirit as in Wiberg and Bränberg (2015). The reason for doing so was to include the case where testing programs register background information only by categories. An example is the variable age that sometimes is recorded according to pre-specified age intervals rather than the actual ages of the test-takers. Lastly, note that with this DGP, it is possible to calculate a true equating function $\varphi(x)$ since data have been generated so that each test-taker has an observation on both test forms, which is never the case in empirical studies. With the generated sample entities, the PSE and CE estimators are calculated as described in Sects. 2 and 4.1.

4.3 Evaluation Measures

To evaluate the PSE and CE estimators, the bias and standard error (SE) as described in Wiberg and González (2016) have been calculated. Let $\hat{\varphi}^{(g)}(x_i)$ denote the estimated equating function (either the PSE- och CE based estimator) for the gth iteration, $g = 1, \ldots, 1000$. Further let $\bar{\varphi}(x_i) = \frac{1}{1000}\sum_{g=1}^{1000}\hat{\varphi}^{(g)}(x_i)$, and $\varphi(x)$ denote the true equating function. Then the bias and SE are calculated as

$$\text{Bias}(\hat{\varphi}(x_i)) = \frac{1}{1000}\sum_{g=1}^{1000}(\hat{\varphi}^{(g)}(x_i) - \varphi(x_i))$$

and

$$\text{SE}(\hat{\varphi}(x_i)) = \sqrt{\frac{1}{1000-1}\sum_{g=1}^{1000}(\hat{\varphi}^{(g)}(x_i) - \bar{\varphi}(x_i))}.$$

4.4 Results

The results are presented for each evaluation measure separately. In Fig. 2a and 2b, the bias of the PSE and CE estimators are presented. What immediately became apparent is that the bias and SE for propensity score models that misspecify the link

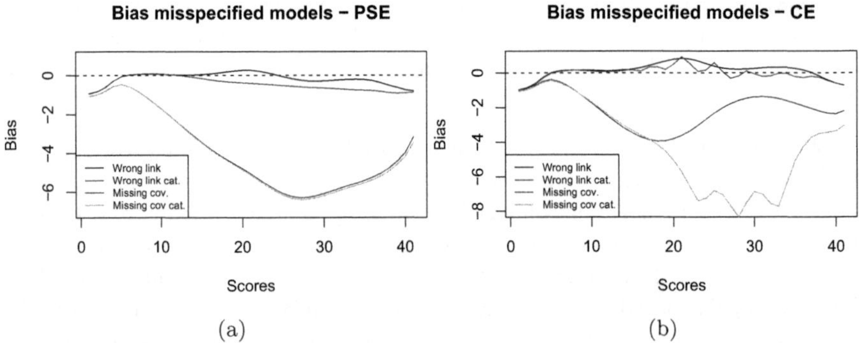

Fig. 2 The bias of the PSE and CE estimators, considering both categorized and uncategorized covariates, and using a misspecified link function and a missing covariate, respectively, in the propensity score estimation model. "Wrong link cat." and "Missing cov cat." refer to propensity score models with a misspecified link function and a missing covariate, respectively, where the covariates have been categorized. (**a**) The bias of the PSE estimator (**b**) The bias of the CE estimator

function and that leave out the second-order term were equal. Furthermore, those biases and SEs were equal to the biases and SEs for correctly specified models. For this reason, the bias and SE curves for the misspecified link function also represents the curves for the missing second-order term of the propensity score.

As seen in Fig. 2a, the bias is very small along the whole score scale for all estimators except for the estimator that misspecifies the propensity score model by leaving out a covariate. It is notable that it does not seem to matter if the covariates are categorized or not, the biases for all misspecifications are very similar regardless. The best performance is given by the estimators that misspecifies the link function (and leaves out the second-order term). Remember that this curve (the black) also represent the bias of a correctly specified model, meaning that the propensity score method of balancing the test groups seems successfull for the PSE estimator.

The bias for the CE is illustrated in Fig. 2b. The pattern is similar to the PSE results, meaning that the bias when misspecifying the link function and leaving out the second order term is small for all score values. The difference between categorized and uncategorized covariates is, as for the PSE case, negligible. When leaving out a covariate however, the bias increases a lot, and is particularly large for categorized covariates.

In Fig. 3a, the SE of the PSE estimator is shown. For all of the misspecified models, the general trend is that the SE is larger in the tails of the score range, which naturally occurs because of the sparse data for the highest and lowest scores. All estimators perform similar, although the model with categorized covariates and a misspecified link function has an increased SE in the middle segment. The SEs of the CE estimators are similar to each other, and similar in quantity compared to the SE values of the PSE estimators.

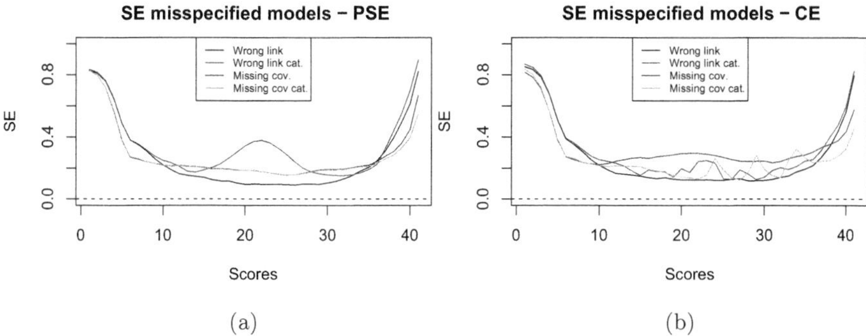

Fig. 3 The SE of the PSE and CE estimators, considering both categorized and uncategorized covariates, and using a misspecified link function and a missing covariate, respectively, in the propensity score estimation model. "Wrong link cat." and "Missing cov cat." refer to propensity score models with a misspecified link function and a missing covariate, respectively, where the covariates have been categorized. (**a**) The SE of the PSE estimator (**b**) The SE of the CE estimator

5 Discussion

This paper expands the study of Wallin and Wiberg (2019) by further exploring the use of propensity scores as a tool to balance nonequivalent test groups before equating their test scores. Since an anchor test can be both difficult and expensive to implement, there is a clear need for other methods that can handle nonequivalent groups. This study assumes that there are a number of covariates available, and for such situations it is natural to want to include as many (relevant) covariates as possible. With the appealing property of being a balancing score, the propensity score has been successfully implemented in a number of different areas of research. The flexibility of the propensity score however opens up many modeling options. It is therefore crucial to assess when the propensity score manages to balance the test groups and when it fails to do so. This study is a first step to get a further understanding of such a question. The results are promising for the propensity score method, since it was not very sensitive to a misspecification of the link function and to leaving out a second-order term in the estimation. The fact that the bias and SE for these two misspecified models were equal to the simulation bias and SE for correctly specified models suggests that the equated scores are robust to model misspecification of the propensity score. Leaving out an important covariate however was negatively affecting the results, which suggests that if the propensity score is going to be used as a proxy for ability, all important information relating to ability needs to be incorporated for it to work as intended. The results of this study relates to those of Waernbaum (2012), where matching estimators of causal effects were found to be robust against model misspecification, including modeling nonlinear relations with linear models.

For future studies, both other kinds of covariates and real testing data should be considered, since this study only considered continuous covariates in a simulation setting. Furthermore, there are testing programs where both an anchor test and covariates are available. It is therefore not unlikely that the precision in the equating can be further increased by incorporating both anchor items and covariates. It also possible to estimate the propensity score in other ways than by logistic regression. Which options are reasonable in an equating context is also subject for future studies.

Acknowledgments The research was funded by the Swedish Wallenberg MMW 2019.0129 grant.

References

Austin, P. C. (2008). Goodness-of-fit diagnostics for the propensity score model when estimating treatment effects using covariate adjustment with the propensity score. *Pharmacoepidemiology and Drug Safety, 17*(12), 1202–1217

Bränberg, K., & Wiberg, M. (2011). Observed score linear equating with covariates. *Journal of Educational Measurement, 48*(4), 419–440

Braun, H., & Holland, P. (1982). Observed-score test equating: a mathematical analysis of some ets equating procedures. In P. Holland, & D. Rubin (Eds.), *Test equating* (vol. 1, pp. 9–49). New York: Academic Press

Cook, L. L., Eignor, D. R., & Schmitt, A. P. (1990). Equating achievement tests using samples matched on ability. *ETS Research Report Series*, 1990(1), i–58

González, J., & Wiberg, M. (2017). *Applying test equating methods using R*. New York: Springer

Haberman, S. J. (2015). Pseudo-equivalent groups and linking. *Journal of Educational and Behavioral Statistics, 40*(3), 254–273

Hsu, T.-C., Wu, K.-L., Yu, J.-Y. W., & Lee, M.-Y. (2002). Exploring the feasibility of collateral information test equating. *International Journal of Testing, 2*(1), 1–14

Invalsi (2013). Rilevazioni nazionali sugli apprendimenti 2012–13. Technical report, Invalsi Publishing

Kolen, M., & Brennan, R. (2014). *Test equating, scaling, and linking: Methods and practices* (3rd ed.). New York: Springer

Kolen, M. J. (1990). Does matching in equating work: A discussion. *Applied Measurement in Education, 3*(1), 97–104

Liou, M., Cheng, P. E., & Li, M.-Y. (2001). Estimating comparable scores using surrogate variables. *Applied Psychological Measurement, 25*(2), 197–207

Livingston, S. A., Dorans, N. J., & Wright, N. K. (1990). What combination of sampling and equating methods works best? *Applied Measurement in Education, 3*(1), 73–95

Longford, N. T. (2015). Equating without an anchor for nonequivalent groups of examinees. *Journal of Educational and Behavioral Statistics, 40*(3), 227–253

Moses, T., Deng, W., & Zhang, Y.-L. (2010). The use of two anchors in nonequivalent groups with anchor test (neat) equating. *ETS Research Report Series, 2010*(2), i–33

Powers, S. J. (2010). Impact of matched samples equating methods on equating accuracy and the adequacy of equating assumptions

Quenette, M. A., Nicewander, W. A., & Thomasson, G. L. (2006). Model-based versus empirical equating of test forms. *Applied Psychological Measurement, 30*(3), 167–182

Rosenbaum, P. R., & Rubin, D. B. (1984). Reducing bias in observational studies using subclassification on the propensity score. *Journal of the American Statistical Association, 79*(387), 516–524

von Davier, A. A., Holland, P., & Thayer, D. (2004). *The Kernel method of test equating*. New York: Springer

Waernbaum, I. (2012). Model misspecification and robustness in causal inference: comparing matching with doubly robust estimation. *Statistics in Medicine, 31*(15), 1572–1581

Wallin, G., & Wiberg, M. (2019). Kernel equating using propensity scores for nonequivalent groups. *Journal of Educational and Behavioral Statistics, 44*(4), 390–414

Wiberg, M., & Bränberg, K. (2015). Kernel equating under the non-equivalent groups with covariates design. *Applied Psychological Measurement, 39*(5), 349–361

Wiberg, M., & González, J. (2016). Statistical assessment of estimated transformations in observed-score equating. *Journal of Educational Measurement, 53*(1), 106–125

Wright, N. K., & Dorans, N. J. (1993). Using the selection variable for matching or equating 1, 2. *ETS Research Report Series, 1993*(1), i–22

Possible Factors Which May Impact Kernel Equating of Mixed-Format Tests

Marie Wiberg and Jorge González

1 Introduction

Test forms may contain either only dichotomously scored items, or only polytomous scored items, or a mixture of both types, which is the case in mixed-format tests (see e.g. Ercikan et al., 1998; Kim et al., 2008, 2010; Kolen & Lee, 2014). Regardless of how the test form is constructed, it may be necessary to compare the scores from different test forms. Test equating is used to compare test scores from different test forms (González & Wiberg, 2017). A number of methods have been proposed to compare scores obtained from binary scored items of different test forms and under different equating designs. When tests are composed of polytomously scored items, the score data are typically analyzed using item response theory (IRT; Lord, 1980) models such as the graded response model or the generalized partial credit model. After modelling the items with IRT, either IRT observed-score equating or IRT true score equating (Lord, 1980) have been used to equate the test scores. Equating of mixed-format tests has received relatively small attention in the literature so far. The aim of this study was to examine the impact of item discrimination, sample size and proportion of polytomously scored items on item response theory (IRT) kernel equating of mixed-format tests under an equivalent groups (EG) design.

M. Wiberg (✉)
Department of Statistics, USBE, Umeå University, Umeå, Västerbottens Län, Sweden
e-mail: marie.wiberg@umu.se

J. González
Faculty of Mathematics, Pontificia Universidad Católica de Chile, Santiago, Chile
e-mail: jorge.gonzalez@mat.uc.cl

M. Wiberg et al. (eds.), *Quantitative Psychology*, Springer Proceedings in Mathematics & Statistics 353, https://doi.org/10.1007/978-3-030-74772-5_18

In the past decade, kernel equating (von Davier et al., 2004) has emerged as an alternative to classical test equating methods as it provides a framework with tools on how to evaluate the performed equating. A large amount of research about kernel equating has focused on extending the method for new situations such as when additional information is available (e.g. Wallin & Wiberg, 2019; Wiberg & Bränberg, 2015) or when it is used within the local equating approach (Wiberg et al., 2014). Regardless of the aim of the study, most research about kernel equating has mainly focused on modelling the sum scores, i.e. scores obtained as the total sum of correctly answered binary scored items. As a matter of fact, the initial step of presmoothing the score distributions before conducting the equating has mainly considered log-linear models for sum score probabilities of binary scored items. Recently, Andersson and Wiberg (2017) proposed to incorporate IRT models within the kernel equating framework as an alternative to the commonly used log-linear models. Polytomous IRT models has also been incorporated within the kernel equating framework (Andersson, 2016).

Previous research on mixed-format test equating has considered classical test equating methods and traditional (observed-score or true-score) IRT equating methods (see e.g. Kolen & Lee, 2014). Some research has also focused on examining and comparing the use of the EG design and the NEAT design including the composition of the anchor test. Kim and Kolen (2006) examined different IRT linking methods with mixed-format tests and Kim et al. (2010) found that using either anchor tests with constructed response items in the NEAT design or in the EG design gave lower bias than if only multiple-choice items were used in the anchor test under the NEAT design. Lee and Lee (2014) examined how dimensionality affected the equating by comparing unidimensional IRT and bi-factor multidimensional equating in mixed-format tests. Wang et al. (2016) examined multidimensionality and classification accuracy of mixed-format tests, and they found that it varied from subject to subject, depending on the disattenuated correlation between scores from multiple-choice and the constructed response subtests. Different psychometric properties of equating of mixed-format tests are summarized in Kolen and Lee (2014) including how the equating is affected by the test dimensionality and the composition of the anchor test. They also included a comparison of unidimensional IRT and multidimensional bi-factor IRT equating, and a section of multidimensional IRT equating. The research in this paper is different from all these studies as none of them explored the possibility of using kernel equating for mixed-format tests. An advantage of using IRT kernel equating for mixed-format test is the beneficiary of using different IRT models within the same equating framework. In addition, using IRT kernel equating for mixed-format tests extends the kernel equating framework by enlarging the situations in which the method can be useful.

The rest of this paper is structured as follows. First, we briefly describe IRT kernel equating and the statistical models used. Next, a simulation study is described followed by the results from the simulations. The paper ends with a discussion with some concluding remarks.

2 IRT Kernel Equating

Kernel equating (von Davier et al., 2004) comprises five steps; (1) presmoothing, (2) estimating score probabilities, (3) continuization, (4) equating and (5) evaluating the equating transformation. In IRT kernel equating, IRT models are used in the presmoothing step instead of the commonly used log-linear models (Andersson & Wiberg, 2017). The IRT models are used to smooth the data and get rid of irregularities. It is possible to use both dichotomous and polytomous IRT models within IRT kernel equating. In this paper we will use the two-parameter logistic (2PL) IRT model to model dichotomously scored items and the generalized partial credit (GPC) model to model the polytomously scored items. Let θ, a_i and b_i be the ability of a test taker, and the item discrimination and difficulty parameter of item i, respectively. The probability to answer an item i correctly with the 2PL model (Lord, 1980) is then defined as

$$P_i(\theta) = \frac{\exp(a_i(\theta - b_i))}{1 + \exp(a_i(\theta - b_i))}.$$

The probability of a test taker with ability θ answering in category l of item i using the GPCM (Muraki, 1992) is defined as

$$P_{il}(\theta) = P_{il}\left(\theta; a_i, b_i, d_{i2,\dots}d_{im_i}\right) = \frac{\exp\left[\sum_{v=1}^{l} a_i(\theta - b_i + d_{iv})\right]}{\sum_{g=1}^{m_i} \exp\left[\sum_{v=1}^{g} a_i(\theta - b_i + d_{iv})\right]},$$

where d_{iv} is a threshold parameter denoting the difficulty of transition between category $l - 1$ and category l for item i, m_i is the number of categories for item i, and a_i and b_i are the item discrimination and difficulty parameters, respectively. Note, $d_{i1} \equiv 0$ is set for model identification purposes.

These IRT models are used in the second step when estimating the score probabilities of a randomly selected test taker in population T scoring x_j on test form X and y_k on test form Y; $r_j = \Pr(X = x_j | T)$ and $s_k = \Pr(Y = y_k | T)$, respectively. Under the IRT framework these probabilities are a function of θ, thus we denote them as $r_j(\theta)$ and $s_k(\theta)$. As it is typically done in IRT observed-score equating, these score probabilities are obtained using the Lord and Wingersky (1984) algorithm, although other methods can also be used to obtain them (González et al., 2016). For details on how the score probabilities are obtained refer to Andersson and Wiberg (2017).

In the third step, the discrete distributions are continuized into continuous distributions using a kernel. Define the cumulative distribution functions (CDFs) of X and Y in T by $F(x) = \Pr(X \leq x | T)$ and $G(y) = \Pr(Y \leq y | T)$, respectively. Here the Gaussian kernel was used although other kernels could have been used (González & von Davier, 2017; Lee & von Davier, 2011). Let $\mu_X = \sum_j x_j r_j$ and σ_X^2 be the mean and variance of X in population T and define $a_X = \sqrt{\sigma_X^2 / \left(\sigma_X^2 + h_X^2\right)}$

where $h_X > 0$ denote the bandwidth parameter which can be selected in several ways (Häggström & Wiberg, 2014; Wallin et al., 2018). Using the Gaussian kernel $\Phi(\cdot)$, the continuized CDF for test form X is defined as

$$F_{h_X}(x; \mathrm{r}) = \sum_j r_j \Phi\left(\frac{x - a_X x_j - (1 - a_X)\mu_X}{a_X h_X}\right),$$

where $\mathbf{r} = (r_1, \ldots, r_J)^t$. Similar definitions lead to $G_{h_Y}(y; \mathbf{s})$ for test score Y. Next, using the continuized score distributions the equating from test form X to test form Y is carried out using the equating transformation function $\varphi_Y(x) = G_{h_Y}^{-1}\left(F_{h_X}(x)\right)$. Finally, the equating transformation is evaluated using different measures (Wiberg & González, 2016). In the simulation study we used standard errors (SE) and percent relative error (PRE). Denote the pth moment of the distribution of test scores Y and that of the equated scores $\varphi_Y(X)$ as $\mu_p(Y) = \sum_k (y_k)^p s_k$ and $\mu_p(\varphi_Y(x)) = \sum_j (\varphi_Y(x_j))^p r_j$, respectively, then the PRE is defined as

$$\mathrm{PRE}(p) = 100\frac{\mu_p(\varphi_Y(X)) - \mu_p(Y)}{\mu_p(Y)}$$

(von Davier et al., 2004).

To evaluate the obtained equated scores, we also used the difference that matters (DTM, Dorans & Feigenbaum, 1994), which was defined here as +/− 0.5 score point difference in equated scores.

3 Simulation Study

We considered an EG design with 1500 test takers for each test form X and Y in three cases depending on the proportion of polytomously scored items. In all three cases, the polytomous items were scored as: 0, 1, and 2. The first case contained 20 dichotomously scored items and 20 polytomously scored items (20D/20P), and thus the score range was 0–60. In the second case, we used 30 dichotomously scored items and 10 polytomously scored items (10P/30D), and thus the score range was 0–50. In the third case, we used 35 dichotomously scored items and 5 polytomously scored items (35D/5P), and thus the score range was 0–45. The dichotomously scored items were modelled with the 2PL IRT model with discrimination parameters drawn from the U(.3,1.3) distribution, whereas the difficulty parameter were drawn from the N(0,1) distribution.

The polytomously scored items were modelled with the GPCM with slope parameters drawn from the U(.3,1.3) distribution and with item location parameters drawn from the N(−.5,1) (first parameter) and N(.5,1) (second parameter) distributions. To examine the condition of more discriminating items we added 0.5 to the discrimination parameter in test form Y, thus drawing them as a ~ U(0.8,1.8). The

Table 1 The PRE in the first 10 moments of the examined conditions

Case	1	2	3	4	5	6	7	8	9	10
20D/20P	−.001	−001	.002	.011	.025	.045	.071	.103	.140	.183
Y disc	−.001	−.001	.002	.010	.024	.044	.069	.101	.138	.181
500	−.001	−.001	.002	.011	.025	.045	.070	.102	.139	.181
500, Y disc	−.001	−.001	.002	.010	.023	.042	.067	.097	.133	.173
30D/10P	.000	.000	.003	.010	,023	.042	.067	.099	.137	.183
Y disc	−.001	.000	.006	.019	.041	.073	.114	.166	.227	.298
500	−.001	−.001	.001	.009	.023	.045	.074	.112	.157	.214
500, Y disc	−.003	−.003	.002	.016	.040	.076	.124	.183	.254	.337
35D/5P	−.001	−.001	.007	.023	.049	.086	.133	.191	.259	.336
Y disc	−.002	.001	.013	.038	.075	.125	.188	.264	.353	.456
500	−.001	−.001	.006	.023	.049	.086	.133	.190	.257	.334
500, Y disc	−.002	−.004	.005	.027	.063	.112	.174	.249	.336	.437

D Dichotomously scored items, *P* Polytomously scored items, *Y disc* Y more discriminating, *500* sample size of 500

baseline sample size case was 3000 test takers. A condition with 500 test takers was also examined. Each condition was replicated 200 times. The Gaussian kernel was used in the continuization step with bandwidths parameters selected using the penalty method. The R package ltm (Rizopoulos, 2006) was used to generate dichotomous and polytomous score responses. The R package mirt (Chalmers, 2012) was used to estimate the IRT models and the R package kequate (Andersson et al., 2013) was used perform the IRT kernel equating.

4 Results

Table 1 display the PRE in the first 10 moments for the three cases (20D/20P, 30D/10P, 35D/5P) in the examined conditions. In general, the PRE were very low, especially for the first four moments. The overall conclusion was that, regardless of case and condition the PRE followed the same pattern in the first 10 moments.

Figure 1 illustrates the three cases with different proportions of polytomous items in the different examined conditions, with equated values in the left column and SE in the right column. It is clear from the left plots in Fig. 1 that the item discrimination has an impact on the equated values. The impact is DTM in the upper score range in the second condition (30D/10P) and over most of the score range in the third case (35D/5P), i.e., that the DTM increases for fewer polytomous items. A reduced sample size of 500 did not yield any large differences in equated values, and thus that line is barely visible in one of the plots and nonexistent in the other plots.

The plots on the right-hand side in Fig. 1 displays the SE for the three examined cases under the examined conditions. As expected, the SE is clearly lower when sample size is larger – which was seen in all cases. Considering a more

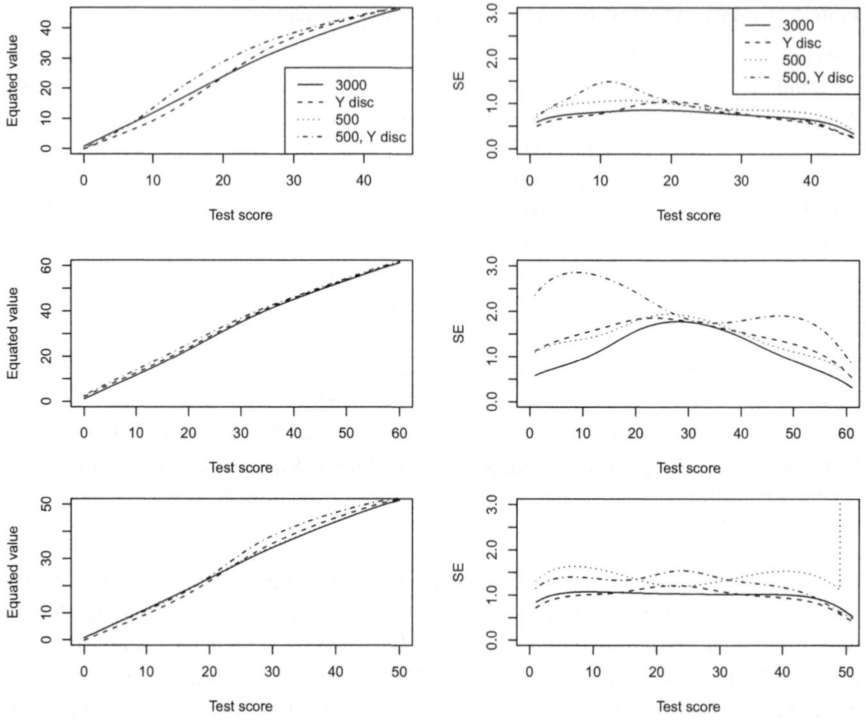

Fig. 1 The first row represents the case with 20D/20P, the second row represent 30D/10P and the third row represents 35D/5P with equated values to the left and SE to the right with respect to the examined conditions

discriminating Y test yields on average higher SE. The SE was also higher when more polytomous scored items were used as was the case for 20D/20P.

5 Discussion

The aim of this paper was to examine the impact of item discrimination, proportion of polytomous items and different sample sizes on equating mixed-format tests with IRT kernel equating. From the simulation study it was evident that the SE were much higher when one test form had items which were more discriminating and, as expected, when a smaller sample size was used. The equated values were however not affected by the smaller sample size – but there were DTM in the equated values especially in the higher score ranges when the proportion of dichotomously scored items were higher. The fact that the degree of item discrimination has an impact on equated values is a result in line with other research in test equating (e.g. van der Linden & Wiberg, 2010). The found DTM in the upper score range should make test developers really aim for test forms which have similar item discriminations.

The SE were higher when more polytomous items were included in the test, a result which should be examined further in the future. A possible reason might be the larger variation of test scores as compared with the other two examined cases. The result that DTM were larger when fewer polytomous items were included in the test was surprising and this result should be examined further in future studies when varying other conditions.

This research focused on the EG design, in the future research one should also examine mixed format tests with IRT kernel equating under the NEAT design and especially examine the impact of the anchor test length and its mixture of binary and polytomous items as well as the item characteristics and relate it to similar research (e.g. Kim et al., 2010; Kolen & Lee, 2014). In addition, one should examine the size of the correlation between the test forms, and how results change if other presmoothing models such as the Rasch or the graded response model are used. The chosen presmoothing model could potentially influence the equated scores as it has recently shown to have an impact on the equating (Wallin & Wiberg, 2020). Summing up, IRT kernel equating seems to be a possible alternative when we have mixed format tests, but more research is needed.

Acknowledgements The research was funded by the Swedish Wallenberg MMW 2019.0129 grant. Jorge González also acknowledges the support by Fondecyt grant 1201129.

References

Andersson, B. (2016). Asymptotic standard errors of observed-score equating with polytomous IRT models. *Journal of Educational Measurement, 53*(4), 459–477.

Andersson, B., & Wiberg, M. (2017). Item response theory observed-score kernel equating. *Psychometrika, 82*(1), 48–66.

Andersson, B., Bränberg, K., & Wiberg, M. (2013). Performing the kernel method of test equating using the package kequate. *Journal of Statistical Software, 55*, 1–25.

Chalmers, R. P. (2012). Mirt: A multidimensional item response theory package for the R environment. *Journal of Statistical Software, 48*(6), 1–29.

Dorans, N. J., & Feigenbaum, M. D. (1994). Equating issues engendered by changes to the SAT and PSAT/NMSQT. In I. M. Lawrence, N. J. Dorans, M. D. Feigenbaum, N. J. Feryok, A. P. Schmitt, & N. K. Wright (Eds.), *Technical issues related to the introduction of the new SAT and PSAT/NMSQT* (ETS research memorandum no. RM-94-10). Educational Testing Service.

Ercikan, K., Schwarz, R. D., Julian, M. W., Burket, G. R., Weber, M. M., & Link, V. (1998). Calibration and scoring of tests with multiple-choice and constructed-response item types. *Journal of Educational Measurement, 35*, 137–154.

González, J., & von Davier, A. A. (2017). An illustration of the Epanechnikov and adaptive continuization methods in kernel equating. In L. A. van der Ark, M. Wiberg, S. A. Culpepper, J. A. Douglas, & W.-C. Wang (Eds.), *Quantitative psychology 81st annual meeting of the psychometric society, Asheville, North Carolina, 2016* (pp. 253–262). Springer.

González, J., & Wiberg, M. (2017). *Applying test equating methods – Using R*. Springer.

González, J., Wiberg, M., & von Davier, A. A. (2016). A note on the Poisson's binomial distribution in item response theory. *Applied Psychological Measurement., 40*(4), 302–310.

Häggström, J., & Wiberg, M. (2014). Optimal bandwidth in observed-score kernel equating. *Journal of Educational Measurement, 51*(2), 201–211.

Kim, S., & Kolen, M. J. (2006). Robustness to format effects of IRT linking methods for mixed-format tests. *Applied Measurement in Education, 19*, 357–381.

Kim, S., Walker, M. E., & McHale, F. (2008). Equating of mixed-format tests in large-scale assessments. In *Technical report (RR-08-26)*. Educational Testing Service.

Kim, S., Walker, M. E., & McHale, F. (2010). Comparisons among designs for equating mixed-format tests in large-scale assessments. *Journal of Educational Measurement, 47*(1), 36–53.

Kolen, M. J., & Lee, W. (Eds.). (2014). *Mixed-format tests: Psychometric properties with a primary focus on equating (volume 3). CASMA monograph no. 2.3*. CASMA. The University of Iowa.

Lee, G., & Lee, W. (2014). A comparison of unidimensional IRT and bi-factor multidimensional IRT equating for mixed-format tests. In M. J. Kolen & W. Lee (Eds.), *Mixed-format tests: Psychometric properties with a primary focus on equating (volume 3)* (CASMA monograph no. 2.3) (pp. 201–234). CASMA. The University of Iowa.

Lee, Y. H., & von Davier, A. A. (2011). *Equating through alternative kernels* (In statistical models for test equating, scaling, and linking (pp. 159–173)). Springer.

Lord, F. M. (1980). *Applications of item response theory to practical testing programs*. Lawrence Erlbaum Associates.

Lord, F. M., & Wingersky, M. S. (1984). Comparison of IRT true-score and equipercentile observed-score "equatings". *Applied Psychological Measurement, 8*, 452–461.

Muraki, E. (1992). A generalized partial credit model: Application of an EM algorithm. *Applied Psychological Measurement, 16*, 159–176.

Rizopoulos, D. (2006). Ltm: An R package for latent variable modeling and item response theory analyses. *Journal of Statistical Software, 17*(5), 1–25.

van der Linden, W. J., & Wiberg, M. (2010). Local observed-score equating with anchor-test designs. *Applied Psychological Measurement, 34*, 620–640.

von Davier, A. A., Holland, P. W., & Thayer, D. T. (2004). *The kernel method of test equating*. Springer.

Wallin, G., & Wiberg, M. (2019). Propensity scores in kernel equating for non-equivalent groups. *Journal of Educational and Behavioral Statistics., 44*(4), 390–414.

Wallin, W., & Wiberg, M. (2020). Selecting a presmoothing model in kernel equating. In M. Wiberg, D. Molenaar, J. González, U. Böckenholt, & S.-J. Kim (Eds.), *Quantitative Psychology – 84th Annual Meeting of the psychometric society, Santiago, Chile, 2019* (pp. 97–105). Springer.

Wallin, G., Häggström, J., & Wiberg, M. (2018). How important is the choice of bandwidth in kernel equating? A simulation study comparing six different methods. In M. Wiberg, S. A. Culpepper, R. Jansen, J. González, & D. Molenaar (Eds.), *Quantitative Psychology – 82nd Annual Meeting of the psychometric society, Zurich, Switzerland, 2017* (pp. 91–100). Springer.

Wang, W., Drasgow, F., & Liu, L. (2016). Classification accuracy of mixed format tests: A bi-factor item response theory approach. *Frontiers in Psychology, 7*(270), 1–11.

Wiberg, M., & Bränberg, K. (2015). Kernel equating under the non-equivalent groups with covariates design. *Applied Psychological Measurement, 39*(5), 349–361.

Wiberg, M., & González, J. (2016). Statistical assessment of estimated transformations in observed-score equating. *Journal of Educational Measurement, 53*(1), 106–125.

Wiberg, M., van der Linden, W. J., & von Davier, A. (2014). Local kernel observed-score equating. *Journal of Educational Measurement, 51*(1), 57–74.

Population Invariance of Equating for Subgroups Differing in Achievement Level

Dongmei Li and Shalini Kapoor

1 Introduction

Test equating is a widely-used methodology to ensure score comparability across test forms that may differ slightly in difficulty. Kolen and Brennan (2014) summarized desirable properties of equating proposed in the research literature. One such property is often referred to as group or population invariance of the equating relationship (e.g. Angoff, 1971; Dorans & Holland, 2000; Kolen, 2004), which means that "the equating relationship is the same regardless of the group of examinees used to conduct the equating" (Kolen & Brennan, 2004, p. 12). Dorans (2004) pointed out that population invariance plays a central role in assessing test equitability, i.e., the extent to which the equating relationship is invariant across important examinee groups determines the extent to which tests are equatable.

Population invariance cannot be assumed to hold in all situations (Flanagan, 1951; Lord, 1980). Whether this property holds can be empirically checked by comparing equating relationships for the different groups of interest in the population. Research has repeatedly demonstrated that equating results are reasonably invariant to the equating sample when test forms are developed according to the same content and statistical specifications. For example, results were similar when equating was conducted using data from different gender, ethnicity, or ability groups (Angoff & Cowell, 1986; Dorans & Holland, 2000; Harris & Kolen, 1986; Kolen, 2004). Yet some research indicated that true-score equating may be more population invariant than observed-score equating (Lord & Wingersky, 1984; van der Linden, 2000), and other studies suggested that population invariance tended to hold less well when equating samples had different achievement distributions (Cook & Petersen,

D. Li (✉) · S. Kapoor
ACT, Inc., Iowa City, IA, USA
e-mail: dongmei.li@act.org; shalini.kapoor@act.org

M. Wiberg et al. (eds.), *Quantitative Psychology*, Springer Proceedings in Mathematics & Statistics 353, https://doi.org/10.1007/978-3-030-74772-5_19

1987; Yi et al., 2008). Moreover, the test population may evolve over time and the population invariance in new subgroups may become of interest. Therefore, it is important for testing programs to continue to evaluate the extent to which the equating relationship is invariant in specific examinee groups of interest.

The purpose of this study was to investigate the extent to which the population invariance property held for subgroups differing in mean achievement levels. Specifically, the study provided an empirical investigation of the following questions under the random groups equating design:

1. How much do equating results differ when equating is conducted using subgroups with known differences in their mean achievement levels as compared with differences expected from randomly selected samples?
2. Is equipercentile equating more or less population invariant than IRT equating?

2 Methodology

2.1 Data and Subgroups

Data used in this study came from two different administrations of the ACT test (ACT, 2020). The ACT test measures students' college readiness in English, math, reading, and science. It is taken by high school students for the purpose of college admission in the United States and is also used for other purposes such as state accountability.

In each administration, three forms were spiraled within schools to obtain randomly equivalent groups. Sample sizes for these forms in each administration are presented in Table 1. Subgroups were created from the total sample in each administration as described below for the purposes of the study. Subgroups were created at the school level so that the randomly equivalent groups within each school were maintained.

Three subgroups with different average achievement levels were created within each administration. First, the schools in each administration were ranked by students' average ACT Composite scores from low to high (ACT Composite = average of English, reading, math, and science scores on a 1–36 scale). Then, the schools were divided into three groups (Low, Medium, and High) with approximately equal

Table 1 Test forms and sample sizes of the total sample

Test administration 1 (269 schools)		Test administration 2 (272 schools)	
Forms	N	Forms	N
Y1	9871	Y2	11,349
A	9694	C	11,432
B	9708	D	11,168
Total	29,273	Total	33,949

Table 2 Sample sizes and descriptive statistics of composite scores by subgroups

		Administration 1			Administration 2		
	Group	N	Mean	SD	N	Mean	SD
	Total	29,273	18.81	5.19	33,949	18.08	4.85
Ranked	1 (low)	9811	15.94	4.03	11,322	15.79	3.95
	2 (medium)	9709	18.71	4.50	11,370	18.17	4.58
	3 (high)	9753	21.79	5.22	11,257	20.29	4.90
Random	1	9811	18.91	5.23	11,322	17.88	4.80
	2	9709	19.35	5.37	11,370	17.75	4.81
	3	9753	18.68	5.31	11,257	17.59	4.81

numbers of students in each group. Students in the "Low" group were designated Group 1, students in the "Medium" group were designated Group 2, and students in the "High" group were designated Group 3. These samples are referred to as the ranked samples in this report.

Three subgroups were also created by randomly sampling schools (without replacement) to serve as a basis for comparison with results from the three ranked groups. First, a random number from 1 to the total number of schools in each administration was created for each school, and then student data were sorted by the random numbers of their schools. To get a sample of size N, student records were selected from the first record to the Nth record in the sorted data. The process was repeated 3 times to get three randomly selected samples. The sample size of each random sample was the same as the sample sizes of the three groups in the ranked samples.

Table 2 presents the sample sizes and the Composite score means and standard deviations of the total group, the three ranked samples, and the three random groups. As expected—considering the manner in which these groups were created—the three ranked groups differed significantly in average achievement, and the three random groups were all similar to the total group in both test administrations.

Table 3 shows the ethnicity distributions of the total group and each subgroup for data from each test administration. The three ranked groups differed from each other and from the total group, and the three random groups were similar to each other and the total group. For example, in Administration 1, the percentage of White examinees in the Low, Medium, and High group was 26%, 65%, and 73%, respectively, but was very similar (57%, 57%, and 54%) in the three random groups.

2.2 *Equating Analysis*

Since the forms were spiraled within each school within each administration, the groups taking each form were randomly equivalent, whether in the total samples, or in each of the ranked or random samples. Following the random groups equating design, equating was conducted using different samples and different statistical

Table 3 Ethnicity distributions by group (in percent)

		Ranked groups			Random groups		
Administration 1	**Total**	**1**	**2**	**3**	**1**	**2**	**3**
Black/African American	18	40	10	5	19	18	19
American Indian/Alaska native	1	1	1	0	0	0	1
White	55	26	65	73	57	57	54
Hispanic/Latino	13	18	12	9	11	12	13
Asian	3	2	2	4	2	4	2
Native Hawaiian/other Pacific Islander	1	1	1	0	1	0	1
Two or more races	7	9	7	5	6	6	7
Prefer not to respond	3	4	3	3	3	3	3
Administration 2							
Black/African American	24	44	21	8	24	25	28
American Indian/Alaska Native	1	2	1	1	1	1	1
White	54	31	59	72	56	53	48
Hispanic/Latino	10	13	9	9	10	11	13
Asian	2	2	2	2	1	2	2
Native Hawaiian/Other Pacific Islander	0	0	0	0	0	0	0
Two or more races	6	6	6	5	6	6	5
Prefer not to respond	3	3	2	2	2	2	3

methods to equate each new form. In Administration 1, Form Y1 was an anchor form, and Forms A and B were equated to Y1. In Administration 2, Form Y2 was an anchor form, and Forms C and D were equated to Y2.

Each form was equated using the 7 different samples in each administration: the total sample, the three ranked samples, and the three random samples. Different statistical methods were used for equating, including equipercentile equating, IRT true score equating, and IRT observed score equating. Cubic spline post-smoothing with a smoothing parameter of 0.05 was used for the equipercentile equating method, and the 3-parameter logistic model (3PL) was used for the IRT equating methods.

2.3 Comparisons of Equating Results

Equating results were examined and compared among different equating samples and different methods from two perspectives: the differences in conversion tables and their impact on group means. Conversion tables are used to convert raw scores (number of items answered correctly) to scale scores (on the 1–36 scale). Equating results tables showed the conversion from raw scores to equated raw scores, unrounded scale scores, and rounded scale scores. Though only the rounded scale scores were used for score reporting, the unrounded scale scores and the equated raw scores were also compared. These conversions were examined graphically through plots of the differences between different conversions in light of the Differences that Matter (DTM) criteria (Dorans et al., 2003), that is, whether the absolute values of the differences were smaller or larger than 0.5 score unit.

A summary statistic, the weighted root mean squared difference (WRMSD), was also calculated for each pair of conversion tables. Let Y_{i1} and Y_{i2} be converted scores associated with raw score i obtained from two equatings, K be the total number of raw score points (or number of items), N be the total number of examinees in a group, and n_i be the number of students with a raw score of i. Then the WRMSD statistic can be expressed as

$$WRMSD = \sqrt{\frac{1}{N}\sum_{i=0}^{K} n_i (Y_{i2} - Y_{i1})^2}.$$

This statistic can be aggregated across different conditions (e.g., test forms, samples, etc.) to get an average WRMSD (AWRMSD).

To examine the impact of the differences in conversion tables on group means, the different conversion tables from the different samples or methods for a test form were applied to all examinees taking that form in the total group and the Low, Medium, and High subgroups.

For both the conversion tables and the group means, the focus of comparison was the differences between results from each of the three ranked samples and those from the total sample, treating results from the total sample as "truth" within each equating method. Several other comparisons were also made, including the comparison of results from the three ranked samples and those from the three random samples, results between each pair within the ranked and random samples, and results between equipercentile equating and IRT equatings.

3 Results

Equipercentile equating, IRT true score equating, and IRT observed score equating were conducted for the total sample and the three ranked samples and the three random samples. Selected results are presented below to address the research questions.

3.1 Comparisons Between Results Based on the Ranked and Random Samples for Equipercentile Equating

Conversion Comparisons Using equating results from selected English forms as an example, Fig. 1 presents the unrounded scale score conversion differences at each raw score point between results from each subgroup and the total group for

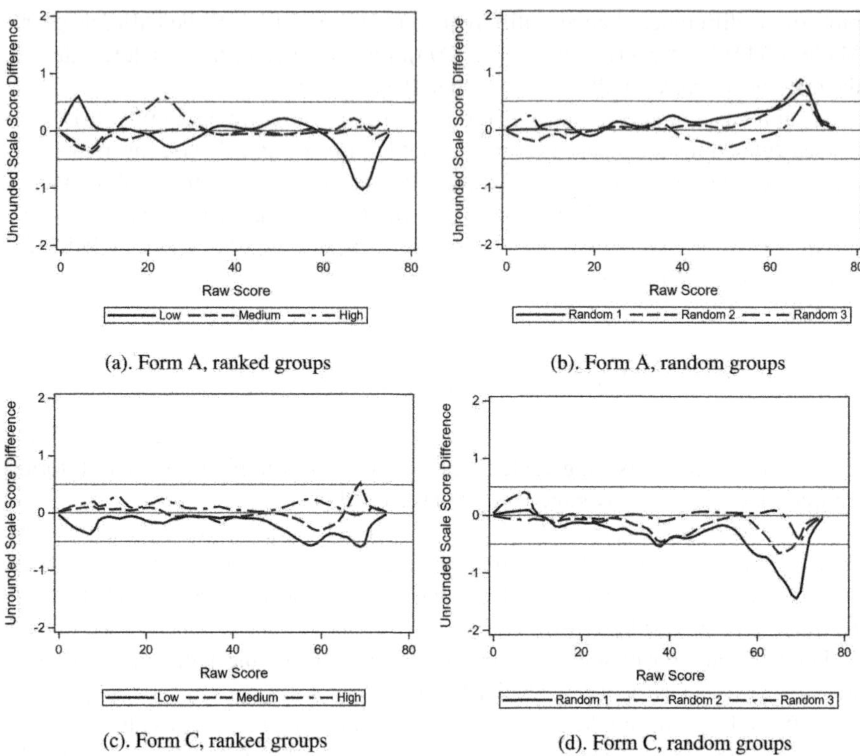

(a). Form A, ranked groups

(b). Form A, random groups

(c). Form C, ranked groups

(d). Form C, random groups

Fig. 1 Unrounded scale score differences between conversions obtained from each subgroup versus those obtained from the total group for equipercentile equating

equipercentile equating. In Fig. 1, the two horizontal reference lines represent the DTM criteria, that is, + 0.5 and - 0.5 score unit. Figures 1a and b are results for Form A equated to Y1, and Figs. 1c and d are for Form C equated to Y2. These plots illustrate that equating results obtained from each subgroup were slightly different from those obtained from the total group, and that the differences for the three ranked samples were similar in magnitude to the differences for the three random groups. Meanwhile, the absolute values of most of the differences along the score scale are smaller than the DTM criteria. Similar observations were made for other subject tests, which are not presented here.

The differences between conversion tables for the equated raw, unrounded, and rounded scale scores were summarized using the WRMSD statistic, which gives an overall indication of the magnitude of differences across conversions. Table 4 presents a comparison of the averages and the standard deviations (SDs) of the WRMSD statistic for the conversion differences between results from the ranked samples and the random samples for each subject test and the averages across subject tests for the equipercentile equating method. The averages of WRMSD were

Table 4 WRMSD mean(SD) of equipercentile equating conversion differences for the ranked and random groups

	Equated raw		Unrounded scale		Rounded scale	
	Ranked	Random	Ranked	Random	Ranked	Random
English	0.45(0.19)	0.41(0.19)	0.22(0.10)	0.19(0.09)	0.37(0.10)	0.39(0.11)
Math	0.43(0.14)	0.34(0.20)	0.24(0.08)	0.18(0.09)	0.42(0.09)	0.36(0.12)
Reading	0.25(0.09)	0.26(0.11)	0.19(0.07)	0.20(0.08)	0.38(0.10)	0.40(0.09)
Science	0.23(0.10)	0.16(0.06)	0.19(0.08)	0.13(0.04)	0.36(0.14)	0.28(0.10)
Average	0.34(0.13)	0.29(0.14)	0.21(0.08)	0.17(0.07)	0.38(0.11)	0.36(0.11)

taken across 24 values: 6 pairs of comparisons (i.e., each subgroup compared with the total group and between each pair of the subgroups) for each of the 4 forms.

On average, the conversion differences from the ranked groups were slightly larger than those from the random groups for all subject tests except for reading. Across all subject tests, the rounded scale score WRMSD were very similar between the ranked (0.38) and the random groups (0.36), indicating that equating results using different groups that had big differences in achievement varied to a similar extent as those using different randomly selected samples for equipercentile equating.

Group Mean Comparisons The raw to rounded scale score conversion of each form was applied to the groups of students taking that form in the total group. The group means were separately calculated for students taking that form in the total group, and those taking that form in the Low, Medium, and High subgroups. For example, within the total group of 29,273 students in Administration 1, there were 9694 students who took Form A (as shown in Table 1), and about one third of these students were in each of the ranked groups. Recall that for each test form, seven different raw-to-scale score conversions were obtained for each equating method: one based on the total group, three based on the ranked groups, and three based on the random groups. Each of these conversions was applied to Form A raw scores in order to calculate group means for students taking Form A in the total group and those in the Low, Medium, and High subgroups. Group mean differences were calculated using different pairs of conversions.

Summary statistics of the absolute group mean differences across all pairs of equipercentile equating conversions from the ranked samples and the random samples across all forms are presented for each subject test and the Composite scores in Table 5. In Table 5, the column "Samples" indicates whether the conversions were obtained using the ranked or the random samples, and the column "Group" indicates to which group of examinees the different conversions were applied. As in other tables, the values outside the parentheses are the averages of the absolute group mean differences across 24 different comparisons (6 pairwise comparison for each of the 4 forms) and the values within the parentheses are the standard deviations of the group mean differences.

Table 5 Mean(SD) of the absolute group mean differences of equipercentile equating for the ranked and random samples

Samples	Group	Composite	English	Math	Reading	Science
Ranked	All	0.07(0.04)	0.10(0.06)	0.11(0.07)	0.10(0.07)	0.10(0.09)
	Low	0.08(0.06)	0.10(0.07)	0.14(0.09)	0.09(0.07)	0.10(0.09)
	Medium	0.07(0.04)	0.10(0.06)	0.11(0.07)	0.10(0.07)	0.10(0.09)
	High	0.07(0.05)	0.10(0.06)	0.11(0.08)	0.12(0.07)	0.10(0.09)
Random	All	0.09(0.07)	0.14(0.09)	0.10(0.08)	0.12(0.09)	0.06(0.04)
	Low	0.07(0.05)	0.09(0.06)	0.10(0.07)	0.10(0.07)	0.07(0.05)
	Medium	0.09(0.07)	0.14(0.09)	0.10(0.08)	0.13(0.09)	0.07(0.05)
	High	0.11(0.09)	0.17(0.12)	0.12(0.10)	0.15(0.11)	0.06(0.05)

The values for the ranked samples in Table 5 tended to be slightly smaller than the random samples for English and reading but tended to be slightly larger than the random samples for math and science. The overall differences across the subject tests (shown in the "Composite" column) were similar for the ranked and random equating samples, indicating that equating using groups differing in achievement levels did not result in greater impact on group means than what would be expected from sampling error.

Comparisons Between Equipercentile and IRT Equating Similar comparisons were made between results from the equipercentile equating method and the IRT true score and IRT observed score equating method for the ranked and the random samples. The IRT true score and IRT observed score equating results were very similar, and the differences between equipercentile equating and IRT equatings were similar for the ranked and the random samples, so only IRT true score equating results from the ranked samples are presented below and are compared with the equipercentile equating results.

Table 6 presents the average WRMSD differences for the comparisons involving the three ranked groups for equipercentile equating and IRT true score equating results. The WRMSD statistics tended to be slightly smaller for the equipercentile equating results than for the IRT results, but on average across all subject tests, they were very similar (0.38 for equipercentile and 0.39 for IRT), indicating that changing the equating method had little impact on the variability of conversion tables across the different samples.

Table 7 presents the descriptive statistics of the absolute group mean differences across the different comparisons for equipercentile and IRT true score equating. The values in Table 7 were very similar between equipercentile and IRT equating except that the group mean differences of IRT true score equating tended to be slightly higher than those of equipercentile equating for science. The Composite score statistics were very similar between equipercentile and IRT true score equating, indicating that equating using samples differing in achievement levels had a similar impact on group means when comparing equipercentile and IRT equating results.

Table 6 WRMSD mean(SD) of conversion differences of equipercentile equating and IRT true score equating using the ranked groups

	Equated raw		Unrounded scale		Rounded scale	
	Equip	IRT True	Equip.	IRT True	Equip.	IRT True
English	0.45(0.19)	0.44(0.17)	0.22(0.10)	0.23(0.11)	0.37(0.10)	0.39(0.09)
Math	0.43(0.14)	0.47(0.20)	0.24(0.08)	0.22(0.10)	0.42(0.09)	0.39(0.11)
Reading	0.25(0.09)	0.28(0.13)	0.19(0.07)	0.22(0.10)	0.38(0.10)	0.37(0.12)
Science	0.23(0.10)	0.33(0.17)	0.19(0.08)	0.33(0.17)	0.36(0.14)	0.43(0.18)
Average	0.34(0.13)	0.38(0.17)	0.21(0.08)	0.25(0.12)	0.38(0.11)	0.39(0.13)

Table 7 Mean(SD) of the absolute group mean differences of equipercentile and IRT true score equating for the ranked groups

	Group	Composite	English	Math	Reading	Science
Equi-percentile	All	0.07(0.04)	0.10(0.06)	0.11(0.07)	0.10(0.07)	0.10(0.09)
	Low	0.08(0.06)	0.10(0.07)	0.14(0.09)	0.09(0.07)	0.10(0.09)
	Medium	0.07(0.04)	0.10(0.06)	0.11(0.07)	0.10(0.07)	0.10(0.09)
	High	0.07(0.05)	0.10(0.06)	0.11(0.08)	0.12(0.07)	0.10(0.09)
IRT true	All	0.08(0.05)	0.10(0.07)	0.10(0.07)	0.09(0.06)	0.14(0.12)
	Low	0.08(0.05)	0.10(0.06)	0.11(0.08)	0.09(0.06)	0.13(0.12)
	Medium	0.08(0.05)	0.09(0.06)	0.10(0.08)	0.09(0.06)	0.14(0.11)
	High	0.09(0.07)	0.12(0.11)	0.13(0.12)	0.12(0.08)	0.17(0.16)

4 Conclusions and Discussion

This study evaluated the extent to which equating relationships were consistent for subgroups differing in achievement levels using empirical data. Results showed that the equating relationships were reasonably consistent, even for groups with large differences in average achievement and demographics. This was apparent from the fact that the magnitude of the differences in conversions and their impact on group means were similar to those solely due to sampling error. The study also showed that there were very small differences between equipercentile equating and the two IRT equating methods in terms of their impact on the population invariance property of equating.

Findings from this study are consistent with similar research (e.g. Harris & Kolen, 1986) and provide additional empirical support for the group or population invariance property of test equating for groups that differ in achievement levels. In practice, the equating sample may be a lower or higher performing group from the test population. Alternatively, even though the equating sample is selected to represent the whole test population, it may be higher or lower in performance compared to different subpopulations, such as students in different states. Results from this study and other empirical studies demonstrated that the equating relationship were reasonably stable whether equating was conducted using a lower performing group or a higher performing group.

These findings can only be generalized to similar situations in which the test forms were developed to be parallel according to detailed test specifications and equating was conducted based on carefully implemented random groups data collection design. Further studies can investigate population invariance in subgroups with different sample sizes or different data collection designs. If smaller sample sizes are used, or when the forms are less parallel, equating relationships might be more group dependent. Equating based on the common item non-equivalent groups design involves more statistical assumptions than equating based on the random equivalent groups design, which might cause the equating relationship to be less population invariant. Because of the potential differences in testing programs in terms of test development, equating sample sizes, and equating data collection designs, we recommend that testing programs conduct their own studies to evaluate the population invariance property of equating for subgroups of interest.

Acknowledgments The authors would like to thank Dr. Jeffrey Steedle for reviewing different versions of the paper and for his insightful comments and edits. The authors would also like to thank Dr. Benjamin Andrews for his inputs and for validating results at the earlier stage of the project.

References

ACT. (2020). *The ACT technical manual*. Author.

Angoff, W. H. (1971). Scales, norms, and equivalent scores. In R. L. Thorndike (Ed.), *Educational measurement* (2nd ed., pp. 508–600). Washington, DC: American Council on Education.

Angoff, W. H., & Cowell, W. R. (1986). An examination of the assumption that the equating of parallel forms is population-independent. *Journal of Educational Measurement, 23*(4), 327–345.

Cook, L. L., & Petersen, N. S. (1987). Problems related to the use of conventional and item response theory equating methods in less than optimal circumstances. *Applied Psychological Measurement, 11*(3), 225–244.

Dorans, N. J., & Holland, P. W. (2000). Population invariance and the equatability of tests: Basic theory and the linear case. *Journal of Educational Measurement, 37*(4), 281–306.

Dorans, N. J., Holland, P. W., Thayer, D. T., & Tateneni, K. (2003). Invariance of score linking across gender groups for three advanced placement program exams. In N. J. Dorans (Ed.), *Population invariance of score linking: Theory and applications to advanced placement program examinations* (pp. 79–118). Research Report 03–27. Educational Testing Service.

Flanagan, J. C. (1951). Units, scores, and norms. In E. F. Lindquist (Ed.), *Educational measurement* (pp. 695–763). American Council on Education.

Harris, J. D., & Kolen, J. M. (1986). Effect of examinee group on equating relationships. *Applied Psychological Measurement, 10*(1), 35–43.

Kolen, M. J. (2004). Population invariance in equating and linking: Concept and history. *Journal of Educational Measurement, 41*(1), 3–14.

Kolen, M. J., & Brennan, R. L. (2014). *Test equating, scaling, and linking: Methods and practices* (3rd ed.). New York, NY: Springer.

Lord, F. M. (1980). *Applications of item response theory to practical testing problems*. Hillsdale, NJ: Erlbaum.

Lord, F. M., & Wingersky, M. S. (1984). Comparison of IRT true-score and equipercentile observed score. "equatings". *Applied Psychological Measurement, 8*, 452–461.

van der Linden, W. J. (2000). A test-theoretic approach to observed-score equating. *Psychometrika, 65*, 437–456.

Yi, Q., Harris, D. J., & Gao, X. (2008). Invariance of equating functions across different subgroups of examinees taking a science achievement test. *Applied Psychological Measurement, 32*(1), 62–80.

Comparison of Outlier Detection Methods in NEAT Design

Chunyan Liu and Daniel Jurich

1 Introduction

von Davier et al. (2004, p.13) emphasized that "current test equating practice requires explicit methods for separating the effects of examinee ability from the assessment of the differences in the difficulty of the two tests". This is accomplished by the equating design used for data collection. The nonequivalent groups with anchor test (NEAT) design is one of the most commonly used equating designs (Kolen & Brennan, 2014; von Davier et al., 2004), where the two test forms share some items in common, called anchor items. Anchor items can be used to equate test forms or create a calibrated item bank in the framework of item response theory (IRT). The anchor items must behave similarly for equating to function. In practice, however, anchor items may function differently across the two test forms and should be eliminated from the anchor item set. These items are referred to as outliers (Kolen & Brennan, 2014) or items with item parameter drift (IPD, Goldstein, 1983; Bock et al., 1988). Failure to pinpoint the outliers from the anchor item set may deteriorate equating accuracy and undermine the validity of test scores (Hu et al., 2008; Huang & Shyv, 2003). Therefore, it is critical to detect the outlier items and exclude them from the anchor item set before conducting equating.

Within the Rasch IRT equating framework, the mean difference of the anchor item difficulties between the two test forms are used to estimate the equating constant or translation constant (*TC*, Wright & Stone, 1979, p.96). Because it is a mean difference, the TC may be greatly impacted by the outliers in the anchor items, especially when the number of anchor items is small or the magnitude of item difficulty drift is large. The most commonly used outlier detection methods are the

C. Liu (✉) · D. Jurich
National Board of Medical Examiners®, Philadelphia, PA, USA
e-mail: CLiu@nbme.org; Djurich@nbme.org

M. Wiberg et al. (eds.), *Quantitative Psychology*, Springer Proceedings in Mathematics & Statistics 353, https://doi.org/10.1007/978-3-030-74772-5_20

logit difference method (Miller et al., 2004) and the robust z statistic method (Hogg, 1979; Huynh & Meyer, 2010), which will be discussed in more detail later. For both methods, a subjective cutoff value (e.g., 0.3 or 0.5 for the logit difference method and 1.65 for the robust z method) is required to be pre-determined in order to identify anomalous behavior of the potential outlier items. Previous research suggests that the logit difference method tends to underestimate the number of outliers and the robust z method with a cutoff value of 1.65 tends to overestimate the number of outliers (Manna & Gu, 2019; Murphy et al., 2010).

A t-test approach was proposed to investigate the presence of items with differential item functioning (DIF) by examining whether the item parameters estimated from two independent calibrations differed significantly (Wright & Stone, 1979). Researchers have recommended a cutoff value of $t = 2$ for identifying DIF items (Muraki & Engelhard, 1989; Smith & Suh, 2003). As other researchers have noted, the problem of detecting outliers in anchor item set is essentially the same as the problem of detecting the presence of DIF items when there are two-time points (Donoghue & Isham, 1998; DeMars, 2004). Thus, the t-test DIF method presents a logical approach for detecting equating outliers as well and we found no research investigating the t-test approach in this context.

The purpose of this study is to investigate the performance of the t-test method, the logit difference method, and the robust z statistic method in detecting outliers in the anchor items under the Rasch framework through a simulation study. More specifically, cutoff value of 2.0 for the t-test approach, 0.3 and 0.5 for the logit difference method, and 2.7 (Huynh & Meyer, 2010) for the robust z method are investigated. In addition, the simulation considered several factors, including sample size, percentage of outlier items, and direction of item drift, and their performances are evaluated using different criteria.

2 Data

This study used empirical data from a medical exam with 200 multiple-choice items, of which 60 (30%) are anchor items. The item difficulties were estimated based on the Rasch model, and linked to a pre-calibrated operational item bank through the anchor items. The item difficulties of the anchor items were considered as true parameters (without estimation error) and used for item manipulation to create different simulation conditions with varying number and magnitude of outliers.

Examinee ability was randomly generated from two normal distribution, $\theta \sim N(0, 1)$ and $\theta \sim N(0.2, 1)$. Item responses were generated for two investigated examinee sample sizes ($N = 500$ and $N = 3000$) based on the manipulated item difficulties and examinee ability distribution for each of the simulated conditions described below. The Rasch item difficulties were estimated using *Winsteps* (Winsteps & Rasch Measurement Software, 2019).

3 Methods

3.1 Outlier Manipulation

The bank values of the anchor item difficulties were considered as the truth and used to simulate different conditions. Four levels of percentages of outliers in the anchor items were investigated: 0% (0 outliers), 10% (6 outliers), 20% (12 outliers), and 30% (18 outliers). In order to mimic a practical situation, most of the outliers were simulated to have small item difficulty drift, and a few of them were simulated to have medium or large drift. Therefore, 1/6 of the outliers were manipulated to be severely drifted (the item difficulties of the outliers were added/subtracted by 1.0, or $\Delta b = 1.0$), 1/6 to be moderately drifted ($\Delta b = 0.5$), and 2/3 to be mildly drifted ($\Delta b = 0.3$).

We also simulated three anchor item difficulty drift directions: positive (outliers become more difficult), negative (outliers become easier), and mixed (some outliers become more difficult and some become easier). Consider the condition of 30% outliers (18 outliers) with positive drift direction as an example. For randomly selected 18 outliers in the anchor items, the item difficulty was added by 1.0 for three of them (1/6 of the 18 outliers), 0.5 for another three (1/6 of the 18 outliers), and 0.3 for the rest of the 12 outliers (2/3 of the 18 outliers). Similarly, the item difficulties were added by -1.0, -0.5, or $-$ 0.3 for the negative drift conditions. For the conditions with mixed drift direction, ± 1.0, ± 0.5, and $\pm$ 0.3 were added to the item difficulties of randomly selected outliers.

3.2 Outlier Detection Methods

Logit Difference Method The logit difference of an anchor item (d_i) is calculated as the difference of item difficulties from the item bank and from the new calibration after scale transformation, and defined as

$$d_i = b_{Bank,i} - \left(\hat{b}_{New,i} + TC\right), \tag{1}$$

where $b_{Bank,\,i}$ and $\hat{b}_{New,i}$ represent the difficulty from the bank and from the new calibration respectively for item i. TC is the translation constant (or equating constant) estimated as the average difference between the bank and the new calibration anchor item difficulties, and is defined as $TC = \frac{\sum_{i=1}^{I}\left(b_{Bank,i}-\hat{b}_{New,i}\right)}{I}$ (Wright & Stone, 1979, p.96), where I is the number of anchor items. For each of the anchor items, if the absolute value of d_i is larger than a pre-determined value, the anchor item is flagged as an outlier and removed from the anchor item set. Both 0.5 logit difference and 0.3 logit difference are considered in this study and are denoted as LogitD_0.5 and LogitD_0.3, respectively.

Robust z Statistic For the vector of logit differences (d) of the anchor items obtained from Eq. (1), the robust z statistic (Hogg, 1979) is defined as

$$Robust\ z = \frac{d - Md}{0.74 \times IQR(d)}, \tag{2}$$

where Md is the median of d, and $IQR(d)$ indicates the inter-quartile range of d. Huynh and Meyer (2010) claim that the robust z statistic follows a standard normal distribution and is not affected by the existence of outliers. A cutoff value of 2.7 was recommended by Huynh and Meyer (2010) and utilized in this study. We term this method and cutoff combination as RobustZ. An item is flagged as a potential outlier if the absolute value of its robust z statistic is larger than 2.7. Please note that the cutoff value of 1.65 is not considered in this study since previous research concluded that the robust z method with cutoff of 1.65 cannot control the Type I error in the baseline conditions where no outliers were simulated (Liu et al., 2020; Manna & Gu, 2019).

***t*-test Approach** In the context of DIF detection, a separate calibration t-test approach was proposed to detect the invariance of the item parameter estimates obtained from two independent Rasch calibrations (Thissen et al., 1992; Wright & Stone, 1979; Smith, 1996; Smith & Suh, 2003). In this approach, the t-statistic for item i is defined as:

$$t_i = \frac{\hat{b}_{Fi} - \hat{b}_{Ri}}{\sqrt{\text{var}\left(\hat{b}_{Fi}\right) + \text{var}\left(\hat{b}_{Ri}\right)}} \tag{3}$$

where $\hat{b}_{Fi}$ and $\hat{b}_{Ri}$ represent the item difficulties for item i estimated from the focal group and reference group respectively, $\text{var}\left(\hat{b}_{Fi}\right)$ and $\text{var}\left(\hat{b}_{Fi}\right)$ are the estimates of the sampling variance associated with the estimated item difficulties. The t statistic approximately follows a standard normal distribution and a cutoff value of 2.0 was recommended for the absolute value of t to yield a Type I error rate of 5% (Muraki & Engelhard, 1989; Smith, 1996).

In the context of outlier detection, Eq. (3) can be modified as follows if we want to flag items that exhibit large differences from the item difficulties in the bank, which are considered as true item difficulties without estimation error:

$$t_i = \frac{b_{Bank,i} - \left(\hat{b}_{New,i} + TC\right)}{\sqrt{\text{var}\left(\hat{b}_{New,i}\right)}}, \tag{4}$$

where $\text{var}\left(\hat{b}_{New,i}\right)$ is the associated estimate of sampling variance of $\hat{b}_{New,i}$. For an item that does not have IPD, we expect the estimated item difficulty, or

$\hat{b}_{New,i} + TC$, to be centered around the bank value with a variance of var$\left(\hat{b}_{New,i}\right)$ and the t statistic approximately follows a standard normal distribution. However, the estimated item difficulty for an outlier with IPD will not center around the bank value and the item will be flagged if t is larger than a pre-determined cutoff value. In this study, the cutoff value of 2.0 is considered and this method is denoted as t_2.0.

3.3 Simulation Procedures

The item difficulties of the 60 anchor items were considered as true parameters and were manipulated to create different scenarios. The investigated factors include, examinee sample size (N = 500 and 3000), group difference (TC = 0 and 0.2), percentage of outliers (0%, 10%, 20%, and 30%), and direction of item difficulty drift (positive, negative, and mixed). The conditions with 0% outliers are considered as the baselines and used to evaluate the performance of these outlier detection methods. The simulation procedures are detailed below:

1. Randomly sample N examinees from the investigated normal distribution;
2. From the anchor items, randomly select outliers with severe, moderate, and mild item difficulty drift, and add/subtract 1.0, 0.5 or 0.3 to/from the item difficulties of these outliers while keeping the rest of the item difficulties unchanged;
3. Simulate 0/1 responses for the 200 items based on the item difficulties from Step 2 and examinee abilities from Step 1;
4. Conduct *Winsteps* calibration;
5. Calculate d_i, Robust z, and t_i for each anchor item based on the calibrated item difficulty and estimation error from Step 4, and their difficulty from the bank;
6. Exclude the item with the largest absolute value of t, z, or logit difference if the considered method falls above the cutoff for this item;
7. Repeat Steps 5 and 6 until no item meets the criteria for removal in Step 6;
   Estimate TC for each outlier detection method based on their corresponding final anchor item set and add it to the estimated examinee abilities from Step 4 to get the final ability estimates;
8. Repeat Steps 2 to Step 8500 times for each of the simulated conditions.

3.4 Evaluation Criteria

Sensitivity and specificity are often considered as ways to evaluate the accuracy of a test or a measure, especially in the medical field. Sensitivity refers to the proportion of correctly identified true positives by the test, and specificity refers to the proportion of correctly identified true negatives by the test (Altman & Bland, 1994). Ideally, we would like both sensitivity and specificity to be 100%. Within the context of outlier detection, mathematically, they are defined as:

$$\text{Sensitivity} = \frac{\text{Number of flagged true outliers}}{\text{Number of true outliers}} \times 100, \tag{5}$$

and

$$\text{Specificity} = \frac{\text{Number of flagged true non} - \text{outliers}}{\text{Number of true non} - \text{outliers}} \times 100. \tag{6}$$

The second criterion used to evaluate the performance of these outlier detection methods is the bias of the estimated *TC*. Since each condition was repeated five hundred times, the bias of the estimated *TC* is defined as

$$Bias_{TC} = \frac{1}{500}\sum_{r=1}^{500} \hat{TC}_r - TC, \tag{7}$$

where $\hat{TC}_r$ is the estimated translation constant obtained from r^{th} replication and *TC* is the true translation constant obtained from the true group difference.

Since the estimated *TC* can directly impact the examinee ability estimation, we also compare the outlier detection methods' performance in recovering examinee ability. We accomplish this through the root mean square error (*RMSE*), which is defined as:

$$\text{RMSE}\left(\hat{\theta}\right) = \frac{1}{500}\sum_{r=1}^{500} \sqrt{\frac{1}{N}\sum_{i=1}^{N}\left(\hat{\theta}_{i,r} - \theta_i\right)^2}, \tag{8}$$

where N is the number of test takers, θ_i and $\hat{\theta}_{i,r}$ represent the true ability and the estimated ability from r^{th} replication respectively for examinee i.

4 Results

In this section, the results for the baseline conditions without outliers are presented first, followed by the results of the simulated conditions with outliers. Our simulation results suggest that the true translation constant has little impact on the performance of these outlier detection methods, so we only provide the results for the conditions where the true $TC = 0$. In addition, the results for the conditions with 20% of outliers (12 items) falls between the reported conditions and can be predicted from the results. Thus, these conditions are also excluded from the paper.

4.1 Baseline Conditions Without Outliers

Table 1 shows the results of specificity, bias of *TC*, and *RMSE* of the estimated examinee ability for the four outlier detection methods for the baseline condition where no outliers are simulated. The results indicate that, on average, the *t*_2.0 correctly identify 96% (SD = 2.8%) of the non-outliers for both sample sizes. The specificity is almost 100% for both LogitD_0.5 and LogitD_0.3 methods, suggesting that the Logit Difference method tends to correctly flag all non-outliers under the baseline conditions. Finally, the specificity is about 97% for the RobustZ method with a standard deviation about 4.0%.

Table 1 also suggests that all outlier detection methods perform similarly in recovering the translation constant and the examinee ability under the baseline conditions without outliers. The bias of *TC* is very close to zero and the *RMSE* of the estimated ability is about 0.173 for all outlier detection methods, even when the sample size is 500.

4.2 Simulated Conditions with Outliers

Sensitivity Table 2 provides the comparison of sensitivity in flagging true outliers for these methods under different simulated conditions.

Table 2 suggests that, on average, the *t*_2.0 method yields a sensitivity ranging from 76% to 84% when the sample size is 500. When the sample size is 3000, the sensitivity is almost 100% for the *t*_2.0 method indicating that the *t*-test approach can accurately flag almost all true outliers when the sample size is large. Comparatively, for the LogitD methods, the sensitivity ranges from 18% to 31% when the cutoff value is 0.5 and from 60% to 75% when the cutoff value is 0.3, which suggests that the LogitD method tends to underestimate the number of true outliers, especially when the cutoff value is 0.5. For the RobustZ method, the sensitivity is about 63% and 100% when the sample size is 500 and 3000 respectively for the simulated conditions with 10% outliers. However, when there are 30% outliers, the sensitivity decreases dramatically to less than 30% when

Table 1 Performance of different outlier detection methods under baseline conditions

	N	*t*_2.0	LogitD_0.5	LogitD_0.3	RobustZ
Specificity	500	96.1 ± 2.8%	100.0 ± 0.2%	99.0 ± 1.7%	97.3 ± 3.5%
	3000	96.0 ± 2.8%	100.0 ± 0.0%	100.0 ± 0.0%	97.2 ± 4.1%
Bias of TC	500	−0.0003	−0.0005	−0.0003	−0.0002
	3000	0.0002	0.0004	0.0004	0.0001
RMSE $\left(\hat{\theta}\right)$	500	0.1734	0.1733	0.1733	0.1734
	3000	0.1725	0.1725	0.1725	0.1725

Note: The value after "±" is the standard deviation of specificity

Table 2 Sensitivity in flagging true outliers under different simulated conditions

N	% of Outliers	Drift Direction	$t\_2.0$	LogitD_0.5	LogitD_0.3	RobustZ
500	10%	Positive	80.5 ± 17.4%	26.3 ± 12.1%	65.4 ± 19.6%	64.3 ± 23.8%
		Negative	80.7 ± 16.2%	26.8 ± 13.0%	64.9 ± 19.6%	62.8 ± 22.7%
		Mixed	84.1 ± 15.9%	27.7 ± 12.9%	66.5 ± 18.1%	66.1 ± 22.7%
	30%	Positive	76.3 ± 13.0%	24.0 ± 8.8%	60.7 ± 15.4%	27.2 ± 14.6%
		Negative	76.2 ± 12.8%	23.3 ± 9.1%	60.8 ± 15.6%	28.3 ± 15.9%
		Mixed	83.0 ± 9.1%	31.1 ± 11.4%	69.8 ± 11.8%	52.4 ± 22.9%
3000	10%	Positive	99.9 ± 1.3%	20.7 ± 7.4%	65.8 ± 22.0%	99.9 ± 1.5%
		Negative	99.9 ± 1.1%	21.9 ± 8.5%	65.2 ± 21.3%	99.9 ± 1.1%
		Mixed	100.0 ± 0.0%	24.8 ± 9.0%	68.2 ± 20.4%	99.9 ± 1.1%
	30%	Positive	100.0 ± 0.4%	17.9 ± 3.9%	65.6 ± 23.8%	29.7 ± 30.2%
		Negative	100.0 ± 0.5%	17.9 ± 3.7%	61.4 ± 23.3%	30.5 ± 31.0%
		Mixed	99.9 ± 0.7%	26.5 ± 8.1%	74.5 ± 15.6%	99.9 ± 0.7%

Note: The value after "±" is the standard deviation of sensitivity

Table 3 Specificity in identifying true non-outliers under different simulated conditions

N	% of Outliers	Drift Direction	$t\_2.0$	LogitD_0.5	LogitD_0.3	RobustZ
500	10%	Positive	95.2 ± 3.0%	100.0 ± 0.3%	98.6 ± 2.3%	97.8 ± 3.7%
		Negative	95.5 ± 3.0%	100.0 ± 0.3%	98.7 ± 2.2%	98.0 ± 3.3%
		Mixed	95.9 ± 2.8%	100.0 ± 0.2%	98.8 ± 2.3%	98.0 ± 3.3%
	30%	Positive	94.5 ± 5.0%	99.9 ± 0.8%	97.3 ± 3.7%	99.4 ± 2.2%
		Negative	94.7 ± 4.9%	99.9 ± 0.6%	97.3 ± 3.7%	99.3 ± 2.0%
		Mixed	96.0 ± 3.6%	100.0 ± 0.2%	98.7 ± 2.5%	99.0 ± 3.3%
3000	10%	Positive	95.6 ± 2.9%	100.0 ± 0.0%	100.0 ± 0.0%	97.7 ± 3.9%
		Negative	95.7 ± 2.8%	100.0 ± 0.0%	100.0 ± 0.0%	97.5 ± 4.2%
		Mixed	96.0 ± 2.5%	100.0 ± 0.0%	100.0 ± 0.0%	97.7 ± 3.1%
	30%	Positive	95.5 ± 3.4%	100.0 ± 0.0%	100.0 ± 0.2%	99.5 ± 2.2%
		Negative	95.8 ± 3.3%	100.0 ± 0.0%	100.0 ± 0.0%	99.2 ± 3.3%
		Mixed	95.9 ± 3.3%	100.0 ± 0.0%	100.0 ± 0.0%	97.3 ± 4.4%

Note: The value after "±" is the standard deviation of specificity

the item difficulties drift to one direction. For all outlier detection methods, the sensitivity tends to be slightly higher when the item difficulty drift direction is mixed.

Overall, the $t\_2.0$ method performs very stable, and outperforms the LogitD methods and the Robust z method in terms of the sensitivity of detecting true outliers under all simulated conditions.

Specificity Table 3 provides the comparison of specificity in correctly identifying true non-outliers for these methods under different simulated conditions.

Table 3 suggests that, on average, the $t\_2.0$ method can correctly identify 94%–96% of the true non-outliers for all simulated conditions. In other words, on average,

2 ~ 3 non-outliers will be flagged as outliers by the *t*_2.0 method for all simulated conditions.

Comparatively, the specificity is almost 100% for LogitD_0.5 and at least 97.3% for LogitD_0.3 method. However, the high specificity likely results from the conservative nature of the LogitD method, as the method also yielded low sensitivity (Table 2). The specificity for the RobustZ method is larger than 97% and 99% when there are 10% and 30% outliers, respectively. As with LogitD, the high specificity under the 30% outlier conditions is mainly because the RobustZ method fails to flag the true outliers.

In general, Table 3 indicates that all outlier detection methods perform very well in correctly identifying the non-outliers.

Bias of Translation Constant Figure 1 illustrates the bias of the estimated *TC* for these outlier detection methods when the sample size is 3000 and 30% of the anchor items are simulated to be outliers. The "No Removal" provides the bias of the estimated *TC* if no outliers are removed from the anchor items before equating and is provided for reference.

For the "Mixed" conditions or when the item difficulties randomly drift in both directions, we can see that the *TC* bias is almost zero for all outlier detection methods even when no outliers are removed. When all item difficulties drift to one direction, we can see that (1) the bias of *TC* is about 0.14 for the negative drift (items become easier) and − 0.14 for the positive drift (items become more difficult) under the "No Removal" conditions; (2) among the four investigated outlier detection methods, this plot indicates that the *TC* bias is almost zero for the *t*-test method indicating that the *t*-test method can recover the true translation constant accurately no matter what the item difficulty drift direction is; (3) the magnitude of the *TC* bias

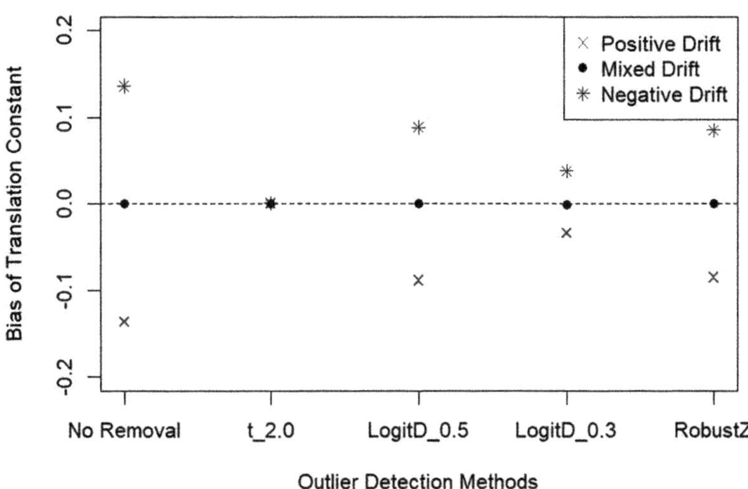

Fig. 1 Comparison of the bias of translation constant (N = 3000 and 30% outliers)

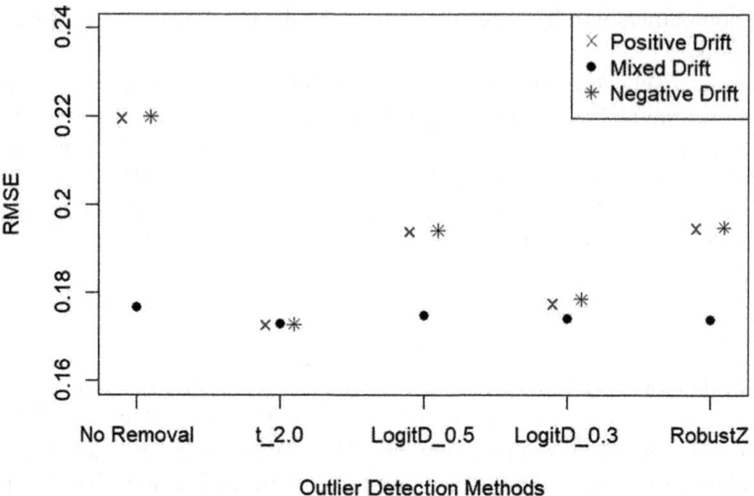

Fig. 2 Comparison of *RMSE* of the estimated abilities (N = 3000 and 30% outliers)

is about 0.09, 0.04, and 0.08 for LogitD_0.5, LogitD_0.3, and RobustZ methods respectively; and (4) for these methods, the *TC* bias tends to be negative when the drift direction is positive and positive when the drift direction is negative.

RMSE Figure 2 provides the comparison of the root mean square error of the estimated examinee ability for these outlier detection methods for the same condition (N = 3000 and 30% outliers). Again, the *RMSE* for the "No Removal" is provided as a reference.

Figure 2 suggests that all outlier removal methods tend to reduce *RMSE* for all simulated conditions, even though the magnitude of reduction is small for the "Mixed" conditions relative to the no removal condition. When all item difficulties drift to one direction (positive or negative), the direction of drift seems have little impact on *RMSE*. The *RMSE* is about 0.220 under positive or negative drift under the "No Removal" conditions. The t-test outperformed the other methods again, yielding an *RMSE* of about 0.173 for all simulated conditions, which is comparable to the baseline conditions provided in Table 1. However, the *RMSE* is about 0.194, 0.178, and 0.195 for LogitD_0.5, LogitD_0.3, and RobustZ methods respectively.

5 Conclusion and Discussion

In NEAT design, the outliers in the anchor items can deteriorate the equating accuracy and undermine score interpretation. This study compares the performance of four outlier detection methods (*t*_2.0, LogitD_0.5, LogitD_0.3, and RobustZ) in flagging outliers through a simulation study. The investigated factors include examinee sample size, group difference, proportion of outliers, and item difficulty drift direction. The *t*-test approach was proposed to evaluate the item difficulty invariance among different examinee groups, but was never used to detect outliers in anchor item equating. However, the logit difference method and the robust z method have been widely investigated and operationally used in flagging outliers in anchor items (He et al., 2013; Huynh & Meyer, 2010; Manna & Gu, 2019; Miller et al., 2004; Murphy et al., 2010).

For the logit difference method, the findings were consistent with previous research that both LogitD_0.5 and LogitD_0.3 methods tend to underestimate the number of outliers (flagging fewer true outliers), yielding a very high specificity (>99%) and small sensitivity in most cases (less than 30% for LogitD_0.5 and less than 70% for LogitD_0.3). However, an important caveat is that the LogitD_0.3 method yielded a higher sensitivity because the magnitude of item difficulty drift was simulated to be 0.3 for the mildly drifted items and most of these outliers were undetected by the LogitD_0.5 method. The robust *z* method with a cutoff value of 2.7 performed very well in most simulated conditions, except when there are 30% outlier and all items drift in one direction. This is probably because the robust *z* statistic is defined as the interquartile range of the difference in item difficulties and it doesn't function well when there are more than 25% outliers in the anchor item set. Comparatively, the *t*-test method outperformed the other methods in terms of detecting true outliers across all simulated conditions, which may be because the *t*-test method utilizes the sampling variance of the estimated item difficulties and the other methods only compare the difference between the newly estimated item difficulties and their corresponding bank values. More specifically, *t*-test method correctly flagged roughly 80% and 100% of the true outliers when the sample size is 500 and 3000 respectively. In addition, this method also correctly identified 95% of the true non-outliers in all simulated conditions, which is consistent with previous research that this approach yields a Type I error rate of 5% (Muraki & Engelhard, 1989; Smith, 1996).

One limitation of the current study is that we did not consider the content representation of the anchor item set to the total test when removing outlier anchor items. Kolen and Brennan (2014, p.287) suggest that the anchor item set should be constructed to the same content and statistical specifications as the total test so that the anchor items can adequately reflect the group differences. Previous research found that lack of content balance in the anchor item set can have a significant negative impact on equating (Harris, 1991; Klein & Jarjoura, 1985). Therefore, dropping outlier items may result in an anchor item set that is not representative of the total test, which, in turn, may negatively impact the equating results and the validity of the test scores. In addition, we tried to manipulate the item difficulty drift for the outlier anchor items to reflect the practical situations. That is, we simulated only a few items that were severely or moderately drifted, whereas most items are mildly drifted. However, there is no empirical evidence or theoretical reason why this distribution of outliers should occur in practice. Different combinations of percentage of outlier items might be investigated in future research.

The importance of equating in educational measurement demands methods and practices that ensure the validity of equated scores. This study examined various outlier detection methods that can help practitioners identify and remove non-invariant anchor items from the equating procedure. The current simulation study demonstrated that the *t*-test approach with a cutoff value of 2.0 can accurately detect true outliers and that removal of these outliers improved examinee ability estimation in terms of the reduction of *RSME* of the estimated examinee ability. Further research on these methods should be conducted, and application of this approach in detecting outliers in practical situations should also be considered.

References

Altman, D. G., & Bland, J. M. (1994). Diagnostic tests. 1: Sensitivity and specificity. *BMJ, 308*, 1552.

Bock, R. D., Muraki, E., & Pfeiffenberger, W. (1988). Item pool maintenance in the presence of item parameter drift. *Journal of Educational Measurement, 25*(4), 275–285.

DeMars, C. E. (2004). Detection of item parameter drift over multiple test administrations. *Applied Measurement in Education, 17*, 265–300.

Donoghue, J. R., & Isham, S. P. (1998). A comparison of procedures to detect item parameter drift. *Applied Psychological Measurement, 22*, 33–51.

Goldstein, H. (1983). Measuring changes in educational attainment over time: Problems and possibilities. *Journal of Educational Measurement, 20*, 369–377.

Harris, D. J. (1991). *Equating with nonrepresentative common item sets and nonequivalent groups*. Paper presented at the annual meeting of the American Educational Research Association, Chicago.

He, Y., Cui, Z., Fang, Y., & Chen, H. (2013). Using a linear regression method to detect outliers in IRT common item equating. *Applied Psychological Measurement, 37*, 522–540.

Hogg, R. V. (1979). Statistical robustness: One view on its use in applications today. *The American Statistician, 33*, 108–115.

Hu, H., Rogers, W. T., & Vukmirovic, Z. (2008). Investigation of IRT-based equating methods in the presence of outlier common items. *Applied Psychological Measurement, 32*, 311–333.

Huang, C. Y., & Shyu, C. Y. (2003, April). *The impact of item parameter drift on equating*. Paper Presented at the Annual Meeting of the National Council on Measurement in Education, Chicago.

Huynh, H., & Meyer, P. (2010). Use of robust z in detecting unstable items in item response theory models. *Practical Assessment, Research and Evaluation, 15*(2).

Klein, L. W., & Jarjoura, D. (1985). The importance of content representation for common-item equating with nonrandom groups. *Journal of Educational Measurement, 22*, 197–206.

Kolen, M. J., & Brennan, R. L. (2014). *Test equating, scaling, and linking*. Springer.

Liu, C., Jurich, D., Morrison, C., & Grabovsky, I. (2020). *Detection of outliers in anchor items using modified Rasch fit statistics*. Paper presented at the annual meeting of the National Council on Measurement in Education, Denver, CO.

Manna, V. F., & Gu, L. (2019). *Different methods of adjusting for form difficulty under the Rasch model: Impact on consistency of assessment results* (Technical report RR-19-08). Educational Testing Service.

Miller, G. E., Rotou, O., & Twing, J. S. (2004). Evaluation of the 0.3 logit screening criterion in common item equating. *Journal of Applied Measurement, 5*, 172–177.

Muraki, E., & Engelhard, G. (1989). *Examining differential item functioning with BIMAIN*. Paper presented at the annual meeting of the American Educational Research Association, San Francisco.

Murphy, S., Little, I., Fan, M., Lin, C., & Kirkpatrick, R. (2010, April). *The impact of different anchor stability methods on equating results and student performance*. Paper presented at the annual meeting of the National Council on Measurement in Education, Denver, CO.

Smith, R. M. (1996). A comparison of the Rasch separate calibration and between-fit methods of detecting item bias. *Educational and Psychological Measurement, 56*(3), 403–418.

Smith, R. M., & Suh, K. K. (2003). Rasch fit statistics as a test of the invariance of item parameter estimates. *Journal of Applied Measurement, 4*, 153–163.

Thissen, D., Steinberg, L., & Wainer, H. (1992). Detection of differential item functioning using the parameters of item response models. In P. W. Holland & H. Wainer (Eds.), *Differential item functioning* (pp. 67–113). Lawrence Erlbaum Associates.

von Davier, A. A., Holland, P. W., & Thayer, D. T. (2004). *The kernel method of test equating*. Springer.

Winsteps & Rasch measurement Software. (2019). *Fit diagnosis: Infit outfit mean-square standardized*. Retrieved from http://www.winsteps.com/winman/misfitdiagnosis.htm.

Wright, B. D., & Stone, M. H. (1979). *Best test design*. MESA Press.

An Illustration on the Quantile-Based Calculation of the Standard Error of Equating in Kernel Equating

Jorge González and Gabriel Wallin

1 Introduction

Equating methods rely on the comparison of score distributions using what is called an equating transformation function. Let F_X and G_Y be the score distributions of the random variables X and Y, corresponding to the test scores on two test forms X and Y, and defined on $\mathcal{X}$ and $\mathcal{Y}$, respectively. The equipercentile equating function $\varphi : \mathcal{X} \mapsto \mathcal{Y}$, computed as

$$\varphi(x) = G_Y^{-1}(F_X(x)), \tag{1}$$

maps the scores from one test form into the scale of the other (Braun & Holland, 1982; González & Wiberg, 2017). The equating transformation is a functional parameter that in practice is estimated using score data. Although various measures for the assessment of equating functions have been proposed (Wiberg & González, 2016), the uncertainty in the estimation of the equating transformation has mainly been measured by the standard error of equating (SEE),

$$\mathrm{SEE}_Y(x) = \sqrt{\mathrm{Var}(\hat{\varphi}(x))}. \tag{2}$$

J. González (✉)
Facultad de Matemáticas, Pontificia Universidad Católica de Chile, Santiago, Chile

Laboratorio Interdiciplinario de Estadística Social, LIES, Pontificia Universidad Católica de Chile, Santiago, Chile
e-mail: jorge.gonzalez@mat.uc.cl

G. Wallin
CNRS, Laboratoire J.A. Dieudonné, team Maasai, Université Côte d'Azur Inria, Nice, France
e-mail: gabriel.wallin@inria.fr

M. Wiberg et al. (eds.), *Quantitative Psychology*, Springer Proceedings in Mathematics & Statistics 353, https://doi.org/10.1007/978-3-030-74772-5_21

Different methods to calculate the SEE include exact formulas (see, e.g., Kolen and Brennan, 2014, Table 7.2); the Delta method (Lord, 1982), (Braun & Holland, 1982, p. 33), (Holland et al., 1989); and the bootstrap (Tsai et al., 2001). Another method proposed in Liou and Cheng (1995) and later extended by Liou et al. (1997) is based on the Bahadur's representation of sample quantiles (Bahadur, 1966; Ghosh, 1971). In this paper, this method will be refereed to as the *Quantile-Based SEE* (QB-SEE).

Liou and Cheng (1995) used the QB-SEE method and obtained results for traditional equipercentile equating under the single group (SG), the equivalent groups (EG), and the nonequivalent groups with anchor test (NEAT) designs. Later, Liou et al. (1997) extended this work to include the kernel equating transformation using Gaussian and Uniform kernels, considering only the NEAT design. These authors did however not make any comparison between the QB-SEE and the more traditionally used Delta method for the estimation of the SEE under the kernel equating framework. In this paper, we aim to fill this gap.

The paper is organized as follows. In Sect. 2 we briefly revise the kernel equating transformation and the way the SEE is calculated using the Delta method. Next, in Sect. 3 we introduce the QB-SEE method and give the details on how it can be used under the kernel equating framework. An illustration of the comparison between the QB-SEE and the delta method applied to the estimated kernel equating transformation is shown in Sect. 4. The paper ends in Sect. 5 summarizing the main results and discussing on future research.

2 Equating and the Standard Error of Equating

In this section we briefly review the basics of kernel equating and the way the SEE has been calculated within this framework. Next, we introduce the QB-SEE method and show how it adapts to be used in KE.

2.1 Kernel Equating

Kernel equating (Holland & Thayer, 1989; von Davier et al., 2004) is a semiparametric method used to estimate the equating function (González & von Davier, 2013). The score distributions are estimated using both kernel density estimation techniques (the nonparametric part) and maximum likelihood estimates of score probabilities (the parametric part).

Let $X(h_X)$ be a continuized version of the discrete score random variable X, defined as

$$X(h_X) = a_X(X + h_X V) + (1 - a_X)\mu_X,$$

where V is a continuous random variable with mean 0 and variance σ_V^2, $a_X^2 = \sigma_X^2/(\sigma_X^2+\sigma_V^2 h_X^2)$, μ_X and σ_X^2 are the mean and variance of X, and h_X is a smoothing parameter. The estimated score distribution of $X(h_X)$ is obtained as

$$\hat{F}_{h_X}(x) = \sum_j \hat{r}_j K(\hat{R}_{jX}(x)),$$

where $r_j = \Pr(X = x_j)$ are score probabilities, typically modelled using log-linear models estimated by maximum likelihood, $\hat{R}_{jX}(x) = \big(x - \hat{a}_X x_j - (1 - \hat{a}_X)\hat{\mu}_X\big)/\hat{a}_X h_X$, and K is a kernel defined by the distribution of V. In this paper we will assume that $V \sim N(0, \sigma_V^2)$ so that $K = \Phi$, the standard normal (or Gaussian) distribution function.

Defining $s_k = \Pr(Y = y_k)$, and with similar expressions for $\hat{R}_{kY}(y)$, a_Y, and $Y(h_Y)$, the score distribution of the continuized Y scores, $\hat{G}_{h_Y}$, is obtained leading to calculate the kernel equating function as

$$\varphi(x, \hat{\mathbf{r}}, \hat{\mathbf{s}}) = \hat{G}_{h_Y}^{-1}(\hat{F}_{h_X}(x)),$$

where $\hat{\mathbf{r}} = (\hat{r}_1, \ldots, \hat{r}_J)^\top$ and $\hat{\mathbf{s}} = (\hat{s}_1, \ldots, \hat{s}_K)^\top$.

Because $\hat{\mathbf{r}}$ and $\hat{\mathbf{s}}$ are maximum likelihood estimates, the Delta method (e.g., Rao, 1973; Lehmann, 1999), described next, has been used to estimate the uncertainty on the estimation of φ.

2.2 SEE in Kernel Equating

The SEE in KE is based on the Delta method. The following theorem from von Davier et al. (2004) formalizes the result.

Theorem 1 (Delta method for the SEE in KE)

If $\begin{pmatrix}\hat{\mathbf{r}}\\ \hat{\mathbf{s}}\end{pmatrix} \dot\sim N\left(\begin{pmatrix}\mathbf{r}\\ \mathbf{s}\end{pmatrix}, \Sigma\right)$, *then*

$$\varphi(x; \hat{\mathbf{r}}, \hat{\mathbf{s}}) \dot\sim N\Big(\varphi(x; \mathbf{r}, \mathbf{s}), J_\varphi \Sigma J_\varphi^\top\Big),$$

where

$$\Sigma = \begin{pmatrix}\Sigma_{\hat{\mathbf{r}}} & \Sigma_{\hat{\mathbf{r}},\hat{\mathbf{s}}}\\ \Sigma_{\hat{\mathbf{r}},\hat{\mathbf{s}}}^\top & \Sigma_{\hat{\mathbf{s}}}\end{pmatrix},$$

and

$$J_\varphi = \left(\frac{\partial\varphi}{\partial\mathbf{r}}, \frac{\partial\varphi}{\partial\mathbf{s}}\right).$$

When the score probabilities are obtained using maximum likelihood estimates from log-linear models and estimated for different equating designs using a design function, $DF(\hat{\mathbf{r}}, \hat{\mathbf{s}})$, von Davier et al. (2004) showed that the asymptotic variance obtained via the Delta method can be written as

$$Var(\hat{\varphi}) = ||J_{\varphi} J_{DF} C||^2$$

where J_{φ} is the Jacobian of the equating function, J_{DF} is the Jacobian matrix of the design function and C is a factor of the covariance matrix such that $\Sigma = CC^{\top}$. From this result, the SEE for the kernel equating function is defined as

$$\text{SEE}_Y(x) = ||J_{\varphi} J_{DF} C||, \tag{3}$$

which in this paper is denoted as $\text{SEE}_Y^{\Delta}(x)$.

3 Quantile-Based Estimation of SEE

The QB-SEE method is based on the so called Bahadur's representation of sample quantiles. The main result is presented in Ghosh (1971) and reproduced here.

Theorem 2 (Ghosh, 1971)

Suppose that G is once differentiable at $\xi_p = G^{-1}(p)$ *with* $G'(\xi_p) > 0$. *If* $0 < p < 1$, *then*

$$\hat{\xi}_p = \xi_p + \frac{p - \hat{G}(\xi)}{G'(\xi)} + o_p\big(N^{-1/2}\big). \tag{4}$$

Liou and Cheng (1995) used this result to derive a formula for the SEE of the equipercentile equating transformation. After replacing p by F_X and checking regularity conditions, these authors took the variance in (4) to obtain

$$Var(\hat{G}^{-1}(F(x))) = \frac{1}{G'(\varphi)^2}\Big\{\text{Var}(\hat{F}_X) + \text{Var}(\hat{G}_Y(\varphi)) - 2\text{Cov}(\hat{F}_X, \hat{G}_Y(\varphi))\Big\}. \tag{5}$$

We call the square root of this expression the QB-SEE and denote it as $\text{SEE}_Y^{B}(x)$. In the next section we describe how the QB-SEE can be used to evaluate the kernel equating transformation under the NEAT design. For a critical review of the NEAT equating design see San Martín and González (2020).

3.1 Quantile-Based SEE in KE

The sample estimates of the score distributions can be replaced by kernel estimates in which case the QB-SEE formula becomes

$$\text{SEE}_Y^B(x) = \frac{1}{G'(\varphi)}\left\{\text{Var}(\hat{F}_{h_X}) + \text{Var}(\hat{G}_{h_Y}(\varphi)) - 2\text{Cov}(\hat{F}_{h_X}, \hat{G}_{h_Y}(\varphi))\right\}^{1/2}. \tag{6}$$

To derive the QB-SEE for the particular case of equating under the NEAT design, we introduce the following additional notation: $t_l = \Pr(A = a_l)$ are the marginal score probabilities for the anchor random variable A, and $r_{j|l}$ and $s_{k|l}$ are the conditional score probabilities of X and Y given A, respectively.

Following Liou et al. (1997), the variances and covariance terms in (6) can be obtained as

$$\begin{aligned}\text{Var}(\hat{F}_{h_X}) &= \text{Var}\left(\sum_j \hat{r}_j K(\hat{R}_{jX}(x))\right)\\ &\approx \sum_j\sum_{j'} K\big(R_{JX}(x)\big)K\big(R_{j'X}(x)\big)\text{Cov}\big[\hat{r}_j, \hat{r}_{j'}\big]\\ &= \sum_j K_{jX}^2\big(R_{JX}(x)\big)\text{Var}\big[\hat{r}_j\big]\\ &+ \sum\sum_{j\neq j'} K_{jX}\big(R_{JX}(x)\big)K_{j'X}\big(R_{JX}(x)\big)\text{Cov}\big[\hat{r}_j, \hat{r}_{j'}\big]\end{aligned}, \tag{7}$$

where

$$\begin{aligned}\text{Var}\big[\hat{r}_j\big] &= \sum_l \left\{\frac{\hat{r}_{j|l}[1-\hat{r}_{j|l}]}{(n_X+1)\hat{h}(a_l)-1}\hat{h}^2(a_l) + \frac{\hat{h}(a_l)[1-\hat{h}(a_l)]}{n_X+n_Y}\hat{r}_{j|l}^2\right.\\ &+ \left.\frac{\hat{r}_{j|l}\big[1-\hat{r}_{j|l}\big]\hat{h}(a_l)\big[1-\hat{h}(a_l)\big]}{\big[(n_X+1)\hat{h}(a_l)-1\big](n_X+n_Y)}\right\} - \sum\sum_{l\neq l'}\frac{\hat{h}(a_l)\hat{h}(a_{l'})}{n_X+n_Y}\hat{r}_{j|a}\hat{r}_{j|a'}\end{aligned}, \tag{8}$$

and

$$\begin{aligned}\text{Cov}\big[\hat{r}_j, \hat{r}_{j'}\big] &= \sum_a \left\{\frac{\hat{h}(a_l)[1-\hat{h}(a_l)]}{n_X+n_Y}\hat{r}_{j|l}\hat{r}_{j'|l} - \frac{\hat{r}_{j|l}\hat{r}_{j'|l}}{(n_X+1)\hat{h}(a_l)-1}\hat{h}^2(a_l)\right.\\ &- \left.\frac{\hat{r}_{j|l}\hat{r}_{j'|l}\hat{h}(a_l)[1-\hat{h}(a_l)]}{\big[(n_X+1)\hat{h}(a_l)-1\big](n_X+n_Y)}\right\} - \sum\sum_{l\neq l'}\frac{\hat{h}(a_l)\hat{h}(a_{l'})}{n_X+n_Y}\hat{r}_{j|l}\hat{r}_{j'|l'}\end{aligned} \tag{9}$$

Replacing terms accordingly, similar derivations lead to obtain the variance of G_Y.

Finally, the covariance term is calculated as

$$\mathrm{Cov}(\hat{F}_{h_X}, \hat{G}_{h_Y}) \approx \sum_j \sum_k K(R_{jX})K(R_{kY}) \Bigg\{ \sum_l \frac{\hat{h}(a_l)[1-\hat{h}(a_l)]}{n_X+n_Y}\hat{r}_{j|l}\hat{s}_{k|l} - \sum\sum_{l \neq l'} \frac{\hat{h}(l)\hat{h}(l')}{n_X+n_Y}\hat{r}_{j|l}\hat{s}_{k|l'} \Bigg\}. \quad (10)$$

In all previous equations either sample estimates or presmoothed score probabilities can be used as weights for the kernel. In the next section, the former case is considered for illustration and to compare the SEE for KE as calculated using the traditional delta method with the QB-SEE method

4 Illustration

4.1 *Data*

We use data described in Kolen and Brennan (2014). The data set consists of two 36-items test forms. Form X was administered to 1,655 examinees and form Y was administered to 1,638 examinees. Also, 12 out of the 36 items are common between both test forms (items 3, 6, 9, 12, 15, 18, 21, 24, 27, 30, 33, and 36). The data come with the distribution of the CIPE software which is freely available at https://education.uiowa.edu/centers/center-advanced-studies-measurement-and-assessment/computer-programs and is also available in the *equate* (Albano, 2016) and *SNSequate* (González, 2014) R packages.

4.2 *Analyses*

To investigate how $\mathrm{SEE}_Y^B(x)$ is related to $\mathrm{SEE}_Y^\Delta(x)$, we compared the SEE for KE under the NEAT-PSE design calculated using the Delta, the QB-SEE, and Bootstrap methods.

The SEE based on the Delta method is calculated using Equation (3), which is implemented in *SNSequate* and appears as one of the output values for a call to the `ker.eq()` function.

The QB-SEE is calculated using Equation (6). The variances and covariance components of the numerator on the right hand side are obtained using Equations 7–10, whereas the denominator corresponds to the derivative of G evaluated in the equated score, which in this case correspond to a Gaussian kernel.

The bootstrap SEE implements the procedure described in Kolen and Brennan (2014, Chap. 7) to compute the SEE using 500 replications.

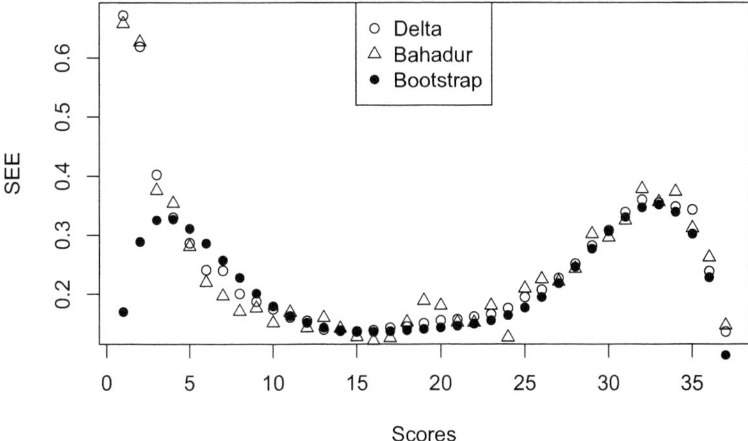

Fig. 1 SEE for the three compared methods

All the analyses were carried out using the R software (R Core Team, 2020) and the code is available from the authors upon request.

4.3 Results

The SEE obtained for the three compared methods are shown graphically in Fig. 1. Except for some score values in the lower range of the score scale, it can be seen that all the methods yielded similar estimations of SEE for the analyzed data.

The results for all SEE methods reflect that there are few test-takers in the tails of the score scale, as illustrated by the increased values of the SEE. The results also suggest that the QB-SEE and the Delta method produce very similar results, although leaning on different asymptotic results. Given that both the QB-SEE and Delta method SEE deviate from the bootstrap SEE in the lower tail, the results also indicate that they might be better approximations when the number of test-takers is large, which is expected given that they both are large-sample approximations.

5 Discussion

In this paper we have revisited the result of Bahadur on the asymptotic representation of sample quantiles and its use in the derivation of what we call the QB-SEE method of estimating the standard error of equating. The method was applied for kernel equating transformations under the NEAT design and compared to the more traditional Delta method of obtaining SEE. Results from a numerical illustration shown that the QB-SEEs are very similar to the SEEs obtained using the Delta method, for the analyzed data set.

An advantage of the QB-SEE method is that it allows to separate sources of uncertainty influencing the SEE, as it can be grasped from (5). A comprehensive simulation study to assess how these variances and covariance terms vary according to different conditions is planned for future research. Another advantage of this method is that, in comparison to the Delta method, it does not rely on normality. This could open room for other models and methods for presmoothing that do not necessarily resort on the normality of parameter estimates, as it is the case of log-linear models estimated using maximum likelihood.

Future work include other methods to estimate the variance-covariance components in the SEE formulas and the evaluation of other kernels and other equating designs.

References

Albano, A. D. (2016). Equate: An R package for observed-score linking and equating. *Journal of Statistical Software, 74*(8), 1–36

Bahadur, R. R. (1966). A note on quantiles in large samples. *The Annals of Mathematical Statistics, 37*(3), 577–580

Braun, H., & Holland, P. (1982). Observed-score test equating: A mathematical analysis of some ets equating procedures. In P. Holland, & D. Rubin (Eds.), *Test equating* (vol 1, pp. 9–49). New York: Academic Press

Ghosh, J. K. (1971). A new proof of the bahadur representation of quantiles and an application. *The Annals of Mathematical Statistics, 42*(6), 1957–1961

González, J. (2014). SNSequate: Standard and nonstandard statistical models and methods for test equating. *Journal of Statistical Software, 59*(7), 1–30

González, J., & von Davier, M. (2013). Statistical models and inference for the true equating transformation in the context of local equating. *Journal of Educational Measurement, 50*(3), 315–320

González, J., & Wiberg, M. (2017). *Applying test equating methods using R*. New York: Springer

Holland, P., King, B., & Thayer, D. (1989). The standard error of equating for the kernel method. Technical Report 89–83, Educational Testing Service

Holland, P., & Thayer, D. (1989). The kernel method of equating score distributions. Technical report, Princeton: Educational Testing Service

Kolen, M., & Brennan, R. (2014). *Test equating, scaling, and linking: Methods and practices* (3rd ed.). New York: Springer

Lehmann, E. L. (1999). *Elements of large-sample theory*. New York: Springer

Liou, M., & Cheng, P. E. (1995). Asymptotic standard error of equipercentile equating. *Journal of Educational and Behavioral Statistics, 20*(3), 259–286

Liou, M., Cheng, P. E., & Johnson, E. G. (1997). Standard error of the kernel equating methods under the common-item design. *Applied Psychological Measurement, 21*(4), 349–369

Lord, F. (1982). The standard error of equipercentile equating. *Journal of Educational and Behavioral Statistics, 7*(3), 165

R Core Team (2020). *R: A language and environment for statistical computing*. Vienna: R Foundation for Statistical Computing, Vienna, Austria

Rao, C. R. (1973). *Linear statistical inference and applications*. New York: Wiley

San Martín, E., & González, J. (2020). A Critical View on the NEAT Equating Design: Statistical Modelling and Identifiability Problems. *Manuscript submitted for publication*

Tsai, T., Hanson, B., Kolen, M., & Forsyth, R. (2001). A comparison of bootstrap standard errors of IRT equating methods for the common-item nonequivalent groups design. *Applied Measurement in Education, 14*(1), 17–30

von Davier, A. A., Holland, P. & Thayer, D. (2004). *The Kernel method of test equating*. New York: Springer

Wiberg, M., & González, J. (2016). Statistical assessment of estimated transformations in observed-score equating. *Journal of Educational Measurement, 53*(1), 106–125

Improving the Measurement Efficiency in Test Construction Related to Cognitive Diagnosis Models

Ya-Hui Su and Ken-Hsien Chu

1 Introduction

Cognitive diagnosis models (CDMs) have been widely used in numerous fields. Many studies have investigated methods of constructing cognitive diagnosis tests (Finkelman et al., 2009, 2010; Henson & Douglas, 2005; Henson et al., 2008; Kuo et al., 2016; Zheng & Chang, 2016). The cognitive diagnostic index (CDI; Henson & Douglas, 2005) and attribute-level discrimination index (ADI; Henson et al., 2008) are commonly used to assemble tests for such models. The CDI is based on Kullback–Leibler (KL; Chang & Ying, 1996) information on all attribute patterns, and the ADI is based on KL information on any attribute patterns that differ one attribute. Studies have revealed that these two indices can be used for constructing cognitive diagnosis tests when attributes have a nonhierarchical relationship. In practice, attributes might have a hierarchical relationship, meaning some are a prerequisite for the presence of others. Furthermore, researchers have not considered the ratio of test length to the number of attributes (RTA) in test construction. Liu et al. (2013) indicated that each attribute must be measured at least three times to obtain favorable attribute correct classification rates (ACCRs).

To include attribute hierarchy and the RTA in test construction, Kuo et al. (2016) proposed the modified CDI and ADI (i.e., MCDI and MADI). They demonstrated that the MCDI and MADI outperformed the CDI and ADI in that they had higher pattern correct classification rates (PCCRs) and ACCRs. However, in their study, when attributes had a nonhierarchical structure, the CDI and ADI tended to select items with one attribute, and the MCDI and MADI tended to select items with one or two attributes, regardless of test length. When attributes had convergent

Y.-H. Su (✉) · K.-H. Chu
Department of Psychology, National Chung Cheng University, Chiayi County, Taiwan
e-mail: psyyhs@ccu.edu.tw

M. Wiberg et al. (eds.), *Quantitative Psychology*, Springer Proceedings in Mathematics & Statistics 353, https://doi.org/10.1007/978-3-030-74772-5_22

and linear structures, the CDI and ADI tended to select items with four and one attributes, respectively. The MCDI and MADI tended to select items with one to seven attributes; however, the MADI did not select more items with attributes that required more prior knowledge, even when the test length was increased to 30 items. Because items with numerous attributes are seldom selected in a hierarchical structure, attributes that required more prior knowledge could not be accurately classified. To select items with various attribute numbers and identify items for measuring each attribute, in this study, attributes used the least were determined to propose revised indices during test construction. When attributes were used more than those with the least uses, items for all attributes that had been selected the least were no longer selected.

1.1 CDM

Many CDMs have been proposed in the literature, including the deterministic input, noisy, and gate (DINA; Haertel, 1989; Junker & Sijtsma, 2001) model; the deterministic input, noisy, or gate (DINO; Templin & Henson, 2006); the noisy input, deterministic, and gate (NIDA; Junker & Sijtsma, 2001) model; the multiple classification latent class model (Maris, 1999); the reduced reparameterized unified model (rRUM; Roussos et al., 2007); and the log-linear CDM (Henson et al., 2009). The present study focused only on the DINA model. A brief introduction of the DINA model is as follows. The probability of obtaining a correct response can be written as

$$P\left(X_{ij}=1|s_j,g_j,\eta_{ij}\right)=\left(1-s_j\right)^{\eta_{ij}}{g_j}^{\left(1-\eta_{ij}\right)}, \tag{1}$$

where $\eta_{ij}=\prod_{k=1}^{K}{\alpha_{ik}}^{q_{jk}}$ represents that examinee *i* has mastered all of the required attributes for item *j*; *K* is the total number of *k* attributes; s_j is the slip parameter, which denotes the probability that examinee *i*, who has all the required attributes, fails to answer item *j* correctly; and g_j is the guessing parameter, which represents the probability that examinee *i*, who lacks at least one of the required attributes, answers item *j* correctly.

1.2 CDI and ADI

Henson and Douglas (2005) proposed the CDI for test construction. The CDI, an alternative to Fisher information, uses the concept of KL information (Chang & Ying, 1996), which is defined as follows:

$$\mathrm{CDI}_j=\frac{\sum_{u\neq v}\left[h(\boldsymbol{\alpha}_u,\boldsymbol{\alpha}_v)^{-1}\boldsymbol{D}_{juv}\right]}{\sum_{u\neq v}\left[h(\boldsymbol{\alpha}_u,\boldsymbol{\alpha}_v)^{-1}\right]}, \tag{2}$$

where

$$h(\boldsymbol{\alpha}_u, \boldsymbol{\alpha}_v) = \sum_{k=1}^{K} (\boldsymbol{\alpha}_u - \boldsymbol{\alpha}_v)^2, \tag{3}$$

and

$$\boldsymbol{D}_{juv} = E\boldsymbol{\alpha}_u \left[\log_e \left[\frac{p_{\boldsymbol{\alpha}_u}(X_j)}{p_{\boldsymbol{\alpha}_v}(X_j)} \right] \right] = p_{\boldsymbol{\alpha}_u}(1) \log_e \left[\frac{p_{\boldsymbol{\alpha}_u}(1)}{p_{\boldsymbol{\alpha}_v}(1)} \right] + p_{\boldsymbol{\alpha}_u}(0) \log_e \left[\frac{p_{\boldsymbol{\alpha}_u}(0)}{p_{\boldsymbol{\alpha}_v}(0)} \right]. \tag{4}$$

In Eqs. (2) to (4), $\boldsymbol{\alpha}_u$ and $\boldsymbol{\alpha}_v$ are $1 \times K$ attribute vectors. In Eq. (4), $p_{\boldsymbol{\alpha}_u}(1)$ and $p_{\boldsymbol{\alpha}_u}(0)$ are the probabilities of a correct and incorrect response given for $\boldsymbol{\alpha}_u$, respectively; and $p_{\boldsymbol{\alpha}_v}(1)$ and $p_{\boldsymbol{\alpha}_v}(0)$ are the probabilities of a correct and incorrect response given for $\boldsymbol{\alpha}_v$, respectively. On the basis of the KL matrix, $\boldsymbol{D}_{juv}$ indicates how well $\boldsymbol{\alpha}_u$ is measured compared with $\boldsymbol{\alpha}_v$. If item j is more useful than other items for discriminating between two attribute patterns, $\boldsymbol{\alpha}_u$ and $\boldsymbol{\alpha}_v$, $\boldsymbol{D}_{juv}$ is larger.

Although the CDI measures an item's overall discriminative power, it is not guaranteed to have the power to discriminate between mastery and nonmastery of a specific attribute. To solve this limitation, Henson et al. (2008) proposed ADI$_j$ to measure the power to discriminate between mastery and nonmastery of a specific attribute. Let $\omega_{k1} = P(\boldsymbol{\alpha}|\,\alpha_k = 1)$ and $\omega_{k0} = P(\boldsymbol{\alpha}|\,\alpha_k = 0)$ represent the joint probability of attribute patterns existing given that the examinee has and has not mastered the kth attribute, respectively. Ω_{k1} and Ω_{k0} are the sets of attribute pattern pairs $(\boldsymbol{\alpha}_u, \boldsymbol{\alpha}_v)$ that differ only in terms of the kth attribute. Distinguishing between mastery and nonmastery is the most difficult when attribute patterns differ only by one attribute. For item j, $d_{jk1} = \sum_{\Omega_{k1}} \omega_{k1} D_{juv}$ is the power to discriminate masters from nonmasters of the kth attribute, and $d_{jk0} = \sum_{\Omega_{k0}} \omega_{k0} D_{juv}$ is the power to discriminate nonmasters from masters of the kth attribute.

$$\text{ADI}_j = \frac{d_{j1} + d_{j0}}{2} = \frac{\sum_{k=1}^{K} d_{jk1} + \sum_{k=1}^{K} d_{jk0}}{2K_j^*}, \tag{5}$$

where $\Omega_{k1} \equiv \{(\boldsymbol{\alpha}_u, \boldsymbol{\alpha}_v)|\,\alpha_{uk} = 1 \text{ and } \alpha_{vk} = 0 \text{ and } \alpha_{um} = \alpha_{vm}\ \forall\ m \neq k\}$, and $\Omega_{k0} \equiv \{(\boldsymbol{\alpha}_u, \boldsymbol{\alpha}_v)|\,\alpha_{uk} = 0 \text{ and } \alpha_{vk} = 1 \text{ and } \alpha_{um} = \alpha_{vm}\ \forall\ m \neq k\}$. The CDI and ADI have been evaluated in the studies of Henson and Douglas (2005) and Henson et al. (2008), respectively.

1.3 MCDI and MADI

MCDI and MADI are defined as follows:

$$\text{MCDI}_j = w_j^L w_j^H \text{CDI}_j \tag{6}$$

and

$$\text{MADI}_j = w_j^L w_j^H \text{ADI}_j, \tag{7}$$

where CDI_j and ADI_j are as defined in Eqs. (2) and (5),

$$w_j^L = \left(1 + \boldsymbol{I}\left(r_L < 3\right) \sum_{v=1}^{V} \boldsymbol{I}\left(\boldsymbol{q}_j^* = \boldsymbol{s}_v\right)\right)^{-1} \tag{8}$$

and

$$w_j^H = \left(1 + r_H \sum_{v=1}^{V} \boldsymbol{I}\left(\boldsymbol{q}_j^* = \boldsymbol{s}_v\right)\right)^{-1}. \tag{9}$$

In Eq. (8), w_j^L is the weight of the RTA. In Eq. (9), w_j^H is the weight of the attribute hierarchy. Let $\text{S} = \{\boldsymbol{s}_1, \ldots, \boldsymbol{s}_v \ldots, \boldsymbol{s}_V\}$ be the set of attribute patterns for items that have been selected and $\boldsymbol{q}_j^*$ be the attribute specification of item *j*, which has not been selected. When $\boldsymbol{q}_j^* = \boldsymbol{s}_v$, both CDI_j and ADI_j are multiplied by the weights of the RTA in Eq. (8) and the attribute hierarchy in Eq. (9); items in the item bank that have the same attribute specifications as the selected items are given a weight that is smaller than 1. By contrast, when $\boldsymbol{q}_j^* \neq \boldsymbol{s}_v$, both weights are equal to 1, and items in the item bank that have different attribute specifications from the selected items are given a full weight (i.e., 1).

Let the RTA be $r_L = I/K$, where I is the test length and K is the total number of attributes. Because Liu et al. (2013) indicated that each attribute must be measured at least three times to obtain favorable ACCR, when $r_L < 3$ and item *j* has the same attribute specification as some of the items already selected, w_j^L is given a weight that is smaller than 1. By contrast, when $r_L \geq 3$, w_j^L is 1. Depending on the attribute hierarchy, Leighton et al. (2004) defined a reachability matrix $\mathbf{R} = [r_{mn}]$ as a $K \times K$ matrix, where $r_{mn} = 1$ when attribute m is a prerequisite to attribute n. Let

$$r_H = \frac{\sum_{m \leq n} r_{mn}}{K\left(K+1\right)\big/_2}, 1 \leq m, n \leq K \tag{10}$$

be a measure of the hierarchical relationship between attributes m and n. The value of this index is between 0 and 1, and the index is larger with a stronger hierarchical relationship between attributes. That is, r_H is 1 when attributes have a linear hierarchy; $r_H = 2K/[K(K+1)]$ when attributes have a nonhierarchical relationship.

2 Method

To select items with various attribute numbers and identify items for measuring each attribute, attributes used the least were determined to propose revised indices during test construction. The purpose of the study was to compare the measurement efficiency of the aforementioned indices (i.e., CDI, ADI, MCDI, and MADI) and revised indices (i.e., rCDI and rADI) during test construction.

2.1 *rCDI and rADI*

Let $\mathrm{C} = \left\lfloor {}^{I}\!/_{K} \right\rfloor$ be the least times each attribute was used, where I is the test length, K is the total number of attributes, and C takes the integer of ${}^{I}\!/_{K}$. When attributes are used less than those with the least uses, w_j^H is used for considering attribute hierarchy, and $\mathrm{rCDI}_j = w_j^H \mathrm{CDI}_j$ and $\mathrm{rADI}_j = w_j^H \mathrm{ADI}_j$. When attributes are used more than those with the least uses, items for all attributes that have been selected the least are no longer selected. That is, $\mathrm{rCDI}_j = 0$ and $\mathrm{rADI}_j = 0$.

2.2 *Simulation Design*

To compare the study results with those of Kuo et al. (2016), the setting of the simulation was similar to that of their study. The number of attributes (K) was fixed at seven. The simulation study investigated three factors: attribute hierarchy (six levels; nonhierarchical, unstructured convergent, unstructured divergent, convergent, divergent, and linear), test construction method (seven levels; Random, CDI, ADI, MCDI, MADI, rCDI, and rADI), and test length (three levels; 10, 20, and 30 items). Six attribute hierarchies H_0, H_1, ..., and H_5 in Fig. 1 were considered to examine how the proposed indices performed when attributes had different hierarchical relationships.

The reduced Q matrix was used for different hierarchies. When the attributes had a nonhierarchical relationship (i.e., H_0), the number of potential item types (i.e., items with unique attribute specifications) was equal to $2^K - 1$ (127 item types). When the attributes had a linear relationship (i.e., H_5), the resulting reduced Q matrix had only seven item types. Regarding the remaining hierarchy levels, the numbers of unique item types were 64 for H_1 and H_2, and 26 for H_3 and H_4. For each item type, 30 items were generated to form different item banks when attributes had different hierarchical relationships. The slip and guessing parameters were set to .05. The number of examinee types is equal to 2^K (128 attribute patterns). For each attribute pattern, 130 examinees were generated when attributes had different hierarchical relationships. The total number of examinees was 16,640

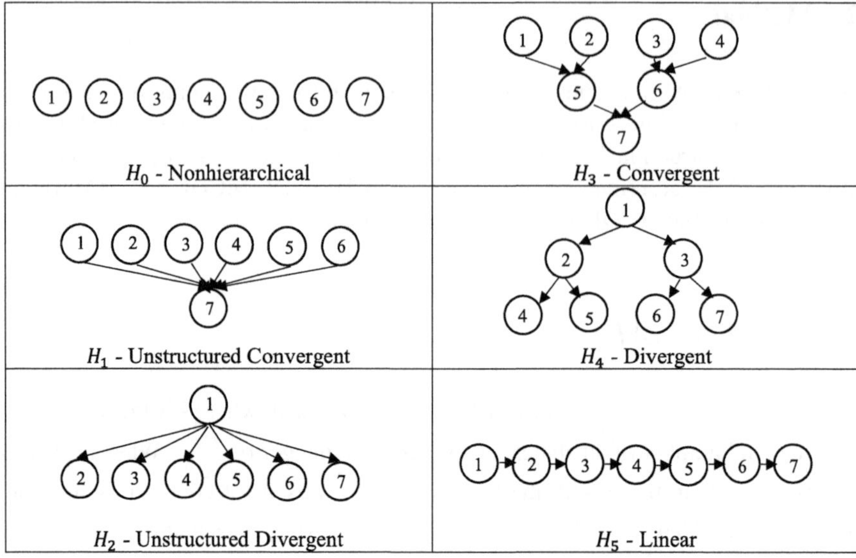

Fig. 1 Attribute hierarchies in the simulation studies

for all conditions. All item responses were generated according to Eq. (1). In the simulation study, different test lengths (i.e., 10, 20, and 30 items) were selected sequentially from hierarchical item banks (i.e., H_0, H_1, ..., and H_5) based on the various test construction methods (i.e., indices). Except for items that were selected randomly (i.e., Random), for all algorithms, items with the largest CDI, ADI, MCDI, MADI, rCDI, or rADI were selected. Each examinee attribute pattern was estimated using expected a posteriori estimation. To minimize the possible impact of Monte Carlo errors, 100 replications were considered for each condition. Finally, the evaluation criteria, including the ACCR, PCCR, and ACCR of the kth attribute, were computed based on 100 replications.

3 Results

Owing to spatial limitations, the results for the 10-item condition under H_0 and H_5 are shown in Tables 1 and 2. The numbers of times k-attribute items were used in the 10-item conditions under H_0 and H_5 are listed in Table 1. Under H_0, Random had an ACCR of 72% and PCCR of 17%; the CDI and ADI had an ACCR of 85% and PCCR of 31%; and the MCDI, MADI, rCDI, and rADI had an ACCR of 95% and PCCR of 70–71%. In line with previous studies, Random tended to select items with different attribute numbers. The CDI, ADI, rCDI, and rADI tended to select items with one attribute. The MCDI and MADI tended to select items with one or two attributes, regardless of test length. Under H_5, Random had an ACCR of 96%

Table 1 Numbers of times k-attribute items were used in the 10-item conditions under H_0 and H_5

				k-attribute items						
Structure	Method	ACCR	PCCR	1	2	3	4	5	6	7
H_0	Random	.72	.17	0.63	1.73	2.73	2.65	1.57	0.62	0.07
	CDI	.85	.31	10	0	0	0	0	0	0
	ADI	.85	.31	10	0	0	0	0	0	0
	MCDI	.95	.70	7	3	0	0	0	0	0
	MADI	.95	.71	7	3	0	0	0	0	0
	rCDI	.95	.70	10	0	0	0	0	0	0
	rADI	.95	.70	10	0	0	0	0	0	0
H_5	Random	.96	.74	1.47.	1.44	1.33	1.43	1.30	1.45	1.58
	CDI	.86	.25	0	0	0	10	0	0	0
	ADI	.79	.25	10	0	0	0	0	0	0
	MCDI	.98	.89	1	1	2	2	2	1	1
	MADI	.98	.89	3	2	1	1	1	1	1
	rCDI	.92	.60	0	0	0	3	3	2	2
	rADI	.98	.88	2	2	2	1	1	1	1

Table 2 Accuracy of the various indices in correctly classifying the kth attribute in the 10-item conditions under H_0 and H_5

		kth attribute						
Structure	Method	1	2	3	4	5	6	7
H_0	Random	.71	.73	.73	.71	.73	.72	.73
	CDI	.88	.84	.87	.83	.88	.88	.81
	ADI	.88	.84	.87	.83	.88	.88	.81
	MCDI	.95	.95	.95	.95	.95	.95	.95
	MADI	.95	.95	.95	.95	.95	.95	.95
	rCDI	.95	.95	.95	.95	.95	.95	.95
	rADI	.95	.95	.95	.95	.95	.95	.95
H_5	Random	.96	.96	.95	.96	.95	.96	.97
	CDI	.88	.75	.87	1.00	.87	.75	.88
	ADI	1.00	.87	.75	.62	.62	.75	.88
	MCDI	.98	.98	.99	.99	.99	.98	.98
	MADI	.99	.99	.99	.98	.97	.97	.98
	rCDI	.88	.75	.87	1.00	1.00	.99	.99
	rADI	.99	.99	.99	.98	.97	.97	.98

and PCCR of 74%; the CDI and ADI had an ACCR of 79%–86% and PCCR of 25%; the MCDI and MADI had an ACCR of 98% and PCCR of 89%; and the rCDI and rADI had an ACCR of 92%–98% and PCCR of 60%–88%. In line with previous studies, Random tended to select items with different attribute numbers. The CDI tended to select items with four attributes, and the ADI tended to select items with one attribute. The MCDI, MADI, and rADI tended to select items with one to seven attributes, and the rCDI tended to select items with four to seven attributes. Generally, all indices had higher ACCRs and PCCRs in the 30-item conditions than in the 10-item conditions. When the test length was 30 items, the MCDI and MADI did not select more items with attributes that required more prior knowledge under H_5.

To reveal the efficiency of the revised indices for item selection, the accuracy levels of the *k*th attribute in the 10-item conditions under H_0 and H_5 are listed in Table 2. Under H_0, Random had an ACCR of over 71% for each attribute; the CDI and ADI had an ACCR of over 81% for each attribute; and the MCDI, MADI, rCDI, and rADI had an ACCR of 95% for each attribute. Under H_5, Random, CDI, and ADI had ACCRs of over 95%, 81%, and 62%, respectively, for each attribute, and the MCDI, MADI, rCDI, and rADI had an ACCR of 97% for each attribute. Generally, all indices had higher ACCRs for each attribute in the 30-item conditions than in the 10-item conditions. When attributes had a linear structure, the rCDI and rADI outperformed the other indices in correctly classifying the seventh attribute that required more prior knowledge than the other attributes.

4 Discussion

Although the rCDI and rADI outperformed the other indices in correctly classifying the attribute that required more prior knowledge than the other attributes when attributes had a linear structure, the rCDI had slightly lower ACCRs for some attributes. Modifying the rCDI and rADI algorithms during item selection is crucial. This study investigated the measurement efficiency of the revised indices in relation to the DINA model. Researchers of previous studies have used numerous CDMs, such as the DINO, the NIDA, and the rRUM. Investigating the performance of the two revised indices in different CDMs is of great interest. In this study, item parameters s and g were equal to .05, indicating that the test was of a high quality. The revised indices might perform differently when s and g are large, indicating that the test was of a low quality. To compare the results with those of Kuo et al. (2016), the number of attributes was set to seven. In practice, an operational test might have a different attribute structure. In the future, the performance of the revised indices in the operational testing environment should be investigated.

References

Chang, H., & Ying, Z. (1996). A global information approach to computerized adaptive testing. *Applied Psychological Measurement, 20*, 213–229.

Finkelman, M., Kim, W., & Roussos, L. A. (2009). Automated test assembly for cognitive diagnosis models using a genetic algorithm. *Journal of Educational Measurement, 46*(3), 273–292. https://doi.org/10.1111/j.1745-3984.2009.00081.x

Finkelman, M. D., Kim, W., Roussos, L., & Verschoor, A. (2010). A binary programming approach to automated test assembly for cognitive diagnosis models. *Applied Psychological Measurement, 34*(5), 310–326. https://doi.org/10.1177/0146621609344844

Haertel, E. H. (1989). Using restricted latent class models to map the skill structure of achievement items. *Journal of Educational Measurement, 26*, 333–352.

Henson, R. A., & Douglas, J. (2005). Test construction for cognitive diagnostics. *Applied Psychological Measurement, 29*(4), 262–277. https://doi.org/10.1177/0146621604272623

Henson, R. A., Roussos, L., Douglas, J., & He, X. (2008). Cognitive diagnostic attribute-level discrimination indices. *Applied Psychological Measurement, 32*(4), 275–288. https://doi.org/10.1177/0146621607302478

Henson, R. A., Templin, J. L., & Willse, J. T. (2009). Defining a family of cognitive diagnosis models using log-linear models with latent variables. *Psychometrika, 74*, 191–210.

Junker, B. W., & Sijtsma, K. (2001). Cognitive assessment models with few assumptions, and connections with nonparametric item response theory. *Applied Psychological Measurement, 25*, 258–272.

Kuo, B.-C., Pai, H.-S., & de la Torre, J. (2016). Modified cognitive diagnostic index and modified attribute level discrimination index for test construction. *Applied Psychological Measurement, 40*(5), 315–330. https://doi.org/10.1177/0146621616638643

Leighton, J. P., Gierl, M. J., & Hunka, S. (2004). The attribute hierarchy model: An approach for integrating cognitive theory with assessment practice. *Journal of Educational Measurement, 41*, 205–236.

Liu, J., Xu, G., & Ying, Z. (2013). Theory of the self-learning Q-matrix. *Bernoulli: official journal of the Bernoulli Society for Mathematical Statistics and Probability, 19*(5A), 1790–1817. https://doi.org/10.3150/12-BEJ430

Maris, E. (1999). Estimating multiple classification latent class models. *Psychometrika, 64*, 87–212.

Roussos, L. A., DiBello, L. V., Stout, W., Hartz, S. M., Henson, R. A., & Templin, J. L. (2007). The fusion model skills diagnosis system. In J. P. Leighton & M. J. Gierl (Eds.), *Cognitive diagnostic assessment for education: Theory and applications* (pp. 275–318). Cambridge University Press.

Templin, J., & Henson, R. (2006). Measurement of psychological disorders using cognitive diagnosis models. *Psychological Methods, 11*(3), 287–305. https://doi.org/10.1037/1082-989X.11.3.287

Zheng, C.-J., & Chang, H.-H. (2016). High-efficiency response distribution–based item selection algorithms for short-length cognitive diagnostic computerized adaptive testing. *Applied Psychological Measurement, 40*(8), 608–624. https://doi.org/10.1177/0146621616665196

Exploring Temporal Functional Dependencies Between Latent Skills in Cognitive Diagnostic Models

Athul Sudheesh and Richard M. Golden

In classroom settings, we often infer changes in a student's abilities by observing their behavior through formative assessments (Black & Wiliam, 1998) and summative assessments. The role of these assessments are to elicit responses from the students for the purpose of determining student knowledge states, ability factors, and skill profiles. Formative assessments are the low-stakes assessment that involve collecting student item responses for improving classroom student learning while summative assessments are the high-stakes assessment events that involve collecting student item responses for evaluating and ranking student learning achievements at the end of an instructional unit (AERA, APA, & NCME, 2014). A recent approach that combines the diagnostic nature of formative assessments with test properties of the high-stakes summative assessments are Cognitive Diagnostic Assessments (Leighton & Gierl, 2007).

Cognitive Diagnostic Assessments (CDAs) are fundamentally different from traditional educational assessments in the way the student's ability parameters are estimated. A traditional educational assessment which follows Classical Test Theory (CTT) or Item Response Theory (IRT) makes the strong assumption that a student's ability may be represented as a number along a one-dimensional proficiency continuum. On the other hand, CDAs uses an alternative psychometric framework referred to as Cognitive Diagnostic Models (CDMs) or Diagnostic Classification Models (DCMs), which assume that a student's ability is not represented as a numerical value but rather as a collection of latent skills that can be either present or absent.

More specifically, Cognitive Diagnostic Models (CDMs) are constrained latent class models that provide diagnostic information about a subject's skill profile

A. Sudheesh (✉) · R. M. Golden
Cognitive Informatics and Statistics Lab, School of Behavioral and Brain Sciences, The University of Texas at Dallas, Richardson, TX, USA
e-mail: Athul.Sudheesh@utdallas.edu

M. Wiberg et al. (eds.), *Quantitative Psychology*, Springer Proceedings in Mathematics & Statistics 353, https://doi.org/10.1007/978-3-030-74772-5_23

Table 1 Sample Q Matrix. The first row of this Q-Matrix specifies that item 95 requires the students to have the skill "Addition" to answer it correctly

ID	Addition	Multiplication	Multiplying-decimals	Pattern-finding
95	1	0	0	0
96	0	0	0	1
133	0	1	0	0
145	0	0	1	0
161	0	1	0	0

by specifying the relationship between the student's latent skill model, test item characteristics, and student's responses to those items as a function of discrete latent variables. A CDM can be formally represented as:

$$P_{ij} = f\left(\alpha_i, \beta_j, q_j\right) \tag{1}$$

where P_{ij} is the probability the ith student answers the jth item correctly. The latent skill vector for the ith student, $\boldsymbol{\alpha}_i = [\alpha_{i1}, \alpha_{i2}, \ldots, \alpha_{ik}]$, is defined such that the kth latent skill, $\alpha_{ik} = 0$ or 1 represents respectively the absence or presence of kth latent skill for ith student. The item specific parameter vector β_j specifies how the ith student's latent skill profile $\boldsymbol{\alpha}_i$ influences the probability the ith student answers the jth item correctly. The jth row vector in the **Q** matrix (Tatsuoka, 1983), $\mathbf{q}_j = \left[q_{j1,}q_{j2}, \ldots, q_{jk}\right]$ specifies the skill requirements for answering the jth item correctly (i.e., $q_{jk} = 1$ if correctly answering the jth question requires the kth latent skill, see Table 1).

Depending on the skill requirement conditions of the model, CDMs can be broadly classified into compensatory, non-compensatory, and general models. Compensatory CDMs are models which assume that some skills can act as proxies for the absence of some other set of latent skills (i.e., a student doesn't require all of the skills as specified by $\mathbf{q}_j$ to correctly answer the jth item). An example compensatory CDM is the DINO (Deterministic Input Noisy "OR" gate) model (Templin & Henson, 2006). Non-compensatory CDMs, on the other hand, assume that all skills as specified by $\mathbf{q}_j$ are required to correctly answer the jth item. For example, the DINA (Deterministic Input Noisy "AND" gate) model is a non-compensatory CDM (de la Torre, 2009). General models like the generalized-DINA (GDINA) models (de la Torre, 2011) are more flexible models that make fewer assumptions regarding how skill requirements impact mastery probability estimation. The mathematical formulations of DINA, DINO & GDINA are listed in Table 2.

Although traditional CDMs like these provide excellent diagnostic information regarding a subject's skill profile, these models often assume that every learning/assessment event is static and independent of each other. However, we know that learning is a latent sequential dynamic process and hence to study such processes we may require statistical models that acknowledge this longitudinal nature.

Table 2 CDMs and their mathematical formulations. The item response probability function (P_{ij}) in DINA, DINO, and GDINA specifies the probability of the ith student answering the jth item correctly. In the DINA and DINO models, the guess parameter g_j and the slip parameter s_j are the item-specific parameters of the jth item. In GDINA model, δ_{j0} is the jth item intercept, δ_{jk} are the main effects due to α_k, $\delta_{jkk'}$ are the two-way interaction effects due to α_k and $\alpha_{k'}$ and $\delta_{j12...K_j}$ are the K_j-way interaction effects due to α_1 through $\alpha_{k'_j}$

Model	Item-response probability function
DINA	$P_{ij} = g_j^{1-\eta_{ij}} (1 - s_j)^{\eta_{ij}}$ where $\eta_{ij} = \prod_k \alpha_{ik}^{q_{ik}}$
DINO	$P_{ij} = g_j^{1-\eta_{ij}} (1 - s_j)^{\eta_{ij}}$ where $\eta_{ij} = 1 - \prod_k (1 - \alpha_{ik})^{q_{jk}}$
GDINA	$P_{ij} = \delta_{j0} + \sum_k \delta_{jk}\alpha_{ik} + \sum_{k'} \sum_k \delta_{jkk'}\alpha_{ik'}\alpha_{ik} + ... + \delta_{j12L...K_j} \prod_k \alpha_{ik}$

Latent Transition Analysis (LTA) uses a special type of statistical model to study latent sequential dynamic processes. LTA was initially developed by Collins & Wugalter (1992) to study stage sequential change in dynamic latent variables like attitudes and personality traits. In a LTA model, three groups of parameters are estimated: (1) transition probabilities, (2) latent skill mastery probability or class membership probabilities, and (3) emission probabilities. The latent transition probability $P(\alpha_{t+1} | \alpha_t)$ specifies the conditional probability of a student transitioning to a future latent class state given the current latent class state. The latent skill mastery probability $P(\boldsymbol{\alpha}_i | X_i)$ specifies the likelihood of mastering the latent skills given the student's item responses. The emission probability $P\left(X_{ij} = 1 | \boldsymbol{\alpha}_i\right)$ specifies the probability, P_{ij}, of the ith student correctly answering the jth item given their latent skill mastery profile vector $\boldsymbol{\alpha}_i$.

Recent approaches which combine LTA with CDMs in the context of an educational setting include Li, Cohen, Bottge, & Templin (2016), Kaya and Leite (2017), and Madison and Bradshaw (2018). Li et al. (2016) combined the LTA model with a DINA model to assess the effect of instructional strategy on transition probabilities. They found that different instructions could have similar or different associated transition probabilities depending on the nature of the instructional strategy. Kaya and Leite (2017) conducted simulation studies using LTA-DINA and LTA-DINO to find the effect of item parameters and sample size on these longitudinal models. They found that sample size didn't affect the classification rates for small values of item parameters (guess and slip) but had a poor classification rate for small sample sizes when the item parameters had values greater than 0.4. Madison and Bradshaw (2018) proposed a more generalized longitudinal CDM called the Transition Diagnostic Classification Model (TDCM) by combining latent transition analysis with the log-linear cognitive diagnostic model.

All these studies (Li et al., 2016, Kaya & Leite, 2017; Madison & Bradshaw, 2018) in general investigated how latent skill mastery probabilities changed from a pre-test scenario to a post-test scenario in a multi-wave experimental design. For computational tractability, all these models assumed that the latent skills evolved independently. In longitudinal studies, latent skills are said to evolve independently when the probability that a latent skill is present at the current assessment time point is functionally dependent only upon whether or not that particular latent skill was present at the previous assessment time point. When one assumes that latent skills evolve independently, one might also implicitly assume that the latent skills within an assessment point are not correlated. While one could argue that these assumptions might be appropriate in a multi-wave pre-test post-test longitudinal analysis like the one conducted in the above studies, they may or may not hold for the longitudinal assessments conducted in a semester-long course. We explore such assumptions with this study.

In this study, we use the ASSISTment Math 2004–2005 dataset accessed via DataShop (Koedinger et al., 2010) to investigate whether latent skill profiles assessed at one time period are predictive of latent skill profiles at a future time period. In addition, we also wanted to investigate the hypothesis that latent skills evolve independently between assessment points and are not correlated within an assessment time point.

1 Methods

1.1 Dataset Description

ASSISTment is an Online Tutoring System (OTS) developed to improve instruction by providing instant, scaffolded feedback to students. ASSISTment Math 2004–2005 is the data collected from 8th-grade students who took tests in the OTS once every two weeks between September 2004 and March 2005. On an average each student was assessed 13 times (*Maximum* =13, *Minimum* =12, *Mode* =13) and each assessment time period assessed different group of latent skills where the number of latent skills in each group was different. The data include the student's ID, item ID, whether their first attempt was correct, whether they used the hint provided by the OTS, and test start and end times. The test items were annotated with 106 latent skills by a subject matter expert.

1.2 Data Preprocessing/Design

The raw data were first grouped by the finish time to separate the assessments at different time points. Data in each group represents the item-response of students for a particular administration week. Each row of the item-response matrix corresponds to whether a student has successfully answered an item, and each column represents the item IDs. For the purpose of reliable parameter estimation, only latent skills that were assessed more than ten times were considered. The **Q** matrix was generated from the skill model annotation document that was provided with the raw dataset. A sample of the extracted **Q** matrix is shown in Table 1.

1.3 Parameter Estimation and Model Selection

The GDINA R package (Ma and de la Torre, 2020) was used to estimate the latent skill profiles of students at four assessment time points: 1 Oct. 2004, 15 Oct. 2004, 19 Nov. 2004 & 10 Dec. 2004. The GDINA R package implements Maximum Likelihood Estimation (MLE) via Expectation Maximization (EM) described in Bock & Aitkin (1981), to handle the latent variable parameter estimation problem in the presence of missing data. The item response data at each assessment point was fitted separately to each of the DINA, DINO, and GDINA models. Then the Bayes Factor (BF) of competing models were calculated using a BIC approximation for each assessment time point using Equation 2 (Jarosz & Wiley, 2014; Kass & Raftery, 1995; Raftery, 1995; Golden, 2020). For all assessment time points, we considered GDINA as the null hypothesis H_0. Raftery (1995) suggests that while BF values in the range of $1-3$ and $3-20$ imply weak and positive evidence in favor of the alternative hypothesis H_1 respectively, values in the range of $20-150$ and values beyond 150 imply strong and very strong evidence in favor of H_1 respectively (Jarosz & Wiley, 2014).

$$BF = \frac{\text{likelihood of data given } H_1}{\text{likelihood of data given } H_0} = e^{0.5\times(BIC_0 - BIC_1)} \tag{2}$$

1.4 Correlation Analysis

The within assessment correlation analysis was conducted by first computing the covariance matrix from the estimated latent skill mastery probability vectors ($P_1,\ P_2, \ldots P_n$, where the jth element of P_i, p_{ij}, represents the estimated probability of ith student mastering jth skill and n is the total number of students e.g., Fig. 1) from DINA and then converting the covariance matrix to a correlation matrix.

To investigate the hypothesis that latent skills evolve independently between assessment points (and hence not correlated between assessment time points), we used a logistic regression model to predict the latent skill MAP (maximum a posteriori) estimate vector of students at a particular time point ($A_i(t) = [\alpha_{i1}(t), \ldots\alpha_{ik}(t)]$, where $\alpha_{ik}(t)$ specifies the presence or absence of kth skill in ith student at time t) from the latent skill MAP estimate vector of students at a previous time point ($A_i(t-1)$). Time periods considered for this analysis include: 1 Oct. - 15 Oct., 1 Oct. - 19 Nov., 1 Oct. - 10 Dec., 15 Oct. - 19 Nov., 15 Oct. - 10 Dec. & 19 Nov. - 10 Dec. The fitted logistic regression models were further tested for model misspecification using the RobustSE R package, which implements the Generalized Information Matrix Test (GIMT) (White, 1982; Golden, Henley, White, & Kashner, 2016) discussed in King & Roberts (2015).

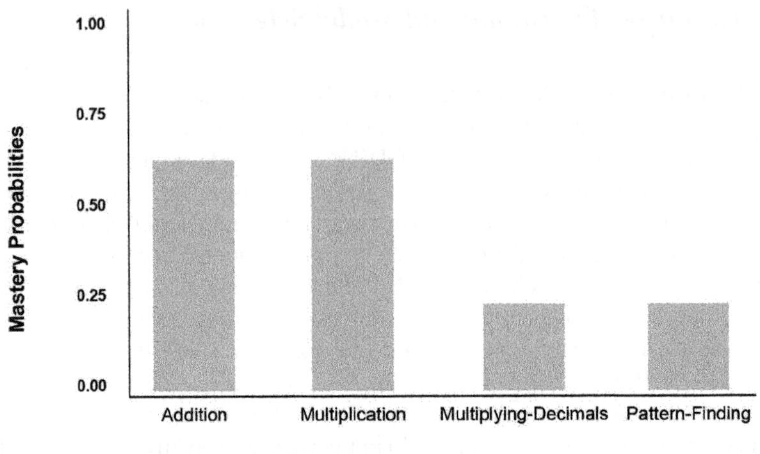

Fig. 1 Probability of skill mastery as a function of latent skill type. In this example, the cognitive diagnostic model estimates the probabilities of the "Addition" and "Multiplication" latent skill to be greater than the other latent skills

2 Results

To estimate the latent skill profile of students at each of the four assessment points considered, the GDINA R package was used to fit the data with all three DINA, DINO and GDINA models. In this analysis, we found that the DINA model had the lowest BIC score for each of the assessment time points but autoGDINA (fitting CDMs on item-level basis) had the highest classification accuracy. In Bayesian hypothesis testing, we found very strong evidence supporting the DINA model for all time points except Oct 1. For Oct 1. assessment data, all models (GDINA, DINA & DINO) were equally preferred. The model fit statistics of DINA, DINO, and GDINA at different assessment time points are listed in Table 3.

In the within assessment correlation analysis, we found that the latent skills are highly correlated regardless of the assessment time point. Figure 2 plots Pearson product-moment correlations between latent skills within an assessment for Oct 15, 2004 and Dec 10, 2004.

In the temporal correlation analysis, we found that a considerable number of latent skills were correlated between two assessment time points. Furthermore, we also found an increase in the number of temporal correlations when the gap between a pair of assessment time points is more than six weeks (i.e., we found considerably more absolute Z scores significant ($p < 0.05$) when predicting 10 Dec. 2004 from 15 Oct. 2004 compared to when predicting 10 Dec. 2004 from 19 Nov. 2004). Figure 3 plots the absolute Z-score of logistic regression models predicting latent skill MAP estimate vectors for 10 Dec. 2004 from 15 Oct. 2004.

Table 3 Model Comparison. The model fit statistics of DINA, DINO, and GDINA at different time points. For Bayesian hypothesis testing, GDINA was considered as the H_0 at all time points

Time point	Model	No. of skills	BIC	BF
1 Oct. 2004	GDINA	4	1255.4	1
	DINA	4	1255.4	1
	DINO	4	1255.4	1
15 Oct. 2004	GDINA	7	3514.15	1
	DINA	7	3446.89	4.03×10^{14}
	DINO	7	3459.37	7.85×10^{11}
19 Nov. 2004	GDINA	13	37544.37	1
	DINA	13	36346.39	1.37×10^{260}
	DINO	13	37416.64	5.44×10^{27}
10 Dec. 2004	GDINA	16	264265.32	1
	DINA	16	264114.55	5.48×10^{32}
	DINO	16	264117.86	1.04×10^{32}

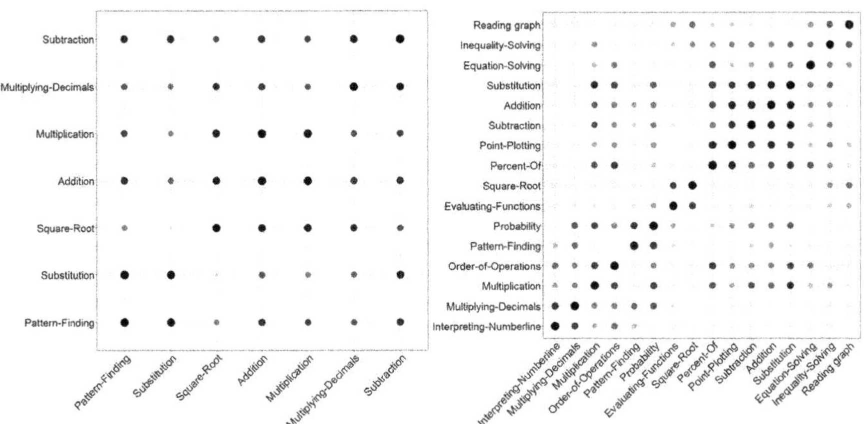

Fig. 2 Pearson product-moment correlation between latent skills within an assessment. The plot on the left shows that the correlation between latent skills at assessment time point 15 October 2004 are prevalent and plot on the right shows that the correlation between latent skills at assessment time point 10 December 2004 are more prevalent. Displayed correlations indicated by darker dots are significant ($p < 0.05$). The size of the dots corresponds to their correlation strength

3 Discussion

In this study, we found that latent skills are correlated not only within assessments but also between assessments. These findings clearly challenge common cognitive diagnostic longitudinal modeling assumptions (e.g., Li et al., 2016; Kaya & Leite, 2017; Madison & Bradshaw, 2018). In particular, it is common in cognitive

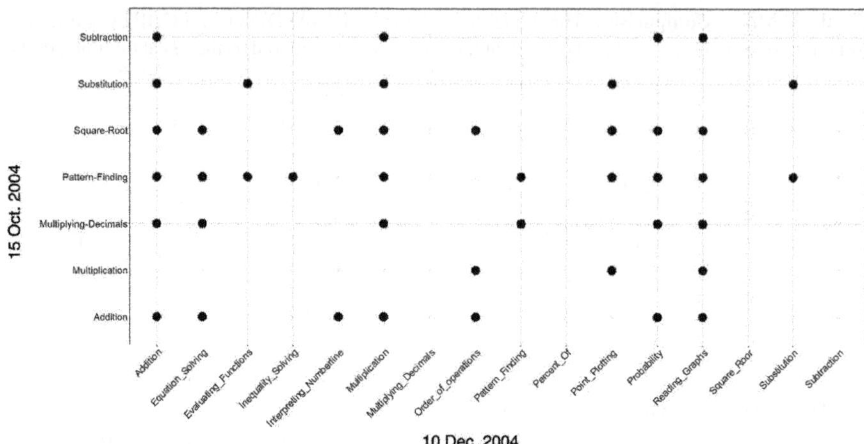

Fig. 3 Effects of estimated latent skills at a prior assessment time period on estimated latent skills at a future assessment time period. The skills listed on the vertical axis were assessed at time point 15 Oct. 2004 and the skills listed on the horizontal axis were assessed at time point 10 Dec. 2004. Displayed dots represent absolute Z-score values that were significant ($p < 0.05$)

diagnostic assessments to assume that one item can only assess one skill. However, the results of the within assessment correlation analysis in this study provide evidence against this assumption.

Furthermore, most current longitudinal CDMs assume that the growth trajectory of each latent skill is independent of each other and measurement invariance is present. The results of this study suggest that the assumption of independent growth trajectories should be more carefully examined in future applications of longitudinal assessments. Longitudinal classroom assessments heavily challenge the measurement invariance assumption, because in a noncumulative assessment series, students will be assessed with a different set of latent skills for each assessment.

One interesting and unexpected result was that the latent skills previously estimated at a prior time period were more predictive of the estimated latent skills at a future time period when the time period was six weeks rather than four weeks or two weeks. One possible explanation might be that for this online learning system, six weeks is an appropriate time period for reliably estimating temporal associations between latent skill profiles estimated at different assessment periods. An alternative explanation is that estimation of temporal associations between latent skill profiles at different assessment periods were confounded because Razzaq et al. (2005) notes that it is possible that students received more difficult items during the first assessment time period.

In this study, we used item response data from an intelligent tutoring system due to the lack of publicly available open traditional-semester-long student response dataset. It would be interesting to replicate the findings in this study with traditional semester/year-long course dataset. Another limitation of this analysis is that temporal dependencies were estimated using a two-stage process. First, MAP estimates of latent skill presence indicators at all time points were estimated. Second, logistic regression analyses were then used to explore temporal dependencies between estimated latent skill presence indicators at different assessment time periods as well as degrees of association between latent skill presence indicators at a particular assessment time period. This type of analysis ignores the presence of sampling error associated with the MAP estimates of the latent skill presence indicators.

On the other hand, despite the deliberate omission of latent skill presence indicator sampling error, the analysis presented here is very straightforward and transparent which makes the results in some cases more interpretable than more sophisticated longitudinal cognitive diagnostic modeling methods. We believe that complementary analyses such as the one presented here are useful for identifying qualitative features of the data generating process without making excessively strong modeling assumptions.

These findings in this paper suggest that it may be helpful to develop longitudinal cognitive diagnostic models that allow for more complex temporal dependencies and possibly more complex skill hierarchies. Another future direction is the development of algorithms to estimate longitudinal cognitive diagnostic model parameters without the assumption of full measurement invariance.

Acknowledgments This project was partially funded by the University of Texas at Dallas Office of Research through the Social Sciences SEED Program.

References

AERA, APA, & NCME. (2014). *Standards for educational and psychological testing*: Washington, DC

Black, P., & Wiliam, D. (1998). Assessment and classroom learning. *Assessment in Education: Principles Policy & Practice, 5*(1), 7–74

Bock, R. D., & Aitkin, M. (1981). Marginal maximum likelihood estimation of item parameters: Application of an EM algorithm. *Psychometrika, 46*(4), 443–459. http://dx.doi.org/10.1007/bf02293801

Collins, L. M., & Wugalter, S. E. (1992). Latent class models for stage-sequential dynamic latent variables. *Multivariate Behavioral Research, 27*(1), 131–157

de la Torre, J. (2009). DINA model and parameter estimation: a didactic. *Journal of Educational and Behavioral Statistics, 34*, 115–130

de la Torre, J. (2011). The generalized DINA model framework. *Psychometrika, 76*, 179–199

Golden, R. M. (2020). *Statistical machine learning: A unified framework*. CRC Press

Golden, R. M., Henley, S. S., White, H., & Kashner, T. M. (2016). Generalized information matrix tests for detecting model misspecification. *Econometrics, 4*(4), 46

Jarosz, A. F. & Wiley, J. (2014). What are the odds? A practical guide to computing and reporting bayes factors. *The Journal of Problem Solving, 7*, 2–9

Kass, R. E. & Raftery, A. E. (1995). Bayes factors. *Journal of the American Statistical Association, 90*(430), 773–795

Kaya, Y. & Leite, W. (2017). Assessing change in latent skills across time with longitudinal cognitive diagnosis modeling: An evaluation of model performance. *Educational and Psychological Measurement, 77*, 369–388

King, G., & Roberts, M. E. (2015). How robust standard errors expose methodological problems they do not fix, and what to do about it. *Political Analysis*, 159–179

Koedinger, K. R., d. Baker, R. S., Cunningham, K., Skogsholm, A., Leber, B., & Stamper, J. (2010). A data repository for the EDM community: The PSLC DataShop. In C. Romero et al. (Eds.), *Handbook of Educational Data Mining*. CRC Press

Leighton, J., & Gierl, M. (2007). *Cognitive diagnostic assessment for education: Theory and applications*. Cambridge University Press

Li, F., Cohen, A., Bottge, B. A., & Templin, J. L. (2016). A latent transition analysis model for assessing change in cognitive skills. *Educational and Psychological Measurement, 76*, 181–204

Ma, W., & Torre, J. de la. (2020). GDINA: An R package for cognitive diagnosis modeling. *Journal of Statistical Software, 93*(14), 1–26

Madison, M. J., & Bradshaw, L. (2018). Assessing growth in a diagnostic classification model framework. *Psychometrika, 83*, 963–990

Raftery, A. E. (1995). Bayesian model selection in social research. *Sociological Methodology, 25*, 111–163

Razzaq, L. M., Feng, M., Nuzzo-Jones, G., Heffernan, N. T., Koedinger, K. R., Junker, B., et al. (2005). Blending assessment and instructional assisting. In *Proceedings of the 12th International Conference on Artificial Intelligence in Education* (pp. 555–562)

Tatsuoka, K. K. (1983). Rule space: An approach for dealing with misconceptions based on item response theory. *Journal of Educational Measurement, 20*(4), 345–354

Templin, J. L. & Henson, R. A. (2006). Measurement of psychological disorders using cognitive diagnosis models. *Psychological Methods, 11*(3), 287–305

White, H. (1982). Maximum likelihood estimation of misspecified models. *Econometrica: Journal of the Econometric Society, 50*(1), 1–25

Sample Size for Latent Dirichlet Allocation of Constructed-Response Items

Jordan M. Wheeler, Allan S. Cohen, Jiawei Xiong, Juyeon Lee, and Hye-Jeong Choi

1 Introduction

Topic models are machine learning algorithms that use a statistical framework to cluster words and documents by deriving latent topics within the underlying semantic space. Topic models were originally developed as an indexing technique to aid information retrieval algorithm and have been used in many disciplines. Topic models work by assuming that documents are a mixture over latent topics where the latent topics are a mixture over words (Steyvers & Griffiths, 2007). Some of the earliest topic models include Latent Semantic Analysis (LSA; Deerwester, Dumais, Furnas, Landauer, & Harshman, 1990), probabilistic Latent Semantic Indexing (pLSI Hofmann, 1999), and Latent Dirichlet Allocation (LDA; Blei, Ng, & Jordan, 2003).

LSA has been used in educational measurement as the basis to many automated essay scoring algorithms due to its high human-machine score agreement (Landauer, Foltz, & Laham, 1998). LDA has been used more recently in educational research to measure the semantic features of a collection of essays that respond to a constructed-response (CR) item (e.g., Buxton et al., 2014; Choi et al., 2019; Xiong, Choi, Kim, Kwak, & Cohen, 2019). Although LDA has shown promising results, it was originally developed for large data sets that contain a large number of latent topics. CR items, especially short answer CR items, typically contain smaller data sets with few words and fewer topics, causing there to be little investigation about LDA's statistical properties when used on CR items.

In this study, we set up a foundation to implement simulation studies using the LDA topic model by presenting the probabilistic and generative LDA models,

J. M. Wheeler (✉) · A. S. Cohen · J. Xiong · J. Lee · H.-J. Choi
The University of Georgia, Athens, GA, USA
e-mail: jmwheeler@uga.edu; acohen@uga.edu; Jiawei.Xiong@uga.edu; juyeon.lee25@uga.edu; hjchoi1@uga.edu

M. Wiberg et al. (eds.), *Quantitative Psychology*, Springer Proceedings in Mathematics & Statistics 353, https://doi.org/10.1007/978-3-030-74772-5_24

discussing how to generate data from an LDA model, and how to evaluate parameter recovery along with potential issues with estimating the LDA model. Then we present a simulation study that investigated the number of documents at varying lengths needed to accurately recover the parameters of the LDA model. Finally, we discuss how this LDA model can be used to enhance educators' understandings of essays written by students.

2 Simulations for Latent Dirichlet Allocation

This section lays out the necessary steps for conducting an LDA simulation study: defining the model and its components, generating the simulated data, estimating the model, and evaluating performance.

2.1 *Latent Dirichlet Allocation (LDA)*

The LDA model estimates three parameters from a corpus of essays: topics $\boldsymbol{\beta}$, topic proportions $\boldsymbol{\theta}$, and topic assignments z. Topics are distributions over the vocabulary V, which is defined as all unique words across all essays. The topic distributions express the probability of each word occurring under the given topic. Topic proportions are distributions over the topics that expresses the proportion of each topic used in a given essay. Topic assignments are the individual topics assigned to each word in every essay.

LDA is considered a hierarchical mixture model. The hierarchical structure is due to the topic distributions being corpus-wide latent parameters (i.e., upper level), and the topic proportions and topic assignments are essay-wide latent parameters (i.e., lower level). The mixture component of LDA is due to the topics being a mixture of words and the essays being a mixture of the latent topics, shown by topic distributions and a document's topic proportions, respectively.

The latent topics identify major themes throughout the corpus. In the case of CR items, the latent topics identify key information seen throughout all responses, which are typical constrained by the item (Kim, Kwak, Cardozo-Gaibisso, Buxton, & Cohen, 2017). The topic proportions cluster the essays in the corpus and identifies which topics each student focused on. Topic proportions can be used aid instructional prescription or to measure the effectiveness of an intervention (e.g., Cardozo-Gaibisso, Kim, Buxton, & Cohen, 2019; Duong, Mellom, & Hixon, 2019).

The latent topics, topic proportions, and topic assignments are estimated through the joint posterior distribution of the LDA model defined as

$$P(\boldsymbol{\theta}, \boldsymbol{\beta}, z, w|\eta, \nu) \propto \prod_{k=1}^{K} P(\boldsymbol{\beta}_k|\nu) \prod_{d=1}^{D} \left(P(\boldsymbol{\theta}_d|\eta) \prod_{n=1}^{N^{(d)}} P(w_{d,n}, z_{d,n}|\boldsymbol{\theta}_d, \boldsymbol{\beta}) \right), \tag{1}$$

where K is the number of topics, D is the number of essays, $N^{(d)}$ is the number of words in essay d, and $\prod_{k=1}^{K} P(\boldsymbol{\beta}_k|\nu)$ is the topic prior distribution, $\prod_{d=1}^{D} P(\boldsymbol{\theta}_d|\eta)$ is the topic proportion prior distribution, and $\prod_{n=1}^{N^{(d)}} P(w_{d,n}, z_{d,n}|\boldsymbol{\theta}_d, \boldsymbol{\beta})$ is the joint likelihood distribution of the topic assignments, $z_{d,n}$, and observed words, $w_{d,n}$. LDA assumes that the topic prior distribution and topic proportion prior distribution follows a Dirichlet distribution with hyper-parameters ν and η, respectively.

The joint likelihood can be further defined by the product of the conditional likelihoods as

$$\prod_{n=1}^{N^{(d)}} P(w_{d,n}, z_{d,n}|\boldsymbol{\theta}_d, \boldsymbol{\beta}) = \prod_{n=1}^{N^{(d)}} \left(P(z_{d,n}|\boldsymbol{\theta}_d) P(w_{d,n}|z_{d,n}, \boldsymbol{\beta}_k) \right), \tag{2}$$

where $P(z_{d,n}|\boldsymbol{\theta}_d)$ is the conditional likelihood of the topic assignments, $P(w_{d,n}|z_{d,n}, \boldsymbol{\beta}_k)$ is the conditional likelihood of the observed word, and $\boldsymbol{\beta_k}$ is the $k = z_{d,n}$ topic distribution. LDA assumes that the conditional likelihood of topic assignments and observed words follow a multinomial distribution with parameters $\boldsymbol{\theta}$ and $\boldsymbol{\beta}$, respectively.

2.2 *Prior Specification*

The LDA model specifies the topic prior and the topic proportion prior as Dirichlet distributions, where the hyper-parameters ν and η impact the density of the distributions. The topic prior distribution hyper-parameter ν is a V-dimensional vector that takes the same value for each position in the vector. Similarly, the topic proportion distribution hyper-parameter η is a K-dimensional vector that takes the same value for each position in the vector.

When ν and η are small (< 1), this indicates that topic distributions consist of a few words (i.e., a few words have high probabilities and the rest have low probabilities) and topic proportions are mainly a few topics (i.e., each essay only uses a select few of the topics). When ν and η are large (> 1), this indicates that the topic distributions are uniformly spread across all words in the vocabulary and that the topic proportions are uniformly spread across all topics. Additionally, when ν and η are equal to 1, it indicates a non-informative prior on topic distributions and topic proportions (Blei & Jordan, 2003).

2.3 Data Generation

The LDA model assumes a generative process for the construction of each essay. Suppose there are D essays and K topics, $\boldsymbol{\beta}_{1:K}$. The LDA model assumes that each essay is generated with the following process (Blei et al., 2003):

1. Choose $N \sim Poisson(\lambda)$
2. Choose $\boldsymbol{\theta} \sim Dirichlet(\eta)$
3. For each word $n \in 1, 2, \ldots, N$:
   i. Choose $z_n \sim Multinomial(\boldsymbol{\theta})$
   ii. Choose $w_n \sim Multinomial(\boldsymbol{\beta_k} | z_n)$

where N is the word length of the essay, λ is the mean length of all essays in the corpus, $\boldsymbol{\theta}$ is the topic proportions of the essay, z_n is the topic assignment for n^{th} word, w_n is the generated observed word for the nth word in the essay, and $\boldsymbol{\beta_k}$ is the topic distribution of the assigned topic z_n, that is $k = z_n$.

The generative model described above is used to generate the simulation data. The latent topics are generated by determining the vocabulary size, V, and the number of topics, K. Since LDA indexes each word in the vocabulary, the actual words do not matter. Therefore, each of the $\boldsymbol{\beta}_{1:K}$ topics are independent random samples from a Dirichlet distribution on the $V - 1$ simplex given the prior hyper-parameter ν, and has a density given by

$$P(\boldsymbol{\beta}_{1:K} | \nu) = \frac{\Gamma(\nu_1 + \nu_2 + \ldots + \nu_V)}{\Gamma(\nu_1)\Gamma(\nu_2)\ldots\Gamma(\nu_V)} \prod_{v=1}^{V} \beta_v^{\nu_v - 1}, \tag{3}$$

where β_v is the probability of word v occurring within the given topic. The topic proportions for each essay are generated after determining the number of topics K and the number of essays D. Each essay's topic proportions $\boldsymbol{\theta}_{1:D}$ are independent random samples from a Dirichlet distribution on the $K - 1$ simplex given the prior hyper-parameter η, and has a density given by

$$P(\boldsymbol{\theta}_{1:D} | \eta) = \frac{\Gamma(\eta_1 + \eta_2 + \ldots + \eta_K)}{\Gamma(\eta_1)\Gamma(\eta_1)\ldots\Gamma(\eta_K)} \prod_{k=1}^{K} \theta_k^{\eta_k - 1}, \tag{4}$$

where θ_k is the proportional usage of topic k within the given essay.

The D essays are generated by giving each essay a length $N^{(d)}$, which is generated from a Poisson distribution given the average length of all essays, λ. The topic assignments for the individual words in each essay are sampled from a multinomial distribution given the essay's topic proportion. The joint density of the topic assignments for a given essay is given by

$$P(z_{1:N^{(d)}}|\boldsymbol{\theta_d}) = N^{(d)}! \prod_{k=1}^{K} \frac{\theta_{d,k}^{|z_{d,k}|}}{|z_{d,k}|!}, \tag{5}$$

where $\theta_{d,k}$ is the topic proportion for topic k of essay d, and $|z_{d,k}|$ is the number of times topic k is assigned to a word in essay d. The individual words in each essay are sampled from a multinomial distribution given the word's topic assignment and the topic distribution of the chosen assignment. The joint density of the words in an essay is obtained by

$$P(w_{1:N^{(d)}}|z_{1:N^{(d)}}, \boldsymbol{\beta_{1:K}}) = N^{(d)}! \prod_{v=1}^{V} \frac{\beta_{d,v}^{|w_{d,v}|}}{|w_{d,v}|!}, \tag{6}$$

where $\beta_{d,v}$ is the probability of word v occurring in essay d given the topic assignment of the word $z_{d,v}$, and $|w_{d,v}|$ is the number of times a word v appears in essay d for the given topic assignment.

2.4 Model Estimation

The joint posterior distribution specified in Equation (1) is intractable, but it can be estimated through various techniques, such as collapsed Gibbs sampling and variational Bayes inference using the Expectation-Maximization (EM) algorithm (Griffiths & Steyvers, 2004; Hoffman, Bach, & Blei, 2010).

The collapsed Gibbs sampling method is easier to implement than variational Bayes, but it is relatively slow. There are two main R packages used to estimate an LDA model: *topicmodels* (Hornik & Grün, 2011) and *lda* (Chang, 2015). Both packages have options to implement the collapsed Gibbs sampling or EM estimation methods.

2.5 Label Switching

A common issue with Bayesian estimated models is label switching, which occurs when latent classes switch during the estimation procedure (Cho, Cohen, & Kim, 2013). In LDA, label switching occurs when one topic switches with another. Label switching is less of a concern in an empirical study where only the final iteration of the estimation procedure is used; however, it is a major issue with simulation studies since keeping track of the latent topics is not trivial.

One way to identify label switching is to calculate the cosine similarity, as shown in Equation (7), between the estimated topics and the known generated topics.

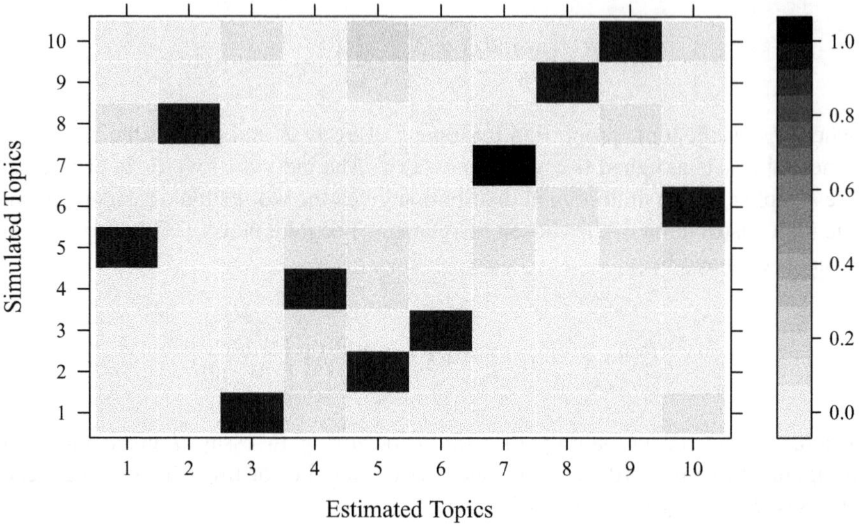

Fig. 1 Lattice plot for identifying label switching using the cosine similarities between the estimated topics and the known simulated topics

$$cos(\hat{\boldsymbol{\beta}}, \boldsymbol{\beta}) = \frac{\sum_{i=1}^{V} \hat{\beta}_i \cdot \beta_i}{\sqrt{\sum_{i=1}^{V} \hat{\beta}_i^{\,2}} \cdot \sqrt{\sum_{i=1}^{V} \beta_i^2}}, \tag{7}$$

where $\hat{\beta}$ is the estimated topic, β is the known generated topic, and V is the length of the vocabulary. The cosine similarity measures the distance between the topics in the underlying semantic space (Singhal, 2001). A cosine similarity closer to 1 indicates the two topics are similar, meaning the estimated topic is the known generated topic. A cosine similarity closer to 0 indicates the two topics are dissimilar, meaning the estimated topic is not the known generated topic.

Figure 1 shows a lattice plot of the cosine similarities between each of the estimated topics and all the known generated topics. The dark blue squares indicate which estimated topics are the known generated topics. For example, the estimated Topic 1 is actually the known generated Topic 5. Addressing label switching allows for accurate evaluation of parameter recovery.

2.6 Evaluation

The cosine similarity measure, Equation (7), is used to assess parameter recovery of the topics and topic proportions. The root mean square error (RMSE), shown in Equation (8), is also used to evaluate the recovery of the topic proportions of each document.

$$RMSE = \sqrt{\frac{\sum_{k=1}^{K} (\hat{\theta_k} - \theta_k)^2}{K}} \tag{8}$$

A larger cosine similarity between the estimated topic and the generated topic indicates that the LDA model successfully recovered the parameters. Additionally, a smaller average RMSE between the estimated topic proportions and the generated topic proportions indicates that the LDA model successfully recovered the topic proportion parameters.

3 Simulation Study

The purpose of this study was to demonstrate how to implement an LDA simulation and to investigate the number of essays needed to recover the latent topics and topic proportions of each essay at varying factor levels.

3.1 Design

A total of 25 replications were used in the study and each replication considered three factors, namely, number of topics (9 levels: 2 to 10 topics), average essay length (10 levels: varied between 10 and 500 words), and number of essays. For each replication, the number of topic factor levels were crossed with the average essay length factor levels and the number of essays were increased until the LDA model was able to accurately recover the model parameters.

Three factors were held constant throughout the entire study, namely, vocabulary size ($V = 3000$ words), topic prior hyper-parameter ($\nu = 1$), and topic proportion prior hyper-parameter ($\eta = 1$).

The latent topics were generated for each replication but held constant throughout the replication. For example, when the number of topics was 3, the three topics were generated once per replication and held constant for the 10 average essay lengths.

Since the purpose of the study was to investigate the number of essays needed to recover the topics and topic proportions an initial 50 essays were generated using the generative process described in the previous section. An initial LDA model was fit to the generated data and estimated the topics and topic proportions. If the estimated parameters did not meet three different stopping criteria, then an additional 5 essays were generated and a new LDA model was fit to the generated data. This process continued until all three stopping criteria were met.

The first stopping criterion was the cosine similarity between each estimated topic and their known generated topic was greater 0.9. The second stopping criterion was the average cosine similarity between the estimated topic proportions and their known generate topic proportions for each essay was greater 0.9. The third stopping criterion was the average RMSE between the estimated topic proportions and their known generate topic proportions for each essay was less than 0.1. These three stopping criteria ensures that the model parameters were accurately recovered.

3.2 *Results*

For each crossed factor, the number of essays needed to pass all three stopping criteria and recover the model parameters were recorded. Table 1 show the average number of essays needed across the 25 replications. The columns of the table represents the 10 levels used for the average document length. The smallest average essay length used was 10, which imitates a short answer CR item. The largest average essay length used was 500, which imitates an essay response to an extended CR item. The rows of the table represents the 9 levels used for the number of topics. The smallest number of topics is 2 and the largest number of topic is 10.

From Table 1, it can be seen that the largest number of essays needed to accurately recover the model parameters was 9, 500, which occurred for the 10-topic model with an average essay length of 10. The smallest number of essays needed to accurately recover the model parameters was 55, which occurred in four different conditions: 2-topic model and average essay length of 200, 2-topic model

Table 1 Documents needed to recover topics and topic proportions

	Average essay length (λ)									
K topics	10	20	25	40	50	75	100	200	250	500
2	800	240	325	220	170	75	85	55	55	55
3	1600	800	750	600	425	240	190	85	95	55
4	2200	1700	1300	950	750	425	425	160	130	65
5	3200	2700	1900	1400	1300	1100	650	325	180	110
6	4400	3000	2500	1800	1500	950	750	350	300	150
7	5000	3700	2900	2200	2000	1500	800	375	350	190
8	6400	4000	4000	2900	2400	1800	1200	600	450	200
9	7200	5500	4500	3300	2700	1600	1600	600	550	275
10	9500	6600	5300	4100	3200	2300	1800	800	600	300

and average essay length of 250, 2-topic model and average essay length of 500, and 3-topic model and average essay length of 500.

The results from Table 1 have two general trends from the number of essays. First, there is a direct relationship between the number of topics and the number of essays needed. That is, as the number of topics increase, so do the number of essays needed. Second, there is an inverse relationship between the average essay length and the number of essays needed. That is, as the average essay length increases, the number of essays needed decreases.

Intuitively, these results are expected. As the number of topics increase, so does the granularity of the model, meaning more data is needed to accurately estimate the parameters. Additionally, as more data becomes available within each essay the number of essays needed to accurately estimate the parameters decreases. Although these general relationships are expected, the results from Table 1 provide an idea about how many essays are actually needed when conducting an empirical study using the LDA model.

4 Discussion

In this article, a guide for simulation studies of LDA topic models was presented. The data generating mechanism relies heavily on the assumed generative process of LDA. The generated topics and prior hyper-parameters are held constant for all simulated essays. Topic proportions are generated for each simulated essay. After fitting an LDA model to the generated essays, the label switching is corrected by computing cosine similarities between each of the estimated topics with the known generated topics. Once the label switching issue is addressed, the LDA model results are compared to the known generated topics to evaluate parameter recovery.

Unlike other topic models, such as LSA and pLSI, the LDA model is computationally expensive due to the number of parameters in the posterior distribution. Multiple estimation algorithms, however, have been developed to reduce the computational costs of LDA, such as the variational Bayes and collapsed Gibbs sampling algorithms. Although these methods speed up the estimation procedure, they remain relatively slow. Therefore, due to the computational cost of estimating the posterior distribution, along with suggested simulation sizes from Cohen, Kane, and Kim (2001), this study used 25 replications.

The results from the simulation study suggest that the number of essays needed to estimate an LDA model depends on the number of latent topics and the average length of each essay. Specifically, the number of essays needed had a direct relationship with the number of topics and an inverse relationship with the average essay length. These results can be used for empirical studies by suggesting the amount of data needed to accurately estimate the latent topics and topic proportions.

Future research can use this guide to investigate other statistical properties of the LDA model, including the investigation of prior specification, effects of vocabulary lengths, and compare differences between estimation algorithms. The LDA model, along with the information presented in this study, can be used in practice to measure the latent structure of CR items, which can be used to evaluate different aspects of student writings, such as the effectiveness of an instructional writing intervention.

References

Blei, D. M., & Jordan, M. I. (2003). Modeling annotated data. In *Proceedings of the 26th Annual International ACM SIGIR Conference on Research and Development in Informaion Retrieval* (pp. 127–134)

Blei, D. M., Ng, A. Y., & Jordan, M. I. (2003). Latent Dirichlet allocation. *Journal of Machine Learning Research, 3*, 993–1022

Buxton, C., Allexsaht-Snider, M., Aghasaleh, R., Kayumova, S., Kim, S., Choi, Y.-J., & Cohen, A. (2014). Potential benefits of bilingual constructed response science assessments for understanding bilingual learners' emergent use of language of scientific investigation practices. *Double Helix, 2*, 1–21

Cardozo-Gaibisso, L., Kim, S., Buxton, C., & Cohen, A. (2019). Thinking beyond the score: Multidimensional analysis of student performance to inform the next generation of science assessments. *Journal of Research in Science Teaching, 1*(57), 856–878

Chang, J. (2015). lda: Collapsed gibbs sampling methods for topic models [Computer software manual]. Retrieved from https://CRAN.R-project.org/package=lda (R package version 1.4.2)

Cho, S.-J., Cohen, A. S., & Kim, S.-H. (2013). Markov chain Monte Carlo estimation of a mixture item response theory model. *Journal of Statistical Computation and Simulation, 83*(2), 278–306

Choi, H.-J., Kwak, M., Kim, S., Xiong, J., Cohen, A. S., & Bottge, B. A. (2019). An application of a topic model to two educational assessments. In M. Wiberg, S. Culpepper, R. Janssen, J. González, & D. Molenaar (Eds.), *Quantitative psychology: 83rd annual meeting of the psychometric society* (Vol. 265, pp. 449–459). New York, NY

Cohen, A. S., Kane, M. T., & Kim, S.-H. (2001). The precision of simulation study results. *Applied Psychological Measurement, 25*(2), 136–145

Deerwester, S., Dumais, S. T., Furnas, G. W., Landauer, T. K., & Harshman, R. (1990). Indexing by latent semantic analysis. *Journal of the American Society for Information Science, 41*(6), 391–407

Duong, E., Mellom, P., & Hixon, R. (2019). Using topic modeling to analyze the effects of instructional conversation on 3rd grade students' writing. *Paper Presented at the Annual Meeting of the American Association for Applied Linguistics, Atlanta, GA*

Griffiths, T. L., & Steyvers, M. (2004). Finding scientific topics. *Proceedings of the National Academy of Sciences, 101* (suppl 1), 5228–5235

Hoffman, M., Bach, F. R., & Blei, D. M. (2010). Online learning for latent dirichlet allocation. In *Advances in neural information processing systems* (pp. 856–864)

Hofmann, T. (1999). Probabilistic latent semantic indexing. In *Proceedings of the 22nd Annual International ACM SIGIR conference on Research and Development in Information Retrieval* (pp. 50–57)

Hornik, K., & Grün, B. (2011). Topicmodels: An R package for fitting topic models. *Journal of Statistical Software, 40*(13), 1–30

Kim, S., Kwak, M., Cardozo-Gaibisso, L., Buxton, C., & Cohen, A. S. (2017). Statistical and qualitative analyses of students' answers to a constructed response test of science inquiry knowledge. *Journal of Writing Analytics, 1*(1), 82–102

Landauer, T. K., Foltz, P. W., & Laham, D. (1998). An introduction to latent semantic analysis. *Discourse Processes, 25*(2–3), 259–284

Singhal, A. (2001). Modern information retrieval: A brief overview. *IEEE Data Engineering Bulletin, 24*(4), 35–43

Steyvers, M., & Griffiths, T. (2007). Probabilistic topic models. *Handbook of Latent Semantic Analysis, 427*(7), 424–440

Xiong, J., Choi, H.-J., Kim, S., Kwak, M., & Cohen, A. S. (2019). Topic modeling of constructed-response answers on social study assessments. In M. Wiberg, S. Culpepper, R. Janssen, J. González, & D. Molenaar (Eds.), *The annual meeting of the psychometric society*. Cham (pp. 263–274)

The Asymptotic Power of the Lagrange Multiplier Tests for Misspecified IRT Models

Lucia Guastadisegni, Silvia Cagnone, Irini Moustaki, and Vassilis Vasdekis

1 Introduction

The power of a test is usually estimated through Monte Carlo simulation methods. However, it can alternatively be computed asymptotically using the distribution of the test statistic under the alternative hypothesis that depends on a noncentrality parameter, often unknown or difficult to compute (Gudicha et al., 2017).

In this work we study the asymptotic power of two test statistics, the Lagrange Multiplier (LM) test and the Generalized Lagrange Multiplier (LM(S)) test, to detect measurement non-invariance under correct model specification and model misspecification.

An item is measurement non-invariant, or biased, if it measures different abilities for different group membership identified by an external variable (Mellenbergh, 1982, 1983). Group differences can be present only on the item intercept or simultaneously on the item intercept and slope.

The Lagrange Multiplier test is used in the IRT context to detect measurement non-invariance (Glas, 1998; Fox & Glas, 2005) and other types of model violations such as local dependence, incorrect specification of the item characteristic curve and a non normal distribution of the latent variables (Glas, 1999; Glas & Falcón, 2003; Liu & Thissen, 2012). Despite its extensive use in IRT models, only in a few studies

L. Guastadisegni (✉) · S. Cagnone
University of Bologna, Bologna, Italy
e-mail: lucia.guastadisegni2@unibo.it; silvia.cagnone@unibo.it

I. Moustaki
London School of Economics and Political Science, London, UK
e-mail: i.moustaki@lse.ac.uk

V. Vasdekis
Athens University of Economics and Business, Athens, Greece
e-mail: vasdekis@aueb.gr

M. Wiberg et al. (eds.), *Quantitative Psychology*, Springer Proceedings in Mathematics & Statistics 353, https://doi.org/10.1007/978-3-030-74772-5_25

the LM test has been applied in the case of model misspecification under the null and the alternative hypothesis (Glas & Falcón, 2003).

In order to take into account possible misspecification in the model, the LM test can be generalized obtaining the so-called Generalized Lagrange Multiplier test (LM(S)), whose expression involves the sandwich variance and covariance matrix (White, 1982). In the IRT context the performance of the LM(S) test under model misspecification has been recently analyzed by Falk and Monroe (2018) through a elaborate simulation study.

The first objective of this paper is to present the theoretical computation of the asymptotic power of these tests using two different approximation methods to obtain the noncentrality parameter. The second objective is to compare the performance of the LM and LM(S) tests through a simulation study to detect measurement invariance under correct model specification and misspecification of the latent variable distribution in terms of asymptotic and empirical power. The model considered under the null and the alternative hypothesis is a classic Multiple Indicator Multiple Causes (MIMIC) model for binary data, based on the assumption of a normal distribution of the latent factor. The misspecification is introduced by assuming a non normal distribution of the latent factor in the data generating model.

The paper is organized as follows; in Sect. 2 we review the theory of the LM test and the procedures to estimate its asymptotic power, in Sect. 3 we describe the LM(S) test and the procedures to estimate its asymptotic power and in Sect. 4 we present a Monte Carlo simulation study. We conclude with some remarks in Sect. 5.

2 The Lagrange Multiplier Test

Consider a sample $\mathbf{y}_1, \ldots, \mathbf{y}_n$ from a model $f(\mathbf{y}, \boldsymbol{\theta})$. Let $\boldsymbol{\theta}_0$ denote the true parameter vector, that can be divided in two subvectors $\boldsymbol{\theta}_0' = (\boldsymbol{\theta}_{01}', \boldsymbol{\theta}_{02}')$. The hypotheses H_0 and H_1 can be formalized as follows:

$$H_0 : \boldsymbol{\theta}_{02}' = \mathbf{c} \qquad vs \qquad H_1 : \boldsymbol{\theta}_{02}' \neq \mathbf{c}, \tag{1}$$

where $\mathbf{c}$ is a vector of constants. The LM statistic is (Engle, 1984):

$$LM = \frac{1}{n} S_2(\tilde{\boldsymbol{\theta}}) A^{22}(\tilde{\boldsymbol{\theta}})^{-1} S_2(\tilde{\boldsymbol{\theta}}), \tag{2}$$

where $\tilde{\boldsymbol{\theta}}' = (\tilde{\boldsymbol{\theta}}_1', \mathbf{c})$ denotes the restricted maximum likelihood estimates of the parameters $\boldsymbol{\theta}$, S_2 is the subset of the vector of score functions $S = \frac{\partial \ln l(\mathbf{y}, \boldsymbol{\theta})}{\partial \boldsymbol{\theta}}$ corresponding to the parameters $\boldsymbol{\theta}_{02}$ evaluated at $\tilde{\boldsymbol{\theta}}$. The matrix A^{22} is the block of the partitioned Fisher information matrix $A = -E\left[\frac{1}{n}\frac{\partial^2 l(\mathbf{y}, \boldsymbol{\theta})}{\partial \boldsymbol{\theta} \partial \boldsymbol{\theta}'}\right]$ defined as:

$$A^{22} = A_{22} - A_{21} A_{11}^{-1} A_{12}, \tag{3}$$

evaluated at $\tilde{\boldsymbol{\theta}}$. The partition of A into $A_{22}, A_{21}, A_{11}, A_{12}$ is derived from the partition of $\boldsymbol{\theta}_0'$ into $(\boldsymbol{\theta}_{01}', \boldsymbol{\theta}_{02}')$. In this study, we consider the LM test computed with the observed Hessian approach, where the Fisher information matrix in formula (2) is replaced by the corresponding observed Hessian matrix

$$\hat{A}(\boldsymbol{\theta}) = -\frac{1}{n}\sum_{i=1}^{n}\frac{\partial^2 l_i(\mathbf{y}_i, \boldsymbol{\theta})}{\partial\boldsymbol{\theta}\partial\boldsymbol{\theta}'} \tag{4}$$

Under a correct specified likelihood and under H_0, the LM statistic is asymptotically distributed as a χ_r^2, where r are the degrees of freedom (df) equal to the dimension of $\boldsymbol{\theta}_{02}$ (Silvey, 1959). When the alternative hypothesis is true but the null is tested, the LM test statistic has an asymptotic noncentral chi-square distribution that depends on two parameters, the df and a noncentrality parameter (Bollen, 1989). To compute the local asymptotic power of the LM test, a standard approach is to consider a set of local alternatives that are close to the null value for large n, $H_1 : \boldsymbol{\theta}_{02} = \boldsymbol{c} + \frac{\boldsymbol{\xi}}{\sqrt{n}}$, where $\boldsymbol{\xi}$ is an arbitrary vector with the same dimension of $\boldsymbol{\theta}_{02}$ (Boos & Stefanski, 2013). Under H_1, the test statistic LM converges in distribution to a $\chi_r^2(\lambda)$ with noncentrality parameter λ equal to (Cox and Hinkley, 1979):

$$\lambda = \boldsymbol{\xi}' A^{22}(\boldsymbol{\theta}^0)\boldsymbol{\xi}, \tag{5}$$

where $\boldsymbol{\theta}^0 = (\boldsymbol{\theta}_{01}, \mathbf{c})$.

The asymptotic local power is computed as $P(\chi_r^2(\lambda) > \chi_r^2(\lambda, 1-\alpha)$.

2.1 *Approximation Procedures for the Asymptotic Power*

The asymptotic distribution of the LM test under the alternative hypothesis as a noncentral chi-square with noncentrality parameter (5) holds when the model defined under the set of local alternatives is true, i.e. when the model under the null hypothesis is barely incorrect for large n (see Agresti 2002 and Reiser 2008). In practice, it is often reasonable to adopt an alternative hypothesis for fixed and finite n (Agresti, 2002), as $H_1 : \boldsymbol{\theta}_{02} = \boldsymbol{c} + \boldsymbol{\xi}$, or to use hypotheses as (1) (Gudicha et al., 2017). We present here two different approximation procedures for the computation of the noncentrality parameter.

The first method extends the approximation procedure for the asymptotic power derived by Gudicha et al. (2017) for the Likelihood-Ratio and the Wald tests to the LM test. It can be summarized in the following steps:

1. From the model defined under the alternative hypothesis, create a large data set (e.g. $N = 10000$ observations).
2. Fit the model under H_0 to the data.

3. Take the value of the LM statistic as the estimate of the noncentrality parameter λ (Satorra, 1989; Bollen, 1989).
4. Compute the noncentrality parameter for a sample of size 1 equal to $\lambda_1 = \frac{\lambda}{N}$.
5. The noncentrality parameter for a sample of size n is $\lambda_n = n\lambda_1$.

The power of the LM test can be determined by comparing the λ_n obtained in step 5 with the tabled values of the noncentral chi-square with df corresponding to the number of parameters constrained under H_0 and significance level α (Bollen, 1989).

We propose a second method, that is also based on some of the steps of the procedure proposed by Gudicha et al. (2017), but the noncentrality parameter is computed according to formula (5). The procedure can be summarized as follows:

1. From the model defined under the alternative hypothesis, create a large data data set (e.g. $N = 10000$ observations).
2. Fit the model under H_0 to the data.
3. Compute $\boldsymbol{\xi} = \sqrt{N}(\boldsymbol{\theta}_{02} - \mathbf{c})$, where $\boldsymbol{\theta}_{02}$ is the vector of the data generating values (values under H_1) of the constrained parameters and $\mathbf{c}$ is the vector of constants under the null hypothesis (Reiser, 2008).
4. Compute the noncentrality parameter according to formula (5) where $A^{22}(\boldsymbol{\theta}^0)$ can be consistently estimated by the corresponding matrix $\hat{A}$, evaluated at $\tilde{\boldsymbol{\theta}}$.
5. Compute the noncentrality parameter for a sample of size 1 as $\lambda_1 = \frac{\lambda}{N}$.
6. The noncentrality parameter for a sample of size n is $\lambda_n = n\lambda_1$

The power is computed as before, using the noncentrality parameter computed at point 5.

3 The Generalized Lagrange Multiplier Test

Consider a sample $\mathbf{y}_1, \ldots, \mathbf{y}_n$ from a model with true density $g(\mathbf{y})$. The model $f(\mathbf{y}; \boldsymbol{\theta})$ is assumed to be true one for the data and differs from $g(\mathbf{y})$. Under the assumptions given in White (1982) the vector of parameter $\hat{\boldsymbol{\theta}}_n$, that maximizes the log-likelihood function based on model $f(\mathbf{y}; \boldsymbol{\theta})$ (Quasi-ML estimator, White 1982), converges in probability to $\boldsymbol{\theta}_*$, the parameter vector that minimizes the Kullback-Leibler information criterion. Moreover the variance and covariance matrix of the Quasi-LM estimator is the sandwich variance and covariance matrix $\hat{C}(\hat{\boldsymbol{\theta}}_n) = \hat{A}^{-1}(\hat{\boldsymbol{\theta}}_n)\hat{B}(\hat{\boldsymbol{\theta}}_n)\hat{A}^{-1}(\hat{\boldsymbol{\theta}}_n)$, where the matrix $\hat{A}$ is defined in formula (4) and $\hat{B} = \frac{1}{n}\sum_{i=1}^{n} \frac{\partial l_i(\mathbf{y}_i,\boldsymbol{\theta})}{\partial \boldsymbol{\theta}} \frac{\partial l_i(\mathbf{y}_i,\boldsymbol{\theta})}{\partial \boldsymbol{\theta}}$ is the observed cross-product matrix (White, 1982).

Under model misspecification, the null and the alternative hypotheses are posed in terms of $\boldsymbol{\theta}_*$. Let $\boldsymbol{\theta}_*$ be divided in two subvectors $\boldsymbol{\theta}'_* = (\boldsymbol{\theta}'_{*1}, \boldsymbol{\theta}'_{*2})$. The hypotheses H_0 and H_1 can be formalized as follows:

$$H_0 : \boldsymbol{\theta}'_{*2} = \mathbf{c} \quad vs \quad H_1 : \boldsymbol{\theta}'_{*2} \neq \mathbf{c}, \tag{6}$$

where $\mathbf{c}$ is a vector of constants.

The Generalized Lagrange Multiplier Test is defined as:

$$LM(S) = \frac{1}{n} S_2(\tilde{\boldsymbol{\theta}}_n)' \hat{A}^{22}(\tilde{\boldsymbol{\theta}}_n)^{-1} \hat{C}_{22}(\tilde{\boldsymbol{\theta}}_n)^{-1} \hat{A}^{22}(\tilde{\boldsymbol{\theta}}_n)^{-1} S_2(\tilde{\boldsymbol{\theta}}_n), \tag{7}$$

where $\tilde{\boldsymbol{\theta}}_n$ is the constrained quasi-ML estimator, $\hat{A}^{22}$ is the block of the partitioned observed Hessian matrix computed as in formula (3), evaluated at $\tilde{\boldsymbol{\theta}}_n$ and $\hat{C}_{22}$ is the block of the matrix $\hat{C}$ corresponding to $\boldsymbol{\theta}'_{*2}$, evaluated at $\tilde{\boldsymbol{\theta}}_n$. Under H_0 the statistic LM(S) is distributed as a χ^2_r, where r are the df equal to the dimension of $\boldsymbol{\theta}_{*2}$ (White, 1982). To compute the local asymptotic power of the LM(S) test, a standard approach is to consider a set of local alternatives $H_1 : \boldsymbol{\theta}_{*2} = \boldsymbol{c} + \frac{\boldsymbol{\xi}}{\sqrt{n}}$, where $\boldsymbol{\xi}$ is an arbitrary vector of dimension $\boldsymbol{\theta}_{*2}$. Under H_1, the test statistic $LM(S)$ converges in distribution to a $\chi^2_r(\lambda)$, where r are the df equal to the dimension of $\boldsymbol{\theta}_{*2}$ and λ is the noncentrality parameter given by Bera et al. (2020):

$$\lambda = \boldsymbol{\xi}' A^{22'} (B_{22} - A_{21} A_{11}^{-1} B_{12} - B_{21} A_{11}^{-1} A_{12} + A_{21} A_{11}^{-1} B_{11} A_{11}^{-1} A_{12})^{-1} A^{22} \boldsymbol{\xi} \tag{8}$$

where A is the Fisher information matrix and B is the expected cross-product matrix, evaluated at $\boldsymbol{\theta}^*$.

If the model is correctly specified, the LM(S) coincides with LM test (White, 1982).

3.1 Estimation Procedure for the Noncentrality Parameter

The estimation method described in Sect. 2.1 to compute the asymptotic power is used here to estimate the asymptotic power for the LM(S) test, with some differences.

In step 3 of the first method, the LM(S) statistic is taken as the estimate of the noncentrality parameter (the proof of this result can be found in Satorra 1989).

In step 4 of the second method, the noncentrality parameter is computed according to formula (8), where the matrices $A(\boldsymbol{\theta}^*)$ and $B(\boldsymbol{\theta}^*)$ are consistently estimated by $\hat{A}$ and $\hat{B}$, evaluated at $\tilde{\boldsymbol{\theta}}_n$.

Moreover, the model fitted under H_0 at step 2 is assumed to be misspecified. Under correct model specification the LM(S) and the LM tests have the same noncentrality parameter and, consequently, the same asymptotic power.

4 Simulation Study

4.1 Simulation Design

The aim of this section is to compare the different procedures described above to estimate the asymptotic and the empirical power of the LM and LM(S) tests to detect measurement non-invariance by means of a simulation study. A MIMIC model for binary data is considered. Both under correct and model misspecification, we consider a binary group variable x because we study measurement non-invariance only in two subgroups of population. Given n individuals and p items, under correct model specification data are generated from the following model, where measurement non-invariance is introduced on the intercept of the last item p through the parameter γ_1 and the group variable x:

$$\begin{aligned} &logit(\pi_{ij}) = \alpha_{0j} + \alpha_{1j} z_i \qquad i = 1, \ldots, n \qquad j = 1, \ldots, p-1 \\ &logit(\pi_{ip}) = \alpha_{0p} + \alpha_{1p} z_i + \gamma_1 x_i \\ &z \sim N(0, 1) \end{aligned} \tag{9}$$

Under misspecification of the latent variable distribution data are generated from the following model, where measurement non-invariance is introduced as before on the intercept of the last item p through the parameter γ_1 and the group variable x:

$$\begin{aligned} &logit(\pi_{ij}) = \alpha_{0j} + \alpha_{1j} z_i \qquad i = 1, \ldots, n \qquad j = 1, \ldots, p-1 \\ &logit(\pi_{ip}) = \alpha_{0p} + \alpha_{1p} z_i + \gamma_1 x_i \\ &z \sim SN(\kappa) \end{aligned} \tag{10}$$

In this case, the latent variable z is generated from a Skew-normal (SN) with skewness parameter κ, with the following probability density function (Azzalini, 1985):

$$\phi(\epsilon; \kappa) = 2\phi(\epsilon)\Phi(\epsilon; \kappa)$$

where ϕ and Φ are the standard normal density and distribution function, respectively. The parameter κ can takes values from $-\infty$ to $+\infty$: when it is equal to 0, the Skew-normal reduces to a Standard normal distribution. In the simulations, we consider two values of κ, 3 and 5. When $\kappa = 3$ the mean and the variance of the latent variable are 0.76 and 0.43, respectively, and when $\kappa = 5$, the mean and the variance of the latent variable are 0.78 and 0.39, respectively. In both models (9) and (10) we consider two possible effect sizes, equal to 0.2 and 0.5, for the parameter γ_1. Moreover, in both cases, the values xs are generated from a Bernoulli distribution with success probability 0.7, the intercepts from a normal distribution with 0 mean and Standard Deviation (SD) 0.1 and the slopes from a normal distribution with 0 mean and SD 0.5.

The following set of hypotheses is being tested:

$$H_0 : \gamma_{1p} = 0 \quad vs \quad H_1 : \gamma_{1p} \neq 0,$$

that implies that the last item is tested for measurement invariance.

Model (9) is fitted to the data with γ_{1p} fixed to 0. When data are generated from model (10) we are working under model misspecification. Indeed, as mentioned before, the true latent variable has mean and variance around 0.7

and 0.4, respectively, and its skewed. Since model (9) is fitted to the data, the misfit is in the mean, assumed to be 0, in the variance, assumed to be 1 and in the distribution of the latent variable, assumed to be symmetric. The following simulation conditions are considered: number of items ($p = 10$) × sample size ($n = 200, 500, 1000, 5000, 10000$) × Test statistic ($LM$, $LM(S)$). Due to the time complexity, the empirical power is computed only for $n = 200, 500, 1000$. 200 replications are considered for each condition of the study. The empirical power $\hat{p}$ is computed as $\hat{p} = \sum_{l=1}^{N_v} \frac{I(T_l \geq c)}{N_v}$, where N_v is the number of valid statistics out of the number of replications, I is the indicator function, T_l is the value of the test statistic evaluated in the l-th replication and c is the theoretical asymptotic critical value corresponding to the 95-th percentile of the χ^2_{df} distribution, with df equal to the number of constrained parameter under H_0. If non valid statistics occur, they are excluded from the analysis. The asymptotic power is computed through methods 1 and 2 described in Sect. 2.1 and 3.1. The nominal level α is equal to 0.05 in all simulations. ML estimates of the parameters are obtained with direct maximization of the likelihood function using 21 Gauss-Hermite quadrature points. Numerical derivatives are used to compute the Hessian and cross-product matrices.

4.2 Results

Table 1 presents the results for the LM and LM(S) tests under correct model specification when γ_1 is equal to 0.2 and 0.5 in the data generating model, $p = 10$, $n = 200, 500, 1000, 5000, 10000$. We can notice that, in general, the differences between the asymptotic and empirical power are small and method 1 is slightly closer to the empirical power than method 2. For what concerns the power to detect measurement non-invariance, the LM test has a slightly higher power compared to the LM(S) tests under all conditions, with the exception of the case $\gamma_1 = 0.5$ and for

Table 1 Asymptotic and empirical power of the LM and LM(S) tests under correct model specification, $\gamma_1 = 0.2, 0.5$, $p = 10$, $n = 200, 500, 1000, 5000, 10000$

			Method 1		Method 2		Empirical	
p	γ_1	n	LM	LM(S)	LM	LM(S)	LM	LM(S)
10	0.2	200	0.086	0.085	0.080	0.079	0.08	0.06
		500	0.144	0.140	0.126	0.122	0.185	0.17
		1000	0.241	0.234	0.204	0.198	0.26	0.25
		5000	0.802	0.785	0.714	0.696	–	–
		10000	0.978	0.973	0.947	0.938	–	–
10	0.5	200	0.240	0.222	0.229	0.211	0.285	0.235
		500	0.508	0.468	0.484	0.445	0.54	0.5
		1000	0.799	0.758	0.775	0.732	0.8	0.78
		5000	1	1	1	1	–	–
		10000	1	1	1	1	–	–

Table 2 Asymptotic power of the LM and LM(S) tests under incorrect distribution of the latent variable, $\gamma_1 = 0.2, 0.5$, $p = 10$, $n = 200, 500, 1000, 5000, 10000$

				Method 1		Method 2		Empirical	
p	ES	α	n	LM	LM(S)	LM	LM(S)	LM	LM(S)
10	0.2	3	200	0.066	0.065	0.071	0.070	0.085	0.04
			500	0.091	0.089	0.104	0.101	0.11	0.075
			1000	0.133	0.129	0.159	0.154	0.185	0.14
			5000	0.464	0.447	0.569	0.550	–	–
			10000	0.753	0.734	0.854	0.839	–	–
		5	200	0.069	0.068	0.071	0.070	0.07	0.055
			500	0.010	0.097	0.102	0.010	0.135	0.085
			1000	0.151	0.146	0.157	0.151	0.145	0.135
			5000	0.538	0.517	0.561	0.540	–	–
			10000	0.828	0.809	0.848	0.829	–	–
10	0.5	3	200	0.158	0.145	0.170	0.155	0.202	0.13
			500	0.325	0.292	0.353	0.317	0.41	0.34
			1000	0.567	0.514	0.609	0.555	0.625	0.585
			5000	0.997	0.994	0.998	0.997	–	–
			10000	1	1	1	1	–	–
		5	200	0.163	0.148	0.168	0.153	0.21	0.15
			500	0.337	0.301	0.347	0.310	0.425	0.345
			1000	0.585	0.529	0.601	0.544	0.61	0.57
			5000	0.998	0.995	0.999	0.996		
			10000	1	1	1	1		

large sample sizes ($n = 5000, 10000$), where the two tests reach the same power, as expected from the theory.

Table 2 shows the results for the LM and LM(S) tests computed under misspecification of the latent variable distribution when γ_1 is equal to 0.2 and 0.5 in the data generating model, $p = 10$, $n = 200, 500, 1000, 5000, 10000$. Also in this case the differences between the asymptotic and empirical power are small. For what concerns the power to detect measurement non-invariance under model misspecification, despite the fact that the LM(S) test is derived under model misspecification, the LM test has the highest power under all conditions. The two tests reach the same power only when $\gamma_1 = 0.5$ and $n = 10000$. In both Tables and for both tests, the power increases with the sample size and the effect size of the parameter γ_1 and decreases when the model is misspecified.

5 Conclusion

In this paper we presented two methods to compute the power of the LM and LM(S) tests, based on their asymptotic distributions under the alternative hypothesis.

Moreover, we assessed the performance of these two tests to detect measurement non-invariance under correct model specification and misspecification of the latent variable distribution. The simulation study highlighted that the asymptotic power, computed through the two different approximation methods for the non-centrality parameter, is very close to the empirical power, also under model misspecification. Small differences between the empirical and asymptotic power have been found also by Gudicha et al. (2017) for the Likelihood-Ratio and Wald tests and by Saris et al. (1987) for the score test.

To compute the noncentrality parameter of the LM and LM(S) tests, we have generated data from the model under the alternative hypothesis considering 10000 observations. Increasing this number could reduce the differences between the empirical and asymptotic power, but it would increase the time burden to obtain the parameter estimates and the numerical derivatives used in the noncentrality parameter approximation procedures.

For what concerns the power of the two tests to detect measurement noninvariance, the LM test has a slightly higher power compared to the LM(S) test under most simulation conditions. The two tests reach the same power only for large sample sizes. A similar behaviour of the power of the LM and LM(S) tests has been found also by Falk and Monroe (2018), under correct model specification and misspecification due to an omitted cross-loading.

From this study we can conclude that the asymptotic power can be a valid alternative to obtain the power of a test, both under the correct model and a model with a misspecified distribution of the latent variable since it allows us to reduced the time complexity compared to the empirical power. Although not shown here, the asymptotic power can be used also to find sample sizes necessary to reach a certain power (Boos & Stefanski, 2013; Gudicha et al., 2017). However, the asymptotic power can be computed only for certain test statistics with known noncentrality parameter.

This work was limited only to one type of misspecification. Further analysis should be carried out on the LM(S) test to evaluate if there might be an improvement in its performance considering different types of model misspecification and different estimation methods.

References

Agresti, A. (2002). *Categorical data analysis*. New York: Wiley

Azzalini, A. (1985). A class of distributions which includes the normal ones. *Scandinavian Journal of Statistics, 12*, 171–178

Bera, A. K., Doğan O., Bilias Y., Yoon M. J., & Taşpınar S. (2020). Adjustments of Rao's score test for distributional and local parametric misspecifications. *Journal of Econometric Methods, 9*(1), 1–29

Bollen, K. A. (1989). *Structural equations with latent variables*. Wiley

Boos, D.D., & Stefanski, L.A. (2013). *Essential statistical inference*. Springer

Cox, D. R., & Hinkley, D. V. (1979). *Theoretical statistics*. CRC Press

Engle, R. F. (1984). Chapter 13 Wald, likelihood ratio, and Lagrange multiplier tests in econometrics. *Handbook of econometrics* (Vol. 2, pp. 775–826). Elsevier

Falk, C. F., & Monroe, S. (2018). On Lagrange multiplier tests in multidimensional item response theory: Information matrices and model misspecification. *Educational and Psychological Measurement, 78*(4), 653–678

Fox, J.-P., & Glas, C. A. (2005). Bayesian modification indices for IRT models. *Statistica Neerlandica, 59*(1), 95–106

Glas, C. A. (1998). Detection of differential item functioning using Lagrange multiplier tests. *Statistica Sinica, 8*, 647–667

Glas, C. A. (1999). Modification indices for the 2-PL and the nominal response model. *Psychometrika, 64*(3), 273–294

Glas, C. A., & Falcón, J. C. S. (2003). A comparison of item-fit statistics for the three-parameter logistic model. *Applied Psychological Measurement, 27*(2), 87–106

Gudicha, D. W., Schmittmann, V. D., & Vermunt, J. K. (2017). Statistical power of likelihood ratio and Wald tests in latent class models with covariates. *Behavior Research Methods, 49*(5), 1824–1837

Liu, Y., & Thissen, D. (2012). Identifying local dependence with a score test statistic based on the bifactor logistic model. *Applied Psychological Measurement, 36*(8), 670–688

Mellenbergh, G. J. (1982). Contingency table models for assessing item bias. *Journal of Educational Statistics, 7*(2), 105–118

Mellenbergh, G. J. (1983). Contingency table models for assessing item bias. In Irvine, S.H., & Berry, J. W. (Eds.), *Human Assessment and Cultural Factors* . NATO Conference Series (III Human Factors). 21. Boston, MA: Springer

Reiser, M. (2008). Goodness-of-fit testing using components based on marginal frequencies of multinomial data. *British Journal of Mathematical and Statistical Psychology, 61*, 331–360

Saris, W., Satorra, A., & Sorbom, D. (1987). The detection and correction of specification errors in structural equation models. *Sociological Methodology, 17*, 105

Satorra, A. (1989). Alternative test criteria in covariance structure analysis: A unified approach. *Psychometrika, 54*(1), 131–151

Silvey, S. D. (1959). The Lagrangian multiplier test. *The Annals of Mathematical Statistics, 30*(2), 389–407

White, H. (1982). Maximum likelihood estimation of misspecified models. *Econometrica, 50*(1), 1–25

Residual Analysis in Rasch Counts Models

Naiara Caroline Aparecido dos Santos and Jorge Luis Bazán

1 Introduction

Count responses are often observed in student achievement testing data, where the responses to the items in an assessment are correct check counts or error counts. Rasch (1960) proposed a model for count data that is now known as the Rasch Poisson count model (RPC).

An example of this type of data was recently shown by (Baghaei & Doebler, 2019), in a dataset of responses of 228 students to 20 blocks, where the task was cross out the digits 2 and 7 in three lines of randomly arranged digits and letters with a 15-second time limit for completing the task. These data were generated by a selective attention test proposed by Beyzaee (2017). An example of a block from the test is given in Fig. 1.

In a recent study, Santos and Bazán (2021) showed that the RPC model presents larger residuals in some items and consequently, is not the best model for this dataset. Additionally, overdispersion and excess zeros were observed in the response, so models considering extensions of the RPC model must be taken into account.

N. C. A. dos Santos (✉)
Instituto de Ciências Matemáticas e de Computação, Universidade de São Paulo – USP, São Carlos/SP, Brasil

Departamento de Estatística, Universidade Federal de São Carlos – UFSCar, São Carlos/SP, Brasil
e-mail: naicaroline2@usp.br

J. L. Bazán
Instituto de Ciências Matemáticas e de Computação, Universidade de São Paulo – USP, São Carlos/SP, Brasil
e-mail: jlbazan@icmc.usp.br

M. Wiberg et al. (eds.), *Quantitative Psychology*, Springer Proceedings in Mathematics & Statistics 353, https://doi.org/10.1007/978-3-030-74772-5_26

2 G O X C 7 M J 7 H Z R N G A S 2 Y W Q 2 L H B Z G J N V 7 E T 2 P R V M J H S T Q 2 C 7 K L W C 7
X M T 7 K T R 2 A V P I W O C 2 G J 7 L S 2 B N V W 7 T O X R 2 P H 7 F D A B M 2 W H K A S T 2 O P
H W E D 2 T R N E Q X 2 P K L 7 P K 7 Z C V 7 2 Z 7 E T G H L K S D I N 7 S 2 W I S N 7 T B M O P W

Fig. 1 Example of a block from the seletive attention test

There are several methods for RPC model estimation (Verhelst & Kamphuis, 2009), such as conditional maximum likelihood (CML), joint maximum likelihood (JML) and marginal maximum likelihood (MML), among others (Baghaei & Doebler, 2019). Also, Baghaei & Doebler (2019) showed that the RPC model can be estimated using the `lme4` package (Bates et al., 2015) in R, considering it as a generalized linear mixed model (GLMM). In this paper, we use frequentist and Bayesian approaches to estimate the Rasch counts model as a GLMM. Thus, we consider the `gamlss` and `INLA` packages using the R software (R Core Team, 2020). In the first case, the specific estimation method is the penalized marginal likelihood (Rigby et al., 2019) and in the second, the estimation method considered is integrated nested Laplace approximation (Wang et al., 2018).

Residual analysis is a useful tool for model diagnostics. It provides an overview in terms of the quality of the model fit (McCullagh & Nelder, 1989). Swaminathan et al. (2006) showed that, since IRT is based on strong mathematical and statistical assumptions, only when these assumptions are met can IRT methods be implemented effectively to analyze data and make inferences. Given that in IRT models the analysis of the residuals can be performed considering the test items, a graphical visualization tool of the residuals can facilitate verification of whether or not an item can be considered as following the proposed model. Detailed descriptions of diagnostic tools for IRT models are shown by Sinharay (2006), Van Rijn et al. (2016) and Bowen (2018). Additionally, the practical advantages of using of residual analysis include the ability to (a) evaluate the impact of misspecification on parameter estimation when the model is wrong; and (b) detect items that do not fit the model.

In the case of Rasch models, Haberman (2009) suggested the use of generalized residuals; and (Baghaei et al., 2019; Holling et al., 2015) considered Pearson residuals to verify the goodness of fit of the models. In this article, we propose the use of randomized quantile residuals (RQR) to assess the fit of model items. This residual was proposed by (Dunn & Smyth, 1996) to handle discrete observations and was applied to evaluate data from mixed generalized linear models (Bai, 2018). However, there is no such work for the evaluation of Rasch counts (RC) models. Thus, implementing model verification for Rasch models is essential, so our objective is to verify that the fitted model is able to explain the data properly.

Motivated by the previous observations, in this work we seek to extend the RPC model considering alternative RC models for the observed response. Initially, we consider the negative Binomial (NB) counts (Hung, 2012) and later we extend this model to consider excess zeros, introducing the zero-inflated Poisson (ZIP) counts (Wang, 2010) and zero-inflated negative Binomial (ZINB) counts models. While the NB IRT and ZIP IRT models were introduced by Hung (2012) and Wang (2010) respectively, the ZINB IRT model is a new contribution to the psychometric literature and includes the previous two models as particular cases. For the ZINB model, we introduce Bayesian and frequentist estimation methods by considering a mixed generalized linear formulation following a recent contribution by Baghaei & Doebler (2019). Additionally, we introduce a new residual analysis considering randomized quantile residuals, which has not been used in the psychometric literature previously and has the advantage of employing graphs to check the residuals.

The article is organized as follows. In Sect. 2, we introduce the Rasch Poisson counts model and present some alternative count models to the RPC model. In Sect. 3, we discuss the estimation methods for the models considered, including model comparison criteria. In Sect. 4, we define residual analysis for items of the test. An application is given in Sect. 5, illustrating the methods presented using a real dataset. Finally, in Sect. 6, we make some concluding remarks.

2 Rasch Counts Model

The RPC model, proposed by Rasch (1960) assumes that count responses Y_{ij} of individual i in item j of a test are conditionally independent in the personal latent trait θ_i and Poisson distributed. Furthermore, it is assumed to have an additive composition, using the *log* link function, expressed by:

$$\begin{aligned} Y_{ij} &\sim Pois(\mu_{ij}) \\ \log\left(\mu_{ij}\right) &= \beta_j + \theta_i + t_j, \end{aligned} \tag{1}$$

with $\theta_i \sim N\left(0, \sigma^2\right)$, $i = 1, \cdots, n$ and $j = 1, \cdots, J$, where, μ_{ij} is the expected latent count for individual i in item j, θ_i is the ability of individual i (latent traits), β_j is the facility of item j, and e^{t_j} is the time limit for item j (offset variable). In case there is no time limit, t_j can be fixed as zero. Additionally, the constraint $\sum_{j=1}^{J} \exp\{t_j + \beta_j\} = 1$ is imposed for model identifiability (Jansen, 1997). Here, $Pois(\mu_{ij})$ denotes the probability mass function of the Poisson distribution with mean $\mu_{ij} > 0$, given by:

$$P_Y(y; \mu_{ij}) = \frac{\mu_{ij}^{y_{ij}} e^{-\mu_{ij}}}{y_{ij}!} \tag{2}$$

where the mean and variance are given by $E[Y] = \mu$ and $Var[Y] = \mu$, respectively.

2.1 Alternative Counts Distribution

The Poisson distribution has the characteristic of equidispersion (mean equal to the variance), and may not adequately model underdispersion or overdispersion of the response variable. Thus, to have greater flexibility in the relationship between the mean and variance the negative Binomial, zero-inflated Poisson and zero-inflated negative Binomial distributions are proposed as alternatives to model count data with these characteristics.

- *Negative Binomial Distribution (NBI)*: The probability function of the negative Binomial distribution, denoted by $NBI(\mu, \phi)$, is given by

$$P_Y(y; \mu, \phi) = \frac{\Gamma\left(y + \frac{1}{\phi}\right)}{\Gamma\left(\frac{1}{\phi}\right)\Gamma(y+1)} \left(\frac{\phi\mu}{1+\phi\mu}\right)^y \left(\frac{1}{1+\phi\mu}\right)^{1/\phi} \tag{3}$$

  where $\mu > 0, \phi > 0$ is the dispersion parameter and $\Gamma(\cdot)$ is the gamma function. The mean and variance of the NBI are $E[Y] = \mu$ and $Var[Y] = \mu + \phi\mu^2$.
- *Zero-inflated Poisson Distribution (ZIP)*: Let $Y = 0$ with probability ω and $Y \sim Pois(\mu)$ with probability $(1-\omega)$. Then we say that Y has a zero-inflated Poisson distribution, denoted by $ZIP(\mu, \omega)$, if its probability function is given by

$$P_Y(y; \mu, \omega) = \begin{cases} \omega + (1-\omega)e^{-\mu} & y = 0 \\ (1-\omega)\dfrac{\mu^y e^{-\mu}}{y!} & y = 1, 2, \cdots \end{cases} \tag{4}$$

  where $\mu > 0$ and $0 < \omega < 1$ is the probability of zeros. The mean and variance of a ZIP random variable can be calculated by $E[Y] = (1-\omega)\mu$ and $Var[Y] = \mu(1-\omega)(1+\mu\omega)$, respectively.
- *Zero-inflated Negative Binomial Distribution (ZINBI)*: Let $Y = 0$ with probability ω and $Y \sim NBI(\mu, \phi)$ with probability $(1-\omega)$. Then we say that Y has a zero-inflated negative Binomial distribution, $ZINBI(\mu, \phi, \omega)$, given by

$$P_Y(y; \mu, \omega, \phi,) = \begin{cases} \omega + (1-\omega)(1+\phi\omega)^{-1/\phi} & y = 0 \\ (1-\omega)\dfrac{\Gamma\left(y + \frac{1}{\phi}\right)}{\Gamma\left(\frac{1}{\phi}\right)\Gamma(y+1)} \left(\dfrac{\phi\mu}{1+\phi\mu}\right)^y \left(\dfrac{1}{1+\phi\mu}\right)^{1/\phi} & y = 1, 2, \cdots \end{cases} \tag{5}$$

  where $\mu > 0, \phi > 0$ is the dispersion parameter, $0 < \omega < 1$ is the probability of zeros and $\Gamma(\cdot)$ is the gamma function. The mean and variance of the ZINBI are $E[Y] = (1-\omega)\mu$ and $Var[Y] = (1-\omega)[1 + (\phi + \omega)\mu]$.

In particular, the most general of these distributions is the ZINBI, while the other distributions are special cases. More details on these models can be seen in Hung (2012), Wang (2010), Magnus and Thissen (2017) and Pineda Gonzalez (2018).

2.2 Alternative RC Models

As an alternative to the Rasch Poisson model, we have that the Y_{ij} count responses follow a NBI, ZIP or ZINBI distribution. For these distributions we consider the additive composition of the Rasch model using the log-link function (Eq. 1). Only the Rasch zero-inflated negative Binomial counts (RZINBIC) model is shown because the other models are special cases of this model.

$$\begin{aligned} Y_{ij} &\sim ZINBI(\mu_{ij}, \phi, \omega) \\ \log\left(\mu_{ij}\right) &= \beta_j + \theta_i + t_j, \end{aligned} \tag{6}$$

with $\theta_i \sim N\left(0, \sigma^2\right)$, $i = 1, \cdots, n$, $j = 1, \cdots, J$, where, θ_i is the ability of individual i, β_j is the facility of item j, t_j is offset variable, ϕ is the dispersion parameter and ω is the probability of zeros. In addition, the same identifiability constraints in (1) can be considered here.

3 Estimation Methods

The estimation of the parameters of the proposed models can be performed considering an equivalent formulation of these models as a GLMM. In other words, the RC models, through their additive specification (Eq. 1), can be viewed as a GLMM considering the latent trait θ_i as a random effect of individual, β_j as a fixed effect associated with items and t_j as an offset variable, that is, a known constant added to the regression equation. By considering this formulation, we propose the use of different estimation methods. In a frequentist approach, we consider the penalized marginal likelihood (PML), using the Rigby and Stasinopoulos (RS) algorithm from the `GAMLSS` package (Rigby et al., 2019). Additionally, in a Bayesian approach and using the GLMM formulation of the RC models, we consider an INLA approach using the `INLA` package (Wang et al., 2018). Prior specification is shown in the application. Details about the estimation methods are omitted here; more details can be seen in Rigby et al. (2019) and Wang et al. (2018).

In order to compare alternative RPC models in the application, under the approaches considered, we make use of some model comparison criteria. Specifically, in the frequentist approach, we consider the Akaike information criterion (AIC) and Schwartz's Bayesian criterion (SBC) defined as $AIC = GD + (2 \times df)$ and $SBC = GD + (\log(n) \times df)$, respectively, where df denotes the total effective degrees of freedom used in the model and $GD = -2\ell(\hat{\theta})$ is the fitted global deviance (Rigby et al., 2019).

In contrast, in the Bayesian approach, we consider the deviance information criterion (DIC), given by $DIC = \bar{D} + p_D$ where $\bar{D}$ is the posterior mean of the deviance of the model and p_D is the effective number of parameters in the model (Wang et al., 2018). In addition, we propose to use the Watanabe-Akaike information criterion (WAIC) defined as $WAIC = -2lppd + 2p_W$, where $lppd$ is the log pointwise predictive density and p_W is the effective number of parameters.

For all the above criteria, smaller values indicate better fit.

4 Residual Analysis

Residual analysis is an important tool to assess a model's fit to a given dataset, where one can identify possible outliers. Among the existing residuals described in the literature, we consider the Pearson residual, defined as:

$$r_{ij} = \frac{y_{ij} - \widehat{E[Y_{ij}]}}{\sqrt{\widehat{V[Y_{ij}]}}} \tag{7}$$

with $r_{ij} \approx N(0, 1)$, where $\widehat{E[Y_{ij}]}$ and $\widehat{V[Y_{ij}]}$ are the estimates of the mean and variance of Y_{ij}, respectively, considering the count distribution adopted (Cordeiro & Simas, 2009).

Feng et al. (2017), using simulation studies, compared the quantile residual with the Pearson residual and concluded that the distribution of the quantile residual is better approximated by the standard normal distribution than the Pearson residual. In addition, the authors showed that the quantile residual is the best for detecting lack of fit. Therefore, we consider the randomized quantile residuals proposed by (Dunn & Smyth, 1996), defined as:

$$q_{ij} = \Phi^{-1}(U_i) \tag{8}$$

with $q_{ij} \sim N(0, 1)$, where $\Phi(\cdot)$ is the standard normal cumulative distribution function and U_i is a uniform random variable in the interval $(a_i, b_i]$ with $a_i = \lim_{y \to y_i^-} F(y; \widehat{\eta})$ and $b_i = F(y_i; \widehat{\eta})$, where $F(\cdot)$ is the cumulative distribution function (cdf) of the corresponding count distribution considered and $\widehat{\eta}$ is the vector of estimated parameters (Dunn & Smyth, 1996).

Table 1 shows how the Pearson and randomized quantile residuals are computed for the different Rasch counts models, where *dpois, dnbinom, dzip and dzinb* denote the probability mass function (pmf) for Pois, NBI, ZIP and ZINBI distributions respectively; and cdf by *ppois, pnbinom, pzip and pzinb* respectively. In the Bayesian

Table 1 Pearson and randomized quantile residuals of the different models

Models	Pearson residuals	Quantile residuals
Pois	$\frac{y_i - \hat{\mu}_{ij}}{\sqrt{\hat{\mu}_{ij}}}$	$\Phi^{-1}\left(ppois(y_i - 1; \hat{\mu}_{ij}) + u_i.dpois(y_i; \hat{\mu}_{ij})\right)$
NBI	$\frac{y_i - \hat{\mu}_{ij}}{\sqrt{\hat{\mu}_{ij} + \hat{\phi}\hat{\mu}_{ij}^2}}$	$\Phi^{-1}\left(pnbinom(y_i - 1; \hat{\mu}_{ij}, \hat{\phi}) + u_i.dnbinom(y_i; \hat{\mu}_{ij}, \hat{\phi})\right)$
ZIP	$\frac{y_i - (1-\hat{\omega})\hat{\mu}_{ij}}{\sqrt{\hat{\mu}_{ij}(1-\hat{\omega})(1+\hat{\mu}_{ij}\hat{\omega})}}$	$\Phi^{-1}\left(pzip(y_i - 1; \hat{\mu}_{ij}, \hat{\omega}) + u_i.dzip(y_i; \hat{\mu}_{ij}, \hat{\omega})\right)$
ZINBI	$\frac{y_i - (1-\hat{\omega})\hat{\mu}_{ij}}{\sqrt{\hat{\mu}_{ij}(1-\hat{\omega})\left[1+(\hat{\phi}+\hat{\omega})\hat{\mu}_{ij}\right]}}$	$\Phi^{-1}\left(pzinb(y_i - 1; \hat{\mu}_{ij}, \hat{\phi}, \hat{\omega}) + u_i.dzinb(y_i; \hat{\mu}_{ij}, \hat{\phi}, \hat{\omega})\right)$

approach, we consider a plug-in estimator for both residuals using the posterior mean of the estimated parameters.

Additionally, we have developed generic R functions that can compute the Pearson and quantile residuals for the different counts models adopted. These functions were implemented based on the fitting outputs of the `gamlss` and `INLA` packages.

In the case of IRT models, we are interested in the residual analysis to test items of the test. Therefore, we consider the Pearson and quantile residuals to estimate the distribution of the residuals for each item j, denoted by r_j and q_j (Pearson and quantile residuals, respectively). Then, for each item j, we have a vector with n values of the Pearson residuals for the individuals $r_{1j}, \cdots, r_{nj}$. Similarly, we have a vector of n values of the quantile residuals for each item, $q_{1j}, \cdots, q_{nj}$. Thus, summary statistics for these residuals, such as the mean, standard deviation, minimum and maximum can be reported.

In order to check the fit of a particular item, we propose the use of violin plots (Hintze & Nelson, 1998). We recommend these plots because they displays the distribution of the residuals along with information about the summary statistics and density shape, providing a useful tool for residual analysis. In the R program, these plots can be obtained using the *ggplot2* package (Wickham, 2016).

5 Application

We illustrate residual analysis for the considered count models (RPC, RNBIC, RZIPC, RZINBIC) with an application to a real dataset. We consider an analysis of the correct verification counts obtained by applying a selective attention test (Beyzaee, 2017) that corresponds to the responses of 228 students to 20 items with a time limit for completing the task of 15 s, where the task is to cross out the digits 2 and 7 in three lines of randomly arranged digits and letters (Baghaei & Doebler, 2019).

For illustration, we only show the hierarchical structure of the RZINBIC model in the Bayesian approach. As already mentioned, the model can be perceived as a GLMM in which the individual is considered a random effect, the item is considered a fixed effect, and priors can be included for the parameters of interest. The priors considered are the default priors using the INLA approach. Thus, the most general model that can be proposed is given by

$$
\begin{aligned}
Y_{ij} \mid \theta_i, \beta_j, t_j, \phi, \omega &\sim ZINBI(\mu_{ij}, \phi, \omega) \\
log(\mu_{ij}) &= \eta_{ij} \\
\eta_{ij} &= \beta_j + \theta_i + t_j \qquad (9) \\
\theta_i \mid \sigma_\theta^2 &\overset{iid}{\sim} \mathcal{N}\left(0, \sigma_\theta^2\right); \ \sigma_\theta^{-2} \sim Gamma\left(1, 10^{-5}\right); \ i = 1, \cdots, n \\
\beta_j &\overset{iid}{\sim} \mathcal{N}(0, 1000); \ j = 1, \cdots, k \\
\phi &\sim \mathcal{N}(0, 0.2) \\
logit(\omega) &\sim \mathcal{N}(-1, 0.2).
\end{aligned}
$$

where $\sigma_\theta^{-2} = \tau_\theta$ is the precision parameter and t_j is a known offset variable.

In the hierarchical formulation of the model above, θ_i is a random effect with hyper priors for the corresponding precision parameter. Also, priors for β_j, ϕ e ω are defined. Special models such as RPC, RZIPC and RNBIC can be obtained by eliminating some lines in the above specification.

Considering the Bayesian and frequentist approaches, we adjusted the proposed Rasch counts models using the `gamlss` and `INLA` packages, respectively. Table 2 shows the fit comparison using the model comparison criteria discussed above. We clearly identified the RZIPC model as the one with the best fit for the data considering all criteria.

In order to verify the fit of the items, considering the RZIPC model, we performed residual analysis. We present the boxplots of these residuals by adding the lines in the value −3 and 3. In Fig. 2 considering the frequentist approach, we can identify three items in Pearson residuals (Fig. 2a) that present a discrepant point, items 5, 13 and 15. Considering the quantile residuals (Fig. 2b), items 4, 5, 13 and 15 are identified. In the Bayesian approach, for Pearson residuals (Fig. 3a), items 5, 13 and 15 were identified as discrepant points (analogous to the frequentist case). Also,

Table 2 Model comparison criteria of Rasch counts models for selective attention test data

	Frequentist approach		Bayesian approach	
Models	AIC	SBC	DIC	WAIC
RPC	24639.39	26146.26	24633.84	24539.88
RNBIC	24641.39	26154.69	25052.45	25154.31
RZIPC	24542.26	25843.72	24589.59	24493.55
RZINBIC	24544.26	25852.14	24592.04	24495.15

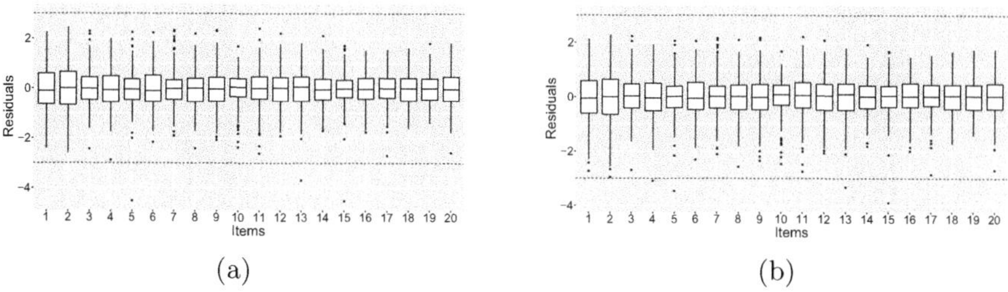

Fig. 2 The frequentist approach. (**a**) Pearson Residuals (**b**) Quantile Residuals

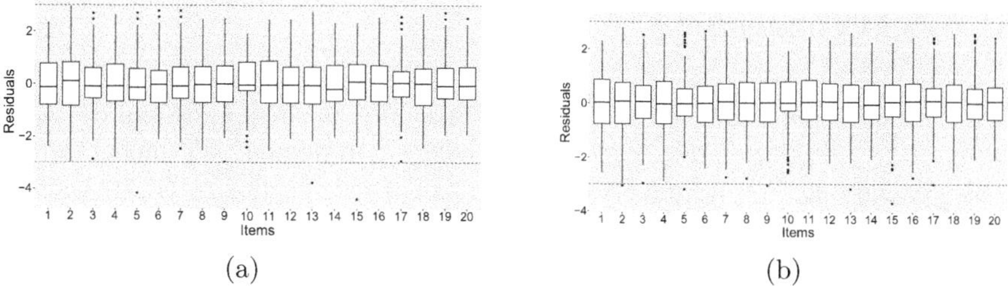

Fig. 3 The Bayesian approach. (**a**) Pearson Residuals (**b**) Quantile Residuals

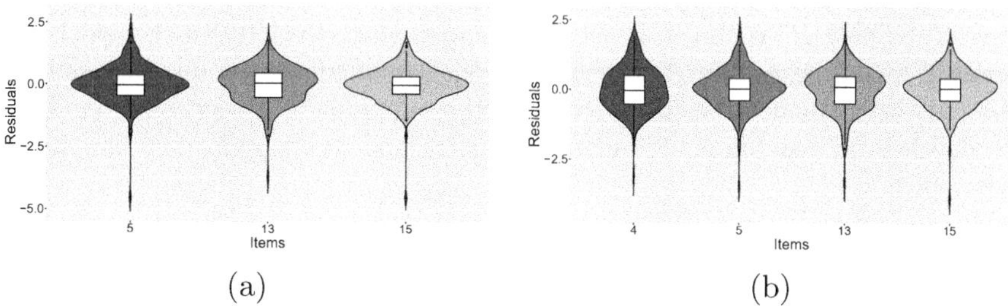

Fig. 4 The frequentist approach. (**a**) Pearson Residuals. (**b**) Quantile Residuals

considering the quantile residuals (Fig. 3b), we identified discrepant points in items 2, 5, 9, 13, 15 and 17.

Thus, in order to clarify the distribution of these items identified as discrepancies in both approaches, we report the distribution of the residuals of these items using a violin plot (Figs. 4 and 5). All items depart from normality, given that in a well-specified item we expect its residuals to exhibit the behavior of a normal distribution. We also note that in quantile residuals, a greater number of items were identified as outliers and a greater number still were identified considering the Bayesian approach. Therefore, these results indicate that the proposed model for the data may still not be the best.

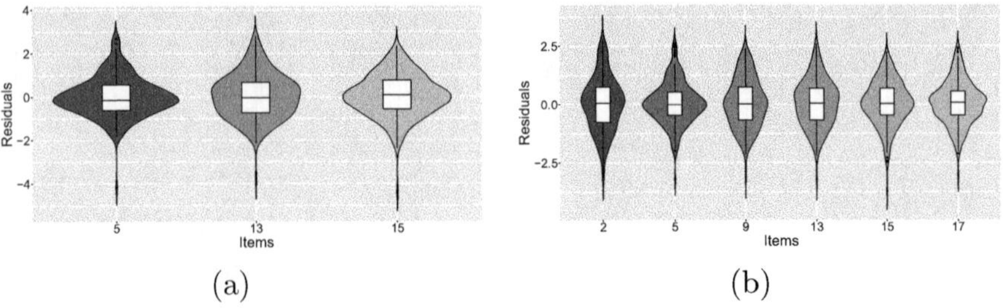

Fig. 5 The Bayesian approach. (**a**) Pearson Residuals (**b**) Quantile Residuals

6 Final Comments

In this paper, we fit four count IRT models considering the frequentist and Bayesian approaches, introducing the zero-inflated negative Binomial IRT model as the most general one. We use the Rasch counts model specification as GLMM, so all models are fitted using the `gamlss` and `INLA` packages in R. We propose the use of the randomized quantile residuals to check the model fit. It is known that these residuals have better performance than Pearson residuals and are normally distributed. Additionally, we show violin plots as an interesting graphical method to analyze the distribution of the residuals for the items of a test.

The models studied are useful alternatives, especially when there are overdispersion in the dataset, as shown in the application, where the ZIP Rasch model was selected as the best model between the models studied but the residual analysis showed that it models no fit still very well to the data and new proposed must be develop on the future. Simulations studies and new applications are being developed.

Acknowledgments The first author would like to thank the Coordenação de Aperfeiçoamento de Pessoal de Nível Superior – Brasil (CAPES) for the financial support. Authors thank reviewer/editor for their comments and suggestions.

References

Baghaei, P., & Doebler, P. (2019). Introduction to the rasch poisson counts model: An r tutorial. *Psychological Reports, 122*(5), 1967–1994

Baghaei, P., Ravand, H., & Nadri, M. (2019). Is the D2 test of attention rasch scalable? Analysis with the rasch poisson counts model. *Perceptual and Motor Skills, 126*(1), 70–86

Bai, W. (2018). *Randomized Quantile Residual for Assessing Generalized Linear Mixed Models with Application to Zero-Inflated Microbiome Data*. Ph.D. thesis, University of Saskatchewan

Bates, D., Mächler, M., Bolker, B., & Walker, S. (2015). Fitting linear mixed-effects models using lme4. *Journal of Statistical Software, 67*(1), 1–48

Beyzaee, S. (2017). A latent variable modeling of verbal reasoning, cognitive flexibility, processing speed, sustained attention, and reading comprehension among iranian efl learners. *Unpublished masters thesis. Mashhad, Iran: Islamic Azad University*

Bowen, B. (2018). *Goodness of Fit via Residual Plots in Item Response Theory*. Ph.D. thesis, University of South Carolina

Cordeiro, G. M., & Simas, A. B. (2009). The distribution of pearson residuals in generalized linear models. *Computational Statistics & Data Analysis, 53*(9), 3397–3411

Dunn, P. K., & Smyth, G. K. (1996). Randomized quantile residuals. *Journal of Computational and Graphical Statistics, 5*(3):236–244

Feng, C., Sadeghpour, A., & Li, L. (2017). Randomized quantile residuals: An omnibus model diagnostic tool with unified reference distribution. *arXiv preprint arXiv:1708.08527*, 7

Haberman, S. J. (2009). Use of generalized residuals to examine goodness of fit of item response models. *ETS Research Report Series, 2009*(1), i–17

Hintze, J. L., & Nelson, R. D. (1998). Violin plots: A box plot-density trace synergism. *The American Statistician, 52*(2), 181–184

Holling, H., Bohning, W., & Bohning, D. (2015). The covariate-adjusted frequency plot for the rasch poisson counts model. *Thailand Statistician, 13*(1), 67–78

Hung, L.-F. (2012). A negative binomial regression model for accuracy tests. *Applied Psychological Measurement, 36*(2), 88–103

Jansen, M. G. (1997). Applications of rasch's poisson counts model to longitudinal count data. *Applications of latent trait and latent class models in the social sciences* (pp. 380–388)

Magnus, B. E., & Thissen, D. (2017). Item response modeling of multivariate count data with zero inflation, maximum inflation, and heaping. *Journal of Educational and Behavioral Statistics, 42*(5), 531–558

McCullagh, P., & Nelder, J. A. (1989). *Generalized linear models* (2nd ed.). London, UK: Chapman and Hall

Pineda Gonzalez, L. F. (2018). Item response models for counting responses. Master's thesis, Universidade Estadual de Campinas, SP

R Core Team (2020). *R: A Language and Environment for Statistical Computing*. R Foundation for Statistical Computing, Vienna, Austria

Rasch, G. (1960). Studies in mathematical psychology: I. probabilistic models for some intelligence and attainment tests. Oxford, England: Nielsen & Lydiche

Rigby, R. A., Stasinopoulos, M. D., Heller, G. Z., & De Bastiani, F. (2019). *Distributions for modeling location, scale, and shape: Using GAMLSS in R*. CRC Press

Santos, N. C. A., & Bazán, J. L. (2021). Residuals analysis in rasch poisson counts models. *Revista Brasileira De Biometria, 39*(1), 206–220

Sinharay, S. (2006). Bayesian item fit analysis for unidimensional item response theory models. *British Journal of Mathematical and Statistical Psychology, 59*(2), 429–449

Swaminathan, H., Hambleton, R. K., & Rogers, H. J. (2006). Assessing the fit of item response theory models. *Handbook of Statistics, 26*, 683–718

Van Rijn, P. W., Sinharay, S., Haberman, S. J., & Johnson, M. S. (2016). Assessment of fit of item response theory models used in large-scale educational survey assessments. *Large-Scale Assessments in Education, 4*(1):10

Verhelst, N., & Kamphuis, F. (2009). A poisson-gamma model for speed tests. *Measurement and Research Department Reports, 2*, 2010–2011

Wang, L. (2010). Irt–zip modeling for multivariate zero-inflated count data. *Journal of Educational and Behavioral Statistics, 35*(6), 671–692

Wang, X., Yue, Y. R., & Faraway, J. J. (2018). *Bayesian regression modeling with INLA*. CRC Press

Wickham, H. (2016). *ggplot2: Elegant graphics for data analysis*. New York: Springer

A Bayesian Solution to Non-convergence of Crossed Random Effects Models

Mingya Huang and Carolyn Anderson

1 Introduction

Crossed random effects models (CREMs) have become the method of choice in studies in which every subject sees every stimulus and every stimulus is viewed by every subject (Baayen et al., 2008). Researchers often encounter a non-convergence problem when fitting CREMs with Maximum likelihood based methods (MLE/REML) because of the complexity of random effects structure and small sample sizes. A common strategy is to simplify models (i.e., using random intercepts only). We conducted an informal survey of articles from the Journal of Memory and Language from 2015 to 2019 citing Baayen et al. (2008) paper, and found that 43% of these articles utilizing CREMs do not include random slopes and/or removed them to achieve convergence. However, improper model structure will impact the parameter estimates as well as their standard errors. Under-parameterization of the covariance structure invalidates inference, and over-parameterization of the covariance structure leads to inefficient estimation (Molenberghs and Verbeke, 2000). If random slopes are removed from a level, the variance(s) related to that level will be redistributed to other levels and therefore result in inaccurate standard errors (Snijders, 2011). Similarly, omitting incorrect fixed effect structures will also lead to incorrect estimates for both random and fixed effects (Raudenbush and Bryk, 2002). To achieve valid inferences, Barr et al. (2013) proposed the maximal model structure for confirmatory factor analysis with every possible random effects rather than simplifying the models so long as the

M. Huang (✉)
University of Wisconsin-Madison, Madison, WI, USA
e-mail: mhuang233@wisc.edu

C. Anderson
University of Illinois Urbana-Champaign, Champaign, IL, USA
e-mail: cja@illinois.edu

M. Wiberg et al. (eds.), *Quantitative Psychology*, Springer Proceedings in Mathematics & Statistics 353, https://doi.org/10.1007/978-3-030-74772-5_27

design justifies. Bates et al. (2015) also argued that the models should not be too simple or too complex, but just right for optimal statistical inference. An advantage of appropriate modeling of the covariance structure is that it can help explain the random variability captured by the fixed effects.

Estimators from both MLE and REML, two typical methods fitting hierarchical linear models, are both consistent and efficient, but these estimation methods often fail to converge as models become more complex (Snijders, 2011). Unlike MLE and REML, Bayesian approaches can be more flexible when dealing with complex models such as CREMs (Snijders, 2011). Therefore, we investigated whether using a Bayesian method is an efficient alternative that can solve non-convergence problems.

2 Crossed-Random Effects Model (CREMs)

CREMs are used to fit the hierarchical data where units are simultaneously nested in multiple types of clusters (Cho & Rabe-Hesketh, 2011). In psycholinguistic research, there is usually one observation/trial per cell in a design crossed by subject and stimuli. An example of a two-level CREM for this type of cross-classification designs is

$$Y_{ij} = \gamma_{00} + \sum_p \gamma_{0p} x_{pi} + \sum_q \gamma_{q0} z_{qj} + U_{0i} + \sum_p U_{pi} x_{pi} + W_{0j} + \sum_q W_{qj} z_{qj} + R_{ij}, \tag{1}$$

3 Bayesian Approach

In Bayesian estimation, samples of parameter estimates are drawn from their posterior distribution, which are proportional to the product of a marginal probability of the parameter and the conditional probability of the data given the parameters. Let $\boldsymbol{\theta}$ be a vector of model parameters and $\boldsymbol{Y}$ represent data. The posterior distribution of parameters conditional on data is

$$f(\boldsymbol{\theta}|\boldsymbol{Y}) \propto f(\boldsymbol{Y}|\boldsymbol{\theta})\, f(\boldsymbol{\theta}), \tag{2}$$

where $f(\boldsymbol{Y}|\boldsymbol{\theta})$ is the likelihood, and $f(\boldsymbol{\theta})$ is the prior distribution which reflects our preceding knowledge of the parameters. We set non-informative priors for both fixed effects (i.e., $N(0, 100)$ which is essentially flat), and variance of the random effects (i.e., Cauchy(0, 5)) based on recommendations from (Gelman, 2006). In simple cases, the posterior distribution can be found analytically (e.g., proportion from a binomial distribution), but for more complex cases, Markov Chain Monte

Carlo (MCMC) is used to sample from the posterior. A Markov chain is a sequence of draws of random variables for which the probability depends only on the previous variable. The sequence of possible estimates for each parameter is known as a "chain," with multiple chains typically run for each parameter. We use Hamiltonian algorithms to iteratively sample the posterior distribution, which is implemented in the brms package (Bürkner, 2017) in R (3.6.2), that function as a wrapper for Stan (Carpenter et al., 2017). Convergence was based on the potential scale reduction factor ($\hat{R}$), which estimates the potential decrease in the between-chains variability relative to the within-chain variability. We expect $\hat{R}$ to be close to 1 at convergence, and Gelman and Rubin (1992) suggests 1.1 as the cutoff value. We also checked the plots of posterior densities, trace plots, and autocorrelation plots to evaluate convergence. The number of Markov chains was set to be 4 with 8,000 iterations per chain where the first 4,000 iterations were warm-ups. The chains were "thinned," a procedure that keeps every k_{th} sample (parameter estimate). We retained every 10th sample, and thus the posterior is only based on 400 sample values for each chain.

4 Simulation

A simulation study with 20 replications was conducted to evaluate the performance of MLE, REML, and Bayesian estimation of CREMs. Data were simulated from CREMs with two or four random slopes and 20 or 50 stimuli and subjects, yielding four conditions (Table 1). For each of the four simulated conditions, we fit an under-specified model (only random intercepts) and the correctly specified model (used to simulate data) using each estimation method. The simplest model fit to data in this study was the random intercepts model,

$$\begin{aligned} Y_{ij} &= \gamma_{00} + \gamma_{01}x_{1i} + \gamma_{10}z_{1j} + \gamma_{02}x_{2i} + \gamma_{20}z_{2j} + \gamma_{03}x_{3i} + \gamma_{30}z_{3j} + \gamma_{04}x_{4i} \\ &\quad + U_{0i} + W_{0j} + R_{ij}. \end{aligned} \tag{3}$$

The model with two random slopes (i.e. condition 1 and 3) was

$$\begin{aligned} Y_{ij} &= \gamma_{00} + \gamma_{01}x_{1i} + \gamma_{10}z_{1j} + \gamma_{02}x_{2i} + \gamma_{20}z_{2j} + \gamma_{03}x_{3i} + \gamma_{30}z_{3j} + \gamma_{04}x_{4i} \\ &\quad + U_{0i} + U_{1i}x_{1i} + W_{0j} + W_{1j}z_{1j} + R_{ij}. \end{aligned} \tag{4}$$

Table 1 Summary of four conditions of simulation study

Conditions	# Subject × # Stimuli	# Random Slopes
Condition 1	20 × 20	2 slopes
Condition 2	20 × 20	4 slopes
Condition 3	50 × 50	2 slopes
Condition 4	50 × 50	4 slopes

Table 2 Models parameters for the fixed effects (left) and distributions (right) from which random effects were drawn for i,j=20,50 on each replication of the simulation study

Fixed effects parameters		Random effects parameters	
Subject-specific	Stimuli-specific	Subject-specific	Stimuli-specific
γ_{0p}	γ_{q0}	U_{ri}	W_{rj}
$\gamma_{00} = 1.00$			
$\gamma_{01} = -2.00$	$\gamma_{10} = 2.00$	$U_{0i} \sim N(0, .16)$,	$W_{0i} \sim N(0, .49)$
$\gamma_{02} = .30$	$\gamma_{20} = 2.00$	$U_{1i} \sim N(0, .04)$,	$W_{1i} \sim N(0, .16)$
$\gamma_{03} = .50$	$\gamma_{30} = .20$	$U_{2i} \sim N(0, .36)$,	$W_{2i} \sim N(0, .81)$
$\gamma_{04} = 1.00$			
		$R_{ij} \sim N(0, 1.00)$	

For the more complex case of 4 random slopes (i.e. condition 2 and 4) was

$$Y_{ij} = \gamma_{00} + \gamma_{01}x_{1i} + \gamma_{10}z_{1j} + \gamma_{02}x_{2i} + \gamma_{20}z_{2j} + \gamma_{03}x_{3i} + \gamma_{30}z_{3j} + \gamma_{04}x_{4i} + U_{0i} + U_{1i}x_{1i} + U_{2i}x_{2i} + W_{0j} + W_{1j}z_{1j} + W_{2j}z_{2j} + R_{ij}. \tag{5}$$

Data from models (4) and (5) were simulated for i, j=20, 50. For each replication of the simulated models, values for x_{pi} and z_{qj} were drawn from the following distributions: $x_{1i} \sim N(0, 2.00)$; $x_{2i} \sim N(0, 3.00)$; $x_{3i} \sim N(0, 1.25)$; $x_{4i} \sim$ Bernoulli (0.1); $z_{1j} \sim N(0, 1.75)$; $z_{2j} \sim N(0, 2)$; and $z_{3j} \sim N(0, 2.25)$. The fixed effects parameters and the distributions for random effects are given in Table 2.

5 Results

5.1 Convergence Rate

Table 3 summarized the convergence rates of each condition out of 20 replications. All models using a Bayesian approach yield convergence rates of 100%. In Condition 1 and MLE, 70% of the under-specified models converged and only 10% of the correctly specified models converged. For REML, 82.5% of the under-specified models converged and only 15% of the correctly specified models converged. In Condition 2, both MLE and REML obtained 100% convergence rates for the under-specified models; however, they both failed to converge even with different optimizers such as NEALTHER-MEAD and BOBYQA in all replications when trying to fit the correctly specified model. In Condition 3, the under-specified models fit by either MLE and REML converged in all cases; however, the convergence rates of the correctly specified model for MLE and REML were only 40% and 45%, respectively. In Condition 4, 100% of the under-specified models converged for both MLE and REML. However, only 20% of the correctly specified models fit by MLE converged, and only 32.5% for REML of the correctly specified models converged.

Table 3 Convergence rates of under-specified models (only random intercepts) and the correctly specified models

Conditions	#Subjects × #Stimuli	# Random slopes	Model fit	MLE	REML	Bayesian
Condition 1	20 × 20	2	Under-specified	70%	82.5%	100%
			Correctly specified	10%	15%	100%
Condition 2	20 × 20	4	Under-specified	100%	100%	100%
			Correctly specified	0%	0%	100%
Condition 3	50 × 50	2	Under-specified	100%	100%	100%
			Correctly specified	40%	45%	100%
Condition 4	50 × 50	4	Under-specified	100%	100%	100%
			Correctly specified	20%	32.5%	100%

With 100% convergence rates, the results indicate that a Bayesian approach is a viable alternative of MLE/REML to deal with convergence problems. Note that as the random effects structure of the model used to simulate data became more complex, it was less likely for the correctly specified model to converge with either MLE or REML. As the number of subjects and stimuli increased, the under-specified model using MLE/REML was more likely to converge. In addition, REML yielded a higher convergence rate than MLE in some conditions, suggesting REML as a useful alternative when MLE encounters non-convergence.

5.2 *Parameter Recovery*

We discuss the efficiency and validity of the Bayesian parameter estimates. Tables 4 and 5 summarize the mean of Bayesian estimates, 95% credible intervals, the scale reduction factor $\hat{R}$, root mean squared error (RMSE), and bias for the 20 replications. In Table 4, the $\hat{R}$s are less than 1.20, indicating convergence. The fixed effects estimates are similar to the values used to simulate the data in both 20 × 20 and 50 × 50 cases. In contrast, the random effects estimates in the under-specified model deviate from the values used to generate the data while the correctly specified model yield similar variance estimates which are close to the true ones. The RMSEs and biases are smaller in the correctly specified models. As the sample size increases from 20 × 20 to 50 × 50, the estimated values become closer to the true values.

Similarly, in Table 5, the fixed effects estimates are close to the true values and are more accurate in the correct model than the under-specified model. For the random effects, the under-specified models yield the variance estimates that deviate from the true values, but they are similar in the correct model. These results are supported by smaller RMSEs and biases for the correctly specified model, with no discernible pattern in the biases. Comparing Tables 4 and 5, we find that as the model become more complex (from two to four slopes), the bias and the RMSEs for random effects also increase. Additionally, the deviations between the estimates and true values are

Table 4 Bayesian parameter estimates, 95% credible intervals, intervals widths, $\hat{R}$ values, RMSE and bias for models fit to simulated data for conditions with 20 subjects × 20 stimuli (top) and 50 × 50 (bottom) and CREMs with 2 slopes

Model		True		95%Credible Intervals		Intervals	$\hat{R}$			
Fit	Param	Value	Est.	Lower	Upper	Width	Min	Max	RMSE	Bias
				Condition 1:	20 × 20					
Under-specified	γ_{00}	1.00	0.96	0.35	1.58	1.23	1.00	1.00	0.26	−0.04
	γ_{01}	−2.00	−2.00	−2.17	−1.84	0.33	1.00	1.00	0.11	−0.00
	γ_{10}	2.00	2.00	1.68	2.32	0.64	1.00	1.00	0.16	−0.00
	γ_{02}	0.30	0.30	0.19	0.41	0.22	1.00	1.00	0.13	−0.00
	γ_{20}	0.20	0.22	−0.05	0.50	0.55	1.00	1.00	0.03	0.02
	γ_{03}	0.50	0.50	0.24	0.76	0.52	1.00	1.00	0.08	−0.00
	γ_{30}	1.50	1.47	1.23	1.72	0.51	1.00	1.00	0.14	−0.03
	γ_{04}	1.00	0.81	−0.19	1.81	2.00	1.00	1.00	0.59	−0.19
	$var(U0)$	0.14	0.35	0.14	0.81	0.67	1.00	1.00	0.25	−0.21
	$var(W0)$	0.04	1.14	0.52	2.42	1.90	1.00	1.00	0.79	−0.53
	$var(Rij)$	1.00	1.14	0.93	1.08	0.15	1.00	1.00	0.46	−0.14
Correctly specified	γ_{00}	1.00	0.99	0.41	1.56	1.15	1.00	1.00	0.25	−0.01
	γ_{01}	−2.00	−1.98	−2.20	−1.75	0.45	1.00	1.01	0.10	0.02
	γ_{10}	2.00	2.01	1.58	2.43	0.85	1.00	1.00	0.17	0.01
	γ_{02}	0.30	0.30	0.20	0.41	0.21	1.00	1.00	0.03	0.00
	γ_{20}	0.20	0.22	−0.04	0.48	0.52	1.00	1.00	0.11	0.02
	γ_{03}	0.50	0.50	0.25	0.75	0.50	1.00	1.00	0.07	−0.00
	γ_{30}	1.50	1.48	1.24	1.71	0.47	1.00	1.00	0.12	−0.02
	γ_{04}	1.00	0.82	−0.25	1.90	2.10	1.00	1.01	0.65	−0.18
	$var(U0)$	0.14	0.18	0.01	0.62	0.61	1.00	1.00	0.09	−0.04
	$var(U1)$	0.04	0.06	0.00	0.30	0.30	1.00	1.02	0.04	−0.02
	$var(W0)$	0.48	0.51	0.05	1.69	1.64	1.00	1.03	0.23	−0.03
	$var(W1)$	0.16	0.27	0.01	1.12	1.11	1.00	1.02	0.18	−0.11
	$var(Rij)$	1.00	1.00	0.93	1.05	0.12	1.00	1.00	0.03	0.00

	γ_{10}	2.00	1.96	1.75	2.16	0.41	1.00	1.00	0.10	−0.04
				Condition 3:	50 × 50					
Under-specified	γ_{00}	1.00	1.03	0.70	1.36	0.66	1.00	1.00	0.18	0.03
	γ_{01}	−2.00	−1.99	−2.07	−1.90	0.08	1.00	1.00	0.06	0.01
	γ_{10}	2.00	1.97	1.80	2.15	0.35	1.00	1.00	0.10	−0.03
	γ_{02}	0.30	0.30	0.25	0.36	0.11	1.00	1.00	0.03	0.00
	γ_{20}	0.20	0.20	0.07	0.34	0.27	1.00	1.00	0.07	0.00
	γ_{03}	0.50	0.50	0.36	0.63	0.27	1.00	1.00	0.06	−0.00
	γ_{30}	1.50	1.49	1.36	1.62	0.26	1.00	1.01	0.05	−0.01
	γ_{04}	1.00	1.05	0.51	1.59	1.08	1.00	1.00	0.29	0.04
	$var(U0)$	0.14	0.32	0.20	0.50	0.30	1.00	1.01	0.18	−0.17
	$var(W0)$	0.04	0.99	0.64	1.49	0.85	1.00	1.00	0.55	−0.82
	$var(Rij)$	1.00	0.99	0.97	1.02	0.05	1.00	1.00	0.28	0.00
Correctly specified	γ_{00}	1.00	1.03	0.73	1.33	0.60	1.00	1.00	0.15	0.03
	γ_{01}	−2.00	−1.98	−2.08	−1.87	0.21	1.00	1.00	0.05	0.02
	γ_{02}	0.30	0.30	0.25	0.35	0.10	1.00	1.00	0.03	0.00
	γ_{20}	0.20	0.21	0.08	0.33	0.24	1.00	1.00	0.06	0.01
	γ_{03}	0.50	0.50	0.37	0.62	0.25	1.00	1.00	0.05	−0.00
	γ_{30}	1.50	1.49	1.37	1.60	0.23	1.00	1.00	0.05	−0.01
	γ_{04}	1.00	1.07	0.57	1.56	0.99	1.00	1.01	0.26	0.0
	$var(U0)$	0.14	0.17	0.07	0.35	0.28	1.00	1.00	0.04	−0.02
	$var(U1)$	0.04	0.04	0.00	0.11	0.11	1.00	1.00	0.02	−0.00
	$var(W0)$	0.48	0.53	0.24	1.00	0.76	1.00	1.00	0.16	−0.08
	$var(W1)$	0.16	0.18	0.02	0.44	0.42	1.00	1.01	0.11	−0.01
	$var(Rij)$	1.00	1.00	0.97	1.00	0.03	1.00	1.00	0.01	−0.01

Table 5 Bayesian parameter estimates, 95% credible intervals, intervals widths, $\hat{R}$ values, RMSE and bias for models fit to simulated data for conditions with 20 subjects × 20 stimuli (top) and 50 × 50 (Bottom) and CREMs with 4 slopes

Model		True		95%Credible intervals		Intervals	$\hat{R}$			
fit	Param	value	Est.	Lower	Upper	Width	Min	Max	RMSE	Bias
				Condition 2:	20 × 20					
Under-specified	γ_{00}	1.00	1.15	−0.26	2.56	2.82	1.00	1.00	0.59	0.15
	γ_{01}	−2.00	−2.01	−2.44	−1.57	0.87	1.00	1.00	0.20	−0.01
	γ_{10}	2.00	2.02	1.33	2.71	1.38	1.00	1.00	.35	0.02
	γ_{02}	0.30	0.37	0.09	0.66	0.57	1.00	1.00	0.19	0.07
	γ_{20}	0.20	0.18	−0.38	0.75	1.13	1.00	1.00	0.37	−0.02
	γ_{03}	0.50	0.57	−0.12	1.24	1.36	1.00	1.00	0.31	0.07
	γ_{30}	1.50	1.50	0.99	2.01	1.02	1.00	1.00	0.19	0.00
	γ_{04}	1.00	0.57	−2.06	3.21	5.27	1.00	1.00	1.97	−0.44
	var(U0)	0.14	2.78	1.23	5.75	4.52	1.00	1.00	3.03	−2.64
	var(W0)	0.04	5.24	2.51	10.83	8.32	1.00	1.00	5.05	−4.77
	var(Rij)	1.00	1.00	0.93	1.08	0.15	1.00	1.00	0.03	0.00
Correctly specified	γ_{00}	1.00	1.26	0.16	2.35	2.19	1.00	1.00	0.43	0.26
	γ_{01}	−2.00	−2.00	−2.46	−1.54	0.92	1.00	1.00	0.19	−0.00
	γ_{10}	2.00	2.06	1.38	2.74	1.36	1.00	1.00	0.26	0.06
	γ_{02}	0.30	0.37	0.01	0.73	0.72	1.00	1.01	0.15	0.07
	γ_{20}	0.20	0.13	−0.57	0.82	0.25	1.00	1.00	0.24	−0.07
	γ_{03}	0.50	0.54	−0.04	1.12	1.16	1.00	1.00	0.27	0.04
	γ_{30}	1.50	1.55	1.12	1.96	0.84	1.00	1.00	0.17	0.05
	γ_{04}	1.00	0.62	−2.24	3.54	5.78	1.00	1.01	1.67	−0.38
	var(U0)	0.14	0.45	0.00	2.51	2.51	1.00	1.00	0.44	−0.31
	var(U1)	0.04	0.14	0.00	0.99	0.99	1.00	1.01	0.14	−0.10
	var(U2)	0.30	0.25	0.02	0.85	0.83	1.00	1.00	0.12	0.05
	var(W0)	0.48	0.62	0.00	3.93	3.93	1.00	1.00	0.41	−0.14
	var(W1)	0.16	0.46	0.00	2.44	2.44	1.00	1.00	0.41	−0.30
	var(W2)	0.81	0.97	0.11	3.02	2.91	1.00	1.00	0.42	−0.16
	var(Rij)	1.00	1.00	0.93	1.08	0.15	1.00	1.00	0.03	0.00

	γ_{10}	2.00	1.97	1.65	2.26	0.61	1.00	1.00	0.17	−0.03
				Condition 4:	50 × 50					
Under-specified	γ_{00}	1.00	1.11	0.28	1.93	1.65	1.00	1.00	0.53	0.11
	γ_{01}	−2.00	−1.99	−2.25	−1.73	0.52	1.00	1.00	0.11	0.01
	γ_{10}	2.00	1.91	1.54	2.28	0.74	1.00	1.00	0.23	−0.09
	γ_{02}	0.30	0.35	0.18	0.52	0.34	1.00	1.00	0.17	0.05
	γ_{20}	0.20	0.14	−0.16	0.44	0.60	1.00	1.00	0.26	−0.06
	γ_{03}	0.50	0.50	0.08	0.91	0.82	1.00	1.00	0.17	−0.00
	γ_{30}	1.50	1.52	1.25	1.79	0.54	1.00	1.00	0.11	0.02
	γ_{04}	1.00	0.90	−0.75	2.54	3.29	1.00	1.00	1.00	−0.10
	var(U0)	0.14	3.19	2.02	4.72	2.70	1.00	1.00	3.33	−3.04
	var(W0)	0.04	4.72	3.07	7.02	3.95	1.00	1.00	4.55	−4.27
	var(Rij)	1.00	1.00	0.97	1.02	0.05	1.00	1.00	0.12	−0.01
Correctly specified	γ_{00}	1.00	1.07	0.57	1.59	1.02	1.00	1.00	0.31	0.07
	γ_{01}	−2.00	−1.98	−2.18	−1.79	0.39	1.00	1.00	0.09	0.02
	γ_{02}	0.30	0.34	0.13	0.54	0.41	1.00	1.00	0.12	0.04
	γ_{20}	0.20	0.23	−0.12	0.58	0.70	1.00	1.00	0.17	0.03
	γ_{03}	0.50	0.52	0.25	0.79	0.54	1.00	1.00	0.11	0.02
	γ_{30}	1.50	1.51	1.34	1.69	0.35	1.00	1.00	0.06	0.01
	γ_{04}	1.00	0.94	−0.26	2.12	2.38	1.00	1.00	0.56	−0.06
	var(U0)	0.14	0.24	0.01	0.93	0.92	1.00	1.00	0.18	−0.09
	var(U1)	0.04	0.05	0.00	0.24	0.24	1.00	1.00	0.04	−0.01
	var(U2)	0.30	0.32	0.13	0.59	0.46	1.00	1.00	0.08	0.00
	var(W0)	0.48	0.31	0.01	1.28	1.27	1.00	1.00	0.23	0.14
	var(W1)	0.16	0.20	0.01	0.68	0.67	1.00	1.01	0.20	−0.03
	var(W2)	0.81	0.95	0.42	1.77	1.35	1.00	1.00	0.26	−0.16
	var(Rij)	1.00	1.00	0.97	1.02	0.05	1.00	1.01	0.12	−0.01

larger in the under-specified models than in the correctly-specified models in all conditions.

Overall, for both under-specified and correctly specified models, the fixed effect parameters were well recovered when using Bayesian estimation. However, differences were found with respect to the 95% credible intervals for the fixed effects. The intervals for the correctly specified models were narrower than the ones from the under-specified model, which was even more prominent with larger sample sizes. Similarly, the random effects variance parameters were recovered better in the correctly-specified models. Also, only the 95% credible intervals in the correctly specified models covered the true values used to simulate the data. The variance estimates for under-specified models have poor performance, and variance parameters were over-estimated such that the 95% credible intervals did not cover the true values used to simulate the data. For correctly specified models, the 95% credible intervals were narrowed for larger sample sizes (and given model complexity) and were narrower for simpler models (for given sample size).

6 Conclusion

Although some previous studies have examined the convergence problems of random effects models and promote a Bayesian approach as a solution (Eager & Roy, 2017), none have specifically considered CREMs. This study is the first to do so, and provides solid evidence for a Bayesian approach when fitting the CREMs to data over MLE/REML. Comparing convergence rates of MLE/REML and Bayesian approaches, the latter obtained 100% convergence rates ($\hat{R}s < 1.1$). As the model became more complex with more random effects, the convergence rates decreased under MLE/REML. Furthermore, the Bayesian estimates of both fixed effects and random effects were valid and efficient in the correctly-specified models but not in the under-specified models. This study highlighted three important points: (1) an improper model structure will result in inefficient estimation and invalid results (2) for more complex random effects structures, the models using Bayesian approach can achieve model convergence but not MLE/REML (3) using Bayesian approach to fit the CREMs can obtain efficient estimates. Future studies will explore whether using a Bayesian approach can select an optimal model.

References

Baayen, R. H., Davidson, D. J., & Bates, D. M. (2008). Mixed-effects modeling with crossed random effects for subjects and items. *Journal of Memory and Language, 59*, 390–412

Barr, D. J., Levy, R., Scheepers, C., & Tily, H. J. (2013). Random effects structure for confirmatory hypothesis testing: Keep it maximal. *Journal of Memory and Language, 68*, 255–278

Bates, D., Kliegl, R., Vasishth, S., & Baayen, H. (2015). Parsimonious mixed models. arXiv preprint arXiv:1506.04967

Bürkner, P. C. (2017). Advanced Bayesian multilevel modeling with the R package brms. arXiv preprint arXiv:1705.11123

Carpenter, B., Gelman, A., Hoffman, M. D., Lee, D., Goodrich, B., Betancourt, M., Brubaker, M., Guo, J., Li, P., & Riddell, A. (2017). Stan: A probabilistic programming language. *Journal of Statistical Software, 76*, 1

Cho, S. J., & Rabe-Hesketh, S. (2011). Alternating imputation posterior estimation of models with crossed random effects. *Computational Statistics & Data Analysis, 55*, 12–25

Eager, C., & Roy, J. (2017). Mixed effects models are sometimes terrible. arXiv preprint arXiv:1701.04858

Gelman, A. (2006). Prior distributions for variance parameters in hierarchical models (comment on article by Browne and Draper). *Bayesian Analysis, 1*, 515–534

Gelman, A., Rubin, D. B. (1992). Inference from iterative simulation using multiple sequences. *Statistical Science, 7*, 457–472

Molenberghs, G., & Verbeke, G. (2000). *Linear mixed models for longitudinal data*. Springer

Raudenbush, S. W., & Bryk, A. S. (2002). *Hierarchical linear models: Applications and data analysis methods* (vol. 1). Sage

Snijders, T. (2011). *Multilevel analysis* (pp. 879–882). Heidelberg: Springer

Priors in Bayesian Estimation Under the Two-Parameter Logistic Model

Seock-Ho Kim, Elaine Duong, Constanza Mardones, Madeline Schellman, Jordan Wheeler, Jiawei Xiong, Guoguo Zheng, Selay Zor, and Allan S. Cohen

1 Introduction

The quality of Bayesian estimates lies in the appropriateness of specifications of the priors. All Bayesian estimation methods should yield comparable item and ability parameter estimates, especially when comparable priors are used or when ignorance or locally-uniform priors are used. This paper was designed to investigate this issue using the two-parameter logistic (2PL) model. Specifically, item and ability parameter estimates from Gibbs sampling using rejection sampling employing different specifications of priors are examined and compared with those from marginal Bayesian estimation (MBE; Mislevy, 1986; Tsutakawa & Lin, 1986). Adopting the presentation in the seminal paper by Swaminathan and Gifford (1985) for Bayesian estimation under the 2PL model, priors in Gibbs sampling are explained below using their framework instead of employing new notation.

For the 2PL model, many estimation methods can be used to obtain item and ability parameter estimates. Item and person parameters can be estimated jointly by maximizing the joint likelihood function. Marginal maximum likelihood estimation using the expectation and maximization algorithm can be used to obtain item parameter estimates (Bock & Aitkin, 1981; du Toit, 2003). In addition, joint Bayes modal estimation (JBME) and MBE can be employed to obtain parameter estimates under the 2PL model (e.g., Birnbaum, 1969; Kim et al., 1994; Mislevy, 1986; Swaminathan and Gifford, 1985; Tsutakawa & Lin, 1986).

S.-H. Kim (✉) · E. Duong · C. Mardones · M. Schellman · J. Wheeler · J. Xiong · G. Zheng
S. Zor · A. S. Cohen
University of Georgia, Athens, GA, USA
e-mail: shkim@uga.edu; eduong@uga.edu; cam04214@uga.edu; mas13@uga.edu; jmwheeler@uga.edu; jx56584@uga.edu; ggzheng@uga.edu; selay.zor25@uga.edu; ascohen@uga.edu

M. Wiberg et al. (eds.), *Quantitative Psychology*, Springer Proceedings in Mathematics & Statistics 353, https://doi.org/10.1007/978-3-030-74772-5_28

Swaminathan and Gifford (1985) described Bayesian estimation for the 2PL model. A number of other papers described Bayesian estimation methods for more general item response theory models (e.g., Leonard & Novick, 1985; Mislevy, 1986; Swaminathan & Gifford, 1986; Tsutakawa & Lin, 1986). Nearly all Bayesian methods in item response theory that are implemented in computer software obtain parameter estimates by maximizing some form of the posterior distribution. More recently, however, Fox (2010), Stone and Zhu (2015), and Levy and Mislevy (2016) presented Bayesian estimation of item and ability parameters based on techniques for the approximation of the posterior distribution. This was not entirely new as Albert (1992) had done the same some time ago. Kim and Bolt (2007) presented an excellent instructional material for the Markov chain Monte Carlo (MCMC) method to estimate parameters in item response theory models. Appendix A contains example code for Gibbs sampling (i.e., the MCMC method in OpenBUGS) used in this study. A summary of priors and their specifications used in the earlier work is presented in Appendix B (i.e., Appendix B Tables 4, 5 and 6, but only portions are shown due to the page limit) in the context of the 2PL model. Papers that presented Bayesian estimation methods for the Rasch model (e.g., Swaminathan & Gifford, 1982; Gonzalez, 2010; Johnson & Sinharay, 2016) or for the limited set of parameters under the 2PL model (e.g., Marcoulides, 2018) were excluded.

1.1 The 2PL Model and Priors

The 2PL model is

$$P_{ij} = P(x_{ij} = 1|\theta_i, \xi_j) = \frac{1}{1 + \exp[-\alpha_j(\theta_i - \beta_j)]}, \tag{1}$$

where θ_i is the ability parameter for person i, $\xi_j \equiv (\alpha_j, \beta_j)$ is the set of item parameters (i.e., α_j is the discrimination parameter and β_j is the difficulty parameter for item j), and x_{ij} is the dichotomous item response.

The posterior distribution for the 2PL model for dichotomous items can be defined as

$$p(\theta, \xi|x) = \frac{p(x|\theta, \xi)p(\theta, \xi)}{p(x)}, \tag{2}$$

where $p(x|\theta, \xi) \equiv l(\theta, \xi) = \prod_i \prod_j p(x_{ij}|\theta_i, \xi_j) = \prod_i \prod_j P_{ij}^{x_{ij}}(1 - P_{ij})^{1-x_{ij}}$ is the likelihood function of a set of parameters θ and ξ with item response data x, $p(\theta, \xi)$ is the prior distribution, and $p(x) = \int\int p(x|\theta, \xi)p(\theta, \xi)d\xi d\theta$.

Following Lindley and Smith (1972) and Novick, Lewis, and Jackson (1973), Swaminathan and Gifford (1985) used independent priors, $p(\theta, \xi) = p(\theta, \alpha, \beta) = p(\theta)p(\alpha)p(\beta)$. The prior for ability can have a hierarchical form as $p(\theta) = \prod_i p(\theta_i|\mu_\theta, \phi_\theta)p(\mu_\theta, \phi_\theta)$. A normal distribution can be used as the prior for ability. For the identification purpose, the specification of $\mu_\theta = 0$ and $\phi_\theta = 1$ can be employed. The prior for discrimination is $p(\alpha) = \prod_j p(\alpha_j|\nu_\alpha, \omega_\alpha)$. The prior for discrimination can be directly specified with a chi distribution $\chi(\nu_\alpha, \omega_\alpha)$, where ν_α is the degrees of freedom and ω_α is a scale parameter. The prior for difficulty can have a hierarchical form as $p(\beta) = \prod_j p(\beta_j|\mu_\beta, \phi_\beta)p(\mu_\beta, \phi_\beta)$, where $p(\mu_\beta, \phi_\beta) = p(\phi_\beta)$ for which $p(\mu_\beta)$ has an improper uniform distribution and $p(\phi_\beta)$ has an inverse chi-square distribution with parameters ν_β and λ_β (i.e., $\phi_\beta \sim \chi^{-2}(\nu_\beta, \lambda_\beta)$). In their paper, the nuisance parameters, μ_β and ϕ_β, were integrated out of the posterior distribution and then the resulting proportional posterior distribution was maximized with the Newton-Raphson scheme to obtain point estimates of the ability and item parameters. An iterative Birnbaum paradigm for the joint Bayes modal estimation was used to obtain a set of ability estimates and followed by a set of item parameter estimates until an overall convergence criterion was met. The specification of the parameters and the hyperparameters (i.e., ν_α, ω_α, ν_β, λ_β) can be a key issue in (hierarchical) Bayesian estimation.

Swaminathan and Gifford (1985) used the scaled chi distribution with the degrees of freedom ν_α and a scale parameter ω_α as a prior for α_j:

$$p(\alpha_j|\nu_\alpha, \omega_\alpha) = \frac{1}{\omega^{\nu_\alpha/2} 2^{(\nu_\alpha/2)-1} \Gamma(\nu_\alpha/2)} e^{-\alpha_j^2/(2\omega_\alpha)} \alpha_j^{\nu_\alpha - 1}. \tag{3}$$

Specifically, they suggested $\chi(\nu_\alpha = 10, \omega_\alpha = 0.1)$ as a prior for α_j. Using a R package, the lower limit of the 99 per cent credibility interval is 0.464312 (i.e., qchi(.005, df=10) * sqrt(0.1)), and the upper limit is 1.587078 (i.e., qchi(.995, df=10) * sqrt(0.1)). A chi distribution is not readily available in OpenBUGS or WinBUGS.

Swaminathan and Gifford (1985, p. 392; 1982, p. 178) used the scaled inverse chi-square distribution for ϕ (cf. without the script β here because the same form of the distribution can also be applied to ability):

$$p(\phi|\nu, \lambda) \propto \frac{1}{\phi^{\frac{1}{2}\nu+1}} \exp\left[\frac{\lambda}{-2\phi}\right], \quad 0 < \phi < \infty, \quad \lambda > 0, \quad \nu > 0 \tag{4}$$

(see Novick & Jackson, 1974, pp. 190–194; Isaacs, Christ, Novick, & Jackson, 1974, pp. 175–196). Such a distribution may not be directly used in available computer software. In OpenBUGS, WinBUGS, as well as BUGS (e.g., Lunn, Jackson, Best, Thomas, & Spiegelhalter, 2013, pp. 345–346), $\phi^{-1} \equiv \tau \sim \text{dgamma}(a, b)$ denotes the density to be

$$p(\tau|a, b) = b^a \tau^{a-1} e^{-b\tau}/\Gamma(a) \quad \text{for} \quad \tau > 0,\ a, b > 0 \tag{5}$$

with mean a/b and variance a/b^2. Note that for OpenBUGS it can be shown that $\nu = 2a$ to be the prior sample size, $\nu/\lambda = a/b$ to be the prior mean of ϕ^{-1}, and $\lambda/(\nu - 2) = b/(a - 1)$ to be the prior mean of ϕ for $\nu = 2a > 2$.

In conjunction with the MCMC method for approximating the entire posterior distribution and in the context of the computer program OpenBUGS (Spiegelhalter, Thomas, Best, & Lunn, 2014) used in this study, either a flat prior or a proper yet noninformative uniform hyperprior distribution for μ_β can be used in addition to employing an independent hyperprior for ϕ_β. A proper yet noninformative uniform prior distribution can also be used directly for β_j.

The specification of the hyperparameters for the hyperprior distributions is an important issue in the hierarchical Bayesian method. A noninformative, diffuse hyperprior distribution can be used for each μ by specifying appropriate hyperparameters, and an informative hyperprior distribution can be used for each ϕ by specifying appropriate hyperparameters. It should be noted that there are other forms of the priors under the 2PL model for Gibbs sampling.

2 Methods

To compare Gibbs sampling with different priors and MBE, the Law School Admission Test-Section 6 (LSAT6; Bock & Lieberman, 1970, p. 188) data and the Knox Cube Test (KCT; Wright & Stone, 1979, p. 31) data were used. The LSAT6 data consisted of 1,000 examinees responses to 5 items. The original responses of 35 students to 18 items on the KCT were analyzed without any modification of data. For Gibbs sampling, OpenBUGS was employed. It may be necessary to present the input lines for an OpenBUGS run, and Appendix A contains such code.

Three sets of prior specifications for items are used for the OpenBUGS runs (i.e., GS1, GS2, and GS3). First in GS1, the informative chi prior on discrimination and the uninformative prior on difficulty were used. Second in GS2, the informative chi prior on discrimination and the hierarchical prior on difficulty were used. The hierarchical prior for difficulty with $a = 2.5$ and $b = 5$ is equivalent to $\nu = 5$ and $\lambda = 10$ in Swaminathan & Gifford (1982) with an uninformative uniform prior for μ. Third in GS3, the lognormal prior on discrimination and the diffuse normal prior on difficulty were used. The lognormal prior on discrimination had mean of 0 and standard deviation of 0.5. The normal distribution on difficulty had mean of 0 and standard deviation of 2.

The MBE of item parameters employed the same prior specifications of GS3. These are the prior specifications available in the computer program BILOG-MG (Zimowski et al., 2002).

Based on the suggestions from Kim and Bolt (2007) and Kim (2001), burn-in was set to 1000 and the next 10,000 iterations were used to construct the posterior distributions for the OpenBUGS runs. To examine the effect of priors, different sets of specifications with varying parameters could be used.

3 Results

Only results from the LSAT6 data are presented here due to the page limit. Results from the KCT data, however, are comparable to those from the LSAT6 data. Results from the KCT are available from the authors.

Using the LSAT6 data, all four methods yielded similar results for the item and ability estimates. Table 1 presents item parameter estimates based on the usual 2PL model scaling (i.e., the ability estimates from the posterior metric based on the prior with mean of zero and standard deviation of unity). GS3 results are very similar to those from MBE because of the use of the same priors.

Intercorrelations and mean absolute deviations (MADs) between estimation methods are presented in Table 2 for the LSAT6 data. Correlations between estimation methods for discrimination are all high among the Gibbs sampling methods (i.e., $r > .93$). GS3 has the highest correlation with MBE among the Gibbs sampling methods as well as the smallest MAD for discrimination. Correlations between estimation methods for difficulty (also for ability) are all near perfect yielding $r = .99$. GS3 has the smallest MAD with MBE among the Gibbs sampling methods for difficulty (also for ability).

Ability estimates and the accompanied posterior standard deviations are reported in Table 3 for each pattern of the item responses. In the Gibbs sampling methods, there were different posterior means for examinees with the same response pattern. In reporting of the ability estimates, the first examinees who got the respective response patterns were used to obtain the estimates (i.e., examinees 1, 4, 10, 12, 23, etc.). Table 3 shows that estimates from the Gibbs sampling methods and MBE/EAP (i.e., expected a posteriori after obtaining item parameter estimates via the method of marginal Bayesian estimation) are similar.

Table 1 LSAT6 item parameter estimates

	GS1		GS2		GS3		MBE	
Item	$\hat{\xi}_j$	(p.s.d.)	$\hat{\xi}_j$	(p.s.d.)	$\hat{\xi}_j$	(p.s.d.)	$\hat{\xi}_j$	(p.s.d.)
Discrimination $\hat{\alpha}_j$								
1	1.09	(0.16)	1.12	(0.16)	0.90	(0.19)	0.81	(0.20)
2	0.95	(0.14)	0.94	(0.36)	0.73	(0.17)	0.75	(0.16)
3	0.99	(0.14)	0.99	(0.42)	0.83	(0.20)	0.86	(0.19)
4	0.94	(0.14)	0.94	(0.14)	0.72	(0.16)	0.72	(0.16)
5	0.98	(0.15)	1.00	(0.15)	0.77	(0.17)	0.71	(0.17)
Difficulty $\hat{\beta}_j$								
1	−2.74	(0.33)	−2.68	(0.30)	−3.26	(0.58)	−3.41	(0.72)
2	−1.12	(0.15)	−1.13	(0.15)	−1.40	(0.30)	−1.34	(0.25)
3	−0.27	(0.08)	−0.27	(0.08)	−0.31	(0.11)	−0.29	(0.10)
4	−1.50	(0.19)	−1.48	(0.19)	−1.87	(0.38)	−1.80	(0.34)
5	−2.29	(0.29)	−2.26	(0.28)	−2.84	(0.56)	−2.93	(0.60)

Note. p.s.d. = posterior standard deviation; GS = Gibbs sampling

Table 2 Intercorrelations and Mean Absolute Deviations between estimation methods for LSAT6

	GS1		GS2		GS3		MBE	
Method	r	(MAD)	r	(MAD)	r	(MAD)	r	(MAD)
Discrimination $\hat{\alpha}_j$								
GS1			.99	(0.01)	.95	(0.20)	.52	(0.22)
GS2					.93	(0.21)	.42	(0.22)
GS3							.73	(0.04)
MBE								
Difficulty $\hat{\beta}_j$								
GS1			.99	(0.02)	.99	(0.35)	.99	(0.37)
GS2					.99	(0.37)	.99	(0.39)
GS3							.99	(0.08)
MBE								
Ability $\hat{\theta}_i$								
GS1			.99	(0.01)	.99	(0.06)	.99	(0.08)
GS2					.99	(0.06)	.99	(0.09)
GS3							.99	(0.04)
MBE/EAP								

4 Discussion

The prior distributions used in GS2 had the chi distribution for discrimination and the hierarchical form for difficulty following (Swaminathan and Gifford, 1985). The hyperparameter mean of the normal prior distribution for difficulty had a noninformative uniform distribution and the inverse of the hyperparameter variance of the normal prior had a gamma distribution. In GS2 with gamma($a = 2.5, b = 5$), the prior sample size of the gamma distribution was specified as $2(2.5) = 5$ and the prior expected value of ϕ^{-1} was $2.5/5 = 0.5$ (i.e., the expected value of the hyperparameter variance ϕ to be $5/1.5 = 3.33$). Note that this prior specification is equivalent to Swaminathan and Gifford's (1985) $\nu = 5$ and $\lambda = 10$. There are also other ways of specifying priors for the 2PL model, instead of using priors used in this paper, as shown in Appendix B Tables 4, 5 and 6.

When difficulty and ability are estimated together in Gibbs sampling, the ability estimate for a specific person is not unique. The same response pattern may yield different ability estimates, and that is not acceptable in practice. In addition, because of employing the exchangeability concept, all ability estimates are estimated simultaneously and there exists some dependency in the resulting estimates. Although estimates are not independent in general, it seems troublesome that estimating ability even with known item parameters may yield different estimates for persons with a specific response pattern. Hence, Gibbs sampling or some other estimation methods based on MCMC may not be seen as viable methods for the usual item and ability parameter estimation for the usual item response theory models for dichotomous items that include the 2PL model.

Table 3 LSAT6 ability estimates

		GS1		GS2		GS3		MBE/EAP	
Pattern	Case	$\hat{\theta}_i$	(p.s.d.)	$\hat{\theta}_i$	(p.s.d.)	$\hat{\theta}_i$	(p.s.d.)	$\hat{\theta}_i$	(p.s.d.)
00000	3	−2.05	(0.72)	−2.05	(0.72)	−1.93	(0.79)	−1.91	(0.79)
00001	6	−1.54	(0.72)	−1.55	(0.72)	−1.46	(0.79)	−1.46	(0.80)
00010	2	−1.56	(0.71)	−1.60	(0.73)	−1.49	(0.79)	−1.45	(0.80)
00011	11	−1.08	(0.73)	−1.07	(0.72)	−1.01	(0.81)	−1.00	(0.80)
00100	1	−1.53	(0.72)	−1.55	(0.72)	−1.43	(0.79)	−1.37	(0.80)
00101	1	−1.05	(0.72)	−1.03	(0.72)	−0.94	(0.81)	−0.91	(0.80)
00110	3	−1.05	(0.72)	−1.07	(0.73)	−0.98	(0.81)	−0.90	(0.81)
00111	4	−0.53	(0.74)	−0.53	(0.74)	−0.50	(0.82)	−0.44	(0.82)
01000	1	−1.56	(0.72)	−1.57	(0.72)	−1.48	(0.79)	−1.44	(0.80)
01001	8	−1.05	(0.73)	−1.06	(0.73)	−1.01	(0.79)	−0.99	(0.80)
01010	0								
01011	16	−0.55	(0.75)	−0.57	(0.74)	−0.56	(0.82)	−0.51	(0.81)
01100	0								
01101	3	−0.53	(0.75)	−0.54	(0.75)	−0.47	(0.82)	−0.42	(0.82)
01110	2	−0.54	(0.74)	−0.59	(0.75)	−0.51	(0.82)	−0.41	(0.82)
01111	15	−0.01	(0.79)	−0.02	(0.78)	−0.01	(0.84)	0.07	(0.83)
10000	10	−1.50	(0.70)	−1.49	(0.72)	−1.39	(0.80)	−1.40	(0.80)
10001	29	−1.00	(0.73)	−0.98	(0.72)	−0.91	(0.80)	−0.95	(0.80)
10010	14	−1.00	(0.73)	−1.00	(0.73)	−0.93	(0.80)	−0.94	(0.80)
10011	81	−0.47	(0.75)	−0.46	(0.75)	−0.44	(0.82)	−0.47	(0.82)
10100	3	−0.98	(0.74)	−0.98	(0.74)	−0.86	(0.82)	−0.84	(0.81)
10100	28	−0.46	(0.75)	−0.45	(0.76)	−0.36	(0.83)	−0.38	(0.82)
10110	15	−0.46	(0.75)	−0.47	(0.75)	−0.41	(0.82)	−0.37	(0.82)
10111	80	0.09	(0.78)	0.10	(0.78)	0.13	(0.85)	0.11	(0.84)
11000	16	−1.00	(0.72)	−0.99	(0.72)	−0.93	(0.81)	−0.92	(0.80)
11001	56	−0.47	(0.75)	−0.48	(0.75)	−0.44	(0.81)	−0.46	(0.82)
11010	21	−0.50	(0.75)	−0.49	(0.75)	−0.47	(0.82)	−0.45	(0.82)
11011	173	0.06	(0.78)	0.07	(0.77)	0.05	(0.83)	0.03	(0.83)
11100	11	−0.46	(0.75)	−0.47	(0.75)	−0.40	(0.83)	−0.36	(0.82)
11101	61	0.09	(0.79)	0.09	(0.78)	0.12	(0.85)	0.13	(0.84)
11110	28	0.08	(0.78)	0.07	(0.78)	0.09	(0.84)	0.13	(0.84)
11111	298	0.69	(0.82)	0.68	(0.83)	0.65	(0.87)	0.65	(0.86)

Note. p.s.d.= posterior standard deviation
GS1 to GS3 estimates were from examinees 1, 4, 10, 12, 23, 24, 25, 28, 32, 33, 41, 57, 60, 62, 77, 87, 116, 130, 211, 214, 242, 257, 337, 353, 409 430, 603, 614, 675, and 703

In this study, the 2PL model was employed without addressing the problem of model selection, choice of link function, or model fit. Kim and Bolt (2007) contains an excellent introductory review of these issues. Interested readers should refer to Kim and Bolt (2007) and other general references including (Lunn et al., 2013).

Although Gibbs sampling and the MCMC methods and some computer programs including OpenBUGS which implemented such procedures have been available for some time, the accuracy of the methods has not been thoroughly studied. Obviously these techniques have been applied to some complicated modeling situations where the traditional maximum likelihood based methods are too difficult to implement, and hence have not been thoroughly tested and compared. Because maximum likelihood based methods have not been implemented at all in such applications, still we need to investigate the relevant estimation procedures. In addition, because there are many different ways of implementing Gibbs sampling in item response theory and many different prior distributions can be employed with many different specifications in Bayesian estimation, the illustrative implementation of Gibbs sampling and comparing results with other existing Bayesian and likelihood based methods may provide measurement specialists and test developers as well as the users of the computer programs with guidelines for using Gibbs sampling under the 2PL model. More cumulative experience with regard to prior specifications for Bayesain estimation is obviously needed.

Appendix A: OpenBUGS Code

```
model {
# 2PL model
  for (i in 1:I) {
    for (j in 1:J) {
      logit(p[i, j]) <- alpha[j] * (theta[i] - beta[j])
      x[i, j] ~ dbern(p[i, j])
    }
# ability prior
    theta[i] ~ dnorm(0, 1)
  }
# item Priors
  for (j in 1:J) {
    a[j] ~ dchisqr(10)
    alpha[j] <- sqrt(a[j] * 0.1)
    beta[j] ~ dunif(-5, 5)
#   beta[j] ~ dnorm(mub, taub) # GS2
#   alpha[j] ~ dlnorm(0, 2) # GS3
#   beta[j] ~ dnorm(0, 0.5) # GS3
  }
# hyperpriors
# mub ~ dflat() # GS2
# taub ~ dgamma(2.5, 5) # GS2
```

```
}
# kct data
list(I = 35, J = 18,
x = structure(.Data = c(
1,1,1,1,1,1,1,0,0,0,0,0,0,0,0,0,0,0,
1,1,1,1,1,1,1,1,1,1,0,0,0,0,0,0,0,0,
1,1,1,1,1,1,1,1,1,0,0,1,0,0,0,0,0,0,
1,1,1,1,0,0,1,0,1,0,0,0,0,0,0,0,0,0,
1,1,1,1,1,1,1,1,1,1,0,0,0,0,0,0,0,0,
1,1,1,1,1,1,1,1,1,0,0,0,0,0,0,0,0,0,
1,1,1,1,1,1,1,1,1,1,1,1,1,0,1,0,0,0,
1,1,1,1,1,1,1,1,1,1,0,0,0,0,0,0,0,0,
1,1,1,1,1,1,1,1,1,1,0,0,0,0,0,0,0,0,
1,1,1,1,1,1,1,1,1,1,1,0,0,0,0,0,0,0,
1,1,1,0,1,1,1,1,1,0,0,0,0,0,0,0,0,0,
1,1,1,1,1,0,1,0,1,1,0,0,0,0,0,0,0,0,
1,1,1,1,1,0,0,1,1,1,1,1,0,0,0,0,0,0,
1,1,1,1,1,1,1,1,1,1,1,0,0,0,0,0,0,0,
1,1,1,1,1,1,1,1,1,1,1,1,1,0,0,0,0,0,
1,1,1,1,1,1,1,1,1,0,1,0,0,0,0,0,0,0,
1,1,1,1,0,1,1,1,1,1,0,0,0,0,0,0,0,0,
1,1,1,1,1,1,1,1,1,1,0,0,1,0,0,0,0,0,
1,1,1,1,1,1,1,1,1,0,0,0,0,0,0,0,0,0,
1,1,1,1,1,1,1,1,1,1,0,0,1,0,0,0,0,0,
1,1,1,1,1,1,1,1,1,1,1,0,1,0,0,0,0,0,
1,1,1,1,1,1,1,1,1,1,1,1,0,0,0,0,0,0,
1,1,1,1,1,1,1,1,1,1,0,0,1,1,0,0,0,0,
1,1,1,1,1,1,1,1,1,1,1,0,1,0,0,1,1,0,
1,1,1,0,1,1,0,0,0,0,0,0,0,0,0,0,0,0,
1,1,1,1,1,1,1,1,1,1,0,0,0,0,0,0,0,0,
1,1,1,1,1,1,1,0,0,0,0,0,0,0,0,0,0,0,
1,1,1,1,1,1,1,1,1,0,1,0,0,0,0,0,0,0,
1,1,1,1,1,1,0,0,1,1,1,0,0,1,0,0,0,0,
1,1,1,1,1,1,1,1,1,0,0,0,0,0,0,0,0,0,
1,1,1,1,1,1,1,1,1,1,0,0,0,0,0,0,0,0,
1,1,1,1,1,1,1,1,1,1,1,0,0,0,0,0,0,0,
1,1,1,1,0,0,1,0,0,1,0,0,0,0,0,0,0,0,
1,1,1,1,1,1,1,1,1,1,0,1,0,1,0,0,0,0,
1,1,1,0,0,0,0,0,0,0,0,0,0,0,0,0,0,0
), .Dim = c(35, 18))
)
# initial values (e.g., GS1)
list(
a = c(
10,10,10,10,10,10, 10,10,10,10,10,10, 10,10,10,10,10,10
),
beta = c(
0,0,0,0,0,0, 0,0,0,0,0,0, 0,0,0,0,0,0
),
```

```
#  mub = 0, taub = 1,
theta = c(
-0.4519851,  0.2231436,  0.2231436, -0.6931472,  0.2231436,  0.2231436,
1.2527630,  0.2231436,  0.2231436,  0.4519851, -0.2231436, -0.2231436,
0.2231436,  0.4519851,  0.9555114,  0.2231436,  0.0000000,  0.4519851,
0.0000000,  0.4519851,  0.6931472,  0.6931472,  0.6931472,  1.2527630,
-0.9555114,  0.2231436, -0.4519851,  0.2231436,  0.2231436,  0.0000000,
0.2231436,  0.4519851, -0.6931472,  0.6931472, -1.6094379
)
)
```

Appendix B: Summary of Priors and Specifications

Papers in Tables 4, 5 and 6 are not exhaustive. Estimation techniques in the tables include JBME, MCMC, and MBE. The acronym BME designates Bayes modal estimation, BE designates Bayes estimation (i.e., posterior mean), EAP designates expected a posteriori (i.e., posterior mean via quadratures), and MAP designates maximum a posteriori (i.e., posterior mode with known item parameters). The types of priors can be classified into two; one without any hierarchical structure and the other with some hierarchical structure for which parameters are modeled with hyperpriors and hyperparameters (i.e., Hierarchical). Priors can also be differentiated as ones with exchangeability for which the same prior will be applied to all items in a test or a subtest (i.e., Exchangeable), others with capability of assigning an individual prior on each parameter (i.e., Individual), and also others obtained with information from the current data (i.e., Empirical). It should be noted that in the tables, the names of the distributions might sound the same but could be mathematically, trivially different. Each paper should be consulted and carefully read before employing the priors in one's research. Also note that several keywords from the computer programs (e.g., SPR, TPR, FLO, AJ, BJ, PA, etc.) are used without any explications.

There are more than six additional, relevant papers that could be included in Tables 4, 5 and 6. The relevant papers are as follows (but without full references): Spiegelhalter et al.'s (1996) "BUGS 0.5 Examples Volume 1"; Johnson and Albert's (1999) "Ordinal Data Modeling"; Curtis's (2010) "Journal of Statistical Software, 36"; Nathesan et al.'s (2016) "Frontiers in Psychology, 7"; Luo and Ziao's (2017) "Educational and Psychological Measurement, Febuary 1"; and Parchev et al.'s (2017) "CRAN Package irtoys". The six papers mentioned in Tables 4, 5 and 6 are representative ones.

Table 4 Priors for discrimination in the Bayesian Estimation Methods under the 2PL model

	Discrimination or Transformed discrimination			
Paper/Technique	Estimation	Category	Prior	Specification
Swaminathan & Gifford (1985) JBME	BME	Exchangeable	$\alpha_j \sim \chi(\nu_\alpha, \omega_\alpha)$	$\nu_\alpha = 10$ $\omega_\alpha = 0.1$ $\chi(10, 0.1)$
Mislevy (1986) MBE	BME	Exchangeable	$\log \alpha_j \sim N(\mu_\alpha, \sigma_\alpha^2)$	$\mu_\alpha = 0$ $\sigma_\alpha^2 = 0.25$
Kim et al. (1994) JBME	BME	Exchangeable Hierarchical	$\log \alpha_j \sim N(\mu_\alpha, \sigma_\alpha^2)$ $\mu_\alpha \sim U(-\infty, \infty)$ $\sigma_\alpha^2 \sim IG(\nu_\alpha, \lambda_\alpha)$	$\nu_\alpha = 4, 11$ $\lambda_\alpha = 1$
Thissen et al. (2002) MBE	BME	Exchangeable	$\alpha_j \sim N(\mu_\alpha, \sigma_\alpha)$	AJ, PA = $(\mu_\alpha, \sigma_\alpha)$
Zimowski et al. (2002) MBE	BME	Exchangeable	$\log \alpha_j \sim N(\mu_\alpha, \sigma_\alpha)$ SPR	SMU = $\mu_\alpha = 0$ SSI = $\sigma_\alpha = 0.5$
	BME	Individual	$\log \alpha_j \sim N(\mu_{\alpha_j}, \sigma_{\alpha_j})$ SPR	SMU = $\{\mu_{\alpha_j}\}$ SSI = $\{\sigma_{\alpha_j}\}$
	BME	Empirical	$\log \alpha_j \sim N(\hat{\mu}_\alpha, \sigma_\alpha)$ SPR, FLO	$\hat{\mu}_\alpha = E(\hat{\alpha}_j)$ $\sigma_\alpha = 0.5$
Stone & Zhu (2015) MCMC	BE	Exchangeable	$\alpha_j \sim \text{lognormal}(0, \sigma_\alpha^2)$	$\sigma_\alpha^2 = 4$

Table 5 Priors for difficulty in the Bayesian Estimation Methods under the 2PL model

	Difficulty or Transformed difficulty			
Paper/Technique	Estimation	Category	Prior	Specification
Swaminathan & Gifford (1985) JBME	BME	Exchangeable Hierarchical	$\beta_j \sim N(\mu_\beta, \phi_\beta)$ $\mu_\beta \sim U(-\infty, \infty)$ $\phi_\beta \sim \chi^{-2}(\nu_\beta, \lambda_\beta)$	$p(\beta_j) \propto 1$
Mislevy (1986) MBE	BME	Exchangeable	$\beta_j \sim N(\mu_\beta, \sigma_\beta^2)$	$\mu_\beta = 0$ $\sigma_\beta^2 = 4$
Kim et al. (1994) JBME	BME	Exchangeable Hierarchical	$\beta_j \sim N(\mu_\beta, \sigma_\beta^2)$ $\mu_\beta \sim U(-\infty, \infty)$ $\sigma_\beta^2 \sim IG(\nu_\beta, \lambda_\beta)$	$\nu_\beta = 4$ $\lambda_\beta = 0.25$
Thissen et al. (2002) MBE	BME	Exchangeable	$\beta_j \sim N(\mu_\beta, \sigma_\beta)$	BJ, PA $= (\mu_\beta, \sigma_\beta)$
Zimowski et al. (2002) MBE	BME	Exchangeable	$\beta_j \sim N(\mu_\beta, \sigma_\beta)$ TPR	TMU $= \mu_\beta = 0$ TSI $= \sigma_\beta = 2$
	BME	Individual	$\beta_j \sim N(\mu_{\beta_j}, \sigma_{\beta_j})$ TPR	TMU $= \{\mu_{\beta_j}\}$ TSI $= \{\sigma_{\beta_j}\}$
	BME	Empirical	$\beta_j \sim N(\hat{\mu}_\beta, \sigma_\beta)$ TPR, FLO	$\hat{\mu}_\beta = E(\hat{\beta}_j)$ $\sigma_\beta = 2$
Stone & Zhu (2015) MCMC	BE	Exchangeable	$\beta_j \sim \text{normal}(0, \sigma_\beta^2)$	$\sigma_\beta^2 = 25$

Table 6 Priors for ability in the Bayesian Estimation Methods under the 2PL model

	Ability			
Paper/Technique	Estimation	Category	Prior	Specification
Swaminathan & Gifford (1985) JBME	BME	Exchangeable Hierarchical	$\theta_i \sim N(\mu_\theta, \phi_\theta)$ $\mu_\theta \sim U(-\infty, \infty)$ $\phi_\theta \sim \chi^{-2}(\nu_\theta, \lambda_\theta)$	$\mu_\theta = 0$ $\phi_\theta = 1$
Mislevy (1986) MBE	EAP	Exchangeable	$\theta_i \sim N(\mu_\theta, \sigma_\theta^2)$	$\mu_\theta = 0$ $\sigma_\theta^2 = 1$
Kim et al. (1994) JBME	BME	Exchangeable Hierarchical	$\theta_i \sim N(\mu_\theta, \sigma_\theta^2)$ $\mu_\theta \sim U(-\infty, \infty)$ $\sigma_\theta^2 \sim IG(\nu_\theta, \lambda_\theta)$	$\mu_\theta = 0$ $\sigma_\theta^2 = 1$
Thissen et al. (2002) MBE	EAP MAP	Exchangeable	$\theta_i \sim N(\mu_\theta, \sigma_\theta)$	$\text{MU} = \mu_\theta = 0$ $\text{SD} = \sigma_\theta = 1$
Zimowski et al. (2002) MBE	EAP MAP	Exchangeable	$\theta_i \sim N(\mu_\theta, \sigma_\theta)$ $\text{IDI} = 0$	$\text{PMN} = \mu_\theta = 0$ $\text{PSD} = \sigma_\theta = 1$
	EAP	Exchangeable	$\theta_i \sim N(\mu_\theta, \sigma_\theta)$ $\text{IDI} = 1, 2$	QUA
	EAP	Empirical	$\theta_i \sim N(\mu_\theta, \sigma_\theta)$ $\text{IDI} = 3$	Phase 2
Stone & Zhu (2015) MCMC	BE	Exchangeable	$\theta_i \sim \text{normal}(0, 1)$	$\sigma_\theta^2 = 1$

References

Albert, J. H. (1992). Bayesian estimation of normal ogive item response curves using Gibbs sampling. *Journal of Educational Statistics, 17,* 251–269.

Birnbaum, A. (1969). Statistical theory for logistic mental test models with a prior distribution of ability. *Journal of Mathematical Psychology, 6,* 258–276.

Bock, R. D., & Aitkin, M. (1981). Marginal maximum likelihood estimation of item parameters: Applications of an EM algorithm. *Psychometrika, 46,* 443–459.

Bock, R. D., & Lieberman, M. (1970). Fitting a response model for *n* dichotomously scored items. *Psychometrika, 35,* 179–197.

du Toit, M. (Ed.). (2003). *IRT from SSI: BILOG-MG, MULTILOG, PARSCALE, TESTFACT.* Chicago, IL: Scientific Software International.

Fox, J.-P. (2010). *Bayesian item response modeling: Theory and applications.* New York, NY: Springer.

Gonzalez, J. (2010). Bayesian methods in psychological research: The case of IRT. *International Journal of Psychological Research, 3*(1), 164–176.

Isaacs, G. I., Christ, D. E., Novick, M. R., & Jackson, P. H. (1974). *Tables for Bayesian statisticians.* The Iowa Testing Program, The University of Iowa, Iowa City, IA.

Johnson, M. S., & Sinharay, S. (2016). Bayesian etimation. In W. J. van der Linden (Ed.), *Handbook of item response theory, Volume 2: Statistical tools* (pp. 237–257). Boca Raton, FL: CRC Press.

Kim, J.-S., & Bolt, D. M. (2007). Estimating item response theory models using Markov chain Monte Carlo methods. *Educational Measurement: Issues and Practice, 26*(4), 38–51.

Kim, S.-H. (2001). An evaluation of a Markov chain Monte Carlo method for the Rasch model. *Applied Psychological Measurement, 25,* 163–176.

Kim, S.-H., Cohen, A. S., Baker, F. B., Subkoviak, M. J., & Leonard, T. (1994). An investigation of hierarchical Bayes procedures in item response theory. *Psychometrika, 59,* 405–421.

Leonard, T., & Novick, M. R. (1985). *Bayesian inference and diagnostics for the three parameter logistic model* (ONR Technical Report Np. 85-5). Iowa City, IA: The University of Iowa, Cada Research Group. (ERIC Document Reproduction Service No. ED261068).

Levy, R., & Mislevy, R. J. (2016). *Bayesian psychometric modeling.* Boca Raton, FL: CRC Press.

Lindley, D. V., & Smith, A. F. (1972). Bayesian estimates for the linear model. *Journal of the Royal Statistical Society, Series B, 34,* 1–41.

Lunn, D., Jackson, C., Best, N., Thomas, A., & Spiegelhalter, D. (2013). *The BUGS book: A practical introduction the Bayesian analysis.* Boca Raton, FL: CRC Press.

Marcoulides, K. M. (2018). Careful with those priors: A note on Bayesian estimation in two-parameter logistic item response theory models. *Measurement, 16,* 92–99.

Mislevy, R. J. (1986). Bayes modal estimation in item response models. *Psychometrika, 51,* 177–195.

Novick, M. R., & Jackson, P. H. (1974). *Statistical methods for educational and psychological research.* New York, NY: McGraw-Hill.

Novick, M. R., Lewis, C., & Jackson, P. H. (1973). The estimation of proportions in *n* groups. *Psychometrika, 38,* 19–46.

Spiegelhalter, D., Thomas, A., Best, N., & Lunn, D. (2014). *OpenBUGS user manual.* Cambridge, UK: MRC Biostatistics Unit, Institute of Public Health.

Stone, C. A., & Zhu, X. (2015). *Bayesian analysis of item response theory models using SAS.* Cary, NC: SAS Institute.

Swaminathan, H., & Gifford, J. A. (1982). Bayesian estimation in the Rasch model. *Journal of Educational Statistics, 7,* 175–191.

Swaminathan, H., & Gifford, J. A. (1985). Bayesian estimation in the two-parameter logistic model. *Psychometrika, 50,* 349–364.

Swaminathan, H., & Gifford, J. A. (1986). Bayesian estimation in the three-parameter logistic model. *Psychometrika, 51,* 589–601.

Thissen, D., Chen, W.-H., & Bock, R. D. (2002). MULTILOG [Computer software]. Lincolnwood, IL: Scientific Software International.

Tsutakawa, R. K., & Lin, H. Y. (1986). Bayesian estimation of item response curves. *Psychometrika, 51,* 251–267.

Wright, B. D., & Stone, M. H. (1979). *Best test design.* Chicago, IL: MESA Press.

Zimowski, M. F., Muraki, E., Mislevy, R. J., & Bock, R. D. (2002). BILOG-MG [Computer software]. Lincolnwood, IL: Scientific Software International.

Increasing Measurement Precision of PISA Through Multistage Adaptive Testing

Hyo Jeong Shin, Kentaro Yamamoto, Lale Khorramdel, and Frederic Robin

1 Introduction

With technology becoming an essential part of learning, problem solving, and daily communication, many international large-scale assessments (ILSAs) are transitioning to computer. For example, the Programme for International Student Assessment (PISA), the world's largest ILSA, switched from a paper-based assessment (PBA) to a primarily computer-based assessment (CBA) in the 2015 cycle, with about 90% of countries choosing CBA in 2018 and almost all selecting CBA in the 2022 cycle. Such a mode change also allows for the implementation of adaptive testing. Adaptive testing has proven advantageous for obtaining precise measurement of examinees compared to traditional linear tests (Wainer, 1990). In particular, multistage adaptive tests (MST) designs "[strike] a balance among adaptability, practicality, measurement accuracy, and control over test forms" (Zenisky et al., 2010) and reduce measurement error at the individual and group levels (Oranje et al., 2014). Likewise, the primary goals of implementing an MST in an ILSA are to reduce measurement error for heterogeneous populations without overburdening individual respondents, to control the content composition of each test form, and to facilitate the use of different item types within specific units to best measure the construct (Yamamoto et al., 2018; Yamamoto & Khorramdel, 2018).

H. J. Shin (✉) · F. Robin
Educational Testing Service, Princeton, NJ, USA
e-mail: hshin@ets.org; frobin@ets.org

K. Yamamoto
Independent Researcher, Princeton, NJ, USA

L. Khorramdel
Boston College, Chestnut Hill, MA, USA

M. Wiberg et al. (eds.), *Quantitative Psychology*, Springer Proceedings in Mathematics & Statistics 353, https://doi.org/10.1007/978-3-030-74772-5_29

In this paper, we focus on PISA 2018 to address two research questions. First, we present what psychometric properties were considered for introducing an MST into PISA, focusing on the invariance of item parameters by unit order. This research question is important because item parameters are estimated using the data collected with the MST design where units were located in different positions across test forms. Second, we evaluate the extent of parameter recovery and measurement precision that can be expected from the PISA 2018 MST compared to the non-adaptive design.

2 Experimental Study: Invariance of Item Parameters by Unit Order

MSTs in ILSAs necessarily place items or units[1] in different orders across test forms, meaning that for an MST to be successfully implemented, psychometric properties of items must hold, regardless of item or unit position across different blocks (i.e., absence of item or unit position effects). Because test forms are assembled at the unit level in PISA, the order of items within a unit does not change, but the position of a unit across blocks does change. Therefore, possible unit order effects have to be examined in order to proceed with the MST. This is particularly important because item parameters for newly developed items need to be estimated under the MST design with proper sampling weights during the main survey. In this section, we describe how we designed an experimental study to investigate unit order effects, and we present the results obtained from PISA 2018 field trial data collected in 217 country-by language groups (165,000 students) and 460 candidate reading items.

2.1 *Methods*

The PISA 2018 field trial used fixed and varying unit positions within 30-minute (intact) blocks, and students were randomly assigned to one of three groups with different unit orders. The field trial study design can be seen as a type of randomized control trial in the sense that the treatment (unit order) was randomly manipulated between groups of students, which allows us to examine whether the same administered units behave differently given unit order.

[1] A set of items (usually ranging from two to eight items) that are designed to share similar or identical content, stimuli, or reading passage. Note that the term "unit" used in this paper is closer to what is called "testlet" in the measurement literature (e.g., Wainer et al., 2007). Wainer and Kiely (1987) described "testlet" as groups of items that relate to a single topic, such as a reading passage.

The unit order design had three different groups: in Group 1, trend Reading items[2] are presented in a fixed unit order (FUO); in Group 2, trend and new Reading items are presented in a variable unit order (VUO); in Group 3, new Reading items are presented in an FUO. Each cluster consisted of multiple units, and the ordering of the units was always fixed and consistent in FUO forms in Groups 1 and 3. In contrast, unit order varied across the VUO forms in Group 2. For example, with three units (A, B, C in the order of easy to hard) per cluster, the order of units in FUO forms was always consistent as ABC, while the ordering of units in VUO forms was one of two alternate orders, either ACB or BAC. More comprehensive sets of ordering were possible (e.g., BCA, CAB, CBA); however, these conditions were not considered. This decision was made because it was expected that test-taking motivation could be negatively impacted by having the most difficult unit (C) appear before relatively easier units (A or B). Each test form contains four clusters, and when the test was initialized for each student, one of the permutations from among the 16 different permutations of the four clusters (4^2; e.g., 1111, 1112, ..., 2222) was randomly assigned.

Because all Reading items were used in both FUO and VUO forms, item performance could be compared between FUO and VUO. Performance of items was investigated based on the percentage correct and response times. To further examine unit order effects, a multiple-group IRT model (Bock & Zimowski, 1997; von Davier & Yamamoto, 2004) based on the 2PL and the generalized partial credit model (GPCM; Muraki, 1992) was characterized with three different unit-order groups (Group 1, Group 2, Group 3). Multiple-group IRT models enable the estimation of item parameters that are common across different populations, as well as unique group means and standard deviations. Let j denote a person responding to item i, so that the pattern of response may be expressed as $\boldsymbol{x}_j = [x_{1j}, x_{2j}, \ldots, x_{nj}]$ when there is a test composed of n items. Assuming conditional independence of responses, the probability of observing the pattern $\boldsymbol{x}_j$ can be written as the multiplication of the probabilities of individual item responses P_i,

$$P\left(\boldsymbol{x}_j|\theta\right) = \prod_{i}^{n} P_i\left(X_i = x_{ij}|\theta\right)$$

which applies to all groups and persons, given the person attribute θ. Based on these IRT models, items are characterized by item slopes and item locations (difficulties), and the item parameters can either be constrained to be the same across different groups or allowed to be unique for each group. A latent person ability, or attribute θ, follows a continuous distribution with a finite mean and variance in the population of persons corresponding to group k. With the probability density function denoted as $g_k(\theta)$, the marginal probability of response pattern $\boldsymbol{x}_j$ in group k can be expressed as

[2]Trend items indicate the items were administered in the previous PISA cycles. In typical PISA design, for the major domain, total item pool comprises one third of trend items and the rest of newly developed items. Trend items provide a stable linking for the trend analysis.

$$\overline{P_k}\left(\boldsymbol{x}_j\right)=\int_{-\infty}^{\infty} P\left(\boldsymbol{x}_j|\theta\right) g_k\left(\theta\right) d\theta.$$

Then, the measurement invariance of items in each group was evaluated through the root mean square deviation (RMSD) with a threshold of 0.15. This threshold value is typically used for checking the item quality in operational settings (OECD, 2020) and is considered acceptable for estimating stable group statistics (Joo et al., 2021). The RMSD statistics are calculated as follows:

$$RMSD_g=\sqrt{\int\left[p_g^{obs}\left(\theta\right)-p_g^{exp}\left(\theta\right)\right]^2 f_g\left(\theta\right) d\theta},$$

where $g = 1, \ldots, G$ is three different unit-order groups (Group 1, Group 2, Group 3); $p_g^{obs}\left(\theta\right)$ and $p_g^{exp}\left(\theta\right)$ are, respectively, the observed and expected probabilities of a correct response given proficiency θ; and $f_g(\theta)$ is the group-specific density distribution on the students' ability scale (Khorramdel et al., 2019; von Davier, 2005). If any significant item-by-unit order interaction existed, item parameter estimation would be affected by the unit order, and the common item parameters would not work for a certain group.

2.2 Results

The left panel in Fig. 1 shows the comparison of the average percentage correct between FUO and VUO per cluster. At the cluster level, the differences in the average percentage correct was less than 2.24 between FUO and VUO for trend items and less than 1.16 for new items. Across clusters, this difference was 0.62 for trend and 0.12 for new items on average. These differences were not statistically significant, and no unit order effect appears to exist for the range of percentage correct.

Similarly, response time spent per cluster was almost identical at the cluster level (right panel of Fig. 1). The differences in average response time were less than 1.33 minutes for trend items and less than 1.41 minutes for new items. Across clusters, the average difference between VUO and FUO was 0.31 minutes for trend items and 0.27 minutes for new items. As seen in Fig. 1, no evidence of interaction by unit order can be found based on the response time average for trend clusters, and deviations are nearly equally distributed above and below the dotted line (indicating equality) for the entire range of cluster-level response times, indicating no unit order effects overall.

Results from the multiple-group IRT model showed that there are no item-by-unit order interactions between any comparable groups with RMSD $\geq$0.15. Figure 2 provides the distribution of RMSD values for trend (left panel) and new items (right panel). The figure shows that the RMSD values for all items (displayed on

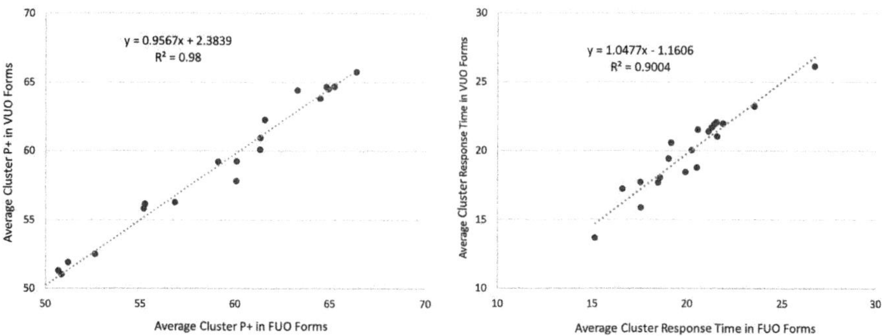

Fig. 1 Comparison of the percentage correct (left panel) and the average cluster response time (right panel)

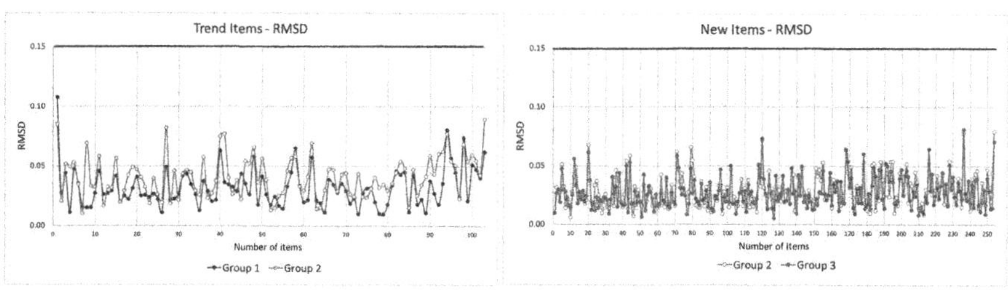

Fig. 2 Distribution of RMSD values for trend items (left panel) and new items (right panel), with the red line indicating a threshold of RMSD = 0.15

the x-axis) are far below this threshold, indicating very good item fit within all unit order groups.

Taken together, the comparison of the percentage correct and response time between FUO and VUO, as well as the evaluation of measurement invariance of item parameters between FUO and VUO, suggests that bias on item parameter estimation due to differential unit order is negligible. If the unit order had shown to significantly impact item parameters and proficiency estimates, an MST design could not be implemented, at least not with the same modeling approach. Therefore, the field trial results confirmed the feasibility of introducing an MST into the main survey, as unit order effects were insignificant.

3 Simulation Study: Parameter Recovery and Measurement Accuracy

A simulation study was designed to evaluate the performance of the PISA 2018 MST in terms of parameter recovery and the expected gains in measurement precision. In this simulation study, the performance of the MST design was evaluated and compared with two other benchmark designs, a complete design (unrealistic) and a random design (non-adaptive, realistic), across 100 replicates.

3.1 Methods

The item pool consisted of the 245 dichotomously and polytomously (three categories except for one item) scored Reading items, and the preliminary item parameter estimates obtained from the PISA 2018 field trial were used as generating values (i.e., item discriminations and difficulties). Details about the implemented MST design in PISA 2018 can be found in Yamamoto, Shin, and Khorramdel (2019). Note that throughout the simulation study, item selection and allocation to units were kept consistent. Next, proficiency distributions for groups were generated reflecting typical past PISA scores on which the scale was constructed to have a mean of 500 and a standard deviation of 100 for the reading domain in 2000 (OECD, 2020). Given that participating populations in PISA are heterogeneous, 12 fictitious countries that vary in performance level were considered, including one reference group that followed the standard normal distribution. This reference group was used to set the constraints to remove the indeterminacy of the IRT scale and allowed all item parameters and group statistics to be estimated. For the remaining 11 groups, proficiency was assumed to be normally distributed with a common standard deviation of 0.76 (100 on the PISA Reading scale), and the mean of the latent ability distribution ranged from −0.29 to 1.23 (400 ~ 600 on the PISA Reading scale), according to the preliminary results obtained from the PISA 2018 field trial. The sample size per country was set to $N = 6300$, which is the standard sample size followed by most PISA participating countries.

Three simulation conditions were considered. First, one complete dataset of item responses was generated using these item parameters and ability distributions. This *complete design* assumes that all students take all 245 items in the item pool. Recognizing this design is not feasible for a population survey, the complete design still provides useful information about estimation errors and sampling errors. As a realistic benchmark, the *random design* was generated by converting valid item responses in the complete design to missing when the items were not taken by students. There can be various ways to represent non-adaptive operational PISA designs, but given that the same number of units are administered to each student, the random design was expected to serve as a realistic operational benchmark for a comparison with the MST design. In this process, each student was assumed to take a randomly selected set of units rather than a pre-determined set of assigned units. Note that matching the student's ability level with the item difficulty level is not considered under this random design. Lastly, the *MST design* was generated by converting valid item responses in the complete design to missing based on the pre-determined MST design structure, including unit selection, unit assignment, and the prespecified sum score ranges (Yamamoto, et al., 2019).

A multiple-group IRT model (Bock & Zimowski, 1997) explained in the previous section (2.1) was fitted for each condition. Note that there are twelve groups with one reference group included for the simulation study. Analyses were conducted using the *mdltm* software that provides marginal maximum likelihood (MML) estimates obtained using customary expectation-maximization methods (von Davier, 2005; Khorramdel et al., 2019). As shown in Glas (1988), Eggen and Verhelst (2011), and Mislevy and Wu (1996), MML estimation enables valid item calibration with MST data, both in the Rasch model and in the 2PL model for the dichotomous and polytomous item responses in an MST design for a single domain.

Two aspects of the simulation study were reported: parameter recovery and measurement precision. In each replication, item parameters (discrimination and difficulties) and group statistics (group means and standard deviations) were estimated under each condition. Concerning the parameter recovery, across 100 replicates, bias and the root mean squared error (RMSE) were calculated. Next, the precision of the person ability estimator was evaluated using the standard errors associated with the weighted likelihood estimates (Warm, 1989). In order to quantify the expected gains, the proportion of standard error of the MST design was calculated against the operational benchmark (random design). The expected gains in precision were averaged over the PISA scale scores, ranging between 200 and 800, where sufficient sample sizes were observed.

3.2 Results

Parameter Recovery Figure 3 shows the distribution of biases and RMSEs across 245 items from each design condition. The MST design yielded absolute biases less than 0.02 for all items, and the magnitude of biases were considered negligible, although they showed slightly larger differences (at the third decimal point) for some items compared to the random design. One outlier item under the MST design (top right panel) had the generating discrimination value of 0.2 with multiple scoring categories. This same item stood out as an outlier in the RMSE under the complete design and the random design; thus, this item was viewed as a special case. The MST design also performed well in terms of recovery of group statistics (means and standard deviations). Both the MST and random design revealed biases in group means ranging from −0.004 to 0.004. RMSE values ranged from 0.015 to 0.020 under the MST design, and this range was narrower than that of the random design. Taken together, the MST design demonstrated an acceptable level of parameter recovery.

Measurement Precision The MST design showed about a 4.2% precision gain on average across 100 replicates, with a minimum gain of 3.2% up to a maximum gain of 5.4%. Most importantly, the MST contributed to the precision of the person ability estimator across all scale scores, particularly at the extreme performance levels of lower than 300 and over 700 with around 10% higher accuracy. This

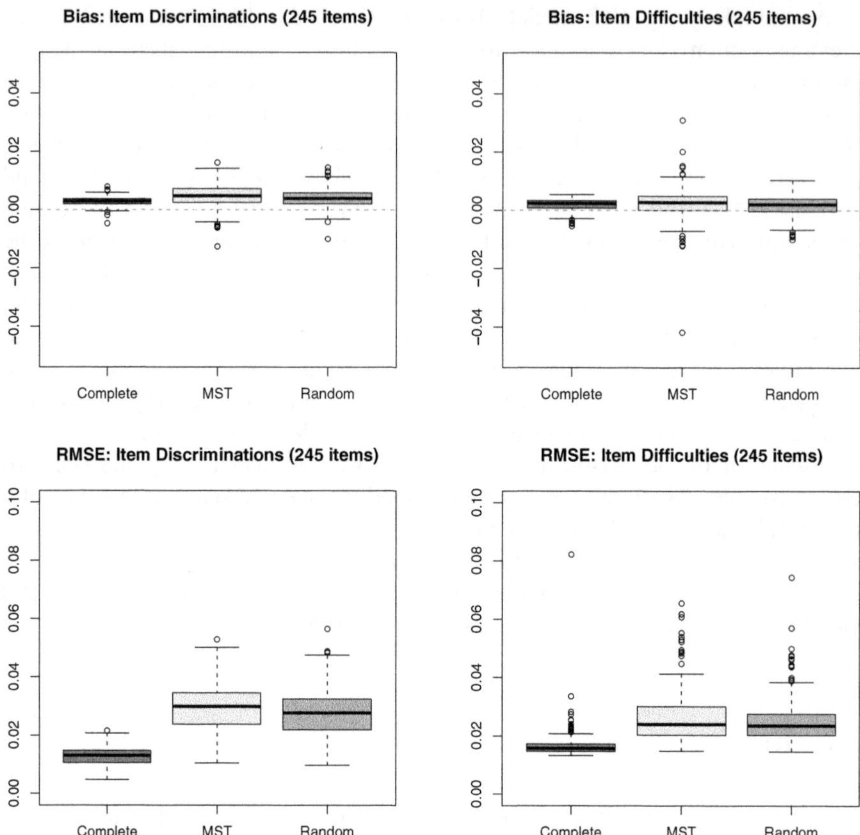

Fig. 3 Bias and RMSE distributions in item parameters

especially helps improve the measurement precision of proficiency estimation when students and countries are located at the extreme level, either high or low. Although the expected 4.2% precision gain of the MST design appears low compared to the expectations from PIAAC and other previous literature, it should be noted that the MST design for PISA 2018 was chosen not only to improve measurement precision but also to ensure a satisfactory level of model parameter recovery, controlling for possible item position effects.

4 Discussion

The MST design in PISA was introduced to provide more accurate and efficient measures when heterogeneous groups of students participate. Other constraints included the number and type of items (automatically vs. human scored) needed to represent the full construct and subscale reporting for the major domain. With these constraints, the MST was designed and investigated through experimental and simulation studies.

The current study is limited to the specific PISA 2018 reading design. However, this paper presents what important psychometric features should be considered and met to introduce the MST design to an ILSA where item parameters are estimated when the data is collected through the MST design. This paper also illustrates how the MST design can be finalized through a simulation study. In the future, more simulation studies that examine the robustness of MST designs in PISA would be useful—for example, effects of the item-by-country interactions and omission rates on parameter recovery. Empirically, item-by-country interactions and omitted responses are often observed (OECD, 2020). Thus, the robustness of the MST design could be investigated through examining the sensitivity of parameter estimation when those factors are taken into account. Also, more flexible and optimized test assembly can be studied through automating the assembly process (e.g., van der Linden, 2005) and relaxing some constraints. Rather than relying on manual effort from content experts conducted during 2018 cycle (OECD, 2020), an automated test assembly procedure that guarantees and balances important aspects (e.g., unit positions, contents, subscale reporting, response times) would further warrant the utility and increase the accuracy of the MST in different domain settings.

References

Bock, R. D., & Zimowski, M. F. (1997). Multiple group IRT. In W. J. van der Linden & R. K. Hambleton (Eds.), *Handbook of modern item response theory* (pp. 433–448). Springer. https://doi.org/10.1007/978-1-4757-2691-6_25

Eggen, T. J., & Verhelst, N. D. (2011). Item calibration in incomplete testing designs. *Psicológica, 32*(1), 107–132. https://ris.utwente.nl/ws/portalfiles/portal/6592241/7EGGEN.pdf

Glas, C. A. W. (1988). The Rasch model and multistage testing. *Journal of Educational Statistics, 13*, 45–52. https://doi.org/10.3102/10769986013001045

Joo, S. H., Khorramdel, L., Yamamoto, K., Shin, H. J., & Robin, F. (2021). Evaluating item fit statistic thresholds in PISA: Analysis of cross-country comparability of cognitive items. *Educational Measurement: Issues and Practice*. https://doi.org/10.1111/emip.12404

Khorramdel, L., Shin, H., & von Davier, M. (2019). GDM software mdltm including parallel EM algorithm. In M. von Davier & Y. S. Lee (Eds.), *Handbook of diagnostic classification models* (pp. 603–628). Springer. https://www.springer.com/gp/book/9783030055837

Mislevy, R. J., & Wu, P. K. (1996). *Missing responses and IRT ability estimation: Omits, choice, time limits, and adaptive testing (Research Report No. RR-96-30-ONR)*. Educational Testing Service. https://www.ets.org/Media/Research/pdf/RR-96-30.pdf

Muraki, E. (1992). A generalized partial credit model: Application of an EM algorithm. *Applied Psychological Measurement, 16*(2), 159–177. https://doi.org/10.1002/j.2333-8504.1992.tb01436.x

Oranje, A., Mazzeo, J., Xu, X., & Kulick, E. (2014). A multistage testing approach to group-score assessments. In D. Yan, A. A. von Davier, & C. Lewis (Eds.), *Computerized multistage testing: Theory and applications* (pp. 371–390). Chapman and Hall/CRC.

Organisation for Economic Co-Operation and Development (2020). *PISA 2018 technical report*. https://www.oecd.org/pisa/data/pisa2018technicalreport/

van der Linden, W. J. (2005). Statistics for social and behavioral sciences. *Linear models for optimal test design*. Springer. doi:https://doi.org/10.1007/0-387-29054-0.

von Davier, M. (2005). *A general diagnostic model applied to language testing data* (Research Report No. RR-05-16). Princeton, NJ: Educational Testing Service. https://www.ets.org/Media/Research/pdf/RR-05-16.pdf

von Davier, M., & Yamamoto, K. (2004). Partially observed mixtures of IRT models: An extension of the generalized partial-credit model. *Applied Psychological Measurement, 28*(6), 389–406. https://doi.org/10.1177/0146621604268734

Wainer, H. (1990). *Computerized adaptive testing: A primer*. Lawrence Erlbaum Associates.

Wainer, H., Bradlow, E. T., & Wang, X. (2007). *Testlet response theory and its applications*. Cambridge University Press. https://doi.org/10.1017/CBO9780511618765

Wainer, H., & Kiely, G. L. (1987). Item clusters and computerized adaptive testing: A case for testlets. *Journal of Educational Measurement, 24*(3), 185–201. https://doi.org/10.1111/j.1745-3984.1987.tb00274.x

Warm, T. A. (1989). Weighted likelihood estimation of ability in item response theory. *Psychometrika, 54*, 427–450. https://doi.org/10.1007/BF02294627

Yamamoto, K., Khorramdel, L., & Shin, H. (2018). Introducing multistage adaptive testing into international large-scale assessments designs using the example of PIAAC. *Psychological Test and Assessment Modeling, 60*, 347–368. https://www.psychologie-aktuell.com/fileadmin/Redaktion/Journale/ptam_3-2018_347-368.pdf

Yamamoto, K., Shin, H., & Khorramdel, L. (2018). Multistage adaptive testing design in international large-scale assessments. *Educational Measurement: Issues and Practice, 37*, 16–27. https://doi.org/10.1111/emip.12226

Yamamoto, K., Shin, H., & Khorramdel, L. (2019). *Introduction of multistage adaptive testing design in PISA 2018*. OECD Education Working Papers No. 209, OECD Publishing, Paris. https://doi.org/10.1787/b9435d4b-en

Zenisky, A. L., Hambleton, R. K., & Luecht, R. M. (2010). Multistage testing: Issues, designs, and research. In W. J. van der Linden & C. A. W. Glas (Eds.), *Elements of adaptive testing* (pp. 355–372). Springer.

Simulation Studies of Item Bias Estimation Accuracy

Ritesh K. Malaiya and Richard M. Golden

1 Introduction

Psychometrics provides various instruments such as Item Response Theory (IRT) and Cognitive Diagnostic Models (CDM) to measure both item-specific parameters and examinee-specific parameters given specific items administered to examinees. Such tools often make the assumption of item invariance which states that item-specific parameter values are the same for different subpopulations. However, smaller population sizes may lead to instability in item and person parameter estimation in CDMs. This presents opportunities to study statistical methods that quantify item parameter invariance in a CDM for large as well as smaller examinee population sizes. This also presents an opportunity to explore item parameter estimation methods suitable for smaller population sizes.

Although, item invariance in CDM models have been extensively studied for large sample sizes and good model fit (Bolt & Kim, 2018; Bradshaw & Madison, 2015; Torre & Lee, 2010; Ravand et al., 2019), most of the studies of item invariance do not account for the presence of missing data. Missing data can happen in scenarios where every examinee is administered a sample of test items from a larger test bank or where examinees can skip an item. In this study, the number of examinees to whom a particular item is administered during an exam is defined as the Item Administered Count (IAC). A typical low-stake college course may see IACs in order of tens even for a large examinee population. This is because college-level exams generate multiple test versions to restrict opportunities for cheating. In such a design, a different set of exam items are distributed to each group of examinees. Low IACs may also be obtained if an examinee does not answer all questions. In both the scenarios, it is assumed that the probability an item is missing

R. K. Malaiya (✉) · R. M. Golden
Cognitive Informatics and Statistics Lab, University of Texas at Dallas, Richardson, TX, USA
e-mail: ritesh.malaiya@utdallas.edu

M. Wiberg et al. (eds.), *Quantitative Psychology*, Springer Proceedings in Mathematics & Statistics 353, https://doi.org/10.1007/978-3-030-74772-5_30

is not functionally dependent upon the item's content, the content of other items, or upon item and examinee parameters.

This simulation study aims to investigate item parameter invariance in the DINA (Deterministic Input Noisy And) CDM model using data from three different data sets having a varying amount of missing data. The original data set is sampled with replacement multiple times to construct multiple bootstrap data sets. Each bootstrapped data set is then split into 2 subpopulations to construct pairs of bootstrapped subpopulations. For both subpopulation members of the bootstrap data sets, the model parameter estimates are obtained using the Expectation-Maximization algorithm implementation in the CDM package in R (George et al., 2016). Also, this study proposes bagging the DINA item-specific parameters to reliably estimate item parameters for smaller examinee populations. This parameter estimation method is similar to the bootstrap aggregating (bagging) method proposed by Breiman (1996).

Because the bootstrap data sets are generated from the same data generating process, violations of the item invariance modeling assumption may be detected by comparing the statistics of the two subpopulations. The item invariance statistics used in this study are bootstrap-AB and bagged-AB. The absolute difference between the item parameter values of the first and the second subpopulation is defined as the parameter bias. The parameter bias is then averaged across all the bootstrapped data sets to calculate the Bootstrap Mean Absolute Bias (bootstrap-AB). The item-specific bagged-AB estimator is defined as the absolute value of the difference between the bagged DINA estimator of the first subpopulation member and the bagged DINA estimator of the second subpopulation member.

2 Related Work

In CDMs, item invariance studies are generally performed by dividing the student population into multiple subpopulations based on either the ability of examinees estimated using other methods or other general properties such as gender (Bolt & Kim, 2018; Bradshaw & Madison, 2015; Torre & Lee, 2010; Ravand et al., 2019). In the simulation study of item invariance properties of the DINA model, Torre and Lee (2010) showed that item invariance depends on model fit. To study item invariance, they calculated Mean Absolute Bias (MAB) by averaging the absolute difference between the true and estimated parameters across items within the same item group. Bradshaw and Madison (2015) performed simulation studies to measure item invariance properties of log-linear CDM over different sample sizes ranging from 500 to 10,000. They showed that scoring accuracy and presence of item invariance improved as the sample size increases but the rate of change differed based on different ability groups. The item invariance was measured using median absolute bias across all items within a specific simulation condition. Both group invariance and item invariance properties were examined. Bolt and Kim (2018) investigated item invariance analysis for single time point exam – Fraction Subtraction Data, longitudinal growth simulation study, and Differential Item Functioning simulation study. For Fraction subtraction data, they compared item parameters between different ability groups to study the item invariance. Ravand et al. (2019) used the global likelihood ratio test on a multi-group GDINA to investigate item parameter invariance. The standard errors were calculated using Jackknife method over 1000 simulations. They showed that for an examinee sample size of 500 per male and female group, not all the G-DINA item parameter estimates were invariant in the Foreign Language test.

3 Data

The three data sets considered in this study are the ECPE (Templin & Hoffman, 2013), the TIMSS (Mullis et al., 2012) and a Social Psychology exam conducted at the University of Texas at Dallas (UTD) (Social-UTD). Both the ECPE and TIMSS data set used in the simulation study were imported from the CDM package in R (George & Robitzsch, 2015). The ECPE data set has 2922 students attempting 28 items with all items administered to all students. The TIMSS data set contains 1010 Austrian fourth-grade students attempting items from a 47 item pool. These 47 items were divided into 3 booklets and each student was given 2 booklets to attempt. The third data set Social-UTD contains 136 students attempting items from a 239 item pool constructed from two trials of the last exam in the semester. Each student is administered 53 items from the 239 item pool in each exam trial. In the TIMSS data set, 48.27% of the item response data is missing and the IAC value can range from 18 to 38. In the Social-UTD data set, 89.53% of the item response data is missing and the IAC can range from 4 to 26. The Social-UTD represents a typical college exam where the number of attempts received per item is comparatively very low despite the total examinee count of 136.

4 Method

In this study, each of the three item-response data sets was represented as $X^{I \times J}$ having I examinees and a pool of total J items. The DINA item-specific guess and slip parameters were estimated using two approaches. First, using Expectation-Maximization estimation method available in the R CDM package (George et al., 2016). Second, using the Bagging approach (Breiman, 1996) over the item-specific parameters estimated using the R CDM package (see Sect. 4.3). A measure of the magnitude of an item-invariance violation was obtained by estimating the bootstrap-AB estimator (see Sect. 4.2) and the bagged-AB estimator (see Sect. 4.3). In a typical exam, the number of examinees I in the exam may not always represent how many times an item was administered (IAC) in that exam. For instance, in the ECPE data set, IAC equals I because each item was administered to each examinee. However for the TIMSS and SP-UTD dataset, IAC $<$ I because each item was

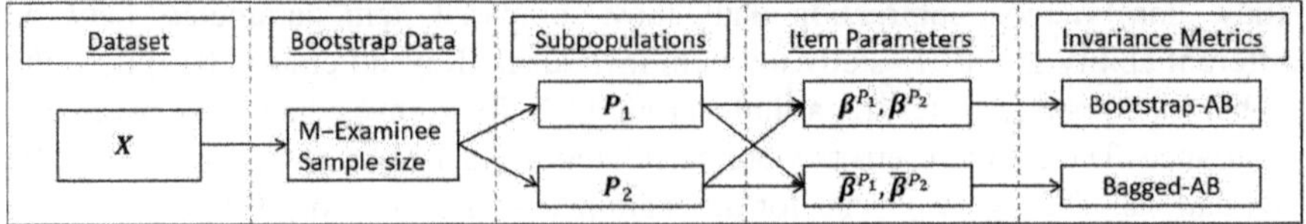

Fig. 1 *This diagram shows how the data set X is sampled to calculate two different item invariance metrics. M* samples of examinees are drawn from the data set X consisting of I examinees. This bootstrap data set is divided in to two $\frac{M}{2}$ size subpopulations P_1 and P_2. The bootstrap-AB (Bootstrap Mean Absolute Bias) and bagged-AB (Bagged Absolute Bias) estimates are then computed for each of the two subpopulations

administered only to a subset of examinees. Hence, item administered count (IAC) was calculated for each item (see Sect. 4.1). IAC represents the examinee population size specific to each item which may be different from the total examinee size in the particular exam. Also, bootstrap-AB and bagged-AB estimators were plotted against IAC to observe the effect of examinee population size on item invariance. To get a large set of IAC values for each item, the bootstrap-AB and bagged-AB estimators were calculated for different examinee sample sizes $M \in \{1 \ldots I\}$ (Fig. 1).

4.1 Bootstrapped Data Set Pairs

Calculation of both bootstrap-AB and bagged-AB estimators required bootstrapped data set pairs for each of the ECPE, TIMSS, and SP-UTD data sets. The first step involved sampling (with replacement) M J-dimensional row vectors from the $X^{I \times J}$ data set. Second, each of the bootstrapped data sets was split into 2 subpopulations. This resulted in two $\frac{M}{2}$ bootstrapped data sets which share the same data generating process. Third, calculate IAC for each item by counting the total number of responses the item received. Fourth, repeat steps one to three 100 times to generate 100 pairs of bootstrapped data sets.

4.2 Bootstrap-AB Estimator

The bootstrapped data set pairs (see Sect. 4.1) were used to calculate the bootstrap-AB for each item using the following procedure. First, the R CDM package was used to estimate item-specific parameters for each of the 100 bootstrapped data set pairs. Second, absolute bias was calculated by computing the absolute magnitude of the difference between the parameter estimates for each of the two subpopulations in each bootstrapped data set pair. This resulted in a distribution containing 100 absolute bias values for each item. Fourth, the mean of this absolute bias distribution was calculated. This mean difference was defined as the bootstrap-AB estimator.

4.3 Bagged Parameter Estimates and Bagged-AB Estimator

First, the average first subpopulation member was computed by averaging the first subpopulation member from each of the bootstrapped data set pairs. These 100 item-specific parameter estimates were then averaged to obtain bagged item-specific parameter estimates. Then, the average second subpopulation member was computed by averaging the second subpopulation member from each of the bootstrapped data set pairs. The absolute difference between the average first subpopulation member and the average second subpopulation member was defined as the bagged-AB estimator.

5 Results

In this study, the item bias distribution is investigated as a function of the Item Administered Count (IAC) value. Each plot is divided into 4 sections representing bootstrap-AB and bagged-AB estimators for Guess and Slip parameters for the given data set. The values in the X-axis represents IAC values starting from 10 examinee count for each data set. The last IAC value ++ represents all the data in the given data set. The Y-axis represents item bias for Guess and Slip probability parameters. For the purpose of this study, an item bias value less than 0.05 is considered as a sufficient presence of item invariance for practical purposes in an educational context.

5.1 ECPE Data Set

Figure 2 shows the distribution of item bias values for ECPE data set. In the bootstrap-AB section of the Fig. 2, for the starting IAC value of 10 examinees, the mean of Guess-specific item bias values is 0.4. Given the guess parameters have a range of [0, 1] the bootstrap-AB value of 0.4 clearly shows a lack of item invariance across subpopulations. Also, the variation in the Guess-specific bootstrap-AB values is large ranging from 0.2 to 0.5. As the IAC value increases the bootstrap-AB values tend to decrease but the variation in bootstrap-AB values remains large till 40 IAC value. At 80 IAC, both the mean and variance of bootstrap-AB sees a rapid decrease. For IAC values higher than 320, all the items show Guess-specific bootstrap-AB values as 0.05 which is the desired criteria for item invariance in this study. Slip-specific bootstrap-AB values are in general lower than Guess-specific bootstrap-AB values even for smaller IAC values. Slip-specific bootstrap-AB values reduces steadily as IAC value increases converging to 0.05 at IAC values higher than 320.

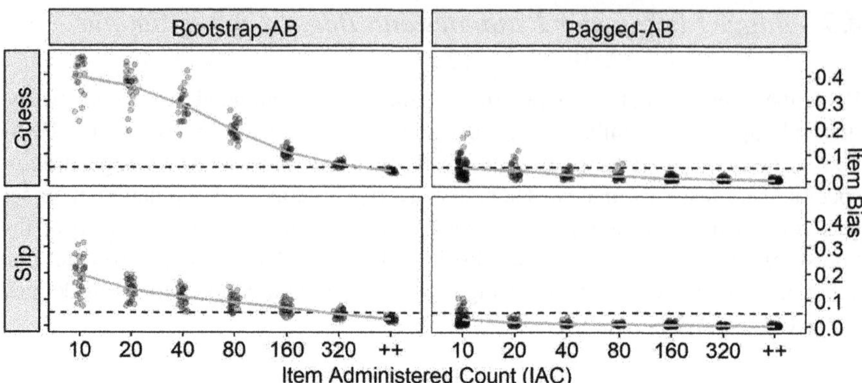

Fig. 2 *DINA Model bootstrap-AB and bagged-AB Item Bias for ECPE data set.* The points are individual bootstrap-AB item bias estimates as a function of IAC. The spread of points shows the distribution of the bootstrap-AB item bias estimates. The line plots the mean of the item bias distribution as a function of IAC. Item bias is dramatically reduced using the bagged-AB estimator relative to the bootstrap-AB estimator across all IAC levels

Interestingly the bagged-AB section of the Fig. 2 shows item bias values lower than 0.1 for most of the items for IAC values as low as 10. Guess and Slip parameters show a similar trend in the reduction of item bias values as IAC value increases. Item bias converges to 0.05 value for most of the items at 40 and larger IAC value.

The ECPE data set has no missing item response, however, in educational scenarios exams may have missing item responses. Hence TIMSS and Social Psychology data set results are reviewed in further sections to observe the effect of IAC on various degrees of missing item response data.

5.2 TIMSS Data Set

Figure 3 represents results of item invariance tests on TIMSS data set. In the bootstrap-AB section of the plot, results show that even for IAC values as small as 10, some items have item bias values lower than 0.05 for both Guess and Slip parameters. However, the count of such items is very small and the majority of items have larger item bias values. As IAC count increases more items start to show item invariance properties for both Guess and Slip parameters. However, even for IAC count more than 320, bootstrap-AB value does not go below 0.05 for both Guess and Slip parameters for some items.

Item bias values in the bagged-AB section of the plot show better results than the DINA model even for IAC values as small as 10. A large number of items start to have item bias values lower than 0.05 for 20 IAC value. Starting from 80 IAC values, guess and slip parameters of all the items have item bias values lower than 0.05.

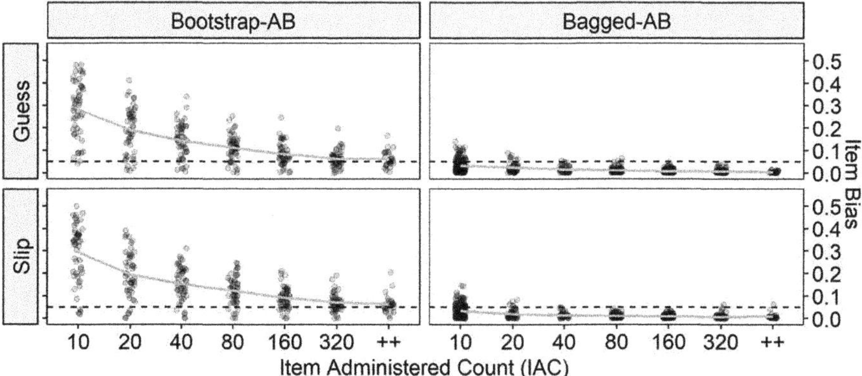

Fig. 3 *DINA Model bootstrap-AB and bagged-AB Item Bias for TIMSS data set.* The points are individual bootstrap-AB item bias estimates as a function of IAC. The spread of points shows the distribution of the bootstrap-AB item bias estimates. The line plots the mean of the item bias distribution as a function of IAC. Item bias is dramatically reduced using the bagged-AB estimator relative to the bootstrap-AB estimator across all IAC levels

It may be concluded that due to the amount of missing response data in the TIMSS data set, bootstrap-AB estimator of DINA model could not show item invariance properties for all the items even when the IAC is greater than 320. However, bagging the item parameters estimated using the Expectation-Maximization algorithm shows promising results for 80 or more examinees in the TIMSS data set.

5.3 *Social Psychology Data Set*

The Fig. 4 shows the item invariance results for the Social-UTD data set. The IAC values for this data set ranges from 2 to 26. However, the count of items that received less than 5 or more than 15 IAC is very small. Hence, for this study's purposes, only the items that have an IAC value between 5 and 15 are shown in Fig. 4. In bootstrap-AB section of the plot, results show that even for such a small IAC range, some of the items have the item bias value smaller than 0.05. However, most of the items show item bias values greater than 0.5 reaching up to 1 for both Guess and Slip parameters. This may suggest a DINA model parameter estimation using the Expectation-Maximization is highly unstable for the data sets having a large amount of missing item response data.

Interestingly, results for Guess and Slip parameters in the bagged-AB section of the plot are very promising. The overall item bias values are smaller than 0.2. And 71% have item bias values are lower than 0.05 for the IAC range of 5 to 15 examinees. These are very encouraging results given the sparsity of Social-UTD item response data set.

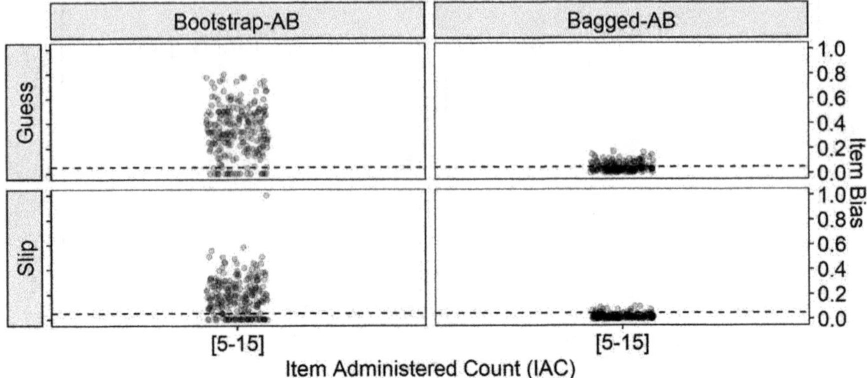

Fig. 4 *DINA Model bootstrap-AB and bagged-AB Item Bias for Social-UTD data set.* This plot contains data only for IAC values between 5 to 15. Item bias is dramatically reduced using the bagged-AB estimator relative to the bootstrap-AB estimator

6 Conclusion

The results show that even though the central tendency of the lack of item invariance reduces as IAC count increases, the spread of the item bias distribution still remains large in the case of data sets with missing item responses for some examinees. As per the current simulation study, more than 300 examinees attempting a particular item are required to reliably estimate item-specific parameters in the DINA model. This makes it infeasible to use the DINA model with standard parameter estimation algorithm for a smaller examinee population typically seen in college courses. However, by bagging item parameters estimated using Expectation-Maximization in the DINA model, the item bias values are closer to 0.05 for most of the items even for IAC values as small as 20. This shows that the bagged estimation approach provides more evidence for item invariance even for smaller IAC values. The bagged estimation approach also seems to be tolerant towards the amount of missing item responses in the TIMSS and the Social-UTD data set.

The bagging method has been theoretically and empirically studied for machine learning algorithms (Domingos, 1997; Friedman, 1997). Also, for the purpose of improving classification accuracy and model selection, model averaging techniques such as Boosting, Bagging, Bayesian Model Averaging has been extensively studied in the machine learning community (Jiang et al., 2020; Posada & Buckley, 2004; Deo, 2015). The impact of such model averaging methods for parameter estimation on other types of CDMs needs to be studied further. The method for checking item invariance proposed in the current study can be utilized to verify the reliability of parameter estimation through model averaging methods. Such studies can promote the adoption of CDM in educational courses seeing various amounts of missing item responses in small and large examinee data sets.

Appendix A: R Code-Snippets for Bootstrap-AB and Bagged-AB Estimators

In this section, R code-snippets representing the methods to calculate item bias (discussed in Sects. 4.1, 4.2, 4.3) are provided. These simplified code-snippets are taken from specific parts of the code written for this study. The full version of the R code is made available at the Open Science Framework repository.[1]

First, 100 bootstrapped data sets of the same size as original data set were generated using the R boot package (Canty & Ripley, 2020). Then only the first M samples from each of the 100 bootstrapped data sets were considered for parameter estimation. These M examinee samples were further divided into 2 subpopulations of size $\frac{M}{2}$.

```
library(boot)
# generating bootstrap indexes
X.bt <- boot(data = df.X ,
           statistic = function(X, i) return(i),
           R = 100, stype = "i");

for (i_val in 1: nrow(X.bt)) {
    X.index <- X.bt[i_val ,]  %>% gather()
    X.index <- X.index$value

    # generating bootstrapped X
    X <- df.X[X.index ,];

    X.s <- head(X, M);
    X.p1.s <- X.s %>% head(round(dim(X.s)[1]/2));
    X.p2.s <- X.s %>% tail(round(dim(X.s)[1]/2));
}
```

Second, the DINA item-specific parameters were estimated using R CDM package (George et al., 2016). These parameter estimates were further used for the calculation of bootstrap-AB estimator, bagged-parameter estimator, and bagged-AB estimator.

```
library(CDM)
function(X.p, Q_reduced, group, Q_names) {
    #Estimating DINA model
    df.cdm <- CDM::din(X.p, Q_reduced, progress=FALSE);

    #Extracting item-specific slip parameter
    df.slip <- tibble("value" = df.cdm$slip$est ,
           "key" = Q_names) %>%
    spread(key = "key", value = "value") %>%
    mutate(parameter = "Slip");
```

[1] *R code is available here:* https://osf.io/naj5t/

```
    #Extracting item-specific guess parameter
    df.guess <- tibble("value" = df.cdm$guess$est,
            "key" = Q_names) %>%
    spread(key = "key", value = "value") %>%
    mutate(parameter = "Guess");
};
```

Third, to estimate the bootstrap-AB for each item, the absolute difference between the item-specific parameters was estimated for each bootstrap represented by *sim_no*. Then the absolute difference is averaged over the bootstraps to get the bootstrap-AB estimator.

```
df %>%
    group_by(parameter, items, IAC, sim_no) %>%

    #Calculating absolute bias
    mutate(d_abs = abs(`Partition 1` - `Partition 2`)) %>%
    group_by(parameter, items, IAC) %>%
    summarise(
            #bootstrap-AB estimator
            MAB = mean(d_abs));
```

Fourth to estimate the bagged parameters for DINA model, average of each item parameter value was calculated over each bootstrapped dataset pair and sampling size. Absolute bias of this bagged parameter was then calculated between bootstrapped data set pairs to get bagged-AB estimator. In below code, *group* variable contains unique id to represent a particular subpopulation and *parameter* variable represents guess or slip item parameter.

```
df %>%
    group_by(group, parameter, items, sampling_size) %>%
    summarise(
            #bagged item-specific parameter estimator
            sampling_mean = mean(item_parameters),
    ) %>%
    spread(key="group", value = "sampling_mean") %>%
    group_by(parameter, items, sampling_size) %>%
    mutate(
        #bagged-AB estimator
        ab_bias = abs(`Partition 1` - `Partition 2`));
```

Acknowledgments This project was partially funded by The University of Texas at Dallas Office of Research through the Social Science Program. We would also like to thank Dr. Karen Huxtable-Jester for contributing the Social-UTD dataset.

References

Bolt, D. M., & Kim, J.-S. (2018). Parameter invariance and skill attribute continuity in the DINA model. *Journal of Educational Measurement, 55*(2), 264–280. https://doi.org/10.1111/jedm.12175

Bradshaw, L. P., & Madison, M. J. (2015). Invariance properties for general diagnostic classification models. *International Journal of Testing, 16*(2), 99–118. https://doi.org/10.1080/15305058.2015.1107076

Breiman, L. (1996). Bagging predictors. *Machine Learning, 24*(2), 123–140. https://doi.org/10.1023/a:1018054314350

Canty, A., & Ripley, B. D. (2020). *Boot: Bootstrap r (s-plus) functions* [R package version 1.3-25]

Deo, R. C. (2015). Machine learning in medicine. *Circulation, 132*(20), 1920–1930. https://doi.org/10.1161/circulationaha.115.001593

Domingos, P. (1997). Why does bagging work? A Bayesian account and its implications. In *KDD'97 Proceedings of the Third International Conference on Knowledge Discovery and Data Mining* (pp. 155–158)

Friedman, J. H. (1997). On bias, variance, 0/1—Loss, and the curse of dimensionality. *Data Mining and Knowledge Discovery, 1*(1), 55–77. https://doi.org/10.1023/a:1009778005914

George, A. C., & Robitzsch, A. (2015). Cognitive diagnosis models in R: A didactic. *The Quantitative Methods for Psychology, 11*(3), 189–205. https://doi.org/10.20982/tqmp.11.3.p189

George, A. C., Robitzsch, A., Kiefer, T., Groß, J., & Ünlü, A. (2016). The R package CDM for cognitive diagnosis models. *Journal of Statistical Software, 74*(2). https://doi.org/10.18637/jss.v074.i02

Jiang, F., Yu, X., Du, J., Gong, D., Zhang, Y., & Peng, Y. (2020). Ensemble learning based on approximate reducts and bootstrap sampling. *Information Sciences, 547*, 797–813. https://doi.org/10.1016/j.ins.2020.08.069

Mullis, I. V. S., Martin, M. O., Foy, P., & Arora, A. (2012). TIMSS 2011 International Results in Mathematics. *International Association for the Evaluation of Educational Achievement*

Posada, D., & Buckley, T. R. (2004). Model selection and model averaging in phylogenetics: Advantages of Akaike information criterion and Bayesian approaches over likelihood ratio tests. *Systematic Biology, 53*(5), 793–808. https://doi.org/10.1080/10635150490522304

Ravand, H., Baghaei, P., & Doebler, P. (2019). Examining parameter invariance in a general diagnostic classification model. *Frontiers in Psychology, 10*, 2930. https://doi.org/10.3389/fpsyg.2019.02930

Templin, J., & Hoffman, L. (2013). Obtaining diagnostic classification model estimates using Mplus. *Educational Measurement: Issues and Practice, 32*(2), 37–50. https://doi.org/10.1111/emip.12010

Torre, J. D. L., & Lee, Y.-S. (2010). A note on the invariance of the DINA model parameters. *Journal of Educational Measurement, 47*(1), 115–127. https://doi.org/10.1111/j.1745-3984.2009.00102.x

Multiple Answer Multiple Choice Items: A Problematic Item Type?

Magdalen Beiting-Parrish, Jay Verkuilen, Sydne McCluskey, Howard Everson, and Claire Wladis

1 Introduction

1.1 Suggestions for MAMC Scoring

Multiple Answer Multiple Choice items (MAMC), also known as pick-N, multiple mark, choose all that apply, or select all that apply questions, are frequently used for large-scale assessments, especially for medical and graduate school entrance examinations (Swanson et al., 2008). These are items that are written similarly to traditional single-answer multiple choice items but they have more than one correct answer; sometimes the amount of correct answers is specified, e.g., "pick the two best answers", or it can be left open-ended, e.g. "select all that apply." Alternatively, these can also be thought of as the examinee choosing a response vector from a number of possible vectors. For instance, if N = 5, the number of statements the examinees must evaluate is 5, meaning there are $2^5 = 32$ possible response patterns, only one of which is the keyed response. For instance, if AB is the keyed response, the examinee could provide 32 possible responses (including the null response), with only one keyed. The following is an exploration of two potential approaches for scoring/analyzing MAMC items. We illustrate using two distinct ability levels of community college students on a sample item from a pilot algebra instrument.

The process for scoring these MAMC items has been hotly debated and there has been much discourse over whether to use a partial credit or dichotomous scoring approach for MAMC (Ripkey & Swanson, 1996). For the partial scoring approach,

M. Beiting-Parrish (✉) · J. Verkuilen (✉) · S. McCluskey · H. Everson
Educational Psychology Department, CUNY Graduate Center, New York, NY, USA
e-mail: mbeiting@gradcenter.cuny.edu; jverkuilen@gc.cuny.edu

C. Wladis
Borough of Manhattan Community College, New York, NY, USA

M. Wiberg et al. (eds.), *Quantitative Psychology*, Springer Proceedings in Mathematics & Statistics 353, https://doi.org/10.1007/978-3-030-74772-5_31

there are multiple methods for how to design and score these items. For example, dichotomous scoring versus partial scoring algorithms was explored on an exam for medical students (Bauer et al., 2010). The two partial scoring methods were one in which the examinee received a static 0.5 points if they chose at least two of the right answers, and one in which the examinee received partial credit in relationship to how many of the correct choices they selected (e.g. examinee selected three of four possible choices resulted in 0.75 credit applied). The authors found that both partial scoring methods resulted in similar psychometric information, were more statistically reliable than single-choice options, and that they awarded more credit overall.

Additionally, the relationship between polytomous and dichotomous scoring was investigated on the American Chemical Society exam using a rubric for assigning partial credit (Grunert et al., 2013). The researchers found that overall average scores increased using the partial credit model, unsurprisingly; however, only the middle performing students really benefitted from partial scoring. Low performers tended not to gain much credit based on strong patterns of mistakes and high performers already received full credit regardless of the scoring model. These results suggest that low performance examinees require a scoring method that awards credit for what these examinees do know that also awards credit for avoiding common mistakes. It also suggests that assigning partial credit provides a useful way to differentiate among different ability levels. This is particularly relevant given the amount of time more complicated items take both to develop and to administer.

Finally, another approach examined the MAMC format through a more thoughtfully designed multiple-true-false method in which the intent was to model partial student knowledge through the pattern of choices and endorsements these students made as compared with traditional single-choice multiple choice items (Brassil & Couch, 2019). The researchers found that the multiple-true-false format allowed the scorers to better understand partial student knowledge as compared with single-choice items. The researchers also posited that these items could provide the test designer with increased content validity because, when properly designed, a single item can address multiple components and false student understandings of a single topic all within one item.

1.2 Local Dependence and Gaming Behavior in MAMC Items

The MAMC format can also induce unpredictable local dependence due to the presence of a common item stem as well as examinees' expectations about how item writers are likely to create items. There is an especially strong dependency between MAMC item choices, especially for mathematics items (Pomplun & Omar, 1997). This is also true for items in which two of the possible choices are direct opposites of each other; an informed examinee would know that logically, only one could be true, creating local dependence. In addition, if the test writer does not specify how many choices are correct (e.g. pick the best two) and leave it open-ended, this can lead to "gaming" on the part of the examinee as they may be unwilling to engage in certain response patterns, especially in cases where all choices are true or none of them are true based on the logic that the item writer would not use such a correct answer. Local dependence greatly complicates modeling such items.

1.3 User Perception of MAMC Items

In addition to the variety of approaches to scoring these items, MAMC items can be difficult for examinees, depending on their skill level. For example, Glasnapp and Poggio (1994) found that young children struggle with the MAMC format, with 25% of third graders who were tested failing to understand the directions and only marking single choices or omitting an answer choice entirely. In addition, Pomplun and Omar (1997) found that third and fourth graders were the most likely to fail to follow the directions for the MAMC items, but this was only 2.61% of fourth grade mathematics students, 4.58% of third grade expository reading students, and only 1.92% of tenth graders failing to follow directions. This suggests that more novice students struggle to answer these questions, but more advanced or experienced students seem to be more successful with this item type. Finally, since MAMC may be an unfamiliar item type, especially for low performance examinees, including more thorough and comprehensive directions, along with the chance to practice the unfamiliar item type may improve student performance (Lakin, 2014).

1.4 Examinee Responses to Novel Item Types

As mentioned above, low ability examinees tend to perform poorly on novel item formats that do not have explicit directions or a chance for the examinee to practice (Lakin, 2014). In general, the low ability examinees may be students with very high math anxiety and very negative preconceived notions about their mathematical ability (Ruff & Boes, 2014). If the student is already experiencing strong negative emotions around the test and their overall mathematical ability, these negative emotions can interfere with higher order thinking which can also impact test performance (Valiente et al., 2012). In addition, these low ability students may also experience stereotype threat in addition to math anxiety which can further stifle higher order thinking, leading to decreased performance (Maloney et al., 2013). Overall, these findings suggest that low ability students may struggle the most with these MAMC items, both because they are a novel format and because of some individual characteristics of these examinees.

2 Method

2.1 Participants

Two samples of students were used. The first sample of participants contained 394 urban community college students who were enrolled in a Basic Arithmetic and Algebra course (57.11%), an Elementary Algebra course (41.37%), or a Statistics with Algebra (1.52%) course in Fall 2016. The second sample of participants contained 628 urban community college students who were enrolled in Precalculus (24.20%), Mathematics for Elementary Education (6.05%), Mathematics for Elementary Education with Algebra (3.82%), Analytic Geometry and Calculus (26.6%), or Intermediate Algebra with Trigonometry (39.33%) in Spring 2018. These two groups made up a low ability group (Fall 2016) and a high ability group (Spring 2018).

2.2 Instrument

The instrument used for this study is the Elementary Algebra Concept Inventory (Wladis et al., 2018). This is a pilot instrument funded through an NSF grant which will eventually replace the current entrance exam with more efficient placement of students in remedial or mainstream community college math classes. The Fall 2016 version of the EACI had 9 single choice multiple choice items and 13 MAMC items. The Spring 2018 version used most of the same items but had 10 single choice multiple choice items and 12 MAMC items. Item A (seen below) is used here (Fig. 1).

Two polynomials have been multiplied together to get $3x^4 - 2x^3 + 5x^2 - 2x + 1$. Which of the following is true? There may be **more than one** correct answer—select **ALL** that are true.

a. $3x^4 - 2x^3 + 5x^2 - 2x + 1$ cannot be factored.

b. $3x^4 - 2x^3 + 5x^2 - 2x + 1$ is factorable.

c. If $3x^4 - 2x^3 + 5x^2 - 2x + 1$ is factorable, then it can be factored into the two polynomials that were originally multiplied together.

d. There is not enough information to determine if $3x^4 - 2x^3 + 5x^2 - 2x + 1$ can be factored.

e. There is not enough information to determine what the factors of $3x^4 - 2x^3 + 5x^2 - 2x + 1$ would be.

Fig. 1 A picture of Item A as it appeared in the EACI. It has two correct keyed responses highlighted in yellow

2.3 Analysis Plan and Justification

A Latent Class Approach This paper suggests an alternative format for item analysis of MAMC items using Latent Class Analysis (Masyn, 2013). Latent Class Analysis (LCA) is a statistical analysis method in which hypothesized latent classes can be observed through covariation that can be measured in the observed variables of interest (McCutcheon, 1987). MAMC items were analyzed individually using LCA with the aim of creating class profiles of latent student knowledge based on the observed patterns of answers for foundational mathematics students (Fall 2016 sample) as compared with the LCA for more advanced mathematics students (Spring 2018 sample). LCA helps reveal homogeneous groupings of item responses within the items.

A Credit-Earned Approach For the purpose of the LCA, a "credit earned" approach was employed in which students received credit for picking the correct keyed responses and for avoiding the distractors. The idea behind this was to award students with the most possible credit, especially since these are foundational mathematics students who likely have at best partial knowledge of these concepts. For example, if the keyed response was AB, a correct response would receive a total of five points, two for selecting the keyed response and three for avoiding the distractors. This awards low ability examinees with more credit than simple dichotomous scoring.

Jaccard's Distance as an Alternative Scoring Method to Number Correct and Binary Credit This paper also explores using Jaccard's distance as an alternative partial scoring method for awarding partial credit to examinees for both groups. Essentially, it can be used to measure how similar or different two words or collections of words are from each other by comparing the letters within the two words of interest or the combinations of words within phrases of interest (Stefanovič & Kurasova, 2019). Jaccard distance between two sets, P, Q can be defined, using set cardinality,

$$d_{Jaccard}\left(\mathrm{P},\mathrm{Q}\right) = 1 - \frac{|\mathrm{P}\cap\mathrm{Q}|}{|\mathrm{P}\cup\mathrm{Q}|} \tag{1}$$

The Jaccard credit function is simply the Jaccard similarity. It compares the number of elements in the intersection between sets to the number in the union and can easily be written as a function of the response coded as a binary vector (in which $\mathrm{x_i}$ is the chosen response and $\mathrm{x_{key}}$ is the keyed response):

$$\gamma_{Jaccard}\left(\mathrm{x_i},\mathrm{x_{key}}\right) = \frac{x_i^T\, x_{key}}{x_i^T x_i + x_{key}^T x_{key} - x_i^T x_{key}} \tag{2}$$

Unlike the other metrics, the Jaccard metric reflects an asymmetry between choice and non-choice. In particular, it does not give an examinee credit for avoiding

Table 1 Credit function for the discrete, Hamming, and Jaccard metrics for N = 3 when A is the keyed response

Response	Discrete	Hamming	Jaccard
∅	0	2/3	0
A	1	1	1
B	0	1/3	0
C	0	1/3	0
AB	0	2/3	1/2
AC	0	2/3	1/2
BC	0	0	0
ABC	0	1/3	1/4

options the key does not call for; this is a particularly useful feature, particularly if N is fairly large and the number of keyed responses is small and thus the number of potential non-choices will dramatically outnumber the number of choices. There are, of course, many other potential *d* functions (Legendre & Legendre, 2012).

In contrast to Jaccard's distance, we also compare it with the Hamming distance. This is typically used for two strings of characters or numbers of equal length to calculate the number of changes needed to go from one to the other (Macleod, 1993). In this case, Hamming distance aligns with the number correct scoring rule. Finally, discrete distance is aligned with dichotomous scoring. In this system, the test taker would get a 1 if they chose the correct keyed response and would get a 0 if they chose any other answer pattern, even if the response contained the keyed response. For the two administrations, 15.7% of the low ability students would have received a 1, if this item were scored with discrete distance, and 32.3% of high ability students would have received a 1.

To understand the difference among these metrics we consider a simple MAMC example where there are N = 3 choices with labels A, B, C in which the participant can choose nothing, one, or more than one choice. In this case, possible responses are ∅, {A}, {B}, {C}, {A,B}, {A,C}, {B,C}, and {A,B,C}. For compactness, we will write these more simply as ∅, A, BC, etc. Assume that the keyed response is A. This is in Table 1. As can be seen, the discrete metric only provides credit for the keyed response. This is a clear scoring metric but loses most of the information about the participant's knowledge state, especially if they have incomplete knowledge that could be revealed by the constellation of responses they did choose. Jaccard is somewhat similar to the discrete metric but provides half credit for responses that include A and have one incorrect choice and quarter credit for the response that includes A and two incorrect choices. All other patterns receive 0 credit. By contrast, the Hamming metric corresponding to total score is markedly different. Nearly all response patterns are given some credit with many receiving 2/3 credit, including the null response. Only failing to choose the correct response A and choosing the incorrect responses BC receives 0 credit—a fact that occurs for all three rules, as seems intuitive. In this context, this has the unfortunate property of giving partial credit to most responses based on avoiding incorrect choices rather than making correct choices.

The three credit functions are reasonably strongly correlated, with Kendall's τ_β near .6. Ordinally they are similar. However, Hamming always assigns higher credit to any response pattern over Jaccard or discrete. This elevation of value is driven primarily by zero-zero matches. As we can see, discrete and Jaccard avoid the problem of zero-zero matches while Hamming suffers greatly from it. This would be particularly true if N is large. In our empirical example, we will show how important this is. As this table shows, the different credit functions assign response patterns to equivalence classes. For instance, the discrete metric, quite obviously, generates only two equivalence classes, while Jaccard generates four, as does Hamming. However, the equivalence classes of Jaccard and Hamming appear to be quite different, with Jaccard overall being much more similar to the discrete metric. To what use should these points be put? They could be used as-is in a total score representing fractional points. Alternatively, they could be used in an ordinal response model, e.g., the generalized partial credit model (GPCM) or a sequential IRT model. The Hamming metric approach would be sensible if the responses were correlated. However, it is quite possible this is not true.

3 Results

3.1 Latent Class Analysis Results

The 13 MAMC items in the Fall 2016 version of the EACI were each treated separately and analyzed using MPLUS (Muthén & Muthén, 2017). For Item A on the Fall 2016 EACI, a four-class model fit best. Class 1 fit 33.16% of the respondents and they were likely to receive credit for avoiding the distractors A, D and E and for correctly picking choice C. Class 2 fit 18.45% of respondents with them most likely receiving credit for avoiding distractor A, D, and E but only picking correct choice B. Class 3 fit 26.74% of the respondents, but these participants were most likely to receive credit for avoiding distractor D and E but not likely to receive credit for correct responses. Finally, Class 4 represented 21.67% of the respondents; they were likely to receive credit for avoiding distractor A and E but were not likely to receive additional credit. Overall, it seems that the low-ability students are receiving the majority of their credit by avoiding the distractors but are not earning credit for choosing the correct answer pattern. Examining other items from the same dataset, however, shows that the number of latent classes identified can differ markedly, suggesting that the idiosyncrasies of individual items remain important.

For the Fall 2018 EACI administration, 59.87% of the participants were placed in Class 1, which showed the examinees both being likely to receive credit for avoiding distractors A, D, E and receiving credit for choosing the correct choices of B and C. This suggests that the Class 1 participants are likely receiving the total amount of points possible between the distractor avoidance and choosing correctly. Class 2 was 23.41% of respondents and represented a class in which the examinee was not likely

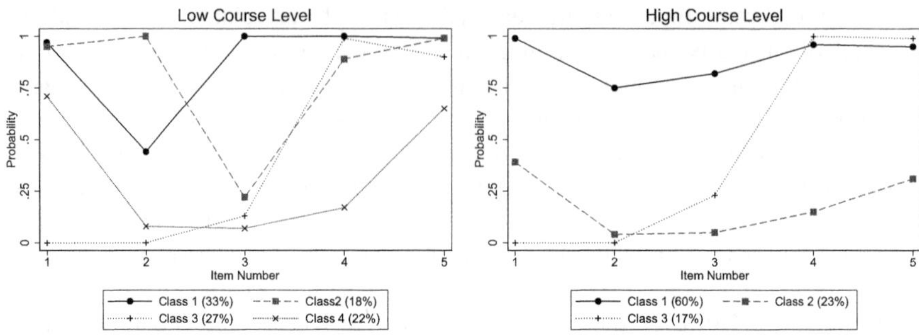

Fig. 2 These diagrams show the probability of the response profiles across both the low and high ability examinees for the LCA for item A

to receive credit for either avoiding the distractors or choosing the correct answer. Finally, 16.72% of respondents were placed in Class 3, which was likely to receive credit for avoiding distractors D and E but did not receive credit for anything else. Overall, for this item, it seems that the high-ability students were able to correctly choose the correct answer pattern, but that one class still benefitted from the credit earned model (Fig. 2).

3.2 *Jaccard's Distance Results*

Item Response Patterns In looking at Item A for the Fall 2106 administration, more participants were likely to select the correct response pattern (15.74%); however, choosing a single answer choice was still very likely with this sample (59.39% of responses). Overall, the low ability sample tends to rely on single choices, despite these being MAMC items. In looking at Item A for the Spring 2018 administration of the EACI, the most popular response pattern is the correct answer choice BC (32.32% of the sample). Next, 41.40% of the response patterns were again single answer choices. Overall, it seems as though the higher-ability sample is more likely to select the right response pattern but is also fairly likely to answer with a single choice, just like the lower-ability sample seen in the 2016 administration.

Jaccard's Distance Results Next, Jaccard's distance was calculated for both administrations and this was plotted against the log frequency of each pattern (Fig. 3). Item A (2016) shows that there are a variety of different patterns for this sample that all occurred with very small frequencies, but that the single answer choices were extremely frequent. In looking at Item A (2018), the correct pattern happened far more frequently, which changes the slope and width of the generated interval. This graph also demonstrates the variety of response patterns, but it seems that the higher ability sample are endorsing single choice patterns and there is higher frequency endorsement of a variety of different patterns.

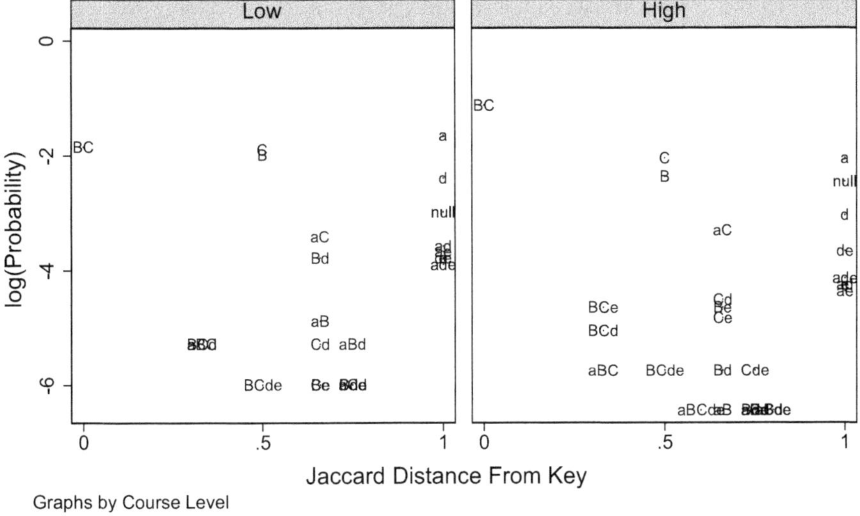

Fig. 3 Log probability of the response patterns of each kind of response plotted against the Jaccard's coefficient

4 Conclusions and Next Steps

This paper aimed to explore two different methods of scoring and analyzing MAMC items using two different samples of data that represented two different examinee groups of varying ability levels. A LCA approach was used to classify learners into different learner profiles which resulted in the lower ability examinee group tending to receive the majority of their points through avoiding distractors. By contrast, the high ability examinee group tended to receive credit through both choosing the correct pattern and avoiding the distractors. Using the credit earned approach to score these items was of strong benefit especially for the lower examinee sample but also for the higher ability group.

Turning to the Jaccard's distance method for scoring these MAMC items, this showed that there were a variety of different patterns for responding to these items and demonstrated that for both ability levels, the examinees were very likely to choose a single choice, despite the item format. The plots of item response distances against log probability demonstrated that there were a wide variety of response patterns, but these varied by examinee group with the higher examinee group having more dispersed probabilities relative to the response patterns. Overall, the majority of the patterns with the smallest Jaccard's distance included one or both pieces of the keyed response, which demonstrates that these students had partial knowledge and were endorsing partial knowledge choices. Across all groups, the most popular choices were single-choice responses, but these frequently included one of the correct answers. In addition, the Jaccard's distance could easily be used as a partial credit scoring algorithm by simply subtracting the Jaccard's distance from 1 to award the partial credit. Using Jaccard's distance also allows the examinee to receive credit for what they do know relative to the correct response pattern such that the test administrator/scorer can better understand the partial knowledge that these examinees may have.

Overall, this item format seemed to be especially difficult for the low ability sample and provoked a lot of anxiety and emotional distress for these examinees, especially as seen through the cognitive interview results. For example, one student said, "It's very confusing to me. ... I don't feel like it really gave me a clear explanation of what it was looking for? . . . So I wasn't sure, so I just didn't pick it, but I tried so I picked E.". Overall, it seems that the lower ability group likely has more math anxiety in general which can impact their performance on any math exam (Maloney et al., 2013), and this item format is especially anxiety inducing, which may have led to the low scores observed here.

Both the credit earned and Jaccard's distance partial scoring algorithm give low level examinees more credit than simple dichotomous scoring. Both models help the test administrator/scorer to better understand the partial knowledge that the examinees do have. In the current format, MAMC items seem to be difficult for all examinees but are especially troublesome for low-ability examinees. One of the largest issues across both ability levels was the examinees' propensity to choose a single choice despite the MAMC format. This may be due to a lack of familiarity with this item type or the entrenched belief that there must be one right answer on a Scantron format answer sheet. These items could be used for this novice population; however, two improvements must be made to use this item format in future research. The first improvement is to include a directions page that has an example question that includes showing the examinee that they can mark multiple responses on their Scantron sheet and that these math questions can have multiple correct responses. Next, the MAMC items need to be written more formally such that different response patterns more intentionally demonstrate shades of partial student knowledge and address the kinds of mistakes students typically make. Since the EACI is intended to ultimately be a pilot instrument for placing community college students into remedial or mainstream math courses, if these items could be designed more intentionally, this could better support educators in meeting these students exactly where they are after being thoughtfully placed in the appropriate course.

There are many implications for this line of inquiry. The largest is that the Jaccard and LCA methods of item analysis could also be used for other novel item types, such as sorting, multiple true false, or even certain kinds of matching items. These analysis approaches could, in fact be used for any keyed response pattern that includes more than one keyed response. This opens up the possibility of more novel item types which can better help educators and test creators to understand the shades of partial knowledge that students may have.

References

Bauer, D., Holzer, M., Kopp, V., & Fischer, M. R. (2010). Pick-N multiple choice-exams: A comparison of scoring algorithms. *Advances in Health Sciences Education, 16*(2), 211–221. https://doi.org/10.1007/s10459-010-9256-1

Brassil, C. E., & Couch, B. A. (2019). Multiple-true-false questions reveal more thoroughly the complexity of student thinking than multiple-choice questions: A Bayesian item response model comparison. *International Journal of STEM Education, 6*(1). https://doi.org/10.1186/s40594-019-0169-0

Glasnapp, D. G., & Poggio, J. P. (1994, April). *Psychometric characteristics of the multiple-correct multiple-choice item*. Paper presented at the annual meeting of the National Council on Measurement in Education, New Orleans.

Grunert, M. L., Raker, J. R., Murphy, K. L., & Holme, T. A. (2013). Polytomous versus dichotomous scoring on multiple-choice examinations: Development of a rubric for rating partial credit. *Journal of Chemical Education, 90*(10), 1310–1315. https://doi.org/10.1021/ed400247d

Lakin, J. (2014). Test directions as a critical component of test design: Best practices and the impact of examinee characteristics. *Educational Assessment, 19*, 17–34. https://doi.org/10.1080/10627197.2014.869448

Legendre, P., & Legendre, L. (2012). *Numerical ecology* (3rd ed.). Cambridge University Press.

Macleod, M. D. (1993). Coding. In *Telecommunications engineer's reference book* (pp. 14-1–14-13). Elsevier. https://doi.org/10.1016/b978-0-7506-1162-6.50020-4

Maloney, E., Schaeffer, M., & Beilock, S. (2013). Mathematics anxiety and stereotype threat: Shared mechanisms, negative consequences and promising interventions. *Research in Mathematics Education, 15*, 115–128. https://doi.org/10.1080/14794802.2013.797744

Masyn, K. E. (2013). Latent class analysis and finite mixture modeling. In *Oxford handbooks online*. Oxford University Press. https://doi.org/10.1093/oxfordhb/9780199934898.013.0025

McCutcheon, A. (1987). *Latent class analysis*. Sage.

Muthén, L. K., & Muthén, B. O. (2017). *Mplus user's guide* (8th ed.). Muthen & Muthen.

Pomplun, M., & Omar, M. H. (1997). Multiple-mark items: An alternative objective item format? *Educational and Psychological Measurement, 57*(6), 949–962. https://doi.org/10.1177/0013164497057006005

Ripkey, D., & Swanson, D. (1996). A "new" item format for assessing aspects of clinical competence. *Academic Medicine: Journal of the Association of American Medical Colleges, 71*(10), S34–S36.

Ruff, S. E., & Boes, S. R. (2014). The sum of all fears: The effects of math anxiety on math achievement in fifth grade students and the implications for school counselors. *Georgia School Counselors Association Journal, 21*(1), 1.

Stefanovič, P., & Kurasova, O. (2019). The n-grams based text similarity detection approach using self-organizing maps and similarity measures. *Applied Sciences, 9*(9), 1870.

Swanson, D., Holtzman, K., & Allbee, K. (2008). Measurement characteristics of content-parallel single-best-answer and extended-matching questions in relation to number and source of options. *Academic Medicine: Journal of the Association of American Medical Colleges, 83*(10), S21–S24.

Valiente, C., Swanson, J., & Eisenberg, N. (2012). Linking students' emotions and academic achievement: When and why emotions matter. *Child Development Perspectives, 6*(2), 129–135. https://doi.org/10.1111/j.1750-8606.2011.00192.x

Wladis, C., Offenholley, K., Licwinko, S., Dawes, D. and Lee, J. K. (2018, February 23). *Development of the elementary algebra concept inventory for the college context*. Mathematical Association of America (MAA) Research in Undergraduate Mathematics Education (RUME) Conference, San Diego, CA.

Modified Method of Drawing Classical ICCs Comparable to IRT-Based ICCs

Sayaka Arai and Gen Hori

1 Introduction

Classical test theory is still widely used in educational settings such as tests in classrooms mainly because it can be applied even if the number of examinees is small as well as its results are easy to interpret. In this study, we focus on line graphs for analyzing the performance of test items based on classical test theory. Hereinafter, we refer to those line graphs as classical item characteristic curves (classical ICCs). Classical ICCs are also called "quintile item response chart" when the examinees are divided into five groups. (cf. Kikuchi, 1999).

1.1 Classical ICCs

Classical ICCs are line graphs showing the correct answer rates to each test item for groups of examinees divided according to the total score. In most cases, examinees are divided into five groups. An example of a classical ICC is shown in Fig. 1. Typically, classical ICCs are drawn as follows:

1. Examinees are divided into five groups (lower(L), lower-middle (LM), middle (M), higher-middle (HM), and higher (H)) based on their total test scores.
2. For each item, the correct answer rates within the groups are plotted.

S. Arai (✉)
National Center for University Entrance Examinations, Meguro-ku, Tokyo
e-mail: sayarai@rd.dnc.ac.jp

G. Hori
Faculty of Business Administration, Asia University, Musashino-shi, Tokyo
e-mail: hori@asia-u.ac.jp

M. Wiberg et al. (eds.), *Quantitative Psychology*, Springer Proceedings in Mathematics & Statistics 353, https://doi.org/10.1007/978-3-030-74772-5_32

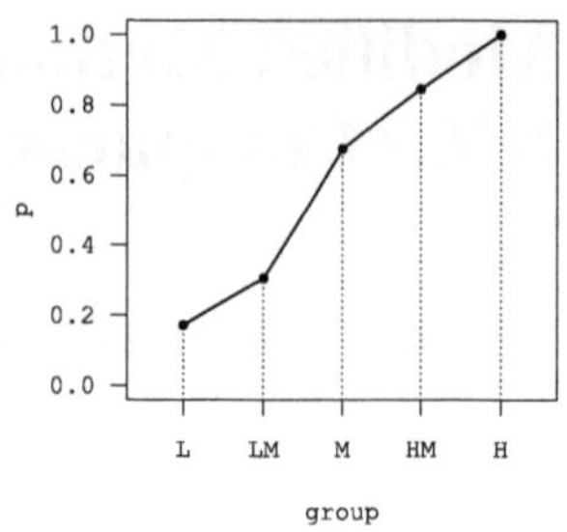

Fig. 1 Classical ICC

When dividing into groups, examinees with the same score are assigned to the same group. Therefore, sometimes it is difficult to divide them into groups of the same size. When drawing a line graph, there is no specific rule about the lateral coordinates of the points indicating each group. Usually, they are set at equal intervals as in the case of drawing a bar graph.

Numerical tables containing the correct answer rates of the items within the groups, from which classical ICCs are drawn, have been in use for a long time (cf. Educational Testing Service, 1963). Also, classical ICCs have been in practical use in actual testing organizations in Japan since the 1980s (Shimizu, 1983).

Several attempts have been made on improving ICCs so far. In addition to widely used ICCs based on parametric IRT models, Ramsay (1991) introduced kernel smoothing approaches to nonparametric item characteristic curves and Ramsay and Wiberg (2017) proposed another method of drawing ICCs based on optimal scores. Classical ICCs, which are the focus of this study, are drawn based on classical test theory. The total test score used for grouping examinees is a test score calculated in classical test theory, i.e. a simple summed score (number-right score) or a weighted summed score, and is not the IRT ability scale.

1.2 Purpose of Study

Since classical ICCs are drawn using classical test theory, they have the same advantages as classical test theory. They do not need to estimate the item parameters, they can be used even for cases where the number of examinees is very small, they can be easily drawn by simply connecting five points, and they are fairly useful for understanding the characteristics of items. On the other hand, the limitations of classical ICCs are that they are difficult to compare to IRT-based ICCs in a common coordinate system and that they do not reflect group sizes even when group sizes are not equal.

To alleviate those limitations, we propose a modified method of drawing classical ICCs in the same coordinate system of IRT-based ICCs. By using the lateral coordinates of the group points for representing the mean scale of the groups, we

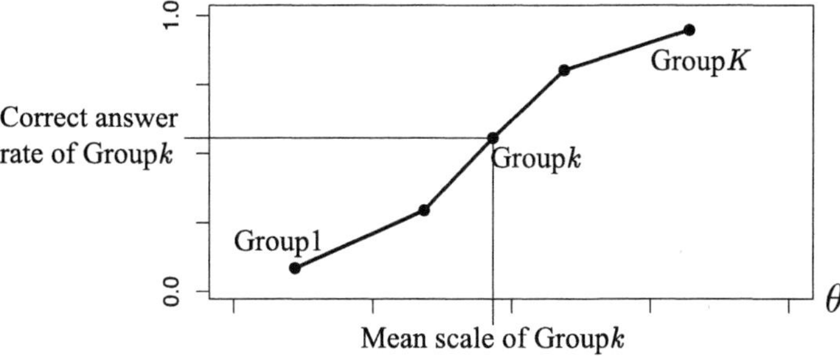

Fig. 2 Coordinates of group points of classical ICC

can draw classical ICCs in the same coordinate system of IRT-based ICCs reflecting group sizes for cases where group sizes are not equal.

The rest of the paper is organized as follows. Section 2 introduces our proposed method and calculates the mean scales of the groups which are required for drawing modified classical ICCs using our proposed method. Section 3 evaluates our proposed method comparing modified classical ICCs with and without information of group sizes. Section 4 concludes the paper.

2 Proposed Method

2.1 *Lateral Coordinates of Group Points*

The purpose of the present work is to introduce a modified method of drawing classical ICCs in the same coordinate system of IRT-based ICCs whose vertical and horizontal axes show the correct answer rate and the scale. A classical ICC has several points on it representing groups of examinees with the vertical coordinates of the points showing the correct answer rates within the groups for the item. When we draw classical ICCs in the coordinate system whose horizontal axis shows the value of the scale, it is quite reasonable to set the lateral coordinates of the group points to the mean scales of the groups. We propose a modified method of drawing classical ICCs in which the lateral coordinates of the group points represent the mean scales of the groups (see Fig. 2).

2.2 *Score-Based Grouping and Scale-Based Grouping*

To draw classical ICCs using the above proposed modified method, we need the actual values of the mean scales of the groups, which are calculated by sorting subjects according to their scores, dividing them into groups, estimating their scales, and averaging the estimated scales for each group. Such a procedure for the score-based grouping requires the estimation of the scales while we aim to develop a method for educators who do not have access to IRT software. Here we note that in most cases, scores and scales are strongly correlated, hence the similarity between the score-based grouping and the scale-based grouping, which is grouping based on sorting according to the scales. As we will see in the following section, the analytical calculation of the mean scales of the groups is tractable for the scale-based grouping. In the present study, we approximate the score-based grouping by the scale-based grouping.

2.3 Mean Scales of Groups for Scale-Based Grouping

In this section, we calculate analytically the mean scales of the groups for the scale-based grouping, that is, we group the examinees based on sorting according to their scales and calculate the mean scale for each group. Such groups correspond to intervals of the scale and the mean scales of the groups are calculated by integration on the intervals. We calculate the mean scales for a general case where the group sizes are not necessarily equal.

We denote the number of the groups by K, the number of the examinees in the k-th group by N_k, and the total number of the examinees by $N = \sum_{k=1}^{K} N_k$. The ratio of the k-th group is then N_k/N and the k-th cumulative ratio is $\sum_{l=1}^{k} N_l/N$. The scale θ is distributed according to the standard normal distribution,

$$\theta \sim N(0, 1), \quad \phi(\theta) = \frac{1}{\sqrt{2\pi}} \exp\left(-\frac{\theta^2}{2}\right).$$

Then the thresholds of the scale dividing the groups are calculated from the cumulative ratios as,

$$t_k = \Phi^{-1}\left(\sum_{l=1}^{k} \frac{N_l}{N}\right), \quad k = 1, \ldots, K-1, \tag{1}$$

using the inverse of the standard normal distribution function,

$$\Phi(\theta) = \int_{-\infty}^{\theta} \phi(z) dz.$$

We put $t_0 = -\infty$ and $t_K = \infty$ for notational convenience. Using the thresholds, the mean scale of the k-th group is defined as,

Table 1 The values of the mean scales of five equal groups

μ_1	μ_2	μ_3	μ_4	μ_5
−1.400	−0.532	0.000	0.532	1.400

$$\mu_k = \frac{\displaystyle\int_{t_{k-1}}^{t_k} \theta \cdot \phi(\theta) d\theta}{\displaystyle\int_{t_{k-1}}^{t_k} \phi(\theta) d\theta},$$

where the numerator is calculated as

$$\int_{t_{k-1}}^{t_k} \theta \cdot \frac{1}{\sqrt{2\pi}} \exp\left(-\frac{\theta^2}{2}\right) d\theta = \left[-\frac{1}{\sqrt{2\pi}} \exp\left(-\frac{\theta^2}{2}\right)\right]_{t_{k-1}}^{t_k} = -(\phi(t_k) - \phi(t_{k-1})),$$

while the denominator is $\Phi(t_k) - \Phi(t_{k-1})$ which leads to

$$\mu_k = -\frac{\phi(t_k) - \phi(t_{k-1})}{\Phi(t_k) - \Phi(t_{k-1})}, \quad k = 1, \ldots, K. \tag{2}$$

With the mean scales of groups μ_k calculated from the group sizes using (1) and (2) being the lateral coordinates of the group points, we draw our proposed modified classical ICC (Fig. 3). In most cases, the group sizes are nearly equal to each other. The values of the mean scales of five equal groups ($N_1 = N_2 = N_3 = N_4 = N_5 = 0.2$) are given in Table 1. We can calculate the functions $\phi(x)$, $\Phi(x)$ and $\Phi^{-1}(x)$ appeared in (1) and (2) using functions of standard spreadsheet softwares. The appendix illustrates how to draw our proposed modified classical ICCs using a standard spreadsheet software.

3 Evaluation

3.1 Performance Index

To evaluate the performance of our proposed method, we define the following performance index,

$$\frac{1}{K} \sum_{k=1}^{K} |p_{\text{irt}}(\mu_k) - p_{\text{prop}}(\mu_k)|, \tag{3}$$

which takes a smaller value when a modified classical ICC is closer to a corresponding IRT-based ICC, meaning that our proposed method is effective.

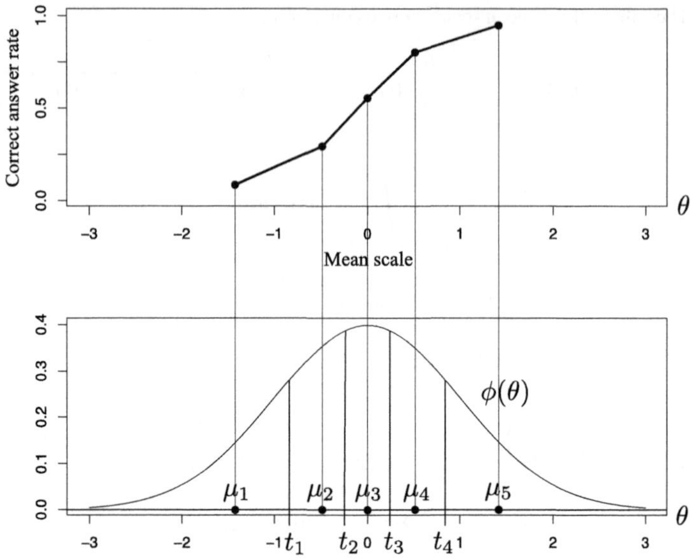

Fig. 3 Modified classical ICC with approximation by scale-based grouping

In the following sections, we compare two variations of our proposed method, which we denote "prop1" and "prop2," to show that our proposed method reflects the information of group size properly in drawing modified classical ICCs.

- Proposed method 1 (prop1) : We set $N_k = \dfrac{1}{K}$ for all the groups, that is, we ignore information of group sizes.
- Proposed method 2 (prop2) : We set N_k to actual group sizes.

We note that we can not compare conventional classical ICCs with our modified classical ICCs because conventional classical ICCs do not have any specifications for the lateral coordinates of their group points. Instead, we compared modified classical ICCs based on equal groups assumption (prop1) and ones based on actual group sizes (prop2) to show that our proposed method properly reflects the information of group sizes.

3.2 Simulation 1: Examples of Modified Classical ICCs

We conducted simulation 1 to illustrate examples of modified classical ICCs using generated response patterns to an example test with 20 items whose characteristics are given by the three-parameter logistic model (3PLM) with item parameters shown in Table 2. These parameters are randomly selected from the 100 items used in Hanson and Béguin (2002).

Table 2 Item parameters (simulation 1)

Item	Parameters			Item	Parameters		
	a	b	c		a	b	c
item1	0.642	−2.522	0.187	item47	1.012	0.421	0.288
item7	0.614	0.037	0.172	item55	0.561	−1.865	0.240
item13	0.839	1.514	0.170	item57	1.665	−0.036	0.109
item14	0.998	1.744	0.057	item61	0.804	−2.283	0.192
item22	0.799	−1.621	0.141	item65	0.892	−0.334	0.211
item36	0.620	−1.208	0.191	item67	0.891	0.157	0.162
item37	0.994	0.189	0.242	item69	1.206	−0.463	0.269
item40	1.715	1.592	0.096	item73	1.613	0.686	0.096
item45	0.953	−0.190	0.212	item81	0.965	−1.862	0.152
item46	1.022	−0.116	0.158	item93	0.893	0.496	0.100

We assumed that the examinees' true score θ follows the standard normal distribution, $\theta \sim N(0, 1)$, and generated a single set of 100 examinees' response patterns using R package "lazy.irt" (Mayekawa, 2018). The test scores (number-right scores) of 100 examinees were calculated based on the response patterns. The correlation coefficient between the test score and the true scale θ was strong ($= 0.897$), supporting our approximation of score-based grouping by scale-based grouping.

We sorted examinees according to the test scores and divided them into five groups , that is, we set $K = 5$. The numbers of examinees in the groups were 23, 22, 24, 16, and 15, respectively. Since we assigned examinees with the same score to the same group, the number of examinees in each group was not exactly 20.

Examples of modified classical ICCs drawn using our proposed method are shown in Fig. 4. As it can be seen from Fig. 4, for some items, the modified classical ICCs are close to the IRT-based ICC (e.g., item 57 and item 61) while for other items, the correct answer rates in each group were not arranged in order (e.g., item 47, item 69, etc.). Although they do not look appropriate, such cases appear where the number of examinees in each group is small.

The values of the performance index (3) of prop1 and prop2 for all the items are given in Table 3. Prop2 performed better for 12 items while prop1 performed better for eight items. Among six items (37, 40, 45, 47, 57, and 65) that differed greatly (more than 0.02) in the values of the performance index, prop2 performed better for five items while prop1 performed better for one item. There was no clear relationship between the performance of the proposed methods and item parameters. The average values of the performance index for prop1 and prop2 were 0.076 and 0.071, respectively. On average, prop2 performed slightly better than prop1 exploiting the information of group sizes.

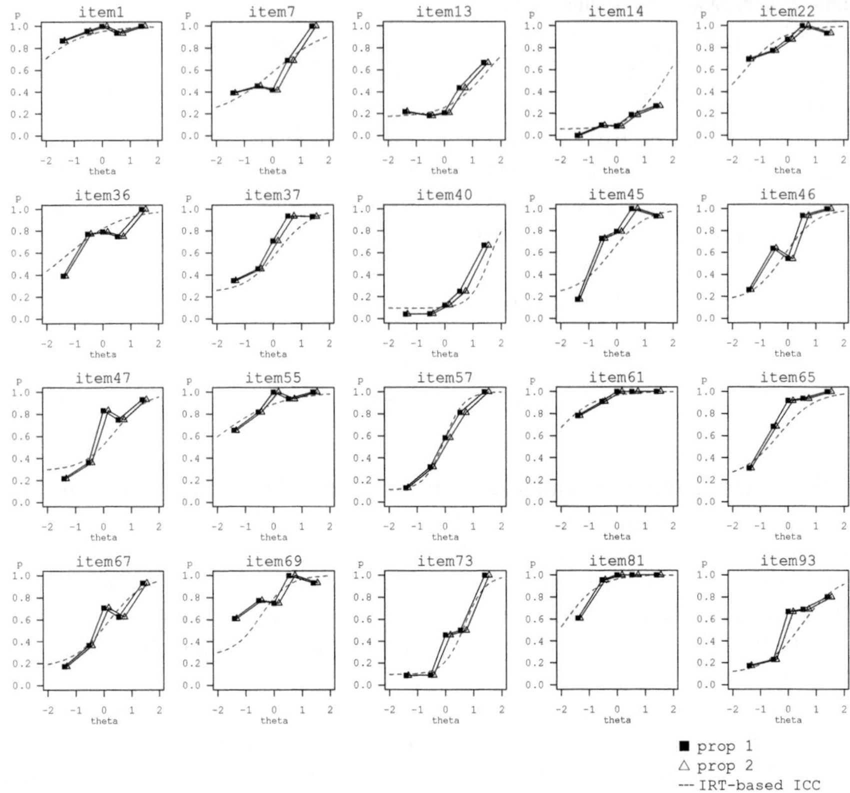

Fig. 4 Examples of modified classical ICCs

Table 3 Performance index (simulation 1)

Item	prop1	prop2	Item	prop1	prop2	Item	prop1	prop2
item1	0.037	0.032	item40	0.096	0.069	item65	0.109	0.085
item7	0.081	0.096	item45	0.137	0.115	item67	0.074	0.078
item13	0.066	0.054	item46	0.101	0.091	item69	0.118	0.112
item14	0.050	0.062	item47	0.114	0.092	item73	0.090	0.081
item22	0.053	0.054	item55	0.043	0.044	item81	0.044	0.043
item36	0.084	0.091	item57	0.019	0.046	item93	0.095	0.080
item37	0.095	0.061	item61	0.022	0.025			

3.3 Simulation 2: Evaluation of Proposed Method

We conducted simulation 2 to investigate the difference in performance between prop1 and prop2 changing the settings such as the number of items and the number of examinees. Simulation 2 is based on the repetition of simulation 1 with randomly selected items and averaging the results for each setting.

We considered two factors (a) the number of examinees (100 and 500) and (b) the number of items (20, 40, and 60) resulting in six settings ($2 \times 3 = 6$) in total as shown in Table 4. For each setting, we repeated trials that are the same as simulation 1 with the number of items and the number of examinees changed. For each trial, a specific number of items are randomly selected from the same set of 100 items used in simulation 1. We repeated the trials 100 times for each setting and averaged the performance index.

The results are shown in Fig. 5 where the left-hand axis shows the average values of the performance index (3) of prop1 and prop2 and the right-hand axis shows the correlation coefficients between the test score (number-right score) and the true score θ for the six settings. In all the settings, the correlation coefficient was greater than 0.89 and prop2 outperformed prop1.

We see that the values of the performance index become smaller for a larger number of examinees. Also, the difference between prop1 and prop2 becomes smaller for a larger number of items. Particularly, the average values of the performance index of prop1 and prop2 are almost the same when the number of items is 80 (settings 3 and 6). These are considered to be because the effect of the group size differences becomes relatively smaller for a larger number of examinees as well as a higher resolution of the score due to a larger number of items.

3.4 Practical Example

This section presents the performance of our proposed method in practice using real data of a mathematics test administered in a university (Hori, 2009). The test consisted of 25 items and the number of examinees was 402. The data were analyzed based on the two-parameter logistic model (2PLM). The item discrimination a ranged from 0.40 to 1.67 and the item difficulty b ranged from -2.19 to 3.99. The

Table 4 Six settings in simulation 2

Setting	# of examinees	# of items
1	100	20
2	100	40
3	100	80
4	500	20
5	500	40
6	500	80

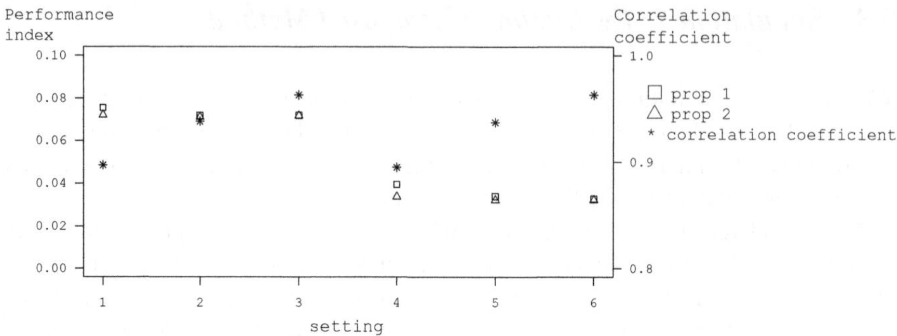

Fig. 5 Comparison of performance index and correlation coefficient

correlation coefficient between the test score (number-right score) and the true score θ was very strong (= 0.993). We sorted examinees according to the test scores and divided them into five groups (L, LM, M, HM, H). The numbers of examinees in the groups were 95, 89, 58, 82, and 78, respectively.

Modified classical ICCs drawn using our proposed method are shown in Fig. 6. The values of the performance index of prop1 and prop2 for all the items were plotted in Fig. 7. Prop2 performed better for 19 items, prop1 performed better for five items, and values of the performance index were almost the same for one remaining item.

As it can be seen in Fig. 6, the modified classical ICCs resemble the 2PLM IRT-based ICCs carrying the features of the curves such as slopes and locations. In Fig. 7, the items are sorted in ascending order of the item difficulty b. We see from Fig. 7 that prop1 performs better for items with low difficulties (items 1–4) while prop2 performs better for items with high difficulties (items 5–23) whereas both methods show almost the same performance for items with very high difficulties (items 24 and 25).

4 Conclusion

We proposed a modified method of drawing classical ICCs in the same coordinate system of IRT-based ICCs. We evaluated our proposed method using numerical simulation that compared modified classical ICCs based on equal groups assumption (prop1) and ones based on actual group sizes (prop2). The results showed that the classical ICCs drawn by prop2 was shown to be closer to the corresponding IRT-based ICC than ones drawn by prop1 and indicated that our proposed method properly reflects the information of group sizes. Through simulation 2, it was shown that prop2 is more effective when the number of items is small.

The main advantage of our proposed method is that it connects the analysis based on the classical test theory to the one based on IRT. Although the modified classical ICCs do not represent the IRT-based ICCs directly, they resemble some features of

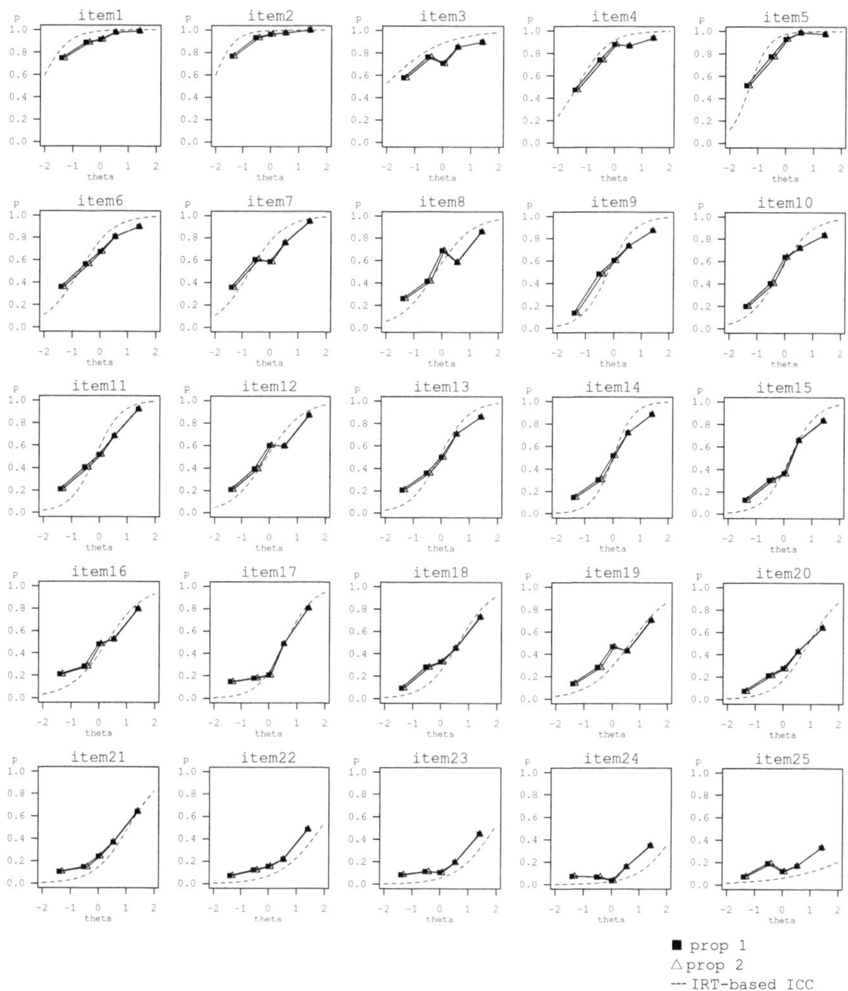

Fig. 6 Modified classical ICCs for real data

the IRT-based ICCs, which allows us to interpret the item characteristics based on IRT even in situations where the number of examinees is limited and therefore only classical ICCs are applicable.

The present study has two limitations. First, we did not compare conventional classical ICCs to our modified classical ICCs because there is no specification for lateral coordinates of group points in conventional classical ICCs, which made a straightforward comparison in our simulations impossible. Second, we did not indicate how small the performance index should be, which we leave to our future study including analysis on the distribution of the performance index. In the present study, we used number-right scores as the test scores, which can be

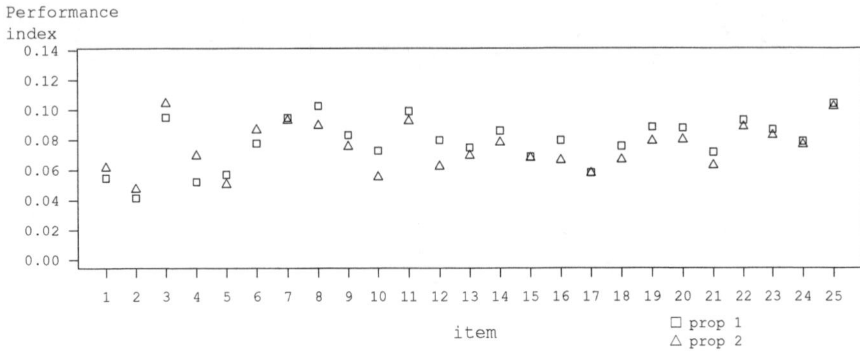

Fig. 7 Comparison of prop1 and prop2 for real data

extended to weighted summed scores as well as optimal scores (Ramsay & Wiberg, 2017; Wiberg, Ramsay, & Li, 2019). Our future study includes the analysis and simulations based on those extended test scores.

Appendix

This appendix illustrates how to draw our proposed modified classical ICCs using a standard spreadsheet software. The figure below gives an example using Microsoft Excel in which columns C and D display the ratios and cumulative ratios of the groups calculated from the group size data entered in column B. According to (1), the first threshold t_1 in cell E2 is calculated from the first cumulative ratio N_1/N in cell D2 using a spreadsheet function `NORM.S.INV(D2)` that calculates $\Phi^{-1}(N_1/N)$, which is then copied to cells E3-E5 for calculation of other thresholds t_2, t_3, and t_4. According to (2), the first mean scale[1] $\mu_1 = -\phi(t_1)/\Phi(t_1)$ in cell F2 is calculated from the first threshold t_1 in cell E2 as `-NORM.S.DIST(E2,FALSE)/NORM.S.DIST(E2,TRUE)` where `NORM.S.DIST(X,FALSE)` and `NORM.S.DIST(X,TRUE)` calculate $\phi(x)$ and $\Phi(x)$, respectively. The second mean scale $\mu_2 = -(\phi(t_2)-\phi(t_1))/(\Phi(t_2)-\Phi(t_1))$ in cell F3 is calculate from the first and second thresholds t_1 and t_2 in cells E2 and E3 as

```
-(NORM.S.DIST(E3,FALSE)-NORM.S.DIST(E2,FALSE))
  /(NORM.S.DIST(E3,TRUE)-NORM.S.DIST(E2,TRUE)),
```

which is copied to cells F4 and F5 for calculation of the mean scales μ_3 and μ_4. The last mean scale[2] $\mu_5 = \phi(t_4)/(1-\Phi(t_4))$ in cell F6 is calculated from the last thresh-

[1] Note that $\phi(t_0) = 0$ and $\Phi(t_0) = 0$ hold since we put $t_0 = -\infty$.

[2] Note that $\phi(t_5) = 0$ and $\Phi(t_5) = 1$ hold since we put $t_5 = \infty$.

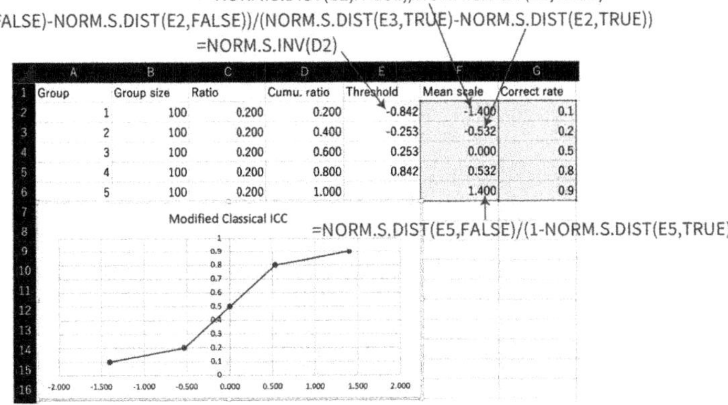

Group	Group size	Ratio	Cumu. ratio	Threshold	Mean scale	Correct rate
1	100	0.200	0.200	-0.842	-1.400	0.1
2	100	0.200	0.400	-0.253	-0.532	0.2
3	100	0.200	0.600	0.253	0.000	0.5
4	100	0.200	0.800	0.842	0.532	0.8
5	100	0.200	1.000		1.400	0.9

Fig. A.1 A modified classical ICC drawn using a spreadsheet software

old t_4 in cell E5 as `NORM.S.DIST(E5,FALSE)/(1-NORM.S.DIST(E5,TRUE))`. The modified classical ICC is drawn by selecting the values of the mean scales and the correct answer rates in F2-G6 and inserting a scatter plot with connecting lines (Fig. A.1).

References

Educational Testing Service. (1963). *Multiple-choice Questions: A Close Look*. Educational Testing Service

Hanson, B., & Béguin, A. (2002). Obtaining a common scale for item response theory item parameters using separate versus concurrent estimation in the common-item equating design. *Applied Psychological Measurement, 26*(1), 3–24

Hori, G. (2009). Exploiting the item response theory in university education. *Journal of the Society for General Academic and Cultural Research, Asia University, 16*, 75–86. (in Japanese)

Kikuchi, K. (1999). Evaluation of quintile item response chart using item response theory. *National Center for University Entrance Examination Research Bulletin, 29*, 1–8. (in Japanese)

Mayekawa, S. (2018, November 15). *Lazy R Packages*. Retrieved from http://mayekawa.in.coocan.jp/Rpackages.html

Ramsay, J. O. (1991). Kernel smoothing approaches to nonparametrci item characteristic curve estimation. *Psychometrika, 56*(4), 611–630

Ramsay, J. O., & Wiberg, M. (2017). A strategy for replacing sum scoring. *Journal of Educational and Behavioral Statistics, 42*(3), 282–307

Shimizu, T. (1983). Analysis of answers in the Joint First-Stage Achievement Test. *University Entrance Examination Forum, 1*, 36–37. (in Japanese)

Wiberg, M., Ramsay, J. O., & Li, J. (2019). Optimal scores: an alternative to parametric item response theory and sum scores. *Psychometrika, 84*(1), 310–322

References

Ontological and Methodological Barriers to the Incorporation of Event Data in Psychometric Models

Tiago Caliço

The increased use of information technologies in education, and particularly educational assessment, has led to the collection of large data sets documenting the actions taken by users of digital platforms in the pursuit of common learning goals, such as navigating a learning management system or completing a digital assessment. Such data are understood to be of interest to research and development in educational assessment, as they have the potential to be evidentiary sources in support of an assessment's validity argument. More crucially, the analysis of data collected on students' task-solving behavior opens the door to the creation of tasks, scoring procedures, and measurement models that focus on task-solving strategies and approaches, rather than on the narrower facet of correctness (Levy, 2012). These data, commonly referred to as "process data", simultaneously hold the potential to fundamentally reconceive the form, focus, practice and use of educational assessments, while challenging the limits of well-established and understood methodological approaches and psychometric methods (Levy, 2020).

However, as every other emergent discipline, research on such behavioral data does not yet benefit from the existence of agreed upon methods, tools or even terminology. Conceptual uncertainty reflects the need to rehearse methods taken from disciplines such as Computer Science, Artificial Intelligence, or Machine Learning, and evaluate their appropriateness to address questions specific to educational assessment and psychometrics. However, the lack of an agreed upon minimal definition of what constitutes "process data", what distinguishes them from other data and what that implies for the design and use of assessments is a barrier to building a shared knowledge base, as well as expectations about what "process data" are and how they should be used.

T. Caliço (✉)
American Institutes for Research, Arlington, VA, USA
e-mail: tcalico@air.org

M. Wiberg et al. (eds.), *Quantitative Psychology*, Springer Proceedings in Mathematics & Statistics 353, https://doi.org/10.1007/978-3-030-74772-5_33

In this paper I argue for necessary, but likely not sufficient, conditions for the advancement of research on the use of behavioral data captured in the context of digital assessments. I reason from the standpoint that the overabundance of terminology in the field is an indicator of conceptual confusion and a hindrance to knowledge accumulation. In the next section I illustrate how the proliferation of terms is at the same time the product of methodological exploration and a reflection of the absence of an ontological foundation. I then propose a general ontology that can easily accommodate behavioral data generated in the context of any educational assessment. In the second and final section, necessary conditions for productive knowledge building and sharing are proposed.

1 Ontological Difficulties: What Is Meant by "Process Data?"

One of the fundamental challenges to the advancement of research on the use of process data is the lack of a clear and well-understood conceptual framework, or ontology, to which practitioners with different methodological backgrounds can refer. The word *ontology* can be used in a broad or restricted sense. In its broader sense, ontology is the branch of philosophy that focuses on the study of the nature and structure of elements of reality. Put another way, ontology studies which elements, or attributes, belong to any given entity because of that entity's very nature (Guarino, Oberle, & Staab, 2009). Of more interest is its restricted sense, commonly used in Computer Science: a way to formally describe which entities compose a system, how they relate to each other, which of these entities and relations are relevant to particular purposes, and how they should be modeled.

A good example of an ontology in the latter sense is the Conceptual Assessment Framework (CAF), proposed by Mislevy, Steinberg, and Almond (2003) on their work on Evidence Centered Design (ECD). The CAF posits that there are five main components that constitute an assessment's design: a competency model, an assembly model, a task model, a presentation model, and, critically, evidence identification and accumulation models. Each of these models provide an abstraction layer, or representation, of artifacts or processes in an assessment blueprint that can be realized in different ways. The existence of a competency model in the CAF prescribes, or reflects, the fact that any assessment begins with a description of what is to be assessed. The theoretical framework which guides that work is beyond the scope of the CAF.

It is this high level of generality at which ECD describes assessment development and deployment cycles that makes it a powerful tool for practitioners with different theoretical backgrounds to productively communicate their experiences and build a common knowledge base. The CAF achieves this goal by abstracting away from individual assessment design practices and collecting those aspects that are common across all instances into a single, general, yet well-defined representation.

Research into process data lacks this ontological clarity and therefore requires specialized conceptual and methodological tools. What uniquely distinguishes such data from more conventional data sets, such as scored item response data? Do process data fit into currently established assessment practices, particularly regarding methods for evidence identification and accumulation? What in process data is germane for assessment purposes and must therefore by judiciously collected and modeled, and what is merely epiphenomenal? The answers to questions such as these will guide the procedures to building an ontology of so-called "process data": a general definition of what data on the behavior of test takers engaged with a digital assessments *are*, in terms of their constituent parts, interplay with other data sources, and analytic use. In the following subsection I present several terms commonly used to refer to such data and explore how they reflect an incomplete understanding of the nature of "process data" while simultaneously providing important clues on its unique nature and use.

1.1 Terminological Overabundance as Evidence of an Emerging Understanding

Because the data commonly referred to as process data are usually of a more complex nature than conventional educational data sets, it is no surprise that inchoative attempts at their definition hinge on research teams' choice of analytic tools, intended uses of the analyses, or data generation mechanisms. The following examples are intended not only to demonstrate how the terminological proliferation came into being but also present good illustrations of the breadth of scope of the content domains and intended use, as well as analytic approaches used in digital assessments, all of which depend in some manner on insights from event data for their value proposition. The interested reader is encouraged to consult the references in this section.

The most commonly used term to refer to these data is of course "process data," which can simultaneously, and ambiguously, refer to the domain to which one wishes to make inferences and the observed data generation process. For example, H. Liu, Liu, and Li (2018) analyzed a "process data file" generated in an interactive problem-solving task in order to make inferences about students' cognitive processes by using a multilevel mixture IRT model. However, if the goal of collecting data on how test-takers interact with an assessment is to make inferences about cognitive processes, no data set by itself will be sufficient. What may provide insights about cognitive processes is the judicious and principled integration of a cognitive model, task specification, behavioral data capture, and its use through appropriate evidence identification and accumulation models.

More recently, there seems to be a move to use the more empirical and less aspirational term "response process data" (Ercikan, 2017; Ercikan, Guo, & He, 2020; Levy, 2020), possibly in an attempt to convey that the data reflect, at best, the *observed* response process and not necessarily the *latent* cognitive process that generated the observed behavior. In either case, the term itself still does not provide clear clues about what such data are, in terms of their nature, content, internal and external relations, or structure. What, if anything, can be inferred from the term is that these are data about observed behavior, which may, under some set of circumstances, provide evidence about unobservable cognitive processes.

Some authors favor terms that reflect the method used to interact with the assessment. One such example is "keystroke data" (von Davier & Mislevy, 2016). It would be expected that, in assessments dependent on keyboards as the main method of interaction, the term "keystroke" would be a substitute for "event". That is the case of the research reported in DeMark and Behrens (2004), in which students had to configure computer network equipment by issuing commands in a simulated terminal. Almond, Deane, Quinlan, Wagner, and Sydorenko (2012) also report on the use of keystroke data to derive inferences about a task that in the modern day is almost exclusively done through a computer keyboard: writing.

A related example is the use of the term "click-stream data" (Owen, Ramirez, Salmon, & Halverson, 2014), as pointing devices are still a privileged method of interaction with computer interfaces. In Mohan, Bergner, and Halpin (2020), students' interactions with a learning management system were analyzed in an effort to elicit evidence of collaborative problem solving. The authors referred to records of these interactions as "click-stream data". Such examples are an attempt to denote a qualitative aspect of process data, that they are the product of recording a specific kind of behavior: the actions taken by the user of a computer system's *interface* in the pursuit of an educational goal. The term does lack in generality however, as in the case of certain simulation applications, the interface may not be a general-purpose computer interface. Take the research reported in Koenig, Lee, and Iseli (2016a,b), in which Navy pilots are trained and assessed on specific tasks by means of a rather complex fac-simile simulator of the interface used in real-world tasks. Even though the actions taken by these students cannot be considered logs of keyboard or mouse use, clearly they have something in common with such data in their ability to provide insights about task-solving behavior in the context of an appropriate interface.

Other terms denote the perspective of monitoring a system's behavior. That is the case of the term "telemetry" (Chung, 2015). As the Greek root of the name indicates, telemetry is the remote monitoring of a system's performance. The system may be subject to the inputs of one or more human agents, but it may also operate autonomously. The purpose of telemetry is to document the system's performance over time and compare it to known operational parameters. The goal in educational assessment is simultaneously broader and more precise. When recording the interactions of a student (the agent) with a digital assessment (the system), it is the behavior of the student that is of interest, whilst the performance of the system itself is assumed to be known or always within parameters. That is not to say the collection of data on the operation of a digital assessment should focus exclusively on the behavior of its human agents at the expense of collecting other information that can inform the system's validation and improvement. Rather, the point is that by using the term telemetry, the focus shifts from the student's behavior to the more general documentation of the system's performance.

Some researchers focus on particular facets, or attributes, of process data. The term "timing data" is one such example. One of many possible attributes of the actions taken within an interactive computer system is the moment of occurrence. Usually this attribute is recorded as either a time stamp, or as the cumulative elapsed time since the beginning of the task and the moment in which the action occurred. Analyses on the time elapsed between actions can potentially inform test developers and users on test- or task-taking strategies. In He, Davier, and Han (2018), event data from two large-scale survey assessments were used to derive feature variables that could be used to sort students into task-solving types. Some of those variables focused exclusively on aspects related to time, such as total time spent on an item, or elapsed time before a specific action was taken. Similarly, Lee and Haberman (2015) distinguished between "timing" and "process" data in their exploration of how examinees behave in a large-scale international language assessment. It is however a rather specific perspective on behavioral data, as it focuses on elapsed time between student actions, or cumulative time spent in a particular item. One can therefore argue that "timing data" are not a category of data per se, but rather a specific perspective on behavioral data, which is of little use without the context that other aspects of the captured behavioral data provide.

Finally, a good example of how the field has tentatively conveyed meaning through sometimes imprecise terms, is the use of the term "log data", and the rather vague "log data analyses". Usually, the performance of a computer system is documented in logs, which may be serialized in files. However, it is important to make a distinction between the conceptual entity (the log and its constituent parts) and its operationalization. Simply, there is a difference between the method "multiple linear regression" and its implementation as a computer routine, like the `lm()` function in the R programming language. Although the latter could not exist without the former, the concept itself can exist and be reasoned about without referring to any particular implementation. Conversely, records of students' behaviors can be collected, stored and transmitted through a multitude of methods, of which individual computer files are but one. The term "log" is ambiguous on its definition of the data's nature. What should be minimally expected of a log [file] and how does that relate to other data and evidentiary sources?

1.2 Towards a General Approach

From the brief review above it is possible to conclude that several of the terms currently used in the literature touch on different aspects of the nature and use of behavioral assessment data, but rather than describing and distinguishing them from more conventional assessment data, these terms focus on aspects of data generation, intended use or analytic method. A more general and descriptive approach is needed, and in fact achievable. It is my belief that researchers should refer to behavioral data collected in the context of digital assessments using terminology that is descriptive, rather than aspirational, general, and precise.

The focus on data collection in any digital assessment is the student's interaction with the interface with the goal of completing a well-defined (set of) goal(s). The interaction consists of discrete actions, which can be executed using distinct means, from a simple mouse and keyboard, to touch-sensitive screens, or interfaces that approximate real-world circumstances. The actions have at the minimum the properties of order and identity. That is to say, for every action, at the very minimum it is necessary to know when it was executed in relation to proceeding and succeeding actions, and what that action was. In almost every application, student actions will be identified and marked with a time stamp that fulfills the order requirement while providing more granular information, as well as with a varying array of descriptive attributes that provide essential semantics to the action. For example, the actions "clicking on a response choice" and "scrolling on a page" will share the minimal properties of identification and moment of occurrence, but will also have action-specific attributes, such as selected option, or final position of the scroll.

2 Moving Forward: Necessary Conditions for Building Shared Knowledge in Process Data Research

What are therefore the necessary conditions for effective, unambiguous, and productive knowledge sharing in the field of process data? As a motivating example, consider the data set at the base of the seminal work reported in Tatsuoka (1985), and its impact on the advancement of Diagnostic Classification Models (DCM) in the past 15 years. Without this well-know and easily accessible data set, much of the literature on DCMs would have been harder to produce and to evaluate. The existence of a "gold-standard" data set not only promoted novel investigations, it simplified its evaluation in relation to previous efforts.

The importance and utility of Tatsuoka's data set stem from four main characteristics. The first is its ontological clarity: the data set is easy to understand, as it records scored answers to items. The only ontological entities are "item", "student", "response" and "correctness". The second characteristic is simplicity of serialization. Because the data set is essentially a two-dimensional array, simple and informal serializations, such as comma-delimited files, were sufficient to economically share it. The third characteristic is freedom, or openness. The data set is popular not only because its contents were made available for free, but also because its form was unencumbered by licensing or patent considerations. Finally, the data set was not only easy to understand and share, its generation mechanism was well understood. The theoretical framework underpinning the items' design was extensively documented, and therefore it was possible to establish the conditions in which its use was defensible. These four characteristics compose the basis for necessary conditions for productive knowledge sharing on process data and its role in educational assessment.

General purpose data ontology. The first condition is a general-purpose data ontology that is general enough to accommodate a vast array of assessment applications, while being flexible enough to incorporate unique aspects of any particular application. The field of Business Process Mining (BPM, van der Aalst, 2011) provides an ontology that can be adapted to educational process data. BPM focuses on the extraction of actionable information on the way business and industrial processes are executed, with the goals of improving efficiency, checking conformance to established parameters, improving process design, or analyzing how individual agents differ in their approach to process execution.

Its data ontology builds on four basic entities: events, traces, logs and attributes, which can be generalized to any kind of process, so long as its execution is done through a computer system that facilitates the process execution while unobtrusively recording the actions of all participating agents. A data ontology that is this general, while precise, is the first conceptual tool for practitioners to build a common knowledge base without sacrificing attention to specific analytic goals, or operational choices. Importantly, the core concept in the BPM data ontology, the event, covers all the important facets identified in Sect. 1. An event is the atomic element that constitutes the log of any process execution. It is a digital translation of an action taken by an agent, human or software logic, engaged in the process' execution. It is multidimensional in the sense that it has several attributes: identity, moment of execution, and event-specific characteristics that expand its semantics.

Applications of the BPM data ontology, as well as of its analytic methods, can be found in fields as diverse as software development (C. Liu, van Dongen, Assy, & van der Aalst, 2018), emergency room administration (Mannhardt, de Leoni, Reijers, van der Aalst, & Toussaint, 2018), or processing traffic violation fines (Mannhardt, de Leoni, Reijers, & van der Aalst, 2017). The BPM ontology provides the minimal conceptual apparatus to reason precisely about "process data".

General purpose data serialization. Once a data ontology is established, it is necessary to operationalize it in some physical format that is suitable for economic transmission. That is to say, it is necessary to have a *data serialization*. Unlike tabular data such as the Tatsuoka data set, event data are multidimensional and nested. Each event exists in the context of a unique process execution. One or more agents may be involved in its execution, for example, in the case of collaborative problem solving. More crucially, each event class holds its own set of attributes. Clearly a simple tabular representation is inadequate, a more formal and complex format is required.

Although some research exists proposing relatively general data serialization formats for the purpose of sharing process data (e.g., Hao, Smith, Mislevy, von Davier, & Bauer, 2016), one should be careful to avoid solutions that impose licensing constraints, such as patented and proprietary data formats. Recall that the Tatsuoka data set is commonly made available through a simple and free data serialization format. Meaningful progress in the sharing of educational assessment event data requires the same degree of freedom, without limiting researchers by having to pay an implicit "data format tax" to the owners of the patents on any specific serialization. Recall that something being made available without there being an explicit charge does not necessarily imply the freedom from commercial licensing terms, or that fees will not be applied in the future, when a proprietary format becomes the de facto standard in the field.

Fortunately, the field of BPM also offers a solution to this problem, in the form of the Extensible Event Stream (XES) data format (IEEE, 2016). This format, adopted as the standard for event data by the Institute of Electrical and Electronics Engineers, establishes the minimal structure for any event log as well as the means to define and expand the semantics of its components.

General purpose, analytic tools. Data sets are of little use without analytic tools, specifically software. It is a common practice for commercial software developers to encourage the use of their products by tying them to proprietary data formats. The use of free and open-source data formats such as XES encourage the development of analytic tools, proprietary or open-source, by providing a level playing field. Consider the developments in CDM modeling and analysis in the past 10 years alone, in which commercial tools such as Mplus (Muthén & Muthén, 2017), or the open-source R package `CDM` (George, Robitzsch, Kiefer, Groß, & Ünlü, 2016), benefited from the existence of a free data format. The XES format has the potential to foster this type of innovation, simplifying data exploration and its inclusion as an evidentiary source in psychometric models. By leveling the playing field with a general data format, researchers can focus on creating tools that simplify common analytic tasks (e.g., computing response times), thereby freeing resources for more foundational research.

Freely available, high-quality "gold-standard" data sets. Finally, high-quality data sets must be made available to the general research community. The existence of a common data format simplifies this goal but is not sufficient by itself. Regulatory and economic considerations complicate data sharing. First, data collection is an expensive and involved process, that occurs in the context of commercial testing, government surveys, or research development. There are few incentives for commercial entities to share event data, as they constitute a competitive edge. Government may have a role in this regard, as event data are now routinely collected in the context of survey assessments such as the National Assessment of Educational Progress (NAEP). The regulatory context may condition data sharing, due to privacy concerns, although these may be addressed through rigorous implementation of data anonymization and other data security procedures.

The field would benefit from the availability of event data sets that reflect a wide variety of assessment practices, such as survey, high-stakes, games- and simulation-based assessments. Such data sets must be complemented with access to their respective student and task models, as well as the specific items that originated the data, providing the necessary context for interpreting results.

3 Conclusion

The first necessary condition for the building of a shared repository of knowledge is the establishment of common terminology. Ontologies are a way to abstract and systematize the essential elements of any field of inquiry, carving out a conceptual space by identifying core elements of interest, characterizing their essential features and establishing basic interrelations. Research on the use of behavioral data generated through digital assessments is still lacking this basic level of systematization. A clear data ontology for event data will open the way for more fruitful foundational research, collaboration, dissemination, and methodological advancement. Simple, yet powerful, ontologies already exist that can be easily adapted and extended to the field of educational testing. Their adoption, alongside principles of openness and collaboration, have the potential to positively impact developments in the field while avoiding risks of market capture by incumbents or technological fragmentation.

It should be noted, however, that the four minimal conditions presented in this paper are not sufficient for there to be meaningful progress in the assessment and psychometrics fields in what relates to the principled use of behavioral data. Although interactive, digital assessments may provide an opportunity to dramatically broaden the nature and scope of what constitutes an educational assessment, they bring their own unique challenges, while reframing old ones. From a practical standpoint, the integration of multidisciplinary teams is of critical importance. Like any other form of assessment, digital assessments can only fulfill their promise when there is a tight coordination between all involved experts. For psychometricians this means that it is necessary to be fluent in concepts and technologies related to Computer Science, in particular data generation and capture. Leaving decisions about instrumentation exclusively to team members who are responsible for their implementation will more often than not result in expensive collection efforts that return data of little to no inferential value.

From a socioeconomic standpoint, other conditions must be met so that data and knowledge can flow relatively unencumbered. Issues of student privacy, as well as of economical equity and fairness, when sharing event data must be urgently addressed in a serious and deliberate manner. Learning and assessment data generated in digital platforms have an inherent monetary value, as they can guide product development and competitiveness. Who gets to extract and benefit from that value is an ethical issue which, particularly in the case of public education, can not be trivially addressed and must be weighed against legitimate business interests. This issue is more pressing as the cost of developing high-quality digital assessments may surpass that of more traditional forms.

References

Almond, R. G., Deane, P., Quinlan, T., Wagner, M., & Sydorenko, T. (2012). A preliminary analysis of keystroke log data from a timed writing task. *ETS Research Report Series, 2012*(2), i–61. https://doi.org/10.1007/978-3-642-13388-6

Chung, G. K. W. K. (2015). Guidelines for the design and implementation of game telemetry for serious games analytics. In C. S. Loh, Y. Sheng, & D. Ifenthaler (Eds.), *Serious games analytics: Methodologies for performance measurement, assessment, and improvement* (pp. 59–79). Cham: Springer International Publishing. Retrieved from https://doi.org/10.1007/978-3-319-05834-4_3

DeMark, S. F., & Behrens, J. T. (2004). Using statistical natural language processing for understanding complex responses to Free-Response tasks. *International Journal of Testing, 4*(4), 371–390. https://doi.org/10.1207/s15327574ijt0404_4

Ercikan, K. (2017). *Validation of score meaning for the next generation of assessments: The use of response processes*. New York, NY: Routledge.

Ercikan, K., Guo, H., & He, Q. (2020). Use of response process data to inform group comparisons and fairness research. *Educational Assessment*, 1–19. https://doi.org/10.1080/10627197.2020.1804353

George, A. C., Robitzsch, A., Kiefer, T., Groß, J., & Ünlü, A. (2016). The R package CDM for cognitive diagnosis models. *Journal of Statistical Software, 74*(2), 1–24. https://doi.org/10.18637/jss.v074.i02

Guarino, N., Oberle, D., & Staab, S. (2009). What is an ontology? In S. Staab & R. Studer (Eds.), *Handbook on ontologies* (pp. 1–17). Berlin: Springer. https://doi.org/10.1007/978-3-540-92673-3_0

Hao, J., Smith, L., Mislevy, R. J., von Davier, A. A., & Bauer, M. (2016). *Taming log les from game/simulation-based assessments: Data models and data analysis tools* (Technical Report No. RR-16-10). Educational Testing Service. https://doi.org/10.1002/ets2.12096

He, Q., von Davier, M., & Han, Z. (2018). Exploring process data in problemsolving items in computer-based large-scale assessments: Case studies in pisa and piaac. In H. Jiao & R. W. Lissitz (Eds.), *Technology enhanced innovative assessment: Development, modeling, and scoring from an inter-disciplinary perspective*. Information Age Publishing.

IEEE. (2016). IEEE approved draft standard for XES – Extensible event stream – For achieving interoperability in event logs and event streams. *IEEE P1849/D03 June 2016*, 1–58.

Koenig, A. D., Lee, J. J., & Iseli, M. R. (2016a). *CRESST shiphandling automated assessment engine: Mooring at a pier* (Technical Report No. 852). Los Angeles, CA: University of California/National Center for Research on Evaluation, Standards, and Student Testing (CRESST).

Koenig, A. D., Lee, J. J., & Iseli, M. R. (2016b). *CRESST shiphandling automated assessment engine: Underway replenishment (UNREP)* (Technical Report No. 853). Los Angeles, CA: University of California/National Center for Research on Evaluation, Standards, and Student Testing (CRESST).

Lee, Y.-H., & Haberman, S. J. (2015). Investigating test-taking behaviors using timing and process data. *International Journal of Testing, 16*(3), 240–267. https://doi.org/10.1080/15305058.2015.1085385

Levy, R. (2012). *Psychometric advances, opportunities, and challenges for simulation-based assessment* (Technical Report). Princeton, NJ: K-12 Center at ETS. Retrieved from http://www.k12center.org/rsc/pdf/session2-levy-paper-tea2012.pdf

Levy, R. (2020). Implications of considering response process data for greater and lesser psychometrics. *Educational Assessment*, 1–18. https://doi.org/10.1080/10627197.2020.1804352

Liu, C., van Dongen, B., Assy, N., & van der Aalst, W. M. P. (2018). A framework to support behavioral design pattern detection from software execution data. In *Proceedings of the 13th International Conference on Evaluation of Novel Approaches to Software Engineering*. SCITEPRESS – Science and Technology Publications. https://doi.org/10.5220/0006688000650076

Liu, H., Liu, Y., & Li, M. (2018). Analysis of process data of PISA 2012 computer-based problem solving: Application of the modified multilevel mixture IRT model. *Frontiers in Psychology, 9*. https://doi.org/10.3389/fpsyg.2018.01372

Mannhardt, F., de Leoni, M., Reijers, H. A., & van der Aalst, W. M. P. (2017). Data-driven process discovery: Revealing conditional infrequent behavior from event logs. In E. Dubois & K. Pohl (Eds.), *Advanced Information Systems Engineering: Proceedings of 29th International Conference, CAiSE 2017* (pp. 545–560). Springer. https://doi.org/10.1007/978-3-319-59536-8_34

Mannhardt, F., de Leoni, M., Reijers, H. A., van der Aalst, W. M. P., & Toussaint, P. J. (2018). Guided process discovery – A pattern-based approach. *Information Systems, 86*, 1–18. Retrieved from https://fmannhardt.de/papers/IS2018-GuidedProcessDiscovery.pdf. https://doi.org/10.1016/j.is.2018.01.009

Mislevy, R. J., Steinberg, L. S., & Almond, R. G. (2003). On the structure of educational assessments. *Measurement: Interdisciplinary Research & Perspective, 1*(1), 3–62. https://doi.org/10.1207/S15366359MEA0101n_02

Mohan, K., Bergner, Y., & Halpin, P. (2020). Predicting group performance using process data in a collaborative assessment. *Technology, Knowledge and Learning*. https://doi.org/10.1007/s10758-020-09439-5

Muthén, L. K., & Muthén, B. O. (2017). *Mplus user's guide. Eighth edition.* Los Angeles, CA: Muthén & Muthén.

Owen, V. E., Ramirez, D., Salmon, A., & Halverson, R. (2014). Capturing learner trajectories in educational games through ADAGE (assessment data aggregator for game environments): A click-stream data framework for assessment of learning in play. In *2014 American Educational Research Association Annual Meeting*, Philadelphia, PA.

Tatsuoka, K. K. (1985). A probabilistic model for diagnosing misconceptions by the pattern classification approach. *Journal of Educational Statistics, 10*(1), 55. Retrieved from https://doi.org/10.2307/1164930

van der Aalst, W. (2011). *Process mining: Discovery, conformance and enhancement of business processes*. Berlin: Springer.

von Davier, A. A., & Mislevy, R. J. (2016). Design and modeling frameworks for 21st century simulations & game-based assessments. In C. S. Wells & M. Faulkner-Bond (Eds.), *Educational measurement: From foundations to future*. New York, NY: Guilford Press.

Psychometrics for Forensic Fingerprint Comparisons

Amanda Luby, Anjali Mazumder, and Brian Junker

1 Introduction

"Forensic science" is a broad field that consists of many different scientific disciplines that are used in a legal context. These scientific disciplines range from highly objective, such as single-source DNA analysis, to highly subjective, such as bite mark analysis. Forensic science relies on forensic examiners, who are responsible for determining whether a piece of evidence left at a crime scene came from a particular source. Depending on the type of evidence, this process may be nearly automatic and consistent across examiners or vary considerably depending on the examiner performing the analysis. For many disciplines, examiners report their results as an expert opinion of one of three outcomes: the suspect is the source of the evidence (known as an identification or individualization),[1] the suspect is not the source of the evidence (known as an exclusion), or that the analysis was inconclusive (Stern, 2017).

This work focuses on fingerprint evidence, in which a forensic examiner compares a *latent* fingerprint (e.g. from a crime scene) to one or more *reference*

[1]An 'individualization' is an 'identification' to the global exclusion of all others (OSAC, 2017). Following Ulery et al. (2011), we use 'individualization' and do not distinguish between 'individualization' and 'identification'.

A. Luby (✉)
Swarthmore College, Swarthmore, PA, USA
e-mail: aluby1@swarthmore.edu

A. Mazumder
The Alan Turing Institute, London, UK

B. Junker
Carnegie Mellon University, Pittsburgh, PA, USA

M. Wiberg et al. (eds.), *Quantitative Psychology*, Springer Proceedings in Mathematics & Statistics 353, https://doi.org/10.1007/978-3-030-74772-5_34

prints to determine whether they came from the same source or not. The standard operating procedure for analyzing fingerprint evidence is a series of steps known as ACE-V (Analysis, Comparison, Evaluation, Verification), but each step in the ACE-V process is a complex task involving many different factors (see, e.g., OSAC, 2019 for details), and forensic examiners may vary in their approach to the ACE-V process. They may have different standards for the quality or clarity of latent fingerprint needed to perform an analysis, may select different fingerprint features (called minutiae) on which to base a comparison, and may have different thresholds for the degree of similarity required to declare an individualization (or exclusion).

The current approach to characterizing uncertainty in examiner decisions has focused on the calculation of aggregated error rates across all examiners and identification tasks. This approach is not ideal for comparing examiner performance, as examiner decisions are not always unanimous, and error rates are likely to vary across identification tasks depending on the difficulty of the comparison. The variation in examiner decisions alongside the variation in task difficulty makes this application conducive for Item Response Theory (IRT) and related psychometric models (Kerkhoff et al., 2015; Luby et al., 2020).

However, standard IRT approaches must be adapted for this type of data. First, responses are not keyed as 'correct' or 'incorrect' by the test provider. While we may infer that an individualization of a same-source print is 'correct', and an exclusion of a same-source print is 'incorrect' (and vice-versa for different-source prints), it is unclear how 'inconclusive' responses should be treated. For example, an inconclusive on a low-quality print may be considered the 'correct' decision, but an inconclusive on a high-quality print may be considered an 'incorrect' decision since a potential individualization or exclusion was missed. Second, fingerprint comparisons consist of a series of sequential steps. Collapsing the decisions made at each of these steps into a single response ignores the conditional structure of the responses and results in the loss of information about variation at each step of the process. We propose the use of the Item Response Trees framework (IRTrees, De Boeck & Partchev, 2012) as a solution to these issues.

The remainder of the paper is organized as follows. In Sect. 2, we introduce the FBI Black Box Study (Ulery et al., 2011), which is the source of the data used throughout the paper. In Sect. 3, we introduce the IRTrees framework and a model for the fingerprint comparison task. Results are briefly described in Sect. 4, and limitations and future work are discussed in Sect. 5.

2 Data

The FBI Black Box study (Ulery et al., 2011) was the first large-scale study performed to assess the accuracy and reliability of fingerprint examiners' decisions in the United States. One-hundred and sixty nine latent print examiners were recruited for the study, and each participant was assigned roughly 100 items from a pool of 744. Each item consisted of a *latent print* (fingerprint of unknown source lifted from, e.g., a crime scene) and a *reference print* (fingerprint of known source taken under idealized conditions). The latent prints were designed to include a range of features and quality similar to those seen in casework and to be representative of searches from an automated fingerprint identification system.

The study provided an estimate of the aggregated false positive rate (0.1%) and false negative rate (7.5%) in casework. In addition, each recorded response to an item consists of results from the following decisions:

1. Latent evaluation: the examiner's evaluation of whether the crime scene print is of *No Value*, *Value for Exclusion Only*, or *Value for Individualization*.
2. Source decision: the examiner's decision of whether the pair of prints is an *Exclusion* (different sources), *Individualization* (same source), or *Inconclusive*.
3. If inconclusive, one of:
   - *Close*: The correspondence of features is supportive of the conclusion that the two impressions originated from the same source, but not to the extent sufficient for individualization
   - *Insufficient Information*: Potentially corresponding areas are present, but there is insufficient information present.
   - *No Overlap*: No overlapping areas between the latent and reference print
4. If exclusion, one of:
   - *Pattern*: The exclusion determination could be made on fingerprint pattern class (the overall shape of the fingerprint ridges) and did not require the use of minutiae (the small details in the fingerprint).
   - *Minutiae*: The exclusion determination required the use of minutiae .
5. Difficulty (Five-point scale)

Note that due to conflicting responses in the latent evaluation stage, we do not distinguish between *value for individualization* and *value for exclusion only* for this analysis, and treat the latent evaluation as a binary response (*Has value* vs *No value*) instead. We also base our analysis on OSAC (2019), and pool the *Insufficient Information* and *No Overlap* inconclusives into one category.

While the study emphasized estimating casework error rates and therefore focused on the source decision, important trends in examiner behavior are also present in the other decisions. For example, latent print examiners vary in their tendencies towards 'no-value' and 'inconclusive decisions'. Figure 1 shows the distribution of the number of inconclusive and no value decisions reported by each examiner. Although most examiners report between 20–40 inconclusives and 15–35 'no value' responses, some examiners report as much as 60 or as few as 5.

Furthermore, there are some items which examiners largely agree on, and other items where there is substantial disagreement. Figure 2 shows an example of one high-disagreement item (left) and one low-disagreement item (right). Each column represents one of the sub-decisions made for each item assessment: (1) latent evaluation, (2) source decision, and (3) reason for the decision. We note that, even

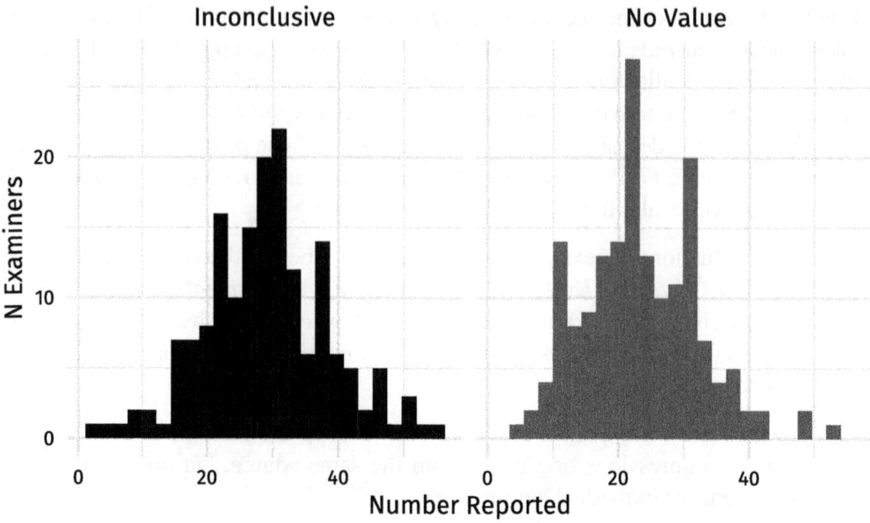

Fig. 1 Number of inconclusive and no value decisions reported by each examiner

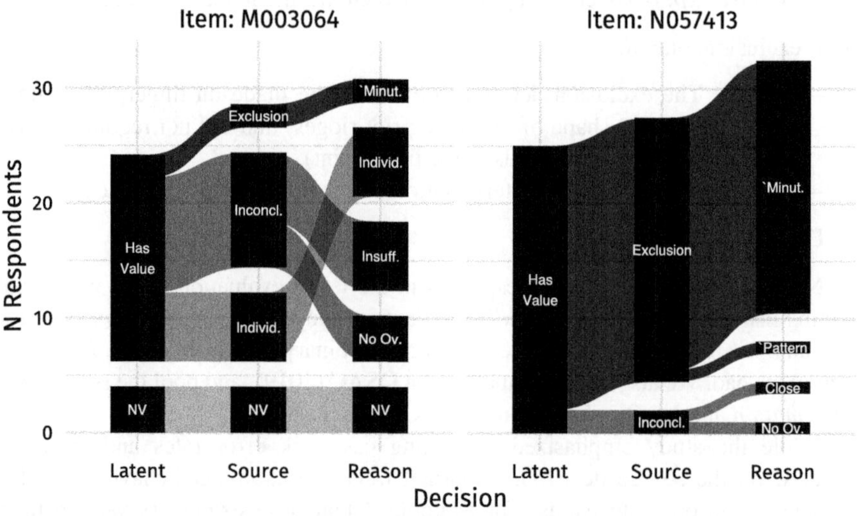

Fig. 2 An illustration of how examiners responded to a high-disagreement item (left) and low-disagreement item (right) for each of three sub-decisions (latent value, source decision, reason for decision)

for the item on the right for which examiners largely agreed, there is still some disagreement in both the source decision and the reason.

By modeling these responses explicitly, we can assess individual differences among examiners in their tendencies to make latent evaluations, source decisions, and reasons for decisions. Similarly, we can measure the variation among items for each stage in the decision-making process.

3 Item Response Trees

Item Response Trees (IRTrees, De Boeck & Partchev, 2012) use decision trees to describe hypothesized cognitive processes, where the leaves are the final observed outcome. The IRTree formulation can represent a wide variety of response formats and response processes, easily adapted for binary responses, unipolar scales, bipolar scales, and Likert responses (Jeon & De Boeck, 2016). In the forensic science setting, IRTrees are useful for representing the sequential decision-making process explicitly (Luby et al., 2020).

Figure 3 illustrates a basic IRTree model for a response with three possible outcome categories (e.g. $Y = 1, 2, 3$), where Y_1^* and Y_2^* are nodes constructed to represent internal decisions that lead to each of three outcomes. If Y_{ij} denotes the response of participant i ($i = 1, \ldots, I$) to item j ($j = 1, \ldots, J$), Y_{1ij}^* denotes the choice of left or right branch at Y_1^* for person i at item j.

The probability of choosing the left branch at node 1 (Y_1^* in Fig. 3) can be modeled using standard IRT models. We use the Rasch model at binary nodes for interpretability and computational convenience: $P(Y_{kij}^* = 1) = \text{logit}^{-1}(\theta_{ki} - b_{kj})$, where θ_{ki} denotes the latent trait involved with choosing the left branch at node k for person i and b_{kj} is the corresponding Rasch parameter for item j. In a standard Rasch model for correct/incorrect outcomes, the item parameters (b_j) correspond to the difficulty of the item, where higher values of b_j decrease the probability that $Y_{ij} = 1$. When IRTree branch decisions do not correspond to incorrect/correct choices, the item parameters represent an "item tendency" towards one branch over the other rather than difficulty.

The model for the probability of choosing the left branch at Y_2^* is similar, except it is conditional on Y_1^* being equal to zero (i.e. we model $P(Y_{2ij}^* = 1|Y_{1ij}^* = 0)$ instead of $P(Y_{2ij} = 1)$). The probability of each observed response (Outcome 1, 2, or 3) is then the product of the probabilities of the internal branches leading to each leaf in the tree (Fig. 3 right).

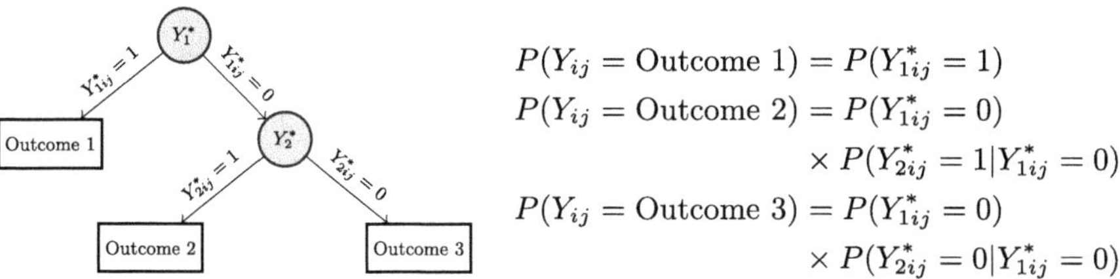

Fig. 3 Example IRTree model tree structure (left) and outcome probabilities (right)

3.1 Model for Fingerprint Comparisons

We use an IRTree model (Fig. 4) constructed using the OSAC Process Map (OSAC, 2019). The constructed IRTree is a necessary simplification of the process map based on the available data in the Black Box study. There are many decisions represented in the Process Map, but there is no way to reconstruct many decisions based on the responses that were recorded in the Black Box study. We also note that not every examiner uses the Process Map for every decision, and that processes may vary by agency.

Each node is parameterized using a Rasch model with $b_{kj} = \beta_{0k} + \beta_{1k} X_j + \epsilon_{kj}$, where $X_j = 1$ if item j is a true same-source pair and 0 if item j is a different-source pair.

We take a Bayesian approach to estimation, which allows us to estimate posterior distributions for all participant and item parameters simultaneously. The IRTree model was implemented in Stan (Stan Development Team, 2018a,b) using R (R Core Team, 2013). Multivariate normal distributions were chosen for $\boldsymbol{\theta}$ and $\mathbf{b}$. Other parameter distributions were chosen based on recommended priors for efficiency, and all code is publicly available.[2]

$$\begin{aligned}
\boldsymbol{\theta}_i &\sim MVN_5(\mathbf{0}, \boldsymbol{\sigma_\theta} L_\theta L_\theta' \boldsymbol{\sigma_\theta}),\\
L_\theta &\sim LKJ(4),\\
\boldsymbol{\sigma_b} &\sim \text{Half}-\text{Cauchy}(0, 2.5),\\
\boldsymbol{b}_j &\sim MVN_5(\boldsymbol{\beta}\mathcal{X}_j, \boldsymbol{\sigma_b} L_b L_b' \boldsymbol{\sigma_b}),\\
L_b &\sim LKJ(4),\\
\boldsymbol{\sigma_b} &\sim \text{Half}-\text{Cauchy}(0, 2.5),\\
\beta_k &\sim N(0, 5).
\end{aligned}$$

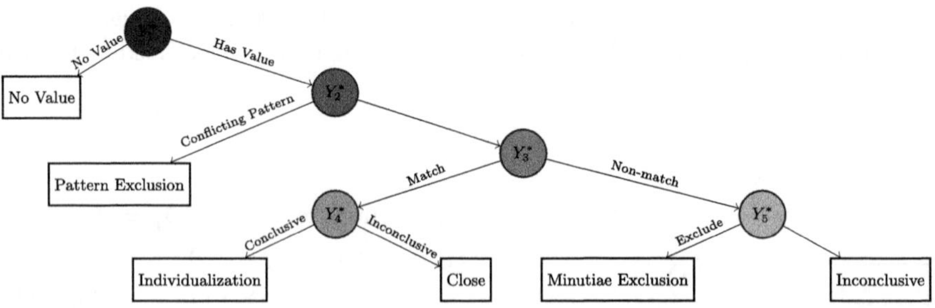

Fig. 4 The *OSAC Process Map* IRTree. Nodes are colored to match the corresponding plots in Fig. 5

[2]github.com/aluby/imps2020

Here $\mathcal{X}_j$ is the column vector $(1, X_j)'$, $\boldsymbol{\beta} = (\boldsymbol{\beta}_1, \ldots, \boldsymbol{\beta}_5)$ is the 5×2 matrix whose k^{th} row is (β_{0k}, β_{1k}), and $\boldsymbol{\sigma_b}$ is a 5×5 diagonal matrix with $\sigma_{1b}, \ldots, \sigma_{5b}$ as the diagonal entries; $\boldsymbol{\sigma_\theta}$ in the previous line is defined similarly. The Stan modeling language does not rely on conjugacy, so the Cholesky factorizations (L_θ and L_b) are modeled instead of the covariance matrices for computational efficiency.

4 Results

The IRTree model introduced in Sect. 3.1 is complex and results in 5 parameters per person and per item, in addition to hyperparameters. We focus on two aspects of the results of the model: (1) the magnitude and uncertainty of participant parameters and (2) using item parameters to generate an "answer key".

4.1 Participant Parameters

For each of the 169 participants (indexed by i), the IRTree model estimates five parameters: a 'no value' tendency (θ_{1i}), a 'pattern exclusion' tendency (θ_{2i}), a 'match' tendency (θ_{3i}), an 'individualization' tendency (θ_{4i}), and a 'minutiae exclusion' tendency (θ_{5i}). Each of these θ estimates correlates with an observed outcome (e.g. θ_{1i} correlates with percent of *No Value* decisions) but also accounts for the corresponding item tendencies. For example, θ_1 represents the tendency of an examiner to choose *no value* after accounting for the subset of items that they were shown. Figure 5 shows the five θ estimates for each examiner (with 95% posterior intervals) as compared to each examiner's proficiency estimate from a Rasch model fitted to scored data.

First, we note that estimated proficiency under a Rasch model is not sufficient for understanding examiner behavior. As outlined in Sects. 1 and 2, fingerprint comparisons are a complex task consisting of a series of steps. Any mapping from the original responses to a binary response necessarily results in the loss of information. Furthermore, there is no designated 'answer key' for the Black Box items, and it is unclear how 'inconclusive' or 'no value' responses should be treated.

Figure 5 demonstrates that even though the IRTree does not require any responses to be scored as correct or incorrect, θ_4 and θ_5 (and to some extent the other parameters) are still correlated with proficiency from a Rasch model. That is, we can still identify examiners who often correctly individualize or exclude (corresponding to more positive θ_4 and θ_5 estimates), as well as those who make more false individualizations and exclusions (corresponding to more negative θ_4 and θ_5 estimates).

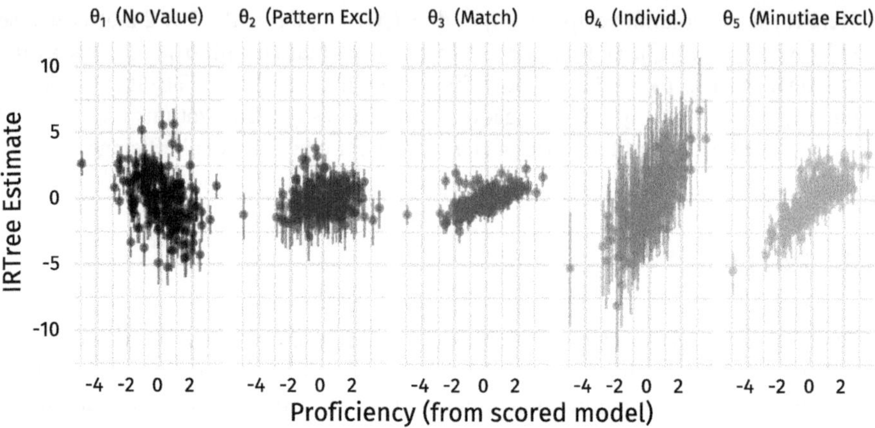

Fig. 5 Number of inconclusive and no value decisions reported by each examiner

Furthermore, the 'match' tendency estimates (θ_3) are the least extreme in magnitude of all of the θ estimates. Examiners are therefore unlikely to disagree on whether a pair of fingerprints is more likely a 'match' or a 'non-match'(the Y_3^* split of the IRTree model in Fig. 4), but *do* disagree on the level of certainty in such a decision (i.e. individualization vs close, Y_4 or minutiae exclusion vs inconclusive, Y_5). This is consistent with previous work that examiners 'willingness to respond' drives much of the disagreement (Dror & Langenburg, 2019).

Finally, we note that there is substantial variation in the 'no value' tendency θ_1. We observe a slight negative correlation between θ_1 and proficiency from a scored model, and that examiners with negative θ_1 estimates (less likely to rate items as *no value*), tend to have positive θ_4 and θ_5 estimates (more likely to rate items as *individualization* or *minutiae exclusion*), providing a link between some of the 'willingness to respond' parameters. The posterior intervals for θ_1 are also noticeably smaller than, e.g., individualization tendency (θ_4), likely due to more observations at earlier nodes in the IRTree.

4.2 Generating an 'Answer Key' from Item Parameters

Using the parameter estimates from each item, we can also estimate the probability of observing each response for a hypothetical "unbiased" examiner. For example, a completely unbiased examiner would have $\theta_k = 0$ for all k nodes in the IRTree, resulting in responses that are totally driven by the item parameters. If such an examiner responded to all 744 items in the FBI "Black Box" study, we can calculate the predicted response to each item. These results could be used as an "answer key" to identify potentially problematic responses since correct and incorrect responses are not keyed by the FBI.

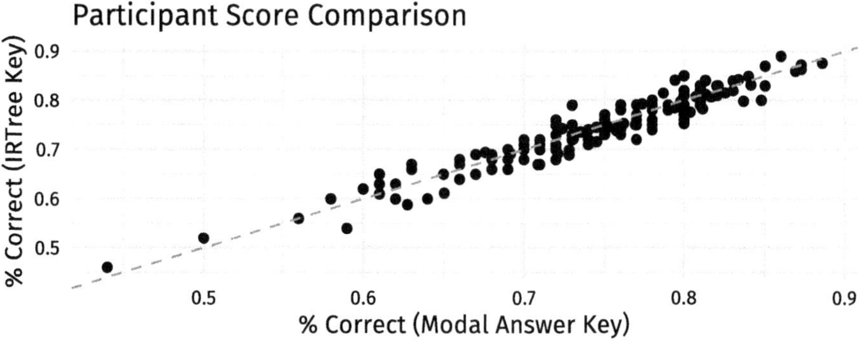

Fig. 6 Each participant's observed score under the IRTree answer key compared to their observed score under the modal answer key. Perfect correspondence is indicated by the dashed line

Table 1 compares the IRTree answer key described above to a modal answer key, where the expected answer to each item is determined by the most popular response to that item. We see that the answer keys largely agree, with both keys labeling very few items as *Pattern Exclusion* or *Close* inconclusive. The most disagreement between the answer keys occurs when the modal answer key predicted a *No Value* or an *Other Inconclusive* and the IRTree model obtained a different label (the first and fourth column, respectively), and when the IRTree model labeled an item with an *Other Inconclusive* (the fourth row).

While Table 1 compares the two answer keys across items, we can also compare the results of the answer keys across participants. Figure 6 shows the observed score (% Correct) for each participant under the IRTree Answer Key and Modal Answer Key. If there was perfect correspondence across the two answer keys, all points would be located on the dashed diagonal line. While some participants receive slightly higher or lower scores under the IRTree answer key than they do under the modal answer key, the scores do not change substantially or in a systematic way. For this setting, we prefer the IRTree framework since the expected responses account for patterns in examiner behavior. For a further discussion of IRTree-generated answer keys and their relationship with other methods such as cultural consensus theory, see Luby (2019).

5 Discussion

The current approach to characterizing uncertainty in forensic decision-making is largely focused on estimating aggregated error rates across examiners and identification tasks. We have proposed a new approach using IRTrees to account for differences in examiner behavior at different points in their decision-making process, and how estimated parameters can be used to generate an answer key to identify potentially problematic responses. Although there are many items with

Table 1 A comparison of how each item was keyed by the IRTree answer key (rows) and the Modal answer key (columns). While the two answer keys agree on most items (corresponding the diagonal entries), there is some disagreement when the modal answer key labeled items as No Value (first column) or inconclusive (fourth column)

		Modal answer key					
		No value	Individualization	Close	Inconclusive	Minutiae exclusion	Pattern exclusion
	No value	175			2		
IRTree	Individualization	1	173		2		
Answer	Close			24	1		
Key	Inconclusive	13		7	170		
	Minutiae exclusion	1			4	154	2
	Pattern exclusion	2					13

substantial variation in the responses, most items were found to have a clear expected answer. Examiners should receive feedback not only when they make a false identification or exclusion, but also when mistaken 'inconclusive' or 'no value' decisions are made. In order to provide such feedback, expected answers must first be generated.

There are, however, limitations to the types of analyses we can perform with this data, particularly in explanatory modeling. For example, rich survey data was collected alongside responses in the Black Box study (e.g. type of training, years of experience, etc.) but survey responses were not linked to test responses to maintain the confidentiality of participants. Furthermore, unlike traditional IRT applications, there are also privacy concerns regarding the items themselves. Each item consists of a pair of images of fingerprints, which by nature are identifiable and cannot be publicly released. This complicates explanatory modeling for participants *and* for items.

Following the Black Box study, there was a series of follow-up studies performed using the same set of participants, and we plan to expand our analyses to include these results. The first was a 'repeatability' study (Ulery et al., 2012), in which 72 participants of the original Black Box study were asked to re-analyze 25 questions seven months after the original study, which provides a unique opportunity to validate conclusions on truly out-of-sample data. The 'White Box' study (Ulery et al., 2014) asked examiners to annotate features, image clarity, and correspondences between latent and reference images when making their determinations. This additional information could be incorporated into a psychometric model to better understand variation in examiner thresholds for making latent evaluation and source decisions.

In addition to research studies, forensic examiners also participate in annual proficiency tests, for which psychometric modeling can also be used (Luby & Kadane, 2018). While current proficiency tests are generally perceived to be easy with high-quality images (Gardner et al., 2020), they can be misinterpreted in legal contexts (Garrett & Mitchell, 2017). IRT-like models should be adopted for all proficiency testing. This would allow for the standardization of examiner scores across multiple years, adjusting for exams that were easier or harder than other exams. Research is also currently being conducted on blind proficiency tests (see Mejia et al. (2020) for overview), in which participants are unaware that they are being tested. This process is more complicated to implement than standard 'open' proficiency tests, as items need to be integrated within regular casework. Psychometrics could provide the methods for validating such tests and comparing results to open proficiency tests.

While we have focused on fingerprint identification throughout this paper, forensic science is a broad term used to describe many scientific fields, each of which relies at least partially on human decision-making. Psychometric models could be applied to each of these scientific areas to better understand the variability in examiner decision-making and potential impacts on final case outcomes.

Forensic science is an area ripe for psychometrics due to variation and uncertainty among forensic examiners, as well as the varying quality of evidence and corresponding difficulty in the analysis task. However, there are also challenges including privacy concerns for participants and for items, responses that are not keyed as correct or incorrect, and the sequential structure of forensic decision-making that must be accounted for. Through complex psychometric modeling, along with domain expertise, we can better understand variation in forensic decision-making and factors that impact that variation.

References

De Boeck, P., & Partchev, I. (2012). Irtrees: Tree-based item response models of the glmm family. *Journal of Statistical Software, Code Snippets, 48*(1), 1–28. https://doi.org/10.18637/jss.v048.c01, https://www.jstatsoft.org/v048/c01

Dror, I. E., & Langenburg, G. (2019). "cannot decide": The fine line between appropriate inconclusive determinations versus unjustifiably deciding not to decide. *Journal of Forensic Sciences, 64*(1), 10–15.

Friction Ridge Subcommittee of the Organization of Scientific Area Committees for Forensic Science. (2017). Guideline for the Articulation of the Decision-Making Process Leading to an Expert Opinion of Source Identification in Friction Ridge Examinations. https://www.nist.gov/system/files/documents/2020/03/23/OSAC%20FRS%20ARTICULATION%20Document%20Template%202020_Final.pdf, online; accessed 15 Sept 2020.

Friction Ridge Subcommittee of the Organization of Scientific Area Committees for Forensic Science. (2019). Friction Ridge Process Map (Current Practice). https://www.nist.gov/system/files/documents/2019/12/10/Friction%20Ridge%20Process%20Map_December%202019.pdf, online; accessed 15 Sept 2020.

Gardner, B. O., Kelley, S., & Pan, K. D. (2020). Latent print proficiency testing: An examination of test respondents, test-taking procedures, and test characteristics. *Journal of Forensic Sciences, 65*(2), 450–457.

Garrett, B. L., & Mitchell, G. (2017). The proficiency of experts. *University of Pennsylvania Law Review, 166*, 901.

Jeon, M., & De Boeck, P. (2016). A generalized item response tree model for psychological assessments. *Behavior Research Methods, 48*(3), 1070–1085.

Kerkhoff, W., Stoel, R., Berger, C., Mattijssen, E., Hermsen, R., Smits, N., & Hardy, H. (2015). Design and results of an exploratory double blind testing program in firearms examination. *Science & Justice, 55*(6), 514–519. https://doi.org/10.1016/j.scijus.2015.06.007

Luby, A. (2019). Accounting for individual differences among decision-makers with applications in forensic evidence evaluation. PhD thesis, Carnegie Mellon University. Available from: http://www.swarthmore.edu/NatSci/aluby1/files/luby-dissertation.pdf

Luby, A., Mazumder, A., & Junker, B. (2020). Psychometric analysis of forensic examiner behavior. *Behaviormetrika, 47*, 355–384.

Luby, A. S., & Kadane, J. B. (2018). Proficiency testing of fingerprint examiners with Bayesian Item Response Theory. *Law, Probability and Risk, 17*(2), 111–121.

Mejia, R., Cuellar, M., & Salyards, J. (2020). Implementing blind proficiency testing in forensic laboratories: Motivation, obstacles, and recommendations. *Forensic Science International Synergy, 2*, 293–298. https://doi.org/10.1016/j.fsisyn.2020.09.002, https://europepmc.org/articles/PMC7552087

R Core Team. (2013). R: A Language and Environment for Statistical Computing. R Foundation for Statistical Computing, Vienna. http://www.R-project.org/

Stan Development Team. (2018a). RStan: The R interface to Stan. http://mc-stan.org/, R package version 2.18.2.

Stan Development Team. (2018b). Stan Modeling Language Users Guide and Reference Manual. http://mc-stan.org

Stern, H. S. (2017). Statistical issues in forensic science. *Annual Review of Statistics and Its Application, 4*, 225–244.

Ulery, B. T., Hicklin, R. A., Buscaglia, J., & Roberts, M. A. (2011). Accuracy and reliability of forensic latent fingerprint decisions. *Proceedings of the National Academy of Sciences, 108*(19), 7733–7738.

Ulery, B. T., Hicklin, R. A., Buscaglia, J., & Roberts, M. A. (2012). Repeatability and reproducibility of decisions by latent fingerprint examiners. *PloS One, 7*(3), e32800.

Ulery, B. T., Hicklin, R. A., Roberts, M. A., & Buscaglia, J. (2014). Measuring what latent fingerprint examiners consider sufficient information for individualization determinations. *PloS One, 9*(11), e110179.

After Thematic Analysis: Introducing the Fuzzy Thematic Network Analysis in Psychological Research

Hojjatollah Farahani, Parviz Azadfallah, and Kazhal Rashidi

1 Introduction

Qualitative researches have a growing and increasing application and popularity in the past decade (Bryman & Burgess, 1994; Denzin & Lincoln, 1994). Thematic analyses can be usefully and effectively aided by and presented as thematic networks. Thematic analysis is a web-like illustration (networks) that summarize the main themes which are extracted from a text. The themes are conceptualized through coding process.

1.1 Structure of a Thematic Network (TN)

Thematic networks are simply used as a way of organizing a thematic analysis of qualitative data. Thematic analyses are to unearth the significant themes in a transcription, and the purpose of thematic networks is to facilitate the structuring and interpreting of these themes. A thematic network starts from the Basic Themes and moves toward a Global Theme (Fig. 1). Braun and Clarke (2006, 2012) describe the thematic networks as follows:

H. Farahani (✉) · P. Azadfallah
Department of Psychology, Tarbiat Modares University, Tehran, Iran
e-mail: h.farahani@mordares.ac.ir; azadfa_p@modares.ac.ir

K. Rashidi
Departyment of Health Psychology, Islamic Azad University, Roudehen, Iran

M. Wiberg et al. (eds.), *Quantitative Psychology*, Springer Proceedings in Mathematics & Statistics 353, https://doi.org/10.1007/978-3-030-74772-5_35

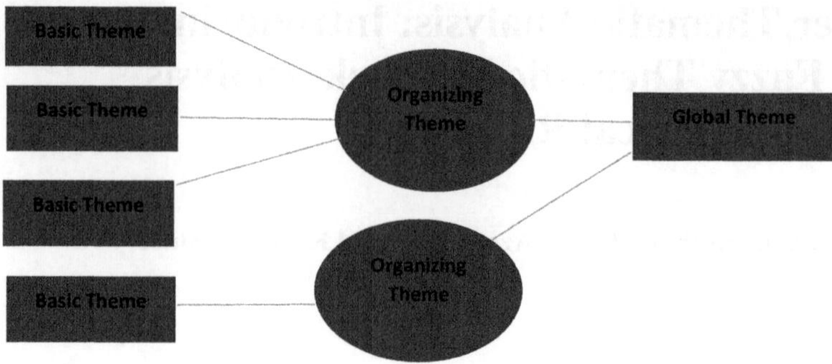

Fig. 1 Structure of a thematic net work

- **Basic Themes** this is the most basic or lowest-order theme that is extracted from the textual data. Basic Themes are simple premises characteristic of the data, and on their own they describe so little about the text or group of texts as a whole.
- **Organizing Themes** this is a middle-order theme that organizes the Basic Themes into categories of similar issues. They are clusters of significations that summarize the principal assumptions of a group of Basic Themes, so they are more abstract and more revealing of what is going on in the texts.
- **Global Themes** super-ordinate themes encapsulating the principal metaphors in the text as a whole. These are then represented as web-like maps depicting the salient themes at each of the three levels, and illustrating the relationships between them.

Each Global Theme is the core of a thematic network; therefore, an analysis may result in more than one thematic network.

1.2 After Thematic Network

In summary, thematic network is a conceptual and interpretive network which is driven from a text such as a transcription of some patients' interviews. What we are introducing here is a method which helps researchers to deepen and expand the obtained results of a thematic network using fuzzy set theory. Although, thematic network analysis and fuzzy set theory are not new, this combination of them are a new direction which can be of interests to all mind researchers and open a new horizon and direction for them. This combination is called here Fuzzy Thematic Network Analysis (FTNA). This method which is based on Mamdani's method described in detail in next section.

2 Fuzzy Thematic Network Analysis (FTNA)

The Polish philosopher Jan Lukasiewicz (1878–1956) was the first to propose a systematic alternative of the bivalued logic (Aristotle's logic) introducing in the early 1900s a three valued logic by adding the term "Possible" between "True" and "False" (Lejewski & Lukasiewicz, 1967). Eventually, an entire notation and axiomatic system was developed by him and he hoped to derive modern mathematics from this development. Later he also extended his logic and proposed four and five valued Logics. Finally, this conclusion came out and he believed that axiomatically nothing could prevent the derivation of an infinite valued Logic. But it was not until relatively recently that an infinite-valued Logic was introduced (Zadeh, 1973), called Fuzzy Logic (FL) by Lotfi. A fuzzy inference system is an inferential system which is based on fuzzy set theory. A fuzzy inference system is a method of the process of formulating the network for a given input to an output using fuzzy logic set theory (Ross, 2010). There is a final decision about given data at the end of this mapping or network. This method combines fuzzy inference system and a thematic network for obtaining a reasonable result (Fig. 2). This type of fuzzy inference systems was introduced by Mamdani (1976) and then extended. Mamdani fuzzy inference was first introduced as a method for fuzzy controller systems. In the article, we use five-input, five-rule and single-output fuzzy inference system (FIS) FTNA is of a 3-stage procedure which is described as follows:

Stage 1 The thematic network obtained from a thematic analysis is given to 5–20 experts and ask them to assign a score to each themes of the network.

Stage2 We ask the experts to assert the rules which describe the relation among the themes in the best way. The amount of the relationships is asserted based on linguistic themes such as high, low .... We aggregate them using max- operator.

Stage3 Applying Fuzzy Inference Fuzzy inference is the process of formulating the mapping from a given input to an output using fuzzy set theory. In the paper, we use five-input, five-rule and single-output fuzzy inference system (FIS) for evaluation of life satisfaction.

Pre-processing Input data are collected from the experts who evaluated the thematic network in a point scale. Then the weights are determined for the edges by them. All inputs are multiplied by their weights and average values are calculated. We need to define five IF-THEN rules for the problem.

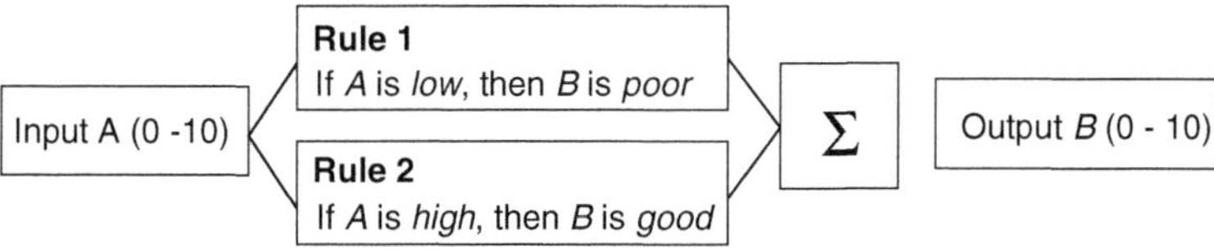

Fig. 2 An illustration of a simple FIS

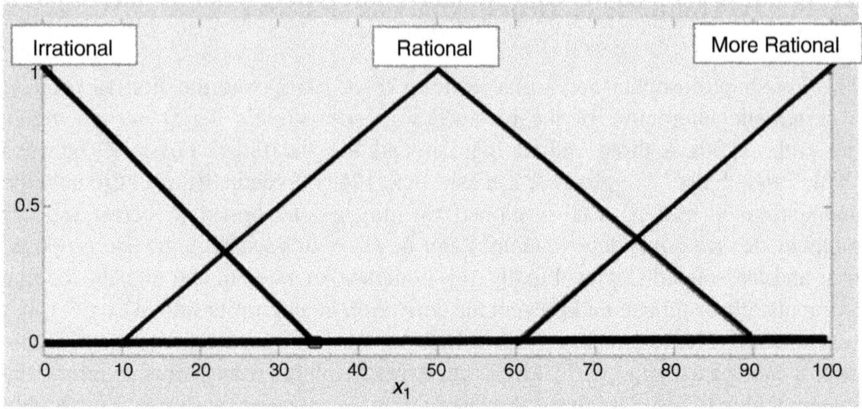

Fig. 3 Triangular Graph of MF of x_1

(a) **Fuzzificating** the input themes. In this step we determine the degree of inputs which they belong to each of the appropriate fuzzy sets via membership functions (MF). Simply, a membership function (MF) is a plot or curve that defines the feature of a fuzzy set by assigning the related membership degree to each element. It depicts each point in the input space to a membership value in interval [0, 1]. There are many membership functions such as Triangular, trapezoidal, Gaussian, Bell-shaped and so on. For example, triangular membership defined as follows. In this equation a, b and c are the parameters of the MF. (Fig. 3)

$$f(x\ ;\ a\ ,\ b\ ,\ c) = \begin{cases} 0 & x \le a \\ \frac{x-a}{b-a} & \le x \le b \\ \frac{c-x}{c-b} & b \le x \le c \\ 0 & C \le x \end{cases}$$

(b) **Using the fuzzy operator in the antecedent**

After the inputs are fuzzified, the degree which each part of the antecedent is satisfied for each rule. If the antecedent of a given rule has more than one part, the fuzzy operator is applied to obtain one number that represents the result of the antecedent for that rule.This number is then applied to the output function. The input to the fuzzy operator is two or more membership values from fuzzified input themes. The output is a single truth value. We used "AND" and probabilistic "OR" operators. The probabilistic "OR" operator is defined as follows:

$$\text{Probor}\ (a, b) = a + b - ab$$

(c) **Implication from the antecedent to the consequent**

Before applying the implication method, every rule is weighted. Every rule has a weight (a number between 0 and 1), which is applied to the number given by the antecedent. In our system, all rules have the same weight and thus have no effect at all on the implication process. After assigning a proper weight to each rule, the implication method is implemented.

(d) **Aggregating the consequents across the rules**

Because decisions are based on the testing of all of the rules in a FIS, the rules must be combined for making a decision. Aggregation is the process by which the fuzzy sets that represent the outputs of each rule are combined into a single fuzzy set.

(e) **Defuzzification**

The input for the defuzzification process is a fuzzy set (the aggregate output fuzzy set) and the output is a single number. We use the Center of Gravity Defuzzification (CoGD) method for the defuzzification.

3 Practical Example

In a qualitative research which has done with us the thematic network was obtained. (Fig. 4)

The thematic network obtained from a thematic analysis is given to at least 20 experts and ask them to assign a score between 0–100 to each themes of the network (Table 1).

We asked the experts to assert the rules which describe the relation among the themes in the best way. The amount of the relationships is asserted based on linguistic themes such as high, low .... We aggregate them using max- operator.

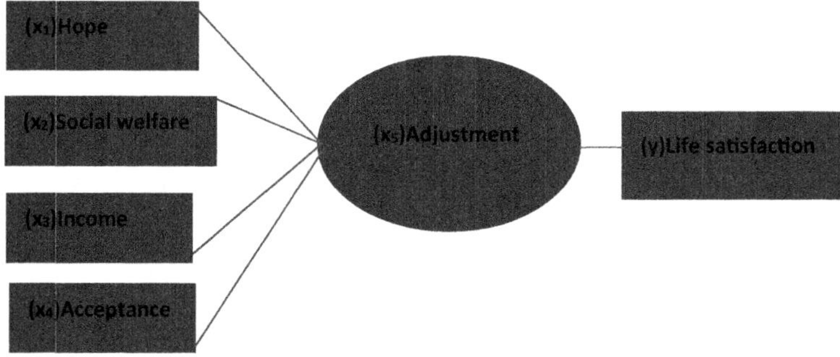

Fig. 4 Thematic network for Life satisfaction

Table 1 The result of the Stage 1

Themes	Mean	SD
Hope	92.68	1.24
Social welfare	91.23	1.63
Income	88.06	2.79
Acceptance	90.27	1.61
Adjustment	88.5	2.08

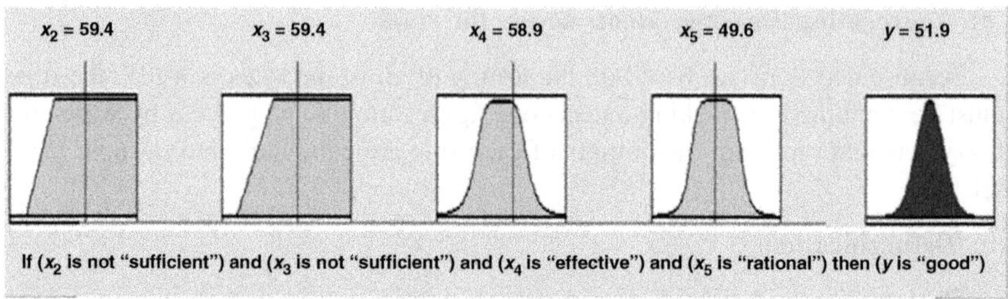
x2 = 59.4
x3 = 59.4
x4 = 58.9
x5 = 49.6
y = 51.9
If (x2 is not "sufficient") and (x3 is not "sufficient") and (x4 is "effective") and (x5 is "rational") then (y is "good")

Fig. 5 The implication process for the IF-THEN rule in the example

Input data are collected from 20 experts who evaluated the thematic network of life satisfaction in 0–100-point scale. Then the weights are determined for the edges by them. All inputs are multiplied by their weights and average values are calculated. We defined five IF-THEN rules for this problem. For example consider this rule:

```
IF social welfare is not "Sufficient" and Income is not
"Sufficient" and Acceptance is "Effective" and Adjustment is
"Rational" THEN Life satisfaction(y) is "Good".
```

The inputs must be fuzzified according to linguistic sets. For example: How effective is "acceptance" in life? If this input is estimated by 60 points in (0–100) scale, the membership degree of the "very effective" linguistic set is 0.4. We use following membership functions for the input data. For each themes we used different membership functions from triangular to Bell-shaped ones. (Fig. 5)

Using the implication process we tested all rules and found the fuzzy output for each of them. Then, we aggregated them for making a combined decision and defuzzification the final result.

We used the Center of Gravity Defuzzification (CoGD) method for the defuzzification. (Figs. 6 and 7)

The crisp value of the aggregated defuzzificated fuzzy output based on fuzzy thematic network analysis is about 52.

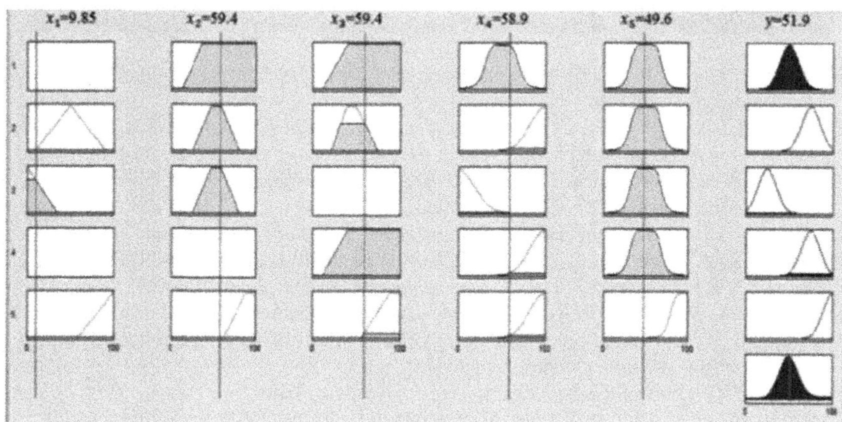

Fig. 6 The aggregation Process for all rules

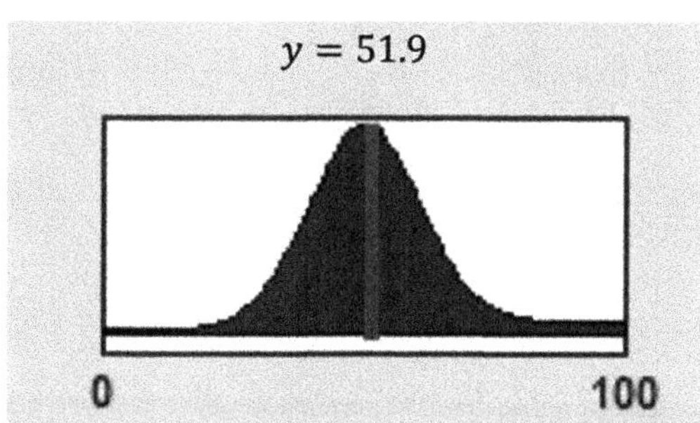

Fig. 7 The defuzzification process

4 Conclusion

Thematic Analysis is a qualitative method. We introduce this method based on the fuzzy theory for providing the rules of the relationships of the themes by interviewing with psychologists having experience in the field. This method is integrating the precision of quantitative methods into the depth of qualitative methods. This integration can be of interest to all psychologists and mind researchers. This paper introduced this new and interesting method and applied a numerical example for testing the degree of accuracy of them using fuzzy set theory. This method can be a turning point in a new methodology which is called it here semi-qualitative methodology.

References

Braun, V., & Clarke, V. (2006). Using thematic analysis in psychology. *Qualitative Research in Psychology, 3*(2), 77–101.

Braun, V., & Clarke, V. (2012). Thematic analysis. In H. Cooper, P. M. Camic, D. L. Long, A. T. Panter, D. Rindskopf, & K. J. Sher (Eds.), *APA handbook of research methods in psychology* (Research designs: Quantitative, qualitative, neuropsychological, and biological) (Vol. 2, pp. 57–71). American Psychological Association.

Bryman, A., & Burgess, R. G. (1994). *Analyzing qualitative data*. Routledge.

Denzin, N. K., & Lincoln, Y. S. (1994). *Handbook of qualitative research*. CA SAGE.

Lejewski, C., & Lukasiewicz, J. (1967). *Encyclopedia of Philosophy, 5*, 104–107.

Mathwork. Fuzzy Inference Process. http://www.mathworks.com

Mamdani, E. H. (1976). Advances in the linguistic synthesis of fuzzy controllers. *International Journal of Man-Machine Studies, 8*, 669–678.

Ross,T. J. (2010). *Fuzzy logic with engineering applications*. Wiley.

Zadeh, L. A. (1973). Outline of a new approach to the analysis of complex systems and decision processes. *IEEE Transactions on Systems, Man, and Cybernetics, 3*(1), 28–44.

Psychometric Models for a New State Science Assessment Aligned to the Next Generation Science Standards

Jing Chen, Jonghwan Lee, Paul Nichols, and M. Christina Schneider

1 Introduction

Unlike traditional unidimensional science standards, the Next Generation Science Standards (NGSS; NGSS Lead States, 2013) emphasize three distinct dimensions: Disciplinary Core Ideas (DCIs), Science and Engineering Practices (SEPs), and Crosscutting Concepts (CCCs). These dimensions are combined to form performance expectations that reflect the inherent complexity in scientific understanding and reasoning. The complexity of the standards and the new task types they require poses significant challenges for psychometric modeling (Gorin & Mislevy, 2013).

The explicit dimensionality in the construct as defined by the NGSS impacts the choice of measurement models for an NGSS assessment. Meanwhile, to measure the NGSS, performance tasks are designed to elicit responses that are more aligned with the targeted reasoning and higher cognitive skills. These tasks often include contextualized and multidimensional items to measure real-world problem-solving skills, which may violate the assumptions of traditional psychometric models (Martineau, 2017). The psychometric challenges introduced by the NGSS require appropriate models to assess the dimensionality and to estimate item and person parameters.

The goal of this study is to identify an appropriate measurement model for an NGSS-aligned state summative science assessment. The assessment was recently created to align to the state's college and career ready standards for science designed around NGSS' three-dimensional science learning. Because of the multidimensional nature of the assessment, the most appropriate measurement model that could be supported by learning theories, capture the patterns within the data, and be

J. Chen (✉) · J. Lee · P. Nichols · M. C. Schneider
NWEA, Portland, OR, USA
e-mail: jing.chen@nwea.org; jay.lee@nwea.org; paul.nichols@nwea.org; christina.schneider@nwea.org

M. Wiberg et al. (eds.), *Quantitative Psychology*, Springer Proceedings in Mathematics & Statistics 353, https://doi.org/10.1007/978-3-030-74772-5_36

feasible to use in an operational setting was investigated. The following sections provide more details about the science assessment and its pilot administration, the dimensionality analyses and results, and a discussion of the findings.

2 Science Pilot Overview

This study was conducted based on data from a pilot test of a new state science assessment administered in Grade 5 and Grade 8 in Spring 2019. The assessment is based on performance tasks, which are phenomena-based scenarios with multiple items to elicit responses that show students' understanding of the DCIs, SEPs, and CCCs. The items are minimally two dimensional. A variety of technology-enhanced item types are used that allow students to show their thinking more fully. For example, the drag-and-drop technology-enhanced item type requires students to drag and drop items into groups. Within each group, students can rank items by dragging and dropping them into place.

Each grade-level pilot test had two test forms (Form A and Form B) that each consisted of two tasks and several items. The two forms at Grade 5 had 11 and 14 items, respectively, and the two forms at Grade 8 had 17 and 18 items, respectively. All items were scored dichotomously. The pilot test was intentionally short to reduce the time students spent away from the classroom.

The student sample for this study was a convenience sample based on schools' availability and willingness to participate. Table 1 presents the total number of students who took the test by grade and form. The student sample's demographic information (including sex and ethnicity) presented in Table 2 suggests that the sample had demographic characteristics similar to the state's general student population at these two grade levels. The differences in percentages between the sample and the general population are all smaller than 5%. In addition, because the two forms at each grade were randomly administered to students within the same school, students were comparable across the forms in terms of their demographics.

Table 1 Pilot sample

	Number of Students		
Grade	Form A	Form B	Total number of students
5	2739	2495	5234
8	3081	2770	5851
Total			11,085

Table 2 Demographic information: Pilot sample vs. general population of the state

		Pilot sample				General population			
		Grade 5		Grade 8		Grade 5		Grade 8	
Demographic variable		N	%	N	%	N	%	N	%
Sex	Female	2351	48.5	2531	48.9	11,789	48.8	11,579	48.9
	Male	2501	51.5	2641	51.1	12,375	51.2	12,117	51.1
Ethn-icity	AIAN[a]	68	1.4	82	1.6	307	1.3	320	1.4
	Asian	144	3.0	111	2.1	664	2.7	638	2.7
	Black	181	3.7	193	3.7	1603	6.6	1654	7.0
	Hispanic	899	18.5	941	18.2	4886	20.2	4660	19.7
	White	3380	69.7	3674	71.0	15,666	64.8	15,513	65.5
	Two or more races	169	3.5	160	3.1	1038	4.3	911	3.8
Total		4841	100.0	5161	100.0	24,164	100.0	23,696	100.0

Note: Around 10% of the students did not have demographic information available and were excluded from Table 2. However, their responses were included in all other analyses
[a]AIAN: American Indian or Alaskan Native

Table 3 Study datasets

	N	Number of tasks	Number of items	Total score points
Grade 5 Form A	2739	2	11	11
Grade 5 Form B	2495	2	14	14
Grade 8 Form A	3081	2	18	18
Grade 8 Form B	2770	2	17	17

3 Dimensionality Analysis

3.1 Description of Four Datasets and Three IRT Models

Four datasets were used in the analyses, one for each form and grade. Table 3 provides the number of students who took the form, the number of tasks and items, and the total score points for each form.

Three IRT models based on content specifications were fit to the data to compare the model fitness and investigate the dimensionality of the assessment: 1) a unidimensional IRT model, 2) a three-dimensional IRT model, and 3) a testlet model. Figure 1 shows a graphic illustration of each model. All the analyses were conducted using the R mirt package (Chalmers, 2012).

3.2 Unidimensional IRT Model (Model 1)

First, unidimensional models were applied to fit the data. Three unidimensional models were examined to determine the best fit: Rasch one-parameter logistic (1PL;

Model 1: Unidimensional IRT Model

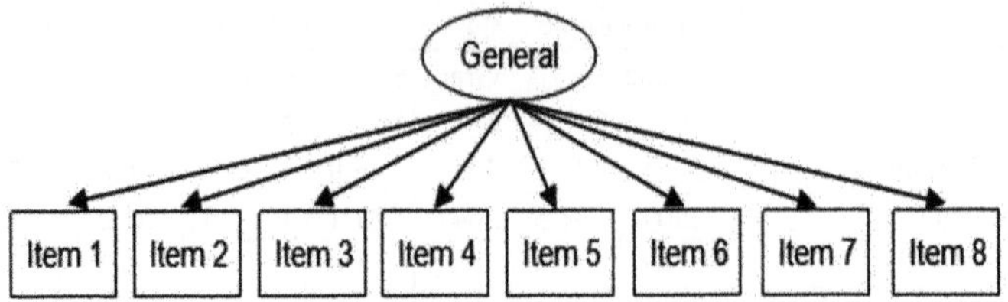

Model 2: Three-Dimensional IRT Model
(SEP, DCI, and CCC)

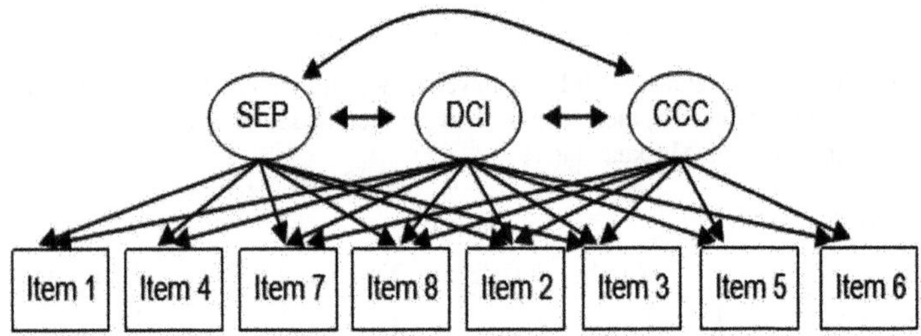

Model 3: Testlet Model
(General, Testlet1, Testlet2)

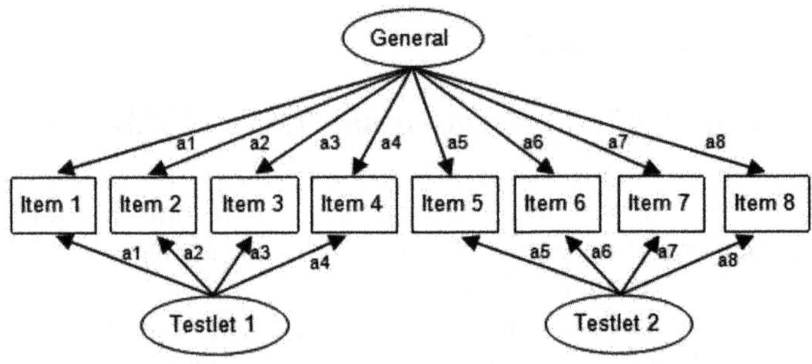

Fig. 1 Graphic illustrations of IRT Models 1, 2, and 3

Rasch, 1960), two-parameter logistic (2PL; Birnbaum, 1968), and three-parameter logistic (3PL; Lord, 1980). The equations for each model are presented below.

$$P\left(U_{ij} = 1|\theta_j, b_i\right) = \frac{e^{\theta_j - b_i}}{1 + e^{\theta_j - b_i}} \quad \text{(1PL)}$$

$$P\left(U_{ij}=1|\theta_j,b_i\right)=\frac{e^{a_i(\theta_j-b_i)}}{1+e^{a_i(\theta_j-b_i)}} \tag{2PL}$$

$$P\left(U_{ij}=1|\theta_j,b_i\right)=c_i+(1-c_i)\frac{e^{a_i(\theta_j-b_i)}}{1+e^{a_i(\theta_j-b_i)}} \tag{3PL}$$

where θ_j, b_i, a_i and c_i are the person, item difficulty, discrimination, and guessing parameters, respectively.

To evaluate model fit, Akaike's Information Criterion (AIC; Akaike, 1973) and the Bayesian Information Criterion (BIC; Schwarz, 1978) were consulted. The better-fitting model is the one with a lower AIC or BIC value. BIC penalizes model complexity more heavily than AIC, which may result in an inconsistent model preference. Table 4 presents the fitting results from the Rasch, 2PL, and 3PL models for each test form. The lowest AIC and BIC values for each dataset are bolded. Though the 3PL model fits the data best for two of the four forms as indicated by the lowest AIC and BIC values, the model has a convergence problem for Grade 8 Form B, and the BIC value indicates that the 2PL model fit better than the 3PL model for the dataset from Grade 5 Form A. Lack of convergence is an indication that the data do not fit the model well because there are too many poorly fitting observations. The 2PL model generally fits much better than the 1PL model. Though it fits the data slightly worse than the 3PL model in some cases, it does not have the same convergence problem as the 3PL model. Thus, a 2PL model was preferred and was selected as Model 1 for the study analyses.

3.3 *Three-Dimensional IRT Model (Model 2)*

Second, a three-dimensional IRT model (Model 2) was applied to fit the data. This model assumes the underlying domains as DCIs, SEPs, and CCCs. This three-

Table 4 Model-fit comparison between unidimensional 1PL, 2PL, and 3PL models

		Form A		Form B	
Grade	Model	AIC	BIC	AIC	BIC
5	Rasch 1PL	23265.85	23337.02	38991.28	39078.74
	2PL	23152.84	**23283.33**	38504.10	38667.36
	3PL	**23136.74**	23332.48	**38327.11**	**38572.01**
8	Rasch 1PL	55042.77	55157.40	51828.75	51935.45
	2PL	53889.39	54106.58	50425.67	50627.22
	3PL	**53341.93**	**53667.72**	NA[a]	NA[a]

Note: The highlighted data indicate the best-fit model
[a]NA indicates that the model did not converge

dimensional model is the multidimensional extension of the 2PL model (Reckase, 2009). The form of the model is given by

$$P\left(U_{ij}=1|\boldsymbol{\theta}_j,\boldsymbol{a}_i,d_i\right)=\frac{e^{\boldsymbol{a}_i\boldsymbol{\theta}'_j+d_i}}{1+e^{\boldsymbol{a}_i\boldsymbol{\theta}'_j+d_i}}$$

where $\boldsymbol{a}$ is a $1\times m$ vector of item discrimination parameters and $\boldsymbol{\theta}$ is a $1\times m$ vector of person coordinates with m indicating the number of dimensions in the coordinate space (i.e., m is 3 in this case). The intercept term, d, is a scalar. The exponent of e in this model can be expanded to show how the elements of the $\boldsymbol{a}$ and $\boldsymbol{\theta}$ vectors interact.

$$\boldsymbol{a}_i\boldsymbol{\theta}'_j+d_i=a_{i1}\theta_{j1}+a_{i2}\theta_{j2}+\cdots+a_{im}\theta_{jm}+d_i$$

The latent traits of this three-dimensional model were set to be correlated because students' abilities in these dimensions are expected to be related to some extent. The empirical results also suggest that the model fits the data better when the latent traits are set to be correlated.

3.4 Testlet Model (Model 3)

A 2PL testlet model (Bradlow et al., 1999) was also applied to fit the data. Because the pilot test was composed of testlet-based items, which may violate the local independence assumption of IRT models, a testlet model was applied to the data to examine the testlet effect. The testlet model assumes a single primary dimension (i.e., general knowledge and abilities in science) and several uncorrelated specific dimensions according to testlets (i.e., tasks) after accounting for the primary dimension. For a testlet model, an item's slope for the specific dimension is constrained to equal the item's slope for the general dimension (Cai, 2010). The 2PL testlet model is given as

$$P_j\left(\theta_i\right)=\frac{1}{1+e^{-a_j\left(\theta_i-b_j-\gamma_{id(j)}\right)'}}$$

where $p_j(\theta_i)$ is the probability of a correct response to item j for examinee i, θ_i is examinee i's latent ability, a_j and b_j are the item discrimination and difficulty parameters, and $\gamma_{id(j)}$ is a person-specific testlet effect that is assumed to follow a distribution $N(0, \sigma^2\gamma id(j))$.

Table 5 Model-fit comparison between Models 1, 2, and 3

			Form A		Form B	
Grade	Model description	Model #	AIC	BIC	AIC	BIC
5	Unidimensional	1	23152.8	23283.3	38504.1	38667.4
	3D (SEP, CCC, DCI)	2	**23074.4**	23317.6	**38206.9**	**38481.0**
	Testlet model	3	23127.6	**23269.9**	38464.3	38639.3
8	Unidimensional	1	53889.4	54106.6	50425.7	50627.2
	3D (SEP, CCC, DCI)	2	**53147.3**	**53521.4**	**49821.7**	**50159.6**
	Testlet model	3	53479.6	53708.8	50399.7	50613.1

3.5 IRT Model-Fit Comparisons

Model fit among Models 1, 2, and 3 was compared. Each model was applied to the four datasets. Table 5 presents the model-fit comparison results for all four datasets. The lowest AIC and BIC statistics are bolded. All the AIC and BIC statistics suggest that Model 2 fits the data best with the exception of the BIC statistics for Grade 5 Form A. Overall, Model 2 (three-dimensional IRT model) provides the best fit across all four datasets.

3.6 Item Fit Statistics

Overall, the three-dimensional IRT model (Model 2) fit the data better than the other two models. To further examine the fitness of the three-dimensional model, the chi-squared-based item-level fit index (S-X^2; Orlando & Thissen, 2000, 2003) was evaluated to see if the model fits the data well at the individual item level. Item fit statistics from the 2PL unidimensional model were used as a baseline for the comparison. The results from the chi-square-based item-level goodness-of-fit tests suggest that more items have bad fit (i.e., p-value <0.05) from the three-dimensional model than from the unidimensional model. For example, four items on Grade 8 Form B showed poor fit to the unidimensional model. However, for the three-dimensional model, these four items and five additional items showed poor model fit. Similar patterns were discovered for the other forms.

All four items that did not fit well to the unidimensional model were technology-enhanced items that required students to enter a short response that is scored as either correct or incorrect. It is possible that students rely on different abilities to respond to these items compared to the abilities measured by the multiple-choice items. A close look of the items by content experts is needed to identify the potential causes of item misfit.

3.7 *Local Dependency Among Items Within a Task*

Although the testlet model fits slightly better than the unidimensional model, the extent to which the local independence assumption is violated was examined using a popular local independence statistic, Yen's Q3 index. Index values greater than 0.20 indicate a degree of local dependence that should be examined by test developers (Chen & Thissen, 1997). Among the 435 item pairs across forms, only two pairs of items had a residual correlation greater than 0.20, suggesting that local item independence generally holds for all forms.

4 Discussion

In general, based on the pilot test data, the model fit statistics suggest that the three-dimensional IRT model that aligns with the DCI, SEP, and CCC dimensions (Model 2) provides slightly better overall fit than the unidimensional model (Model 1) and the testlet model (Model 3). However, the fit of the three-dimensional model at the item level is poor. Another issue to consider for this model is that the NGSS dimensions may not be conceptualized in the same manner that test score dimensionality has been conceptualized, which may create some confusion (Martineau, 2017). The use of the term "dimensionality" in NGSS may be better described as "complex" performance (Dunbar et al., 1991), which involves knowledge and skills across a number of domains or subjects.

Local independence is a fundamental assumption of unidimensional models. Fitting a unidimensional model in the presence of local dependencies may result in biased item parameters and standard errors of measurement (Yen, 1993). The American Institute of Research (AIR) applied a Rasch testlet model (Wang & Wilson, 2005) to calibrate NGSS-aligned science assessments for multiple states (Rijmen, 2018). However, for the new science assessment used in this study, the local independency assumption still generally holds and the testlet model only provides slightly better fit than the unidimensional model.

It is important to note that the data used in this study were collected from a pilot test, so the quality of some items may be low. These items may impact the model fitness results. Students' low motivation for the pilot test may also have affected the quality of the data. The relatively short test length compared to a regular state assessment limited the number of items to be administered for each dimension. All these factors may cause the structure of the pilot data to not strongly resemble the structure of data from operational assessments. It will be worth conducting the dimensionality analysis again using data from the operational test to identify the most appropriate measurement model for the assessment.

Unidimensional IRT models are widely used in testing programs. In contrast, MIRT models are rarely implemented in any state testing program due to its complexity. They require a large sample size to obtain accurate parameter estimates and take a much longer estimation time, which pose challenges in an operational setting. The sample size of an operational test will be much larger than the sample size of this study that used pilot data. Applying a multidimensional model will significantly increase computation time. Implementing MIRT models in operation will likely be a new practice for most vendors working with states. The need for more complex measurement models needs to be further evaluated. Data from the operational test will be collected to further evaluate the need of using MIRT models and examine the robustness of the unidimensional model under various test conditions in future studies.

References

Akaike, H. (1973). Information theory and an extension of the maximum likelihood principle. In B. N. Petrov & F. Caski (Eds.), *Proceedings of the second international symposium on information theory* (pp. 267–281). Akademiai Kiado.

Birnbaum, A. (1968). Some latent trait models and their use in inferring an examinee's ability. In F. M. Lord & M. R. Novick (Eds.), *Statistical theories of mental test scores* (pp. 397–479). Addison-Wesley.

Bradlow, E. T., Wainer, H., & Wang, X. (1999). A Bayesian random effects model for testlets. *Psychometrika, 64*, 153–168.

Cai, L. (2010). A two-tier full-information item factor analysis model with applications. *Psychometrika, 75*, 581–612.

Chalmers, P. R. (2012). mirt: A multidimensional item response theory package for the R environment. *Journal of Statistical Software, 48*(6), 1–29.

Chen, W. H., & Thissen, D. (1997). Local dependence indices from item pairs using item response theory. *Journal of Educational and Behavioral Statistics, 22*, 265–289.

Dunbar, S. B., Koretz, D. M., & Hoover, H. D. (1991). Quality control in the development and use of performance assessments. *Applied Measurement in Education, 4*(4), 289–303.

Gorin, J. S., & Mislevy, R. J. (2013). *Inherent measurement challenges in the Next Generation Science Standards for both formative and summative assessment.* Commissioned paper presented at the K–12 Center at ITS Invitational Research Symposium on Science Assessment, Washington DC.

Lord, F. M. (1980). *Application of item response theory to practical testing problems*. Lawrence Erlbaum Associates.

Martineau, J. (2017). *The intersection of measurement model, equating, and the Next Generation Science Standards*. Center for Assessment. https://www.nciea.org/sites/default/files/inline-files/Martineau_RILS%20-%20Brief%20on%20NGSS%20Measurement%20Models%20and%20Equating%20-%20Final.pdf

NGSS Lead States. (2013). *Next generation science standards: For states, by states*. The National Academic Press. https://www.nextgenscience.org/search-standards

Orlando, M., & Thissen, D. (2000). New item fit indices for dichotomous item response theory models. *Applied Psychological Measurement, 24*, 50–64.

Orlando, M., & Thissen, D. (2003). Further investigation of the performance of S-X^2: An item fit index for use with dichotomous item response theory models. *Applied Psychological Measurement, 27*, 289–298.

Rasch, G. (1960). *Probabilistic models for some intelligence and attainment tests*. Danish Institute for Educational Research (Expanded edition, 1980. University of Chicago Press).

Reckase, M. (2009). *Multidimensional item response theory*. Springer.

Rijmen, F. (2018). *Scoring and reporting for assessments developed for the new science standards*. Paper presented at the National Conference on Student Assessment.

Schwarz, G. (1978). Estimating the dimension of a model. *The Annals of Statistics, 6*, 461–464.

Wang, W. C., & Wilson, M. (2005). The Rasch testlet model. *Applied Psychological Measurement, 29*, 126–149.

Yen, W. M. (1993). Scaling performance assessments: Strategies for managing local item dependence. *Journal of Educational Measurement, 30*(3), 187–213.

Diagnostic Classification Using a Polytomous Measure of Korean Organizational Commitment

Jungwon Rachael R. Ahn and Leah Feuerstahler

1 Introduction

Diagnostic classification models (DCMs; Rupp et al., 2010) use individuals' responses on a series of items to estimate whether individual respondents possess or lack one or more latent attributes. To date, most DCMs have been developed in the context of dichotomous item responses. As such, many applications of DCMs to rating scale data have dichotomized polytomous responses in order to use existing dichotomous DCMs (e.g., Johnson et al., 2013; Su, 2013; cited in Ma & de la Torre, 2016). However, the process of dichotomization leads to a loss of information and may make meaningful interpretations difficult (Chen & de la Torre, 2018). Other DCMs have been developed to directly model polytomous Likert scale data, including the nominal response diagnostic model (NRDM; Templin et al., 2008), the partial-credit DINA model (PC-DINA; de la Torre, 2010), and the sequential DCM (Ma & de la Torre, 2016). However, these polytomous DCMs tend to require large sample sizes to accurately estimate the large number of parameters defined by these models (Liu & Jiang, 2020).

1.1 Recent Polytomous DCMs

Recently, several DCMs for polytomous responses have been proposed that apply different modeling processes and estimation methods (Chen & de la Torre, 2018; Culpepper, 2019; Liu & Jiang, 2018, 2020). Chen and de la Torre's general polytomous diagnosis model (GPDM) was developed by combining a general

J. R. Ahn (✉) · L. Feuerstahler
Fordham University, Bronx, NY, USA
e-mail: jahn20@fordham.edu; lfeuerstahler@fordham.edu

M. Wiberg et al. (eds.), *Quantitative Psychology*, Springer Proceedings
in Mathematics & Statistics 353, https://doi.org/10.1007/978-3-030-74772-5_37

DCM model for dichotomous responses with an item-splitting process similar to the graded response model (Samejima, 1969). Culpepper (2019) proposed an exploratory diagnostic model (DM) for ordinal data that does not require a pre-defined latent structure. Culpepper's exploratory DM extends Chen and de la Torre's confirmatory GPDM to the exploratory setting, using a cumulative probit link and Bayesian variable selection techniques to estimate the latent structure. Liu and Jiang (2018) developed the ordinal response diagnostic model (ORDM) and the modified ORDM (MORDM) by applying constraints to the NRDM (Templin et al., 2008). The ORDM constrains the NRDM by specifying an overall main effect parameter for each item that is shared across the item's response options. The MORDM applies further constraints to the intercept parameters of the ORDM, forcing the same set of the intercept parameters for each response option to be shared across items within the same trait. Lastly, Liu and Jiang (2020) proposed the rating scale diagnostic model (RSDM) which further modifies the MORDM by constraining both the intercept and main effect parameters for each response option to be shared across items within the same trait. Liu and Jiang used Bayesian estimation with a variant of Markov chain Monte Carlo (MCMC) estimation in stan (Carpenter et al., 2017) to estimate parameters for all the three models. They concluded that all the models performed as well as the traditional NRDM but with fewer parameters.

The present study examines the usefulness of the MORDM in modeling responses to a survey of organizational commitment in Korean workers. The application of the model to another ordinal dataset with similar properties to Liu and Jiang's study (e.g., latent structure, number of items, sample size) contributes to evaluating the usefulness of the model.

2 MORDM

The MORDM defines the probability of an individual in latent class c selecting response option m, $m = 0, \ldots, M - 1$, on item i as follows:

$$P\left(X_i = m \mid \alpha_c\right) = \frac{\exp \sum_{l=0}^{m} \left[\lambda_{0,i} + \sum_{v=1}^{V} \lambda_{0,l_v} w_{iv} + \lambda_i^T \mathrm{h}\ (\alpha_c, q_i) \right]}{\sum_{s}^{M-1} \exp \sum_{l=0}^{s} \left[\lambda_{0,i} + \sum_{v=1}^{V} \lambda_{0,l_v} w_{iv} + \lambda_i^T \mathrm{h}\ (\alpha_c, q_i) \right]}$$

where M is the number of response options, $\alpha_c = \{\alpha_1, \ldots, \alpha_k\}$ is the attribute profile for class c, and k is the total number of attributes. In addition, $\lambda_{0,\,i}$ is an item intercept parameter, w_{iv} is an indicator variable of whether item i measures attribute combination v, and λ_{0,m_v} are step parameters for each response option that are shared across all items that measure attribute set v. Finally, the term $\lambda_i^T \mathrm{h}\ (\alpha_c, q_i)$ adds a parameter for each unique attribute and combination of attributes required by item i. Specifically, a parameter is included in the expression only if the item requires that (combination of) attribute(s) and the examinee possesses that (combination of) attribute(s).

The MORDM is a divide-by-total model that takes a function of the sum of terms corresponding to a certain response option over the sum of these expressions over all response options. Compared to the NRDM, the MORDM reduces the number of parameters drastically by constraining step parameters to be shared within each attribute set and by requiring the overall main effect parameter to be shared across response options in each item. For example, for the data analyzed in this study, the NRDM requires 80 item parameters, whereas the MORDM requires only 24 item parameters, reducing the number of parameters by 70%.

3 Analysis of Data

The data used in this study reflect organizational commitment (OC) in Korean bank employees and were originally analyzed by Ahn and Lee (2018). Ahn and Lee conceptualized and validated the construct of OC reflecting organizational culture in Korea, addressing the problems of the three-component model of OC (Allen & Meyer, 1990) commonly used in organizational research. The data analyzed in the current study are a subset of Ahn and Lee's data and include eight items from 519 individuals, of which four questions ask about employees' affective commitment (AC; Ahn & Lee, 2018) and four other questions ask about continuance commitment (CC; Allen & Meyer, 1990). Each item was validated to measure the intended attribute with item complexity equal to one (Ahn & Lee, 2018). AC measures employees' loyalty to their organizations in terms of a positive emotional bond to the organizations, whereas CC measures "maintaining employment", that is, organizational commitment motivated by considering the costs that might be accrued by turnover rather than a mindset of commitment. All the items allowed responses of 1 (*Strongly Disagree*) through 5 (*Strongly Agree*). Table 1 presents the item-attribute relationship and frequencies of each response option. Overall, the response data is negatively skewed with most responses occurring in the highest two categories.

3.1 Specification of the MORDM

Based on Table 1, each item represents only one attribute, either AC or CC. Therefore, the fitted model does not require any terms corresponding to higher-order interactions. In this case, the MORDM simplifies to the following form:

$$P\left(X_i = m|\alpha_c\right) = \frac{\exp\sum_{l=0}^{m}\left[\lambda_{0,i} + \lambda_{0,l_v}w_{iv} + \lambda_{1,i}\text{h}\ (\alpha_c, q_i)\right]}{\sum_{s}^{M-1}\exp\ \sum_{l=0}^{s}\left[\lambda_{0,i} + \lambda_{0,l_v}w_{iv} + \lambda_{1,i}\text{h}\ (\alpha_c, q_i)\right]},$$

Table 1 Item text and descriptive statistics

Translated items		Attribute	Strongly disagree		Disagree		Neutral		Agree		Strongly agree	
1	I am happy being a member of this organization	AC	4	(0.8%)	14	(2.7%)	80	(15.4%)	249	(48.0%)	172	(33.1%)
2	This organization has a great deal of personal meaning for me	AC	2	(0.4%)	14	(2.7%)	69	(13.3%)	210	(40.5%)	224	(43.2%)
3	My organization deserves my loyalty because of its treatment toward me	AC	2	(0.4%)	29	(5.6%)	108	(20.8%)	253	(48.8%)	127	(24.5%)
4	This organization has a mission that I believe in and am committed to	AC	5	(1.0%)	24	(4.6%)	132	(25.4%)	258	(49.7%)	100	(19.3%)
5	If I decide to quit the company, much of my life will be difficult	CC	9	(1.7%)	57	(11.0%)	129	(24.9%)	178	(34.3%)	146	(28.1%)
6	If I quit the company right now, great economic difficulties will come	CC	14	(2.7%)	45	(8.7%)	110	(21.2%)	141	(27.2%)	209	(40.3%)
7	If I leave the company, I have few other options	CC	26	(5.0%)	107	(20.6%)	152	(29.3%)	154	(29.7%)	80	(15.4%)
8	One of the serious consequences of my leaving the company is that there won't be many places to go	CC	28	(5.4%)	73	(14.1%)	113	(21.8%)	175	(33.7%)	130	(25.1%)

where v represent an attribute and h (α_c, q_i) equals one if an examinee possesses the attribute and zero otherwise. Therefore, fitting this model requires only 24 item parameters: eight item intercepts $\lambda_{0,\,i}$, eight item main effect parameters $\lambda_{1,\,i}$, and four step parameters λ_{0,m_v} for each of the two attributes.

3.2 *Fitting the Model*

Following Liu and Jiang's procedure, a two-dimensional MORDM was specified with the stan software (Carpenter et al., 2017) using the default algorithm. Stan is open-source software for Bayesian analysis using a variant of MCMC sampling of the joint posterior distribution (Gelman et al., 2015). The priors were set to $N(0, 20)$ for each item parameter, and *Dirichlet*(2) for each of the four attribute profiles (i.e., combinations of possessing/lacking AC and CC). Four chains of 3000 iterations per chain were run with random starting values, generating 6000 posterior samples after discarding the first 1500 for burn-in for each chain. Parameter estimates and standard errors were obtained as the mean and standard deviation of the 6000 posterior samples for each parameter. To assess the convergence of parameters, the $\hat{R}$ statistic (Gelman & Rubin, 1992) was used. $\hat{R} < 1.1$ suggests that all chains are approximating the same posterior distribution regardless of the initial arbitrary starting values of the chains. However, $\hat{R} < 1.1$ for every item parameter is not a sufficient condition for inferring convergence (Gelman, 1996). If the posterior samples are highly autocorrelated within a chain (as typically they are), this can lead to slower exploration of the posterior distribution, indicating the need for additional posterior samples (Geyer, 2011). Therefore, the effective number of samples, n_{eff}, for each parameter was also examined. The ratio n_{eff}/S was used to gauge the extent of autocorrelation, where S indicates the number of posterior samples. Values of n_{eff}/S greater than 0.1 imply negligible autocorrelations among samples (Gelman et al., 2013, Sec 11.5).

Model fit was assessed in terms of the root mean square error of approximation (RMSEA) item fit (Robitzsch et al., 2020) and posterior prediction model checking (PPMC; Guttman, 1967). Liu and Jiang did not discuss or apply any item fit measures to the MORDM and few papers have evaluated the performance of item fit statistics in the context of polytomous DCMs. Thus, RMSEA item fit and PPMC were used to evaluate item fit in this study. The former is commonly used to evaluate item fit in DCMs for dichotomized or non-ordered polytomous data (Kunina-Habenicht et al., 2009), and the latter is commonly used to evaluate the fit of Bayesian models. All analyses were conducted in R.

3.3 *RMSEA Item-Fit*

For item i, RMSEA item fit is calculated as follows (Robitzsch et al., 2020):

$$\mathrm{RMSEA}_i = \sqrt{\sum_m \sum_c \pi\left(\theta_c\right)\left(P_i\left(\theta_c\right) - \frac{n_{imc}}{N_{ic}}\right)^2}$$

where $\pi(\theta_c)$ is the estimated proportion of examinees with attribute combination θ_c, n_{imc} is the expected number of respondents with attribute combination θ_c responding in category m to item i, N_{ic} is the total expected number of examinees with attribute combination θ_c responding to item i, and all other notation is as previously defined. In words, the RMSEA compares the observed and model-predicted item response frequencies, weighted by the proportion of respondents in each latent class. To calculate the RMSEA, maximum a priori (MAP) estimates of the attribute profile for each examinee were calculated based on the posterior mean of item parameter estimates and observed data. It has been suggested that RMSEA < .05 indicates good fit, RMSEA < .10 indicates moderate fit, and RMSEA > .10 indicates poor fit (Kunina-Habenicht et al., 2009).

3.4 Posterior Prediction Model Checking

In the present study, posterior predictive modeling checking (PPMC) was used to further evaluate RMSEA item fit for the observed data. We evaluated the degree of plausibility for each item's RMSEA under perfect model fit by simulating the model-based *posterior predictive distribution* for each item's RMSEA. For this, 6000 new data sets (y^{rep}, ω^s) were simulated based on the 6000 draws from the posterior distribution of the fitted model $P(\omega^s \mid y)$, where ω^s represents parameter estimates from draw s, $s = 1, \ldots, 6000$, of the posterior distribution. Then, from each ω^s and corresponding (y^{rep}, ω^s), MAP estimates of individuals' latent classes and the corresponding item fit RMSEAs were estimated to construct a *posterior predictive distribution* of the RMSEA for each item. This process resulted in 6000 new draws from the joint posterior distribution $P(y^{rep}, \omega^s|y)$. Lastly, a posterior predictive p-value (PPP), a tail posterior probability of an item's replicated RMSEA distribution from the model, was obtained by its comparison with the observed item's RMSEA from the data. The PPP, a Bayesian p-value, is different than a classical p-value in that it is properly used as a diagnostic rather than as part of a formal test, and can be calculated as follows:

$$\mathrm{PPP}_i = P\left(\mathrm{RMSEA}_i\left(y^{rep}, \omega^s\right) \geq \mathrm{RMSEA}_i\left(\mathrm{y}, \omega\right)\right).$$

PPP values will be clustered around .5 under perfect model fit, and values close to 0 or 1 indicate misfit (Sinharay, 2003).

4 Results

The MCMC algorithm resulted in 6000 draws from the posterior distribution for each parameter. The model converged as the highest $\hat{R}$ equaled 1.004 (<1.1), and all n_{eff}/S ratios were > 0.1 indicating negligible autocorrelations among samples.

4.1 Item Parameters

In total, 28 item parameters were estimated under the MORDM, including 24 item parameters and four class probabilities corresponding to the four combinations of possessing or not possessing AC and CC. Out of 519 bank employees, 83 (16%) were classified as having neither commitment, 138 (27%) as possessing AC only, 44 (8.5%) as possessing CC only, and 254 (49%) as possessing both types of commitments. In other words, the model estimated that 76% of respondents possess AC, whereas only 8.5% possess CC only, a smaller proportion than that proportion estimated to have neither commitment. The estimated distribution of attribute profiles is consistent with the results of Ahn and Lee's study. In particular, Ahn and Lee found that the concept of CC is difficult to establish as an aspect of organizational commitment in Korean organizational culture, where unity and loyalty toward groups are emphasized. Table 2 presents the item parameter estimates and associated standard errors for this fitted model.

Items with larger $\lambda_{0,i}$ values imply that individuals lacking the requisite attribute will have an increased probability of endorsing a higher response option than items with smaller $\lambda_{0,i}$ values. Items with larger $\lambda_{1,i,}$ values imply greater differences in the probability of a response in each category for individuals possessing versus lacking the requisite attribute. Note that the item step parameters $\lambda_{0,m}$ are shared across items that measure the same attribute.

Table 2 Item parameter estimates and standard errors

Items	$\lambda_{0,i}$ *(SE)*	$\lambda_{0,m=1}$ *(SE)*	$\lambda'_{0,m=2}$ *(SE)*	$\lambda'_{0,m=3}$ *(SE)*	$\lambda'_{0,m=4}$ *(SE)*	$\lambda_{1,i}$ *(SE)*
1	8.90 (0.15)	−6.40 (0.15)	−0.01 (0.00)	−0.26 (0.00)	−2.78 (0.00)	2.64 (0.00)
2	9.73 (0.15)	*	*	*	*	3.10 (0.00)
3	9.73 (0.15)	*	*	*	*	2.15 (0.00)
4	8.67 (0.15)	*	*	*	*	1.83 (0.00)
5	9.02 (0.16)	−6.76 (0.16)	−0.02 (0.00)	−0.58 (0.00)	−1.85 (0.00)	2.04 (0.00)
6	8.52 (0.16)	*	*	*	*	2.61 (0.00)
7	7.89 (0.16)	*	*	*	*	1.31 (0.00)
8	7.76 (0.16)	*	*	*	*	1.76 (0.00)

Note. $\lambda_{0,i,}$: intercept parameters, λ': step parameters, $\lambda_{1,i}$: main effect parameters. "*" indicates that the item shares the same values of the step parameters with the cell above it

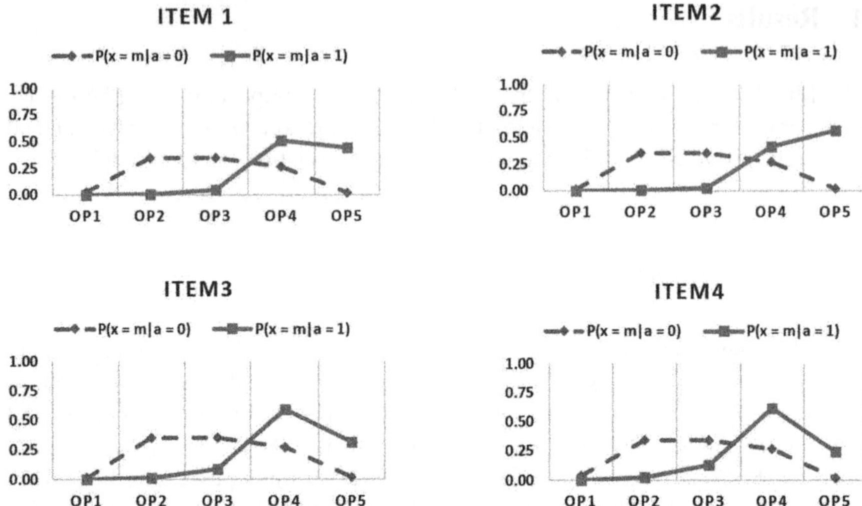

Fig. 1 Response option curves for AC items

Figures 1 and 2 present the estimated probability of a response in each category for all eight items. In each plot, the lines with squares represent the probability that an individual with the requisite attribute will select each response option, and the lines with diamonds represent these probabilities for that an individual lacking the requisite attribute. Overall, the plots suggest that individuals with the requisite attribute are highly likely to endorse the *Agree* or *Strongly Agree* categories, whereas the category probabilities are more spread out for individuals lacking the requisite attribute.

4.2 Fit Indices

The RMSEAs and PPP values are displayed in Table 3. Item fit RMSEAs were calculated based on MAP estimates of each individual's latent class. According to the previously stated cutoffs, seven items showed poor fit, and only item 8 showed moderate fit. These results suggest that the MORDM does not adequately represent the response process underlying these data. The PPMC results reinforced this conclusion as the PPP values for the first seven items equaled 0. Item 8 had a PPP value of 0.08, which is closer to zero than is typically recommended (Sinharay, 2003).

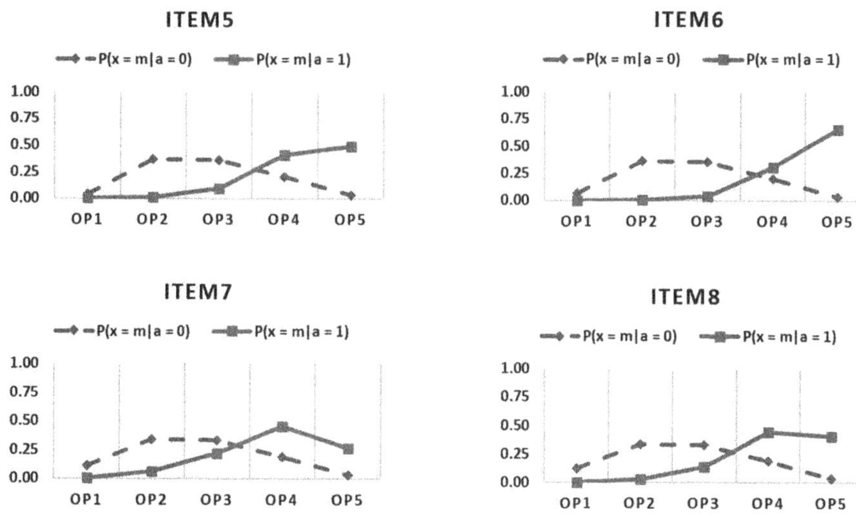

Fig. 2 Response option curves for CC items

Table 3 RMSEA item fit indices and PPP values

	Item1	Item2	Item3	Item4	Item5	Item6	Item7	Item8
RMSEA	0.18	0.17	0.14	0.15	0.14	0.15	0.12	0.09
PPP	0.00	0.00	0.00	0.00	0.00	0.00	0.00	0.08

5 Discussion

This study applied the newly developed MORDM to data reflecting organizational commitment in Korean bank employees and evaluated model-data fit with the RMSEA (Robitzsch et al., 2020) and PPMC (Guttman, 1967) measures. Although the MORDM led to reasonable parameter estimates and a plausible attribute profile distribution, both types of fit indices indicated poor model-data fit. Although these results suggest that the MORDM is not appropriate for these data, they also highlight several avenues for future research.

One interpretation of these results is that the MORDM may not be flexible enough to adequately describe these data. Namely, the simplifying assumptions made by the MORDM may not be realistic for these data. For example, it may be that models which freely estimate different main effects for each step parameter (Liu & Jiang, 2020) are more appropriate for these data. Not only this, but other model modifications may also lead to a better representation of the response process. Based on the distribution of data in Table 1, it may be appropriate to collapse the lowest two response categories. Particularly for the items measuring AC, the first response category (*Strongly disagree*) was endorsed in less than 1% of respondents, and there may not be enough information in these data to meaningfully distinguish between the *Strongly disagree* and *Disagree* responses. Finally, it may be that dichotomous latent attributes are inadequate to describe the latent structure of these data. Models with more than two latent classes per attribute or models with continuous latent traits may be necessary to describe the underlying response processes. Although this study did not compare the MORDM to any alternative models, this is a natural next step in understanding the structure of these data.

Another interpretation of these results is that the fit indices are not performing as expected for this model. For instance, the RMSEA may be overly sensitive to small deviations of fit in the model and may signal misfit even when deviations from perfect fit are inconsequential. One clear limitation of the RMSEA fit statistic is that it uses point estimates of the latent class attributes. Although the PPMC of the RMSEA better accounts for the variability in latent class probabilities, it still relies on point estimates of the latent classes for each iteration. A thorough evaluation of fit indices applied to DCMs for ordered polytomous data would improve the usefulness of these models for applied researchers.

One major limitation of the current study is that it applies only one model to one data set. However, the challenges encountered in modeling these data suggest directions for future research on DCMs using both real and simulated data. One future direction is to develop more computationally efficient estimation methods to fit these models. Although MCMC is a flexible estimation method, it is computationally intensive and may be impractical when working with larger data sets (Huo & de la Torre, 2014). The application of faster estimation methods such as the EM algorithm may make these models more accessible to applied researchers. In addition, more research is needed to evaluate which DCMs for ordered polytomous responses best balance model flexibility with model parsimony. As new DCMs are developed, we encourage researchers to simultaneously evaluate the appropriateness of fit indices for these models.

References

Ahn, J., & Lee, S. (2018). Conceptualization and validation of organizational commitment: Focused on full time workers of domestic banks in Korea. *Korean Journal of Industrial and Organizational Psychology, 31*(2), 459–497.

Allen, N. J., & Meyer, J. P. (1990). The measurement and antecedents of affective, continuance and normative commitment to the organization. *Journal of Occupational Psychology, 63*(1), 1–18.

Carpenter, B., Gelman, A., Hoffman, M. D., Lee, D., Goodrich, B., Betancourt, M., ... Riddell, A. (2017). Stan: A probabilistic programming language. *Journal of Statistical Software, 76*(1).

Chen, J., & de la Torre, J. (2018). Introducing the general polytomous diagnosis modeling framework. *Frontiers in Psychology, 9*, 1474.

Culpepper, S. A. (2019). An exploratory diagnostic model for ordinal responses with binary attributes: Identifiability and estimation. *Psychometrika, 84*(4), 921–940.

de la Torre, J. (2010, July). *The partial-credit DINA model.* Paper presented at the international meeting of the Psychometric Society, Athens, GA.

Gelman, A. (1996). Inference and monitoring convergence. *Markov Chain Monte Carlo in Practice*, 131–143.

Gelman, A., Carlin, J. B., Stern, H. S., Dunson, D. B., Vehtari, A., & Rubin, D. B. (2013). *Bayesian data analysis*. CRC Press.

Gelman, A., Lee, D., & Guo, J. (2015). Stan: A probabilistic programming language for Bayesian inference and optimization. *Journal of Educational and Behavioral Statistics, 40*(5), 530–543.

Gelman, A., & Rubin, D. B. (1992). Inference from iterative simulation using multiple sequences. *Statistical Science, 7*(4), 457–472.

Geyer, C. J. (2011). Introduction to Markov Chain Monte Carlo. In S. Brooks, A. Gelman, G. L. Jones, & X.-L. Meng (Eds.), *Handbook of Markov Chain Monte Carlo* (pp. 3–48). Chapman; Hall/CRC.

Guttman, I. (1967). The use of the concept of a future observation in goodness-of-fit problems. *Journal of the Royal Statistical Society: Series B (Methodological), 29*(1), 83–100.

Huo, Y., & de la Torre, J. (2014). Estimating a cognitive diagnostic model for multiple strategies via the EM algorithm. *Applied Psychological Measurement, 38*(6), 464–485.

Johnson, M., Lee, Y.-S., Sachdeva, R. J., Zhang, J., Waldman, M., & Park, J. Y. (2013, April). *Examination of gender differences using the multiple groups DINA model.* Paper presented at the annual meeting of the National Council on Measurement in Education, San Francisco, CA.

Kunina-Habenicht, O., Rupp, A. A., & Wilhelm, O. (2009). A practical illustration of multidimensional diagnostic skills profiling: Comparing results from confirmatory factor analysis and diagnostic classification models. *Studies in Educational Evaluation, 35*(2–3), 64–70.

Liu, R., & Jiang, Z. (2018). Diagnostic classification models for ordinal item responses. *Frontiers in Psychology, 9*, 2512.

Liu, R., & Jiang, Z. (2020). A general diagnostic classification model for rating scales. *Behavior Research Methods, 52*(1), 422–439.

Ma, W., & de la Torre, J. (2016). A sequential cognitive diagnosis model for polytomous responses. *British Journal of Mathematical and Statistical Psychology, 69*(3), 253–275.

Robitzsch, A., Kiefer, T., George, A. C., & Uenlue, A. (2020). CDM: Cognitive diagnosis modeling (R package version 7.5-15). Retrieved from https://CRAN.R-project.org/package=CDM

Rupp, A. A., Templin, J. L., & Henson, R. A. (2010). *Diagnostic measurement: Theory, methods, and applications*. Guilford Press.

Samejima, F. (1969). *Estimation of latent ability using a response pattern of graded scores* (Psychometrika Monograph No.17). Psychometric Society.

Sinharay, S. (2003). Practical applications of posterior predictive model checking for assessing fit of common item response theory models. *ETS Research Report Series, 2003*(2), i-38.

Su, Y.-L. (2013). *Cognitive diagnostic analysis using hierarchically structured skills.* Unpublished doctoral dissertation, University of Iowa.

Templin, J., Henson, R. A., Rupp, A. A., Jang, E., & Ahmed, M. (2008, March). *Cognitive diagnosis models for nominal response data.* Paper presented at the annual meeting of the National Council on Measurement in Education, New York, NY.

An Empirical Study of Developing Automated Scoring Engine Using Supervised Latent Dirichlet Allocation

Jiawei Xiong, Jordan M. Wheeler, Hye-Jeong Choi, Juyeon Lee, and Allan S. Cohen

1 Introduction

1.1 Constructed Response Items and Its Scoring

Each item in an educational test has its well-designed purpose such as assessing an examinee's reading skills, inference abilities, or writing efficiencies. Constructed response (CR) items are believed to be more effective than multiple choice items in measurement (Chan & Kennedy, 2002; Nickerson, 1989) and have been applied across various areas in both high- and low-stakes assessments. Constructed responses may be scored by human raters or through an automated essay scoring algorithm. Conventional human rater scoring typically requires a rubric that clearly defines scoring procedures to maximize the reliability and ensure the validity and fairness of the final scores (Hogan & Murphy, 2007). Sometimes, several groups of raters are involved to avoid individual scoring bias. The ratings from different raters, however, could be subjective due to the variation and discrepancies in rater training from one testing time to another (Ercikan et al., 1998). To minimize the differences between individual raters, this process usually requires high quality rater training and monitoring of the score accuracy. Consequently, the associated time and expense involved in the scoring process are two of the primary problems in human scoring.

Compared with human raters, the automated essay scoring algorithms have attracted many researchers due to its stable scoring results and economical property. Accuracy and reliability of automated scores for writing assessments have been found to have high agreement with human raters (Attali, 2004; Landauer, Laham,

J. Xiong (✉) · J. M. Wheeler · H.-J. Choi · J. Lee · A. S. Cohen
University of Georgia, Athens, GA, USA
e-mail: jiawei.xiong@uga.edu

M. Wiberg et al. (eds.), *Quantitative Psychology*, Springer Proceedings in Mathematics & Statistics 353, https://doi.org/10.1007/978-3-030-74772-5_38

Rehder, & Schreiner, 1997; Nichols, 2004; Sebrechts, Bennett, & Rock, 1991). Traditional automated essay scoring algorithms depend on carefully designed linguistic features of the response content to evaluate the composition (Dzikovska, Nielsen, & Brew, 2012; Livingston, 2009). Although they make reliable scores in application, some of the statistical latent semantic features in the responses may not be well recognized by the scoring algorithms and therefore cannot replace human raters in its current rubric design (Dikli, 2006; Liu et al., 2014).

1.2 Topic Models and Supervised Latent Dirichlet Allocation

Topic models provide a tool for mining textual data in an effort to detect the latent semantic structures. Topic modeling approaches based on Latent Dirichlet Allocation (Blei, Ng, & Jordan, 2003) were originally established to evaluate the text of large corpora.

The supervised Latent Dirichlet Allocation (sLDA; Mcauliffe & Blei, 2008) model is commonly used in text analysis. It includes a dependent variable as the supervisor for the topic modeling. In the context of analyzing constructed responses, a variable such as the rubric-based scores of examinees' answers can be used for the supervisor. As an example, sLDA has been used for detecting the latent topic structure from a corpus of CR answers on two social study tests (Xiong, Choi, Kim, Kwak, & Cohen, 2019).

This study uses sLDA as a statistical model to detect the latent semantic structure of empirical data from an English and Language Arts assessment. Different n-grams were used as tokens to build distinct sLDA models. Response length was used as additional covariate to the topic proportions in the final sLDA model. Finally, a comparison and discussion is presented among the performance of the models.

2 Methods

2.1 Supervised Latent Dirichlet Allocation

Parameter Estimation. sLDA is different from the unsupervised LDA model in that it jointly models the text with the associated supervisor label to estimate appropriate latent topics which can predict the label for future documents. The label could be various response types such as real values or ordered class.

Suppose there are K topics $\beta_{1:K}$ in the documents. With the Dirichlet parameter α, response parameter η and σ^2, the sLDA model generalizes the document and response label in the following steps (Mcauliffe & Blei, 2008):

1. The topic proportions $\theta|\alpha$ are drawn from $Dir(\alpha)$.
2. The topic assignments $z_n|\theta$ are drawn from $Mult(\theta)$.
3. The word $w_n|z_n$ is drawn from each topic z_n, where $\beta_{1:K}$ follows $Mult(\beta_{z_n})$.
4. The response variable $y|z_{1:N}, \eta, \sigma^2$ is then drawn from $N(\eta'\bar{z}, \sigma^2)$.

where the $\bar{z}$ here is defined as $\frac{1}{N}\sum_{n=1}^{N} z_n$.

The response label used in this study has 5 ordered categories and an exponential dispersion link was used. The natural parameter ζ and dispersion parameter σ were used in the canonical link function under the generalized linear model. Therefore, the response variable has the following distribution under the general version of sLDA (Mcauliffe & Blei, 2008).

$$p(y|z_{1:N}, \eta, \delta) = h(y, \delta)exp\{\frac{\eta'(\bar{z}y) - A(\eta'\bar{z})}{\delta}\} \tag{1}$$

where $\eta'\bar{z}$ is the linear predictor and is set to be identical to the parameter ζ; $h(y, \delta)$ is the base measure; y is a sufficient statistic; and $A(\eta'\bar{z})$ is the log-normalizer. A variation expectation-maximization (EM) algorithm from LDA (Blei, Ng, & Jordan, 2003) can be used to estimate sLDA model parameters and yields an expected response given a new document as:

$$E[Y|w_{1:N}, \alpha, \beta_{1:K}, \eta, \delta] \approx E_q[\mu(\eta'\bar{z})] \tag{2}$$

where $\mu(\eta'\bar{z}) = E_{GLM}[Y|\zeta = \eta'\bar{z}]$ follows the exponential family properties.

N-gram models. Different n-grams were used as tokens in building up the various sLDA models. In this study we estimated four sLDA models using four different n-gram sizes, namely, unigram, bigram, trigram, and mixgram models, where the mixgram model used a combination of unigrams and bigrams. Each model's performance was compared over real data. The response length was also included in each of the four models as a covariate. These four grams were evaluated in terms of accuracy to predict the response label in sLDA.

2.2 Data

Description. The data used in this study were written responses from a narrative writing extended response (ER) item in an English American Literature assessment administered to high school examinees (n = 1,273). The human rater scores are used as the supervisor variable for each document. The scores for this item were ordered categorically and summarized in Table 1.

Preparation. Students' responses to the ER item were cleaned and the effective documents were used in the sLDA model. The effective documents are non-empty documents and contain at least 10 words. The data cleaning process includes

Table 1 Extended CR item score categories

	0	1	2	3	4
Count	351	221	273	318	109

Table 2 Descriptive statistics before and after data preparation

	Effective documents	Total words	Unique words
Before preparation	1,070	312,226	11,752
After preparation	1,061	131,659	6,544

removal of non-alphanumeric symbols, switching upper case letters to lower case, stemming of words and removal of stop words. Table 2 shows descriptive statistics for the valid number of words before and after the data cleaning process. The valid number of words drastically declined, however, only 9 effective documents were dropped.

2.3 Evaluation Criteria

Classification Accuracy. The classification accuracy (CA) is used for evaluating classification results in many machine learning classifiers (Kotsiantis, Zaharakis, & Pintelas, 2007). It is defined as the fraction of correct predictions from the model. For a classifier with N classes, a $N \times N$ confusion matrix is created and a CA measure is calculated by:

$$CA = \frac{\sum_i^N \sum_j^N n_{ij(i=j)}}{\sum_i^N \sum_j^N n_{ij}} \tag{3}$$

where the n_{ij} means the counts of the ith row and jth column in the matrix. In this study, the accuracy of the predicted scores by sLDA for the human raters' scores was of primary interest.

Quadratic-Weighted Kappa. The classical Kappa coefficient (Cohen, 1960) has been used to indicate the agreement between two ratings. Landis and Koch (1977) proposed divisions on the Kappa coefficient and verified they are useful by giving the following suggested intervals: poor ($\leq$0.00), slight (0.00–0.20), fair (0.21–0.40), moderate (0.41–0.60), substantial (0.61–0.80), almost perfect (0.81–1.00). The quadratic-weighted kappa (QWK; Fleiss & Cohen, 1973), which varies from 0 (trivial agreement between ratings) to 1 (complete agreement between ratings), was then developed to quantify the amount of agreement among multiple raters. For a given $N \times N$ confusion matrix, the QWK score can be represented as:

$$K_w = \frac{\sum_i \sum_j w_{ij} P_{ij} - \sum_i \sum_j w_{ij} P_{i.} P_{j.}}{1 - \sum_i \sum_j w_{ij} P_{i.} P_{j.}} \quad (4)$$

where $w_{ij} = 1 - \frac{(i-j)^2}{(N-1)^2}$ are the quadratic weights and $P_{i.}$ and $P_{j.}$ are marginal probabilities of the ith row and jth column of the matrix, respectively.

In machine learning, the QWK is typically used to measure the agreement between a human rater's label and an algorithm's prediction on the same observation. This paper adopted a determinant QWK threshold of 0.70 which suggests high human machine score agreement (Williamson, Xi, & Breyer, 2012).

3 Results

3.1 Topic Numbers Selection

One important step in fitting a sLDA model is to determine the number of topics. More topics do not always indicate better model accountability and precision. There are many model selection methods, such as the log-likelihood, deviance information criterion and harmonic mean (Griffiths & Steyvers, 2004; Wallach, Murray, Salakhutdinov, & Mimno, 2009; Xiong et al., 2019). However, there is no standard method of selecting the number of topics in advance. Since the ultimate goal of the sLDA is prediction, this study considered the CA as a measurement criterion of selecting the optimal number of topics.

Figure 1 presents CA results for each condition. It shows the optimal number of topics are not identical across the different n-gram models. The CA selects three topics for the unigram and bigram model, six topics for the trigram model, and five topics for the mixgram model.

3.2 Classification Results

After determining the number of topics, four separate augmented n-gram sLDA models were estimated using the sLDA topic proportions and scaled response length. The response length is the length of an examinee's response after data cleaning. The sample of examinees' responses were split into five folds (i.e., subsets). For each model, four of the five folds were used as the training set and the remaining fold was used as the test set to measure the model's performance. This process was used repeatedly so that each fold was used as the test set once. Figure 2 presents the accuracy and QWK scores from the 5-fold cross validation in the four n-gram augmented models. All models reported improved accuracy when using the response length as a covariate (Fig. 2), although some of them are better than others.

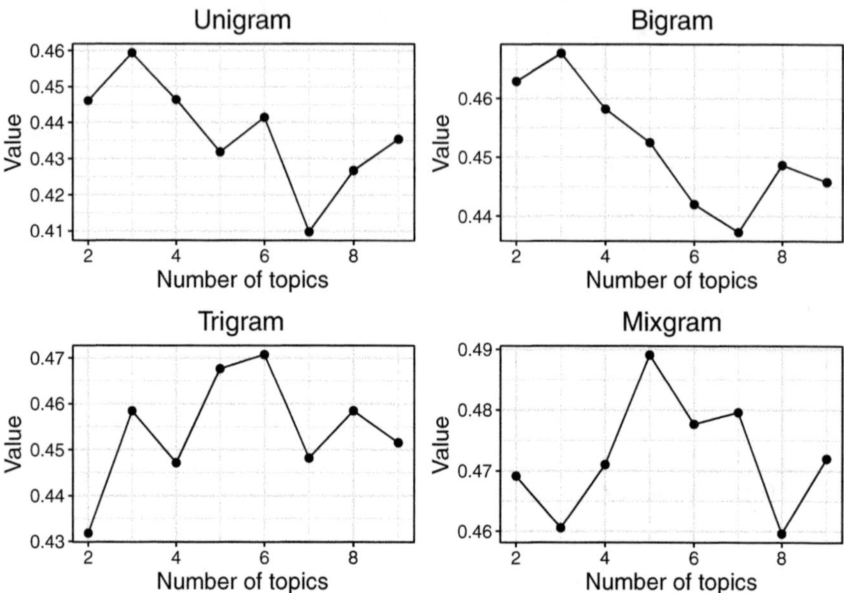

Fig. 1 Classification accuracy given by number of topics under each n-gram condition

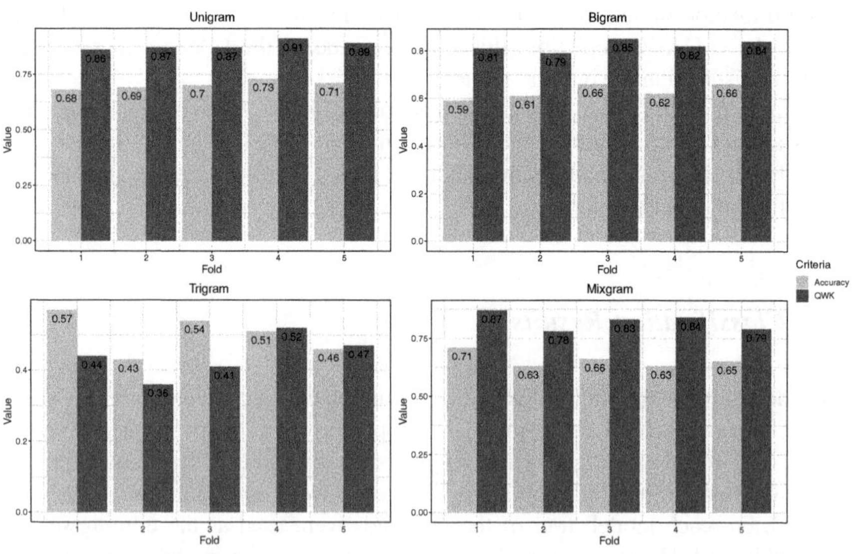

Fig. 2 Different model classification accuracy and QWK scores under optimal topic numbers

Table 3 Average of classification accuracy and quadratic-weighted kappa for different n-grams

Models	Classification accuracy	Quadratic weighted kappa
Unigram	0.702	0.880
Bigram	0.628	0.822
Trigram	0.502	0.440
Mixgram	0.656	0.822

The average CA and QWK scores from the five folds for each of the four models are summarized in the Table 3. The unigram model shows the highest CA and QWK and the trigram model shows the lowest CA and QWK scores. The lower CA and QWK scores from the trigram model indicate that model might be over fitting to the data.

3.3 Unigram Model

The classification accuracy indicated the unigram model was optimal, so the augmented unigram sLDA was fitted to all of the response data. The results from the multi-category sLDA model provided the following logits for each score category:

$$\log\left(\frac{\pi_1}{\pi_0}\right) = -1.49l + 1.98\theta_1 + 0.93\theta_2 - 1.99\theta_3 \tag{5}$$

$$\log\left(\frac{\pi_2}{\pi_0}\right) = 2.19l + 7.09\theta_1 + 3.60\theta_2 - 2.78\theta_3 \tag{6}$$

$$\log\left(\frac{\pi_3}{\pi_0}\right) = 4.99l + 8.73\theta_1 + 3.06\theta_2 - 9.76\theta_3 \tag{7}$$

$$\log\left(\frac{\pi_4}{\pi_0}\right) = 6.53l + 7.92\theta_1 - 1.67\theta_2 - 16.65\theta_3 \tag{8}$$

where $\pi_i (i = 0, 1, 2, 3, 4)$ is the probability of getting score i; l is the scaled valid response length; and $\theta_j (j = 1, 2, 3)$ are the topic proportions for each response. The overall accuracy from the unigram model is 0.69. This means on 69% of all responses, the unigram model agrees with the human rater score. The QWK score is 0.86, which surpasses the 0.70 threshold adopted for this study.

The confusion matrix in Table 4 shows the predictions against the human rater scores for each score category. The cells on the diagonal show the number of cases where the unigram model and human raters are in prefect agreement. We were also interested in the off diagonal cells because it can provide information beyond the model precision, such as categorical sensitivity and specificity. For example, for documents that received a score of 3 by the human rater, the unigram model predicts 240 correctly, which indicates a 76% sensitivity for score 3. The unigram

Table 4 The confusion matrix predicted by the unigram 3-topic sLDA model

	Human rater scores				
Prediction	0	1	2	3	4
0	84	43	3	0	0
1	38	147	23	0	0
2	8	31	197	56	0
3	4	0	50	240	49
4	0	0	0	21	59

Table 5 Top 10 words for each topic for the unigram 3-topic sLDA model

Topic 1		Topic 2		Topic 3	
Clock	0.018	Paint	0.024	Paint	0.064
See	0.016	See	0.021	Art	0.027
Around	0.013	Know	0.014	Surrealist	0.022
Walk	0.010	Think	0.012	World	0.017
Eye	0.009	Wake	0.011	Artist	0.015
Feel	0.009	Ask	0.010	Feel	0.013
Melt	0.008	Start	0.010	Mean	0.012
Begin	0.007	Walk	0.009	Movement	0.010
Myself	0.007	Come	0.008	Time	0.010
Open	0.007	Dream	0.008	Surrealism	0.009

model classifies 49 documents into score 3 when the human-rater score equals 4, so sensitivity for score 4 is only 55% ($\frac{59}{59+49} = 55\%$), which means the unigram model is conservative on assigning high scores to responses.

Examinee's responses can also be reflected from the unigram model topic structures. Table 5 summarizes the top 10 words from each of the three topics in the unigram model. Topic 1 could be identified as a topic related with narrator body movement under the item's scenario, while Topic 2 and Topic 3 could be identified as different art content topics.

4 Discussion and Conclusion

This study proposed an automated scoring engine using the sLDA as the foundation. A critical question in this study was to find the appropriate token dimension to represent the item response. Four different n-gram tokens, namely, unigram, bigram, trigram and mixgram were used to compare model performance. The classification accuracy was used as criterion to select the best number of topics for each sLDA model, and four augmented sLDA models corresponding to n-gram tokens were built.

The results from the empirical data showed that the sLDA with unigram performed best with the highest human-machine score agreement. The models were tested further using the 5-fold cross-validation. Each model incorporated a covariate for the response length, which improved the models' performance. Among these four models, the unigram, bigram and mixgram models yield similar model precision. whereas, the trigram model appeared to over-fit the data due to the complex token dimensions. The unigram sLDA model showed the highest classification accuracy based on a 0.880 QWK score. The overall CA from the unigram model was 0.69. However, the score sensitivity for the perfect scores was not ideal, which suggests the unigram model might be conservative to assign perfect scores.

The sLDA uses a supervisor variable that estimates latent topics to help understand an examinee's writings with relation to the supervisor label. Some problems exist such as the model dimensionality caused by over-complex tokens. Future studies could consider word embedding, hash featuring or suchlike to overcome the problem. The model could be further pruned to yield higher accuracy by adding effective features in the sLDA model as well.

References

Attali, Y. (2004). Exploring the feedback and revision features of Criterion. *Journal of Second Language Writing, 14*, 191–205.

Blei, D. M., Ng, A. Y., & Jordan, M. I. (2003). Latent dirichlet allocation. *Journal of Machine Learning Research, 3*, 993–1022.

Chan, N., & Kenedy, P. E. (2002). Are multiple-choice exams easier for economics students? A comparison of multiple choice and "equivalent" constructed response exam questions. *Southern Economic Journal, 68*(4), 957–971.

Cohen, J. (1960). A coefficient of agreement for nominal scales. *Educational and Psychological Measurement, 20*(1), 37–46.

Dikli, S. (2006). An overview of automated scoring of essays. *The Journal of Technology, Learning, and Assessment, 5*(1), 1–35.

Dzikovska, M. O., Nielsen, R., & Brew, C. (2012). *Towards effective tutorial feedback for explanation questions: A dataset and baselines*. Paper presented at the Proceedings of the 2012 Conference of the North American Chapter of the Association for Computational Linguistics: Human Language Technologies.

Ercikan, K., Sehwarz, R. D., Julian, M. W., Burket, G. R., Weber, M. M., & Link, V. (1998). Calibration and scoring of tests with multiple-choice and constructed-response item types. *Journal of Educational Measurement, 35*(2), 137–154.

Fleiss, J. L., & Cohen, J. (1973). The equivalence of weighted kappa and the intraclass correlation coefficient as measures of reliability. *Educational and Psychological Measurement, 33*(3), 613–619.

Griffiths, T. L., & Steyvers, M. (2004). *Finding scientific topics*. Paper presented at the Proceedings of the National Academy of Sciences.

Hogan, T. P., & Murphy, G. (2007). Recommendations for preparing and scoring constructed-response items: What the experts say. *Applied Measurement in Education, 20*(4), 427–441.

Kotsiantis, S. B., Zaharakis, I., & Pintelas, P. (2007). Supervised machine learning: A review of classification techniques. *Emerging Artificial Intelligence Applications in Computer Engineering, 160*(1), 3–24.

Landauer, T. K., Laham, D., Rehder, B., & Schreiner, M. E. (1997). *How well can passage meaning be derived without using word order? A comparison of Latent Semantic Analysis and humans.* Paper presented at the Proceedings of the 19th Annual Meeting of the Cognitive Science Society.

Landis, J. R., & Koch, G. G. (1977). The measurement of observer agreement for categorical data. *Biometrics, 33*(1), 159–174.

Liu, O. L., Brew, C., Blackmore, J., Gerard, L., Madhok, J., & Linn, M. C. (2014). Automated scoring of constructed-response science items: Prospects and obstacles. *Educational Measurement: Issues and Practice 33*(2), 19–28.

Livingston, S. A. (2009). Constructed-Response Test Questions: Why We Use Them; How We Score Them. R&D Connections. Number 11. *Educational Testing Service*.

Mcauliffe, J. D., & Blei, D. M. (2008). Supervised topic models. In *Advances in neural information processing systems* (pp. 121–128). Red Hook, NY: Curran Associates, Inc.

Nichols, P. (2004). *Evidence for the interpretation and use of scores from an automated essay scorer.* Paper presented at the Annual Meeting of the American Educational Research Association.

Nickerson, R. S. (1989). New directions in educational assessment. *Educational Researcher, 18*(9), 3–7.

Sebrechts, M. M., Bennett, R. E., & Rock, D. A. (1991). Agreement between expert-system and human raters' scores on complex constructed-response quantitative items. *ETS Research Report Series, 1991*(1), 856–862.

Wallach, H. M., Murray, I., Salakhutdinov, R., & Mimno, D. (2009). *Evaluation methods for topic models.* Paper presented at the Proceedings of the 26th Annual International Conference on Machine Learning.

Williamson, D. M., Xi, X., & Breyer, F. J. (2012). A framework for evaluation and use of automated scoring. *Educational Measurement: Issues and Practice, 31*(1), 2–13.

Xiong, J., Choi, H.-J., Kim, S., Kwak, M., & Cohen, A. S. (2019). *Topic modeling of constructed-response answers on social study assessments.* Paper presented at the The Annual Meeting of the Psychometric Society.

Where the Choice of Model Leads Us: An Empirical Comparison of Dyadic Data Analysis Frameworks

Hanna Kim and Jee-Seon Kim

1 Introduction

Dyads refer to small groups of two members each, where the persons share the same environment and actively interact with one another. Complexities arise from such data, where the inter-personal influence of the members within a dyad is essential, just as much as the individual, intra-personal effects. Such inter-personal effects cannot be addressed by conventional models designed for random samples assuming independence or for clustered data summarizing within-group influences through group-level means and residual variances. The high degree of dependence between the members of the same dyad, often addressed as 'interdependence' (Galovan et al., 2017), reflects the mutual influence that members of a dyad share over time.

Dyadic data analysis models have been developed and used for decades, among which the Actor-Partner Interdependence Model (APIM; Kenny, 1996) and the Common Fate Model (CFM; Kenny & La Voie, 1985) have gained popularity as unique approaches to modeling dyadic data. The APIM disentangles interdependence as direct individual influences that members project onto their partners, whereas the CFM synthesizes interdependence at the dyadic level.

However, choosing among the models when analyzing dyadic data is not clear-cut. Rather, it is often a matter of theory-based decisions, considering the research questions and data characteristics. Generally, it is recommended that the CFM be utilized instead of the APIM when we assume the variables are purely dyadic (Cook, 1998) or the measures are moderately to highly correlated ($r > .20$) (Ledermann &

H. Kim (✉) · J.-S. Kim
University of Wisconsin-Madison, Madison, WI, USA
e-mail: hanna.kim@wisc.edu

M. Wiberg et al. (eds.), *Quantitative Psychology*, Springer Proceedings in Mathematics & Statistics 353, https://doi.org/10.1007/978-3-030-74772-5_39

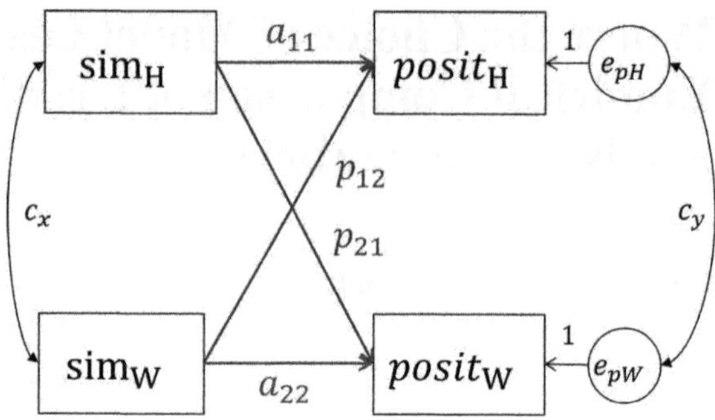

Fig. 1 The basic Actor-Partner Interdependence Model

Kenny, 2012).[1] Still, the appropriate level of analysis is often not easily discerned (Cook, 1998) and the APIM is frequently used over the CFM simply as a "default" choice in applied research (Galovan et al., 2017; Ledermann & Kenny, 2012).

Given that the choice of model may not only convey different theoretical implications, but also produce distinct results, this study aims to compare the two modeling frameworks in an empirical setting. We first review the models, referring to their characteristics and use in related fields. We then provide an empirical data analysis using the Wisconsin Longitudinal Study[2] to illustrate the research questions that each model addresses and to discuss their respective strengths.

2 Overview of Dyadic Data Analysis Models

2.1 Actor-Partner Interdependence Model

The APIM (Kenny, 1996) models dyadic interdependence as a combination of explicit and direct paths between the predictors and outcomes of members in a dyad. These paths are called 'actor effects' and 'partner effects' as reflected in the name, Actor-Partner Interdependence Model. Figure 1 depicts the structure of a basic APIM with a single predictor (similarity; sim_H, sim_W) and outcome (positive affect; $posit_H$, $posit_W$) for both members (husband and wife).

Actor effects (the horizontal arrows denoted as a_{11} and a_{22}) show the impact of one's own predictor on their own outcome for each person as a typical regression

[1]A higher correlation of indicators is required to ensure a strong measurement model with only one pair of indicators for a given construct. However, weak loadings cannot be compensated by obtaining additional indicators (Ledermann & Kenny, 2012).

[2]Wisconsin Longitudinal Study (WLS) [graduates, siblings, and spouses]: 1957–2019 Version 13.07. [machine-readable data file] / Hauser, Robert M., William H. Sewell, and Pamela Herd. [principal investigator(s)]. Madison, WI: University of Wisconsin-Madison, WLS. [distributor]; http://www.ssc.wisc.edu/wlsresearch/documentation/

model would do. On the other hand, partner effects (the diagonal arrows denoted as p_{12} and p_{21}) assess the influence on one's outcome coming from their partner's predictor level.[3] It is by these partner effects that APIM captures interdependence. Residual covariance between the residual terms of the two members' outcomes ($c_y = cov\ (e_{pH}, e_{pW})$) indicate any covariances not captured by the model, so that their outcome values are still correlated after removing the variance explained by the partner effects (Cook, 1998). The APIM also allows for a covariance between the predictor variables (c_x), reflecting the belief that the predictors of members within a dyad are not independent.

Within APIM, we can consider the following research questions. First, we can examine if one's predictor level is associated with their own outcome by estimating corresponding actor effects for both members. We can evaluate if there is a significant difference between the actor effects by comparing models with and without an equality constraint on the actor effects. Next, we investigate if one's predictor level affects their partner's outcome level by estimating partner effects. The difference in the partner effects can also be tested by the fit of models with and without equality constraints (Maroufizadeh et al., 2018). Additionally, we can compute the ratio (k) of each member's partner effect to their actor effect to identify the 'dyadic pattern' of the relationship, such as the actor-only pattern ($k = 0$), couple pattern ($k = 1$), and the contrast pattern ($k = -1$) (Kenny & Ledermann, 2010).

The APIM has been widely used in psychological studies involving families and close relationships, and is increasingly being used to better understand intra- and inter-personal dynamics in various fields including education and health management.

2.2 *Common Fate Model*

On the other hand, the CFM (Kenny & La Voie, 1985) focuses on modeling the interdependence as a joint process, a relationship occurring at the dyadic level rather than as a set of separate individual paths. As its name indicates, the CFM assumes that members in a dyad demonstrate interdependence due to a shared external factor, namely the 'common fate' variable. It can be an environmental factor, a cultural background, or even a shared experience of the members. Since interdependence occurs due to the 'common fate', the outcome of interest is also analyzed at the dyadic level. In order to form a dyadic predictor and outcome, CFM utilizes both members' responses as measurements of dyadic constructs. By doing so, we are able to account for measurement errors, but at the same time, it may be more difficult to estimate the CFM with small samples as compared to the APIM.

[3] Note the convention to label the partner effect of person 1 (the path of X_2 to Y_1) as p_{12}, and vice versa (Garcia et al., 2015). To whom the outcome variable belongs, in other words who receives the partner effect, matters in naming the partner effects.

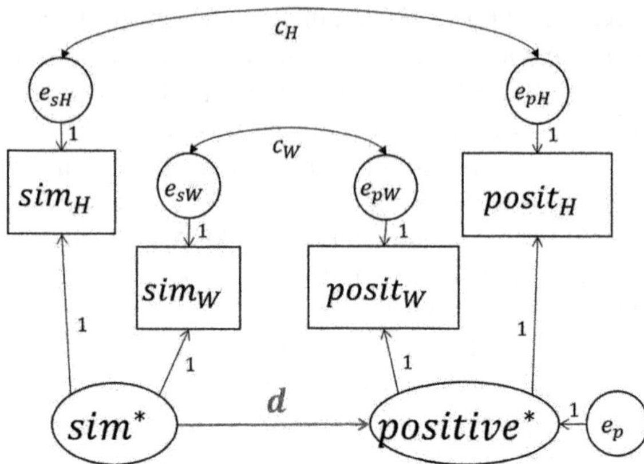

Fig. 2 The basic Common Fate Model

Figure 2 depicts the structure of a basic CFM with a single latent predictor (similarity; *sim**) and outcome (positive affect; *positive**). The ultimate goal is to estimate the influence of the 'common fate' predictor on the latent outcome, which is called the 'direct effect' (*d*) (Loeys & Molenberghs, 2013). Covariances between the residual variances of the manifest variables ($c_H = cov\ (e_{sH}, e_{pH})$, $c_W = cov\ (e_{sW}, e_{hW})$) are set for each member to model the residual individual relationships not fully explained by the dyadic direct effect. Consequently, the dyad members do not directly impact one another but instead exact effects through the latent factors (Maroufizadeh et al., 2018).

With CFM, we can examine if the dyadic predictor affects the outcome at the dyadic level. This implies that interdependence occurs because both members are affected by a common variable. Therefore, it is generally advised that CFM be used in cases where the variables measure a truly dyadic relationship, so that the associations between the variables can be analyzed at the dyadic level (Ledermann & Macho, 2009). It is also recommended that the variables form a reliable measurement model. When a CFM fails to provide good fit to the data, it could indicate that the member's scores are not equally affected by the dyadic effect (Cook, 1998). It may be that the loadings on the latent variables are not equal, or that the relationship of interest in fact cannot be well-summarized by an overall 'direct effect'.

3 Empirical Analysis

3.1 Research Questions

For illustration, APIM and CFM models were applied to data from the Wisconsin Longitudinal Study (WLS) to understand how marital quality affects happiness in married couples. The association between marital quality and happiness in married couples (Russel & Wells, 1994), as well as the relationship of similarity between spouses in multiple domains and the positive affect of spouses (Gaunt, 2006) have been reported. Based on a previous study that measured marital quality with the similarity of outlook on life and closeness between spouses (Moorman, 2011), we aimed to investigate the following research questions through dyadic data analyses:

- How does marital quality affect happiness in married couples?
- Do similarity and closeness differently impact positive and negative affect?
- If significant influences exist, are they better understood as combinations of individual influences or couple-level joint processes?

3.2 Data and Variables

The WLS tracks 10,317 Wisconsin high school graduates from 1957.[4] Survey data were collected from the graduates in 1957, 1964, 1975, 1993, 2004, and 2011, and from selected siblings in 1977, 1994, 2005, and 2011. Spouses of the graduates (in 2004) and siblings (in 2006) were invited to participate in the study as well. Although the WLS is a longitudinal data set, data from married couples were collected only for a single wave, making the present study a cross-sectional investigation. In this study, we focused on *6012* graduates and siblings who (a) participated in the 2004 wave of the WLS, (b) completed at least a part of the telephone interview, (c) were currently married, (d) had spouses that were heterosexual and participated at least partially in a parallel telephone interview.[5] Missing data (less than 5%) were imputed, using one of 20 multiple imputation sets in further analyses. The variables of analysis and their descriptive statistics are presented in Table 1.

3.3 Analysis Models and Results

APIM and CFM models were fit to understand how marital quality affects happiness of married couples.[6] First, single sets of indicators were used for the predictor and outcome as in the basic form of APIM (Fig. 1) and CFM (Fig. 2), resulting in models 1–4 and 6–9. Next, multiple sets of indicators were used to form a comprehensive APIM (Fig. 3) and CFM (Fig. 4), resulting in models 5 and 10.

[4]WLS Homepage, https://ssc.wisc.edu/wlsresearch/, last accessed 2020/9/1.

[5]This was done for the purpose of testing the difference in influences that wives had on husbands and vice versa. One respondent was eliminated from subsequent analyses because both she and her spouse were female.

[6]R (version 4.0.3; R Core Team, 2020) codes for APIM and CFM analyses can be provided upon request.

Table 1 Descriptive statistics of variables used in analysis

Variable	Question contents	Scale	Husbands			Wives		
			n	Mean	SD	n	Mean	SD
Similarity (*sim*)	How similar do you find your outlook on life is with that of your spouse?	1 = not at all similar 2 = not very similar 3 = somewhat similar 4 = very similar	6012	3.59	0.55	6012	3.56	0.59
Closeness (*close*)	How close are you with your current spouse?	1 = not at all close 2 = not very close 3 = somewhat close 4 = very close	6012	3.84	0.39	6012	3.81	0.45
Positive affect (*posit*)	How happy have you been during the past four weeks?	1 = so unhappy that life is not worthwhile 2 = very unhappy 3 = somewhat unhappy 4 = somewhat happy 5 = happy and interested in life	6012	4.80	0.51	6012	4.79	0.56
Negative affect (*nonneg*)	How often did you feel fretful, angry, irritable, anxious, or depressed in the past four weeks?	1 = almost always 2 = often 3 = occasionally 4 = rarely 5 = never (reverse-coded)	6012	4.33	0.87	6012	4.09	0.93

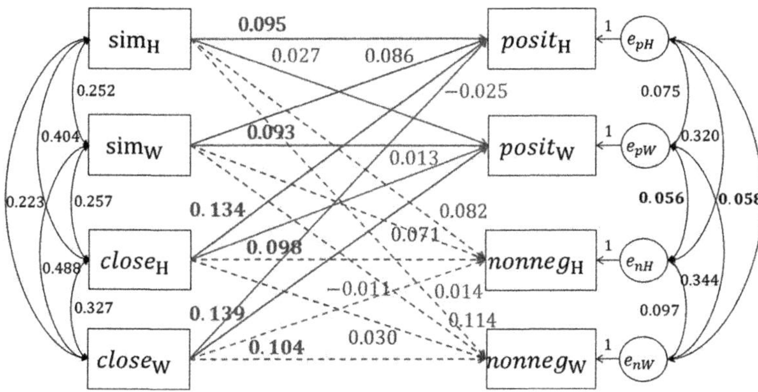

Fig. 3 The Actor-Partner Interdependence Model with Multiple Indicators (Model 5). (Note. Standardized estimates with equality constraints are in bold, insignificant estimates are marked in grey)

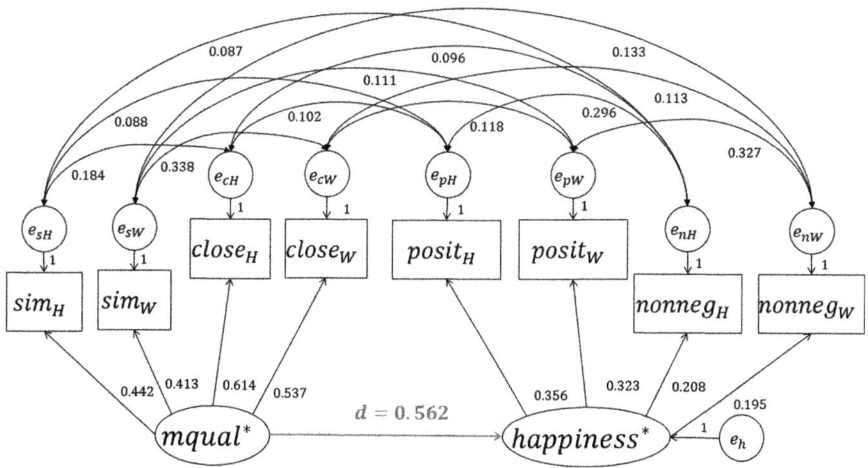

Fig. 4 The Common Fate Model with Multiple Indicators (Model 10). (Note. Standardized estimates are provided)

Model fit statistics provided in Table 2 show that the APIM with single indicators is saturated with zero degrees of freedom unless additional constraints are applied. In contrast, goodness of fit statistics can always be calculated for the CFM with single indicators and no constraints. Fit statistics for Model 5 and Model 10 indicate that the fit for more complex models with multiple indicators tends to worsen, with APIM being relatively stable.

The parameter estimates for APIM with a single set of indicators reveal that one's own perception on the similarity or closeness to one's spouse has significant positive effects on one's positive or negative affect (Table 3). The actor effects were not significantly different among husbands and wives, except that wife level of

Table 2 Goodness of fit statistics

Type	Model	Equality constraints	χ^2 (df, p)	CFI	RMSEA	AIC	BIC
APIM with single indicators	Model 1	$a_{11} = a_{22}$	2.235 (1, 0.135)	0.999	0.014	38724.807	38785.120
	Model 2		0.000 (0, NA)	1.000	0.000	51431.383	51498.399
	Model 3	$a_{11} = a_{22}, p_{12} = p_{21}$	2.221 (2, 0.329)	1.000	0.004	31034.722	31088.334
	Model 4	$a_{11} = a_{22}, p_{12} = p_{21}$	3.323 (2, 0.190)	0.999	0.010	43808.726	43862.339
APIM with multiple indicators	Model 5	$a_{11} = a_{22},\ a_{13} = a_{24},\ a_{31} = a_{42}, c_{y5} = c_{y6}$	2.823 (4, 0.588)	1.000	0.000	78282.536	78946.984
CFM with single indicators	Model 6		6.021 (1, 0.014)	0.994	0.029	38728.592	38788.906
	Model 7		3.680 (1, 0.055)	0.997	0.021	51433.064	51493.377
	Model 8	$c_H = c_W$	3.198 (2, 0.202)	0.999	0.010	31035.699	31089.311
	Model 9		1.514 (1, 0.219)	1.000	0.009	43808.918	43869.231
CFM with multiple indicators	Model 10		144.513 (13, 0.000)	0.979	0.041	78406.226	78560.361

similarity had a stronger effect on reducing negative affect compared to husband. The positive and negative affect felt by married persons were also subjected to their spouse perception of similarity and closeness. These partner effects were relatively weak compared to actor effects. It is notable that wife emotion was more impacted by husband similarity, than was husband being impacted by wife perceived level of similarity. Such a difference did not hold for closeness, where the amount of partner effect was not significantly different among husbands and wives.

The analysis results of CFM with single sets of indicators summarize the interdependence between spousal perceptions and emotions into a direct effect at the dyadic level (Table 4). Overall, the perception of married couples on their similarity or closeness positively affects their positive and negative affect. The differences in the effects of husbands and wives is no longer addressed and is mixed in the direct effect of the CFM. This is suitable for modeling the relationship between closeness and positive or negative affect (Models 8 & 9) because the spouses do not exhibit disparate actor and partner effects. However, modeling the influence of similarity on the positive or negative affect of married couples by CFM could obscure the difference in the amount of impact that wives and husbands receive from one another.

As similarity and closeness measure marital quality while positive and negative affects reflect happiness, APIM and CFM with multiple indicators (Models 5 & 10) were fit to jointly model the dyadic relationships among the variables. In Model 5, the actor effects were all significantly positive and mostly indifferent across husbands and wives as in the APIMs with single indicators (Fig. 3). However, after simultaneously accounting for the variables, some partner effects no longer persisted, such as the effect of closeness on positive affect. As the number of indicators increases, a joint APIM will become more complicated with added actor- and partner effects affecting each other. Model 10 synthesizes the overall effect of 'marital quality' on 'happiness' as 0.562, which means when a couple's marital quality is 1 SD higher than the average couple, their happiness as a married couple will be about 0.562 SD higher than the average (Fig. 4). As more indicators with high reliability are added, CFM will provide stronger evidence on a composite dyadic relationship.[7]

4 Discussion

In this study, we examined the two dyadic data analysis frameworks, APIM and CFM, with respect to their conceptual focuses and empirical implications. The illustrative example applying both APIM and CFM to the WLS data confirmed the positive relationships between marital quality and happiness of married couples

[7]The reliability was 0.644 for 'marital quality' and 0.477 for 'happiness' within our empirical example.

Table 3 Summary of APIM estimates (Models 1–4, n = 6012)

	Model 1: similarity → positive affect			Model 2: similarity → negative affect			Model 3: closeness → positive affect			Model 4: closeness → negative affect		
	Est.	s.e.	Std. est.	Est.	s.e.	Std. est.	Est.	s.e.	Std. est.	Est.	s.e.	Std. est.
Actor effects												
a_{11}	*0.140**	0.009	0.151*	0.182*	0.021	0.115*	*0.229**	0.012	0.179*	*0.315**	0.020	0.143*
a_{22}	*0.140**	0.009	0.149*	0.264*	0.021	0.168*	*0.229**	0.012	0.184*	*0.315**	0.020	0.152*
Partner effects												
p_{12}	0.080*	0.011	0.093*	0.121*	0.019	0.082*	*0.035**	0.012	0.031*	*0.078**	0.020	0.040*
p_{21}	0.051*	0.013	0.050*	0.060*	0.022	0.035*	*0.035**	0.012	0.024*	*0.078**	0.020	0.033*
Covariances												
c_x	0.082*	0.004	0.252*	0.082*	0.004	0.252*	0.058*	0.002	0.327*	0.058*	0.002	0.327*
c_y	0.021*	0.004	0.076*	0.078*	0.010	0.099*	0.023*	0.004	0.084*	0.082*	0.010	0.104*

*$p < 0.05$

Note. Numbers in italic indicate parameter estimates with equality constraints

Table 4 Summary of CFM estimates (Models 6–9, n = 6012)

	Model 6: similarity → positive affect			Model 7: similarity → negative affect			Model 8: closeness → positive affect			Model 9: closeness → negative affect		
	Est.	s.e.	Std. est.	Est.	s.e.	Std. est.	Est.	s.e.	Std. est.	Est.	s.e.	Std. est.
Factor loadings (predictor/outcome factor → husband/wife)												
l_1(pred. H)	*1*	–	0.521*	*1*	–	0.522*	*1*	–	0.609*	*1*	–	0.611*
l_2(pred. W)	*1*	–	0.485*	*1*	–	0.485*	*1*	–	0.537*	*1*	–	0.535*
l_3(outc. H)	*1*	–	0.336*	*1*	–	0.358*	*1*	–	0.335*	*1*	–	0.358*
l_4(outc. W)	*1*	–	0.304*	*1*	–	0.333*	*1*	–	0.306*	*1*	–	0.335*
Direct effect (predictor factor → outcome factor)												
d	0.405*	0.036	0.684*	0.590*	0.059	0.546*	0.337*	0.035	0.477*	0.567*	0.061	0.437*
Covariances (predictor indicator ~ outcome indicator)												
c_H	0.011*	0.004	0.049*	0.015*	0.007	0.040*	*0.022**	0.002	0.150*	0.021*	0.005	0.084*
c_W	0.025*	0.004	0.092*	0.050*	0.007	0.111*	*0.022**	0.002	0.112*	0.035*	0.005	0.104*

$^{*}p < 0.05$

Note. Numbers in italic indicate parameter estimates with equality constraints

found in previous studies. However, in APIM, separating out the individual impacts on each other was emphasized, whereas CFM focused more on a composite, joint effect at the couple-level. Depending on the dyadic relationship of interest, the individual differences could be overlooked by only utilizing CFM. On the other hand, when measuring dyadic constructs and jointly modeling a dyadic relationship is required, CFM can better suit the purpose. It should be noted though that strong measurement models based on theory are needed in order to fully benefit from the latent structure of CFM.

The exact relationship between APIM and CFM parameters deserve theoretical investigation, and simulation studies can help provide detailed guidance on choosing the right dyadic data analysis model depending on the research question and characteristics such as dyadic patterns. Future research could also examine the impact of additional covariates or sample size, and may extend the models to cover closely related groups of three or more members, with increasing availability of quality data.

Acknowledgments This research uses data from the Wisconsin Longitudinal Study, funded by the National Institute on Aging (R01 AG009775; R01 AG033285). Support for this research was provided by the Office of the Vice Chancellor for Research and Graduate Education and a Vilas Faculty Mid-Career Investigator Award from the University of Wisconsin-Madison.

References

Cook, W. L. (1998). Integrating models of interdependence with treatment evaluations in marital therapy research. *Journal of Family Psychology, 12*(4), 529–542. https://doi.org/10.1037/0893-3200.12.4.529

Galovan, A. M., Holmes, E. K., & Proulx, C. M. (2017). Theoretical and methodological issues in relationship research: Considering the common fate model. *Journal of Social and Personal Relationships, 34*(1), 44–68. https://doi.org/10.1177/0265407515621179

Garcia, R. L., Kenny, D. A., & Ledermann, T. (2015). Moderation in the actor-partner interdependence model. *Personal Relationships, 22*(1), 8–29. https://doi.org/10.1111/pere.12060

Gaunt, R. (2006). Couple similarity and marital satisfaction: Are similar spouses happier? *Journal of Personality, 74*(5), 1401–1420. https://doi.org/10.1111/j.1467-6494.2006.00414.x

Kenny, D. A. (1996). Models of nonindependence in dyadic research. *Journal of Social and Personal Relationships, 13*, 279–294. https://doi.org/10.1177/0265407596132007

Kenny, D. A., & La Voie, L. (1985). Separating individual and group effects. *Journal of Personality and Social Psychology, 48*(2), 339–348. https://doi.org/10.1037/0022-3514.48.2.339

Kenny, D. A., & Ledermann, T. (2010). Detecting, measuring, and testing dyadic patterns in the actor-partner interdependence model. *Journal of Family Psychology, 24*(3), 359–366. https://doi.org/10.1037/a0019651

Ledermann, T., & Kenny, D. A. (2012). The common fate model for dyadic data: Variations of a theoretically important but underutilized model. *Journal of Family Psychology, 26*(1), 140–148. https://doi.org/10.1037/a0026624

Ledermann, T., & Macho, S. (2009). Mediation in dyadic data at the level of the dyads: A structural equation modeling approach. *Journal of Family Psychology, 23*(5), 661–670. https://doi.org/10.1037/a0016197

Loeys, T., & Molenberghs, G. (2013). Modeling actor and partner effects in dyadic data when outcomes are categorical. *Psychological Methods, 18*(2), 220–236. https://doi.org/10.1037/a0030640

Maroufizadeh, S., Hosseini, M., Rahimi Foroushani, A., Omani-Samani, R., & Amini, P. (2018). Application of the dyadic data analysis in behavioral medicine research: Marital satisfaction and anxiety in infertile couples. *BMC Medical Research Methodology, 18*(1), 1–10. https://doi.org/10.1186/s12874-018-0582-y

Moorman, S. M. (2011). The importance of feeling understood in marital conversations about end-of-life health care1. *Journal of Social and Personal Relationships, 28*(1), 100–116. https://doi.org/10.1177/0265407510386137

Moorman, S. M. (2016). Dyadic perspectives on marital quality and loneliness in later life. *Journal of Social and Personal Relationships, 33*(5), 600–618. https://doi.org/10.1177/0265407515584504

Russel, R., & Wells, P. (1994). Predictors of happiness in married couples. *Personality and Individual Differences, 17*(3), 313–321.

R Core Team. (2020). R: *A Language and Environment for Statistical Computing*. https://www.r-project.org/

Wisconsin Longitudinal Study (WLS) [graduates, siblings, and spouses]: 1957–2019 Version 13.07. [machine-readable data file] / Hauser, Robert M., William H. Sewell, and Pamela Herd. [principal investigator(s)]. Madison, WI: University of Wisconsin-Madison, WLS. [distributor]; http://www.ssc.wisc.edu/wlsresearch/documentation/

Generalized Additive Modeling for Learning Trajectories in E-Learning Environments

Jung Yeon Park, JinHo Kim, Dries Debeer, and Wim Van den Noortgate

1 Introduction

1.1 Technology-Enhanced E-Learning

Adaptive E-learning is growing in popularity. It allows teachers to track individual student's learning needs and to provide timely personalized support (Klinkenberg et al., 2011). In educational testing environments, high-stakes computerized assessments typically do not provide feedback during the test, and the test-taker's proficiency is expected to be stable during the assessment. In contrast, an a priori expectation of the adaptive E-learning environments is that the learners' learning performance may change in real time as the learners complete a sequence of practice items. In addition, often timely and personalized feedback is included in the environment (Park et al., 2019). To be specific, the individuals' learning (performance) trajectories may be irregularly shaped. Because there is freedom for

J. Y. Park
College of Education and Human Development, George Mason University, Fairfax, VA, USA

Faculty of Psychology and Educational Sciences and itec, imec Research Group, KU Leuven, Campus KULAK, Kortrijk, Belgium

J. Kim (✉)
Faculty of Psychology and Educational Sciences and itec, imec Research Group, KU Leuven, Campus KULAK, Kortrijk, Belgium

Graduate School of Education and Urban Bigdata·AI Institute, University of Seoul, Seoul, South Korea
e-mail: jinhokim@uos.ac.kr

D. Debeer · W. Van den Noortgate
Faculty of Psychology and Educational Sciences and itec, imec Research Group, KU Leuven, Campus KULAK, Kortrijk, Belgium

M. Wiberg et al. (eds.), *Quantitative Psychology*, Springer Proceedings in Mathematics & Statistics 353, https://doi.org/10.1007/978-3-030-74772-5_40

each learner to access E-learning platforms and choose their own study session, the learning trajectories may change within a single study session (i.e., while the learner is engaged in the E-learning environments). It is also necessary to consider that the trajectories may change between study sessions (i.e., while they are not engaged in the E-learning environments). It is probably because the learner could experience some constructive learning through other mechanisms or simply forget things they learned in previous study sessions.

Therefore, it is desirable to use a statistical modeling approach that enables one to flexibly examine the learner's learning change. Kadengye et al. (2015) used a type of generalized linear mixed models (GLMM) in order to estimate the learner trajectory over time within- and between-study sessions in the E-learning environments. Park et al. (2018) proposed using the GLMM with learner explanatory variables for the purpose of alleviating the cold-start in adaptive learning systems – the problem that for new learners we do not have an idea of their ability and therefore the adaptive learning environment might not perform well until the learner completed a substantial number of items. As an extension to those successful endeavors, this study aims to demonstrate the potential of a different modeling approach that could enhance the predictive capability to infer the dynamics of learners' performance in an E-learning environment.

1.2 Generalized Additive Mixed Model

In this study, we employ a generalized additive mixed model (GAMM; Hastie & Tibshirani, 1990; Wood, 2017) to examine the learner trajectory in the E-learning environments by considering the within- and between-session time trend variables. The GAMM is an extended variant of GLMM in which a linear predictor includes a sum of smooth functions of covariates (e.g., time). The model has the following structure:

$$g\left(E\left(Y_i\right)\right)=A_i\xi+f_1\left(x_{1i}\right)+f_2\left(x_{2i}\right)+f_3\left(x_{3i},x_{4i}\right)\ldots,\ f\left(x_i\right)=\sum_{j=1}^{q} b_j\left(x_i\right)\ \gamma_{ji} \tag{1}$$

where A_i is a row of the model matrix for the parametric terms, ξ is the corresponding parameter vector, $f_m(x_i)$ is the m-th function of its covariate(s), $x_i^{'}s$ for the smooth terms, $b_j(x)$ is the j-th basis function, where $j = 1, \ldots, q$, γ_{ji} is the unknown parameter which can include random effects, and $g(.)$ is a link function that maps the expected outcome $E(Y_i)$ on the right-hand-side of the equation. Because we focus on binary outcomes, we will assume $g(.)$ is the logit function.

As can be seen in Eq. (1), the relationship between item responses and predictor variables in the GAMM is flexible via the semi-parametric modeling approach. In contrast, in the GLMM this relationship is predetermined to be linear or linear with respect to a predefined transformation of the predictor. For the choice of basis function, $b_j(x)$, the cubic regression spline and thin plate were explored; however, other basis functions are also possible.

1.3 Purpose of Study

In this study, first, we investigate the applicability of a GAMM, a semi-parametric modeling approach to examine the real-time learner performance in an item-based E-learning environment. This study aims to consider within-session time (i.e., the time spent while they are engaged in the learning environment) and also between-session time (i.e., the time spent outside the learning environment) to estimate the learning (performance) trajectories in a more precise and practical manner. Second, we investigate whether, using this method, the learning trajectories can be better estimated than using a GLMM. We demonstrate its applicability to log data generated by a real-life E-learning environment.

2 Application to Real-Life Data

2.1 Statistics Online Data

A subset of the data collected from a web-based learning platform, 'Statistics-Online' was used for this study. This platform was designed as an item-based, E-learning environment to supplement the classroom learning of undergraduate students in the Educational Sciences and the Speech Therapy & Audiology Sciences at the University of Leuven (a.k.a. KU Leuven). Learners were allowed to log in at the time of their choice outside the classroom-based lecture times. A total of 145 multiple-choice items from the "regression analysis" module were presented in a random order across study sessions. Data from the 2011–2012 academic year was used for the current analysis. Students' responses to the items (i.e., scores) were dichotomous (0 = incorrect answer; 1 = correct answer). In addition to the item responses, the dataset contains timestamps recording when each student started and finished each item. We refer to the spacing time between two consecutive study sessions of a student as the between-session time. In this example, the between-session time is defined by the time between two consecutive item responses that is longer than 24 h, and the within-session time is defined by the time that the student is logged in, excluding the between-session time. Based on this information, we computed the amount of time spent within ('wtime') and between ('btime') the study sessions. In particular, the 'wtime' indicates cumulative learning time in hours within study sessions, and the 'btime' represents cumulative spacing time in days between study sessions. Table 1 shows an example of the structure of the data. To secure a stable and valid estimation of fitting the GAMMs, only the data of students

Table 1 Structure of statistics online data

Student	Session	Item	Score	wtime	btime
1	1	1	1	0.000	0.000
1	1	2	1	0.002	0.000
1	1	3	1	0.005	0.000
1	1	4	1	0.008	0.000
1	1	5	1	0.009	0.000
1	...	...	...	...	...
1	1	20	1	0.245	0.000
1	2	21	1	0.246	119.707
1	2	22	1	0.249	119.707
1	2	16	1	0.251	119.707
1	2	23	1	0.254	119.707
1	2	24	1	0.257	119.707
1	...	...	...	...	...
1	2	15	1	0.400	119.707
1	3	17	1	0.401	143.821
1	3	37	1	0.403	143.821
1	3	38	1	0.406	143.821
1	3	39	0	0.411	143.821
1	3	5	1	0.414	143.821
1	...	...	...	...	...
1	3	43	1	0.432	143.821
1	4	44	1	0.433	167.920
1	4	6	1	0.436	167.920
1	...	...	...	...	...

who responded to at least five items, engaged in at least two study sessions (that resulted in 64 learners in total) were considered for analysis.

2.2 *Models and Methods*

In order to infer the learner's learning performance within study sessions after controlling for the spacing times between study sessions, we used two models. First, we used the GLMM with parametric terms associated with the within-session time (*wtime*) and between-session time (*btime*) as follows:

$$logit\left(E\left(Y_{pi(t)}=1\right)\right)=\left(\alpha_{00}+\theta_{0p}\right)+\left(\alpha_{10}+\theta_{1p}\right)wtime_{p(t)}+\left(\alpha_{20}+\theta_{2p}\right)btime_{p(t)}+\beta_i. \quad (2)$$

In the equation, α_{00}, α_{10}, and α_{20} refer to the expected initial performance, the expected rate of performance change within sessions, and the expected effect of the spacing time between sessions on the within-session performance, respectively. Similarly, θ_{0p}, θ_{1p}, and θ_{2p} are the random deviations of the learner p estimates for each term related to the learning performance. Also, β_i is the random effect (or item difficulty) of item i.

Table 2 Model fits of GLMM and GAMM

Criterion	GLMM	GAMM
AIC	3641.58	3640.42
MSE	0.260	0.257

Secondly, we fit the GAMM to the data which incorporates both the within-session and between-session times into the smooth functions as below:

$$logit\left(E\left(Y_{pi(t)}=1\right)\right)=\left(\alpha_{00}+\theta_{0p}\right)+f_1\left(wtime_{p(t)}\right)+f_2\left(wtime_{p(t)},\theta_{1p}\right) + f_3\left(btime_{p(t)}\right)+f_4\left(btime_{p(t)},\theta_{2p}\right)+\beta_i, \quad (3)$$

where $f_m(.)$ denotes the m-th smooth function, and other terms are defined as in Eq. (2), but the effects of within-session time (i.e., $f_1(wtime_{p(t)})$) and between-session time (i.e., $f_3(btime_{p(t)})$) are in the smooth terms. $f_2(wtime_{p(t)}, \theta_{1p})$ and $f_4(btime_{p(t)}, \theta_{2p})$ indicate the learner-specific random deviations from their overall effects. Note that if $f_m(.)$ is just a linear function, it reduces to the GLMM. To fit the GAMMs, the *bam* function in the *mgcv* R package (Wood, 2017, 2020) was used for this study.

For a smoothing parameter estimation, the restricted maximum likelihood method (REML) was used. In order to evaluate and compare the model fits and prediction accuracy between the two modeling approaches, we considered information criterion such as the Akaike Information Criterion (AIC) as well as the Mean Squared Error (MSE) for item responses. For the models fitted by the *mgcv* R package, the AIC was computed based on the effective degrees of freedom (edf; Wood, 2020).

2.3 Results

As seen in Table 2, results suggest that the GAMM has lower values in AIC and MSE than the GLMM, indicating a better model-data fit. Therefore, including the smooth functions to estimate the learners' unique learning trajectories over time (within- and between-study sessions) performs better than merely assuming the linear trajectories as in the GLMM. Note that given the specific data, the gap of model fits appeared not to be dramatically noticeable but it still implies the potential of using the GAMM.

Table 3 shows the significance of the two smooth terms over time for within- and between-study sessions, the learner-specific random effects for the intercept and the slopes, and the item-specific random effect of GAMM (see Eq. 3). The greater the effective degrees of freedom (edf), the wigglier the smooth function becomes. Specifically, an edf > 2 indicates a highly non-linear relationship (note that an edf $= 1$ indicates a linear relationship). Results of the edf values corresponding to both within- and between-session time trends ensure that the expected logit and

Table 3 Approximate significance of smooth terms of GAMM

	edf	X^2
$f_1(wtime_{pi})$	2.46	9.51*
$f_3(btime_{pi})$	1.00	0.12
θ_{0p}	40.83	399.31***
$f_2(wtime_{p(t)}, \theta_{1p})$	0.00	0.00
$f_4(btime_{p(t)}, \theta_{2p})$	0.00	0.00
β_i	105.90	662.94***

Note. edf = effective degrees of freedom; $* = p < .05$; $*** = p < .001$

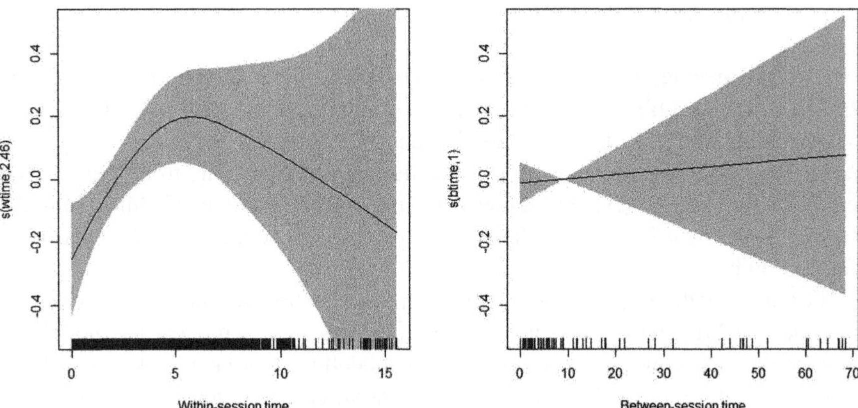

Fig. 1 General time trends within and between sessions

the *wtime* variable is not linearly related, suggesting that the GAMM provides more information than the GLMM in this regard.

Figure 1 visualizes the general within- and between-session learning trajectories (*wtime* and *btime*) of an average learner where the other terms are held constant in Eq. (3). The 95% confidence intervals indicated by the shaded region on the plots reflect the uncertainty around the estimated smooth functions. The estimated trajectory within sessions (left panel in Fig. 1) was significant. Specifically, the trajectory appears to increase monotonically for the first fifth and seventh hours during the course of learning, and then starts to decrease. Similarly, the confidence interval widens as the within-session time gets longer. The general learning trajectory for between-session time only slightly increases. As also implied by the edf value in Table 3, the relationship between the expected logit and the *btime* variable appears to be linear.

Figure 2 visualizes the learning trajectories of a randomly selected learner. Specifically, the panel on the left shows the learner's within-session trajectory and the panel on the right shows his or her between-session trajectory. Note that the two functions in this figure represent the summed effects including the intercept and other predictors in the GAMM. The plots currently give the impression that the

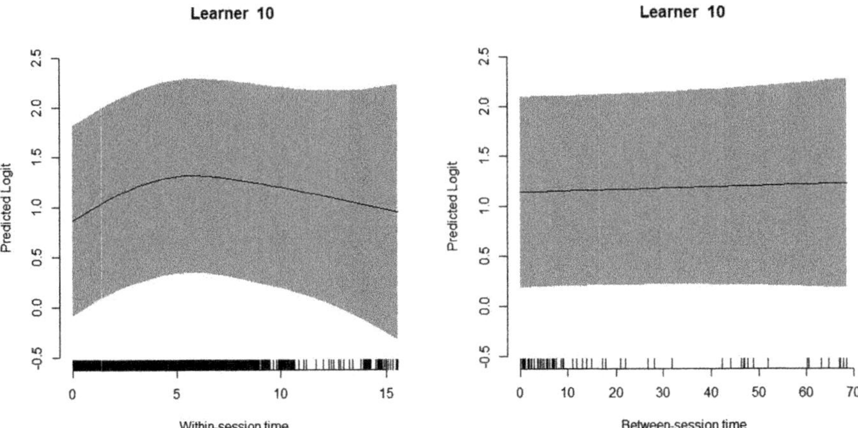

Fig. 2 An individual learner's learning trajectories within (left) and between (right) sessions

learner's performance is expected to increase right up to fifth hour within the study sessions, and then gradually decreases for the next 10 h.

3 Conclusion and Implication

The present study explored the capability of a GAMM to examine learners' real-time performance in the E-learning environments. Smoothing splines were used for the nonparametric functions to estimate changeable learning trajectories. This flexible approach was compared with a more traditional approach such as a GLMM. We demonstrated its applicability and potentiality to log data available from an item-based, E-learning assessment for learning statistics online. We found that the GAMM was able to estimate both linear and non-linear learning trajectories for the within-session and between-session times. However, we acknowledge that the data used in this study is relatively small with regard to the number of items and learners to be able to illustrate advantages of the GAMM over the GLMM substantially. Nevertheless, we found that the GAMM has shown methodological values for modeling the learner trajectory and improving the response prediction, using the semi-parametric approach based on smooth functions. As future work, one could investigate its added values through bigger data examples that allow to explore comprehensive and meaningful learning trajectories over a longer period of time in similar E-learning environments.

Appendix

```
library(mgcv)
library(itsadug)

# Model 1. Generalized linear mixed model (GLMM) estimating within
and between learning trajectories

glmm.wt.bt <- bam(grade ~ 1 + s(iduser,bs="re") + wtime +
s(wtime,iduser,bs="re") + btime + s(btime,iduser,bs="re")
                 + s(iditem,bs="re"), family = binomial(link =
"logit"),
                data = math.sub)
summary(glmm.wt.bt)
gam.vcomp(glmm.wt.bt)
AIC(glmm.wt.bt)
BIC(glmm.wt.bt)


# Model 2. Generalized additive mixed model (GAMM) estimating within
and between learning trajectories

gamm.wt.bt <- bam(grade ~ 1 + s(iduser,bs="re") + s(wtime,bs="cr") +
s(wtime,iduser,bs="re") + s(btime,bs="cr") + s(btime,iduser,bs="re")
                 + s(iditem,bs="re"), family = binomial(link =
"logit"),
                data = math.sub)
summary(gamm.wt.bt)
gam.vcomp(gamm.wt.bt)
AIC(gamm.wt.bt)
BIC(gamm.wt.bt)


par(mfrow=c(1,2))
plot.gam(gamm.wt.bt,select=2,scale = 0,
         xlab="Within-session time",shade = TRUE,col ="blue")
plot.gam(gamm.wt.bt,select=4,scale = 0,
         xlab="Between-session time",shade = TRUE,col ="blue")


user_vec=c("5","10","25")
par(mfrow=c(2,3))

for(i in user_vec){
  plot_smooth(gamm.wt.bt, view =
"wtime",cond=list(iduser=i),rm.ranef=FALSE,col = "blue",
              xlab = "Between-session time",ylab=paste("Predicted
Logit"),ylim=c(0,2),main=paste("Learner ",i), h0=-1)
}
for(i in user_vec){
  plot_smooth(gamm.wt.bt, view =
"btime",cond=list(iduser=i),rm.ranef=FALSE,col = "blue",
              xlab = "Between-session time",ylab=paste("Predicted
Logit"),ylim=c(0,2),main=paste("Learner ",i),h0=-1)

}
```

References

Hastie, T. J., & Tibshirani, R. J. (1990). *Generalized additive models*. Chapman and Hall.

Kadengye, D. T., Ceulemans, E., & Van den Noortgate, W. (2015). Modeling growth in electronic learning environments using a longitudinal random item response model. *The Journal of Experimental Education, 83*(2), 175–202.

Klinkenberg, S., Straatemeier, M., & van der Maas, H. L. J. (2011). Computer adaptive practice of Maths ability using a new item response model for on the fly ability and difficulty estimation. *Computers & Education, 57*(2), 1813–1824.

Park, J. Y., Joo, S., Cornillie, F., Van der Maas, H. L. J., & Van den Noortgate, W. (2018). An explanatory item response theory method for alleviating the cold-start problem in adaptive learning environments. *Behavior Research Methods, 51*(2), 895–909.

Park, J. Y., Cornillie, F., van der Maas, H. L. J., & Van den Noortgate, W. (2019). A multidimensional IRT approach for dynamically monitoring ability growth in computerized practice environments. *Frontiers in Psychology, 10*, 620. https://doi.org/10.3389/fpsyg.2019.00620

Wood, S. N. (2017). *Generalized additive models: An introduction with R* (2nd ed.). Chapman and Hall/CRC.

Wood, S. N. (2020). *mgcv*. R Package Version 1.8-33. Available from: https://cran.r-project.org/web/packages/mgcv/mgcv.pdf

Students Ratings Their Open Classroom Discussion

Diego Carrasco, Ernesto Treviño, Natalia López Hornickel, and Carolina Castillo

1 Introduction

Past research in civic education has positioned open classroom discussion of political and social issues (OPD) as an essential factor for different citizenship outcomes, including civic knowledge (Isac et al., 2014), support of egalitarian values (Carrasco & Torres Irribarra, 2018), political efficacy (Knowles & McCafferty-Wright, 2015), among others. At the same time, it present hostile relations with youth alienation (Torney-Purta, 2009), authoritarianism endorsement (Hahn & Tocci, 1990), and tolerance of corruption (Carrasco et al., 2020).

OPD is a reflective measure of the learning environment and not a classical individual difference measure. It allows capturing students' experience as a collective (at the school level) through students' perceptions as individuals. Student responses are the source of information about their school practices, were students rate their learning environments (Carrasco & Torres Irribarra, 2018). OPD items are reference-shift items, and if their rating response nature is ignored, the compositional models can lead to the wrong conclusions. It is argued that compositional model specification produce an unnecessary correction of level 2 estimates for reference shift scale scores (Lüdtke et al., 2009). Additionally, OPD scores of schools are subject to students' inter-rater variability. As such, two different schools may receive the same OPD mean score, yet the students' OPD ratings can vary broadly (Schweig, 2016). How much students' rating variability is tolerable? Cut off scores may not be easily determined. Common advice in the organizational literature is to exclude

D. Carrasco (✉)
Centro de Medición MIDE UC, Pontificia Universidad Católica de Chile, Santiago, Chile
e-mail: dacarras@uc.cl

E. Treviño · N. López Hornickel · C. Castillo
Facultad de Educación, Pontificia Universidad Católica de Chile, Santiago, Chile
e-mail: ernesto.trevino@uc.cl; nvlopez@uc.cl; carolina.castillo@uc.cl

M. Wiberg et al. (eds.), *Quantitative Psychology*, Springer Proceedings in Mathematics & Statistics 353, https://doi.org/10.1007/978-3-030-74772-5_41

aggregated measures with a low inter-rater agreement (> 0.70) (Lüdtke et al., 2006; Woehr et al., 2015). However, these inter-rater agreement indexes are subject to uncertainty, which depends on group size and intraclass correlations of the rating scores (Lüdtke & Robitzsch, 2009). Therefore, the recommended cut scores may not be generalizable to all scenarios.

In the present work, we address these two problems. The current manuscript consists of five sections. Firstly, a literature review is included to situate the problems under study. Second, a methodology section describes the observed data to illustrate the problems here presented. Then, each problem is presented separately, with its respective analytical strategy. Finally, a conclusion and discussion section are included to present a summary of the presented findings and its implications for large scale studies.

2 Referent Shift Items

Educational research uses students' responses to assess the learning environments students are in. According to Lüdtke et al. (2009), there are three areas where it is possible to find student questionnaires that collect information about learning environments, including climate research, teacher effectiveness, and students' motivational development. In this sense, using students' responses to describe learning environment features is a recurrent practice in educational research.

Reference shift items ask persons in a group about their perceptions concerning a group attribute, or a context factor that affect them collectively. Then, their responses are aggregated at the group level, assuming that group members develop shared perceptions as a function of the attributes of the context (Lang et al., 2018). According to Lüdtke students' ratings represent the individual students' perception of these attributes, and their aggregated scores at the classroom or school level represent shared perceptions of the learning environment, corrected for individual idiosyncrasies (Lüdtke et al., 2006, p. 216).

The OPD scale is an example of these reference shift item scale. All of its item's referred to the school, including what teachers do and what students can do. For example, 'Teachers encourage students to make up their minds' and 'Students bring up current political events for discussion in class' are items that elicit response referring to a learning environment feature. These are not individual differences between students. However, researchers include OPD scores in different ways in their models (Carrasco & Torres Irribarra, 2018), including individual scores, school means, or by including OPD scores of students and school means, as in standard compositional models (Caro & Lenkeit, 2012). This latter practice is troublesome when comparing learning environments using reference shift item scales, because the generated estimates do not directly produce the parameter of interest and may lead to wrong conclusions (Lüdtke et al., 2009).

When students respond to reference shift items, their responses can be considered a particular case of rater mediated measures (Engelhard & Wind, 2018). When their rating nature is recognized, two elements are more easily represented: the scores reference and its rater agreement variability. Two methodological problems are presented here in this regard. The first problem concerns what model specification is more interpretable, when comparisons of learning environments are of interest, but scores were generated using reference-shift item scales. The second pertains to the varying inter-rater agreement between students from different schools. These can vary greatly, and the sole exclusion of low agreement schools as a solution leads to considerable loss of sample (Lüdtke et al., 2006). The present study is an effort to respond to these two methodological challenges. In the following sections, we describe the data we used to illustrate these two problems, and for each problem, we propose an alternative model specification.

3 Methods

3.1 Selected Data and Measures for Illustrations

We used data from the International Civic and Citizenship Education Study from 2016 (ICCS 2016). This study collects responses from intact classrooms, using a two-stage sampling design, where schools are selected using a stratified design in each participating country. These are representative samples of eighth grade students. To illustrate the two identified problems, we use data from Italy (problem 1), and Perú (problem 2), as these two countries are ideal examples for the methodological challenges here discussed. The observed data includes 3450 students and 170 schools from Italy, and 5166 students and 206 schools from Perú.

Dependent variable. Civic Knowledge (y_{ij}) scores represent students' political sophistication that reflects their understanding of political issues. It consists of five plausible values, generated with IRT Rasch model (Rasch, 1960) over a random booklet design of 87 item-test. It presents an international mean of 500 points and a standard deviation of 100 points.

Independent variables. To illustrate the presented problems, we are using two variables. Socioeconomic Status (ses_{ij}), is a score created based on the Parents Education level, Parents Occupation, and number of books at home, reduced via principal components and standardized in each country. OPD scores (opd_{ij}) is a reflective measure of the school environment. This score represents the responses to six reference shift items (e.g., "Teachers encourage students to express their opinions"). OPD scores are IRT scores, generated with a partial credit model (Masters, 2016). More details of regarding the selected variables and the study design can be found in its technical report (Schulz et al., 2018).

In the following sections, the two problems are illustrated and addressed separately. All estimates are pseudo maximum likelihood estimates, where survey design weights and plausible values are accommodated accordingly. Survey weights were partitioned into students and school levels and scaled to their effective samples while including pseudo strata in the estimates. Plausible Values of civic knowledge scores are treated as imputed values and estimates are generated following Rubin-Schaffer rules (Rutkowski et al., 2010).

4 Problem 1: Wrong Inference Model

To illustrate the problem of wrong model specification, we will fit a compositional model over civic knowledge, using the OPD scores (see Eq. 1). This model is equivalent to a Mundlak specification (Bell et al., 2018), and is commonly used to get compositional effects of socioeconomic status over educational outcomes (Caro & Lenkeit, 2012). In this application of the model, y_{ij} stand for the civic knowledge scores of student $_i$ from school $_j$ and is modeled with the overall mean α, and each school specific intercept u_{oj} and a random error ε_{ij}. Additionally, we conditioned y_{ij} with students OPD scores (opd_{ij}) by including its respective centered versions. $\left(opd_{ij} - \overline{opd}_{..}\right)$ are OPD scores centered to the grand mean, while $\left(\overline{opd}_{.j} - \overline{opd}_{..}\right)$ are school level OPD scores centered to the grand mean.

$$y_{ij} = \alpha + \gamma_{w}^{cgm}\left(opd_{ij} - \overline{opd}_{..}\right) + \gamma_{c}\left(\overline{opd}_{.j} - \overline{opd}_{..}\right) + u_{oj} + \varepsilon_{ij} \tag{1}$$

In this model, γ_c would be interpreted as the school level effect of OPD. However, this model does not retrieve the relationship of interest. When we want to compare learning environments, we are interested in the difference between school environments as a whole. This is different from γ_c, which is the relationship of OPD school scores $\left(opd_{.j} - \overline{opd}_{..}\right)$, that cannot be accounted by OPD student scores $\left(opd_{ij} - \overline{opd}_{..}\right)$. Thus, γ_c is a partial effect. A more appropriate parametrization of the model, is the fully disaggregated model (Rights et al., 2019), or also called the within-between model (Bell et al., 2018) (see Eq. 2). In this later model γ_{w}^{cwc} is obtained by centering OPD scores with their respective school means $\left(opd_{ij} - \overline{opd}_{.j}\right)$, or centering within cluster. This centering specification changes the meaning of the between school estimate γ_b. This latter estimate is not a partial effect, but an overall relationship between school means of OPD scores, and civic knowledge scores school random intercepts.

$$y_{ij} = \alpha + \gamma_{w}^{cwc}\left(opd_{ij} - \overline{opd}_{.j}\right) + \gamma_{b}\left(\overline{opd}_{.j} - \overline{opd}_{..}\right) + u_{oj} + \varepsilon_{ij} \tag{2}$$

To illustrate the risk of such a wrong model specification, we use data from Italy from ICCS 2016, and fit both mixed model specifications. In this current application, we have standardized OPD scores. Therefore, OPD coefficient estimates can be interpreted as the expected change in civic knowledge scores, per one standard deviation of OPD scores between students (Table 1).

Table 1 Effects of students' rating of OPD on civic knowledge

	Compositional model			Within-between model		
Fixed effects		E	S.E.		E	S.E.
Intercept	α	521.74	(4.22)***	α	521.73	(4.22)***
Open classroom discussion						
Student level	γ_w^{cgm}	20.63	(1.90)***	γ_w^{cwc}	20.63	(1.90)***
School level	γ_c	−0.11	(8.16)	γ_b	20.53	(8.65)**
Random effects						
var(u_j)		1174.97	(266.59)***		1184.53	(269.11)***
var(ε_{ij})		5769.262	(202.60)***		5767.69	(203.12)***

Note: *E* unstandardized estimate, *S.E.* standard error, *var.* variance component, γ_w^{cgm} OPD scores centered to the grand mean, γ_w^{cwc} OPD scores centered within cluster. ***p < 0.001, **p < 0.01, *p < 0.05

In the case of Italy, γ_w and γ_b are of similar size. Thus, this example renders the extreme case, where the compositional model specification erases the effect of interest. As such, the compositional model can lead to the wrong conclusion that OPD has null effects on civic knowledge between schools ($\gamma_c = -0.11$ (8.16), $p = 0.99$), if and only if, γ_c is interpreted as a learning environment effect. In contrast, the recommended model specification supports the interpretation that students who attend schools with higher OPD are expected to present higher levels of civic knowledge ($\gamma_b = 20.53$ (8.65), $p < 0.001$).

In this latter model, γ_b capture the relationship between OPD scores and civic knowledge, between schools. Whereas, γ_c is an overcorrected estimate of the relationship of interest (Lüdtke et al., 2009). In fact, γ_c is γ_b minus γ_w from Eq. 2. We express this later interpretation with a diagram (Fig. 1). In Fig. 1, γ_b and γ_w are of different size. This latter feature allows us to represent γ_c as the remainder of γ_b if we subtract γ_w from γ_b. In the y axis we are depicting the location of civic knowledge scores, a learning outcome. In the x axis we include OPD scores, which depicts students' ratings of a learning environment attribute. With circles we represent the observations of three different ideal schools. From left to right, these are a school with low, average, and high levels of OPD scores at the school level. In the center of each circle, we have placed a black dot, which represent the schools means of the OPD scores. The line across these black dots, represents the between school relations between the learning outcome and the OPD scores at the school level. In Eq. 2, the inclination of this line is capture by γ_b. Finally, the line within each circle, represents the relationship between the student's ratings of the learning environment, centered at the school level and civic knowledge scores. The inclination of this line is capture by γ_w. With this diagram, we express what γ_c is: the portion of the between school relation of OPD scores and the learning outcome, minus the relationship of the student's ratings of OPD across schools.

When γ_w is of similar size to γ_b, the compositional effect γ_c is close to zero. In general, γ_c is an underestimate version of γ_b, regardless of the relative sizes of γ_b

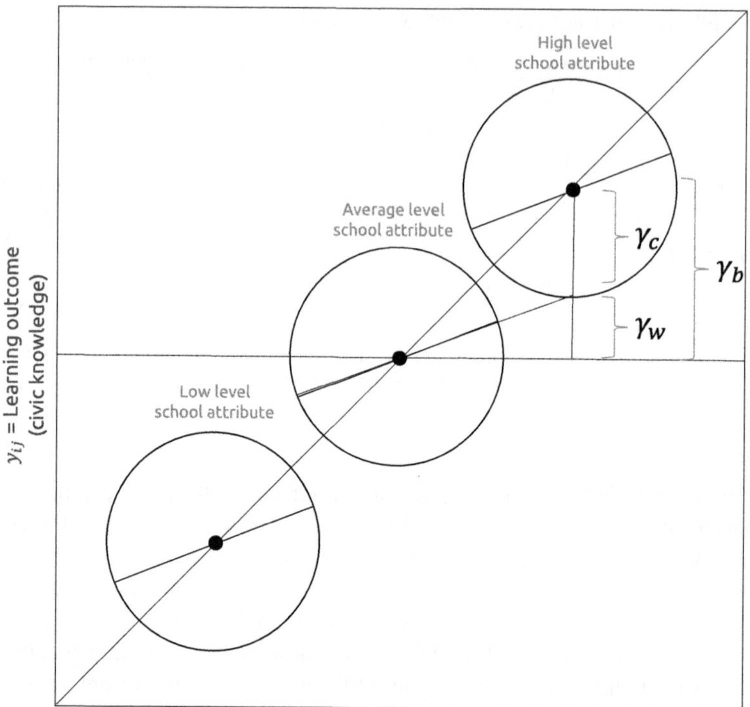

Fig. 1 Graphical representation of $\gamma_c = \gamma_b - \gamma_w$

and γ_w. In Table 2 we include the estimates of γ_b, γ_w and γ_c for all participating ICCS 2016 samples, using the disaggregated model.

In total 6 out of 24 countries, present a similar scenario of Italy. In Italy, Slovenia, Russia, Latvia, Norway, and Belgium, there is a risk of making the conclusion that OPD school levels are not relevant to explain civic knowledge between schools, if γ_c is wrongly interpreted as a learning environment effect.

5 Problem 2: Students Rating Agreement Variability

Group members rating agreement variability is considered a source of concern when building aggregated scores. When different members of the same group do not show similar rating scores regarding the level of a group attribute or context factor, then it is difficult to consider the group mean score as a convincing representation of the rated attribute. In this regard, a common advice found in the organizational behavior literature is to assure a certain level of inter rater cluster agreement ($r_{wg(j)} >$

Table 2 Estimates of OPD scores relations to civic knowledge for all ICCS 2016 samples

ICCS 2016 samples	γ_b	γ_w	$\gamma_c = \gamma_b - \gamma_w$
Lithuania	−0.58 (15.93)	5.42 (2.45)*	−6.00 (16.66)
Italy	20.53 (8.65)*	20.63 (1.90)***	−0.10 (8.16)
Slovenia	23.30 (6.94)**	21.86 (2.01)***	1.45 (6.90)
Finland	15.10 (8.81)	12.76 (2.96)***	2.34 (8.68)
Latvia	28.20 (12.41)*	20.10 (2.21)***	8.10 (12.12)
Russia	23.05 (8.67)**	14.77 (2.05)***	8.29 (8.61)
Norway	29.93 (7.96)***	19.86 (2.01)***	10.07 (8.72)
Croatia	32.23 (7.23)***	15.20 (1.82)***	17.04 (7.57)*
Belgium	32.12 (12.68)*	12.90 (2.31)***	19.23 (12.05)
Korea	28.74 (16.41)	7.82 (2.21)***	20.92 (17.06)
Sweden	42.28 (9.14)***	21.35 (2.64)***	20.93 (9.62)*
Dominican	50.23 (10.00)***	22.20 (1.94)***	28.03 (9.96)**
Denmark	52.39 (9.64)***	22.80 (1.42)***	29.59 (9.91)**
Chinese Taipei	44.26 (11.97)***	14.37 (1.98)***	29.89 (12.26)*
Mexico	49.56 (12.49)***	13.64 (2.57)***	35.92 (12.50)**
Estonia	50.41 (8.12)***	11.28 (1.75)***	39.13 (8.18)***
Chile	61.39 (11.03)***	13.78 (1.26)***	47.61 (10.97)***
Colombia	65.02 (9.89)***	16.43 (1.56)***	48.59 (9.56)***
Hong Kong	71.47 (18.38)***	12.26 (2.17)***	59.22 (18.33)**
Bulgaria	87.02 (10.01)***	19.73 (2.58)***	67.29 (10.33)***
Peru	88.70 (9.96)***	14.59 (2.02)***	74.11 (10.15)***
NRW	97.75 (18.24)***	13.95 (1.87)***	83.80 (18.72)***
Netherlands	106.81 (14.97)***	8.54 (1.82)***	98.28 (14.75)***
Malta	129.45 (19.03)***	19.65 (1.53)***	109.80 (18.91)***

Note: Unstandardized estimates, standard errors in parenthesis, ***p < 0.001, **p < 0.01, *p < 0.05. *NRW* North Rhine-Westphalia, Germany. Estimates are ordered by γ_c size, from low to high. Random effect estimates are omitted and are available upon request from the corresponding author

0.70) (Woehr et al., 2015). However, the uncertainty around the agreement indexes depends on the intraclass correlation and the clusters' group size. As such, cut off scores are not easily generalizable to different studies (Lüdtke & Robitzsch, 2009). Then, how much agreement is needed among students when these are rating their learning environment?

To illustrate the following problem, we select Perú data from ICCS 2016. This is an ideal example because OPD scores present enough variability of students rating. Under the standard recommendation, of discarding all schools below the $r_{wg(j)} >$ 0.70 threshold, we would need to discard 23 of 206 schools from the peruvian sample. Accounting for survey design, this implies discarding 18% schools of the projected population of schools. In turn, we propose to keep all generated scores, and assess what is the relationship of OPD school mean scores, conditional to a dispersion score.

We can express the proposed model, in the following way. The civic knowledge scores of student $_i$ from school $_j$ is represented by y_{ij}. These scores are modelled in a mixed model where the grand mean of y_{ij} is represented by α, each school specific intercept is represented by u_{oj} and random error ε_{ij} when conditioned by the included terms of the equation: socioeconomic status of each student (ses_{ij}), and OPD realizations (θ_w, θ_b). ses_{ij} is included in the model, as in the disaggregated model, first centered at the cluster level $\left(ses_{ij} - \overline{ses}_{.j}\right)$, and then including its school means centered at the grand mean $\left(\overline{ses}_{.j} - \overline{ses}_{..}\right)$. OPD scores are represented in this model as realizations of a multilevel partial credit model, similar to the one presented by Kamata and Vaughn (2011), yet with factor loadings fix to one, and using adjacent category logits to model item responses. Realizations of this later latent variable model generates two orthogonal components θ_w and θ_b. The sum of these components, θ_w and θ_b yields θ_p which represents the propensity of students to report high level of OPD. θ_w is the propensity of students to report a high level of OPD across schools. Thus, is centered within school score. θ_b is the OPD school level generated by the response model, and is a grand mean centered score by definition. These two components are logits scores. Thus, ses_{ij} and OPD realizations are included in the disaggregated model as within and between components. Coefficients in the model are depicted as $_w$ to represent within school estimates, and as $_b$ to represent between school estimate. Additionally, we estimate $\delta_{.j}$, which represents the school level standard deviation of θ_p. This later variable is a dispersion score. The dispersion score is a measure of how much students vary in their ratings in each school. Thus, schools with more disagreement (i.e. lack of consensus), will present higher values, and schools with less disagreement (i.e. stronger consensus) will present lower values. The proposed model is defined as:

$$\begin{aligned} y_{ij} &= \alpha + \pi_w \left(ses_{ij} - \overline{ses}_{.j}\right) + \pi_b \left(\overline{ses}_{.j} - \overline{ses}_{..}\right) \\ &+ \gamma_w \theta_w + \gamma_b \theta_b + \beta_b \left(\delta_{.j} - \overline{\delta}_{..}\right) + \lambda_b \theta_b \left(\delta_{.j} - \overline{\delta}_{..}\right) + u_{oj} + \varepsilon_{ij} \end{aligned} \quad (3)$$

In essence this model is similar to a climate strength model, where the withing group variability of common perceptions of a group attribute is considered a moderator of the group attribute effects (Schneider et al., 2002). However, in the present model specification dispersion scores are in the reverse direction of a climate strength index. As such, the interaction term needs to be interpreted accordingly. We will call this model specification, a dispersion effect model. The parameter of interest is γ_b. γ_b expresses the relationship OPD score realizations between schools, at average values of students' socioeconomic background, at average levels of OPD logit scores, and at the average level of disagreement between regarding the OPD levels. In Table 3, we fit three versions of the proposed model in a stepwise fashion. Model 1, where only ses_{ij} and OPD logits scores are included. Model 2, where, in addition to terms included in Model 1 the dispersion score included to assess its main effect. And Model 3, where the dispersion score is included, and the interaction term between θ_b and $\left(\delta_{.j} - \overline{\delta}_{..}\right)$ is also included.

Table 3 Effects of students' rating of OPD on civic knowledge

	Model 1		Model 2		Model 3	
Fixed effects	E	p<	E	p<	E	p<
α Intercept	427.81	***	427.83	***	428.98	***
Socioeconomic Index						
π_w student deviations	13.81	***	13.81	***	13.8	***
π_b school means	48.45	***	48.31	***	45.98	***
Open classroom discussion						
γ_w student deviations	26.03	***	26.03	***	26.04	***
γ_b school means	81.31	***	81.51	***	89.58	***
β_b dispersion			−2.41		−24.26	
λ_b school means × Dispersion					−237.13	**
Random effects						
var($u_{.j}$)	4401.68	***	4399.69	***	4397.39	***
var(ε_{ij})	1089.53	***	1096.82	***	1002.91	***

Note: *E* unstandardized estimate, *var.* variance component, ***p < 0.001, **p < 0.01, *p < 0.05

In Model 1 presents a positive relationship to civic knowledge scores of the students ($\gamma_b = 81.31$ (12.24), $p < 0.001$). Thus, students in schools with 1 standard deviation of more OPD are expected to present gains of 81% of standard deviations in civic knowledge scores. When the dispersion score of students rating is included in Model 2, we observed similar results ($\gamma_b = 81.51$ (12.71), $p < 0.001$), while the dispersion score alone presents small point estimate ($\beta_b = -2.41$ (29.11), $p = 0.93$). In Model 3, dispersion scores are allowed to condition the relationship of OPD scores to civic knowledge. In this model γ_b represents the expected change in civic knowledge scores at average levels of students' lack of inter-rater agreement on OPD scores ($\overline{\delta}_{..} = 0.53$). In this model, the expected change in civic knowledge scores is of similar size as in Model 1 ($\gamma_b = 89.58$ (10.17), $p < 0.001$, CI95[69.64, 109.52]). However, the interaction term λ_b tells us these values are expected to be lower when there is less agreement between students (more dispersion) regarding how frequent OPD occurs in their schools ($\lambda_b = -237.13$ (73.46), $p < 0.01$).

For example, if OPD rating scores present 1SD above the average of dispersion ($\overline{\delta}_{..}$ + 1SD = 0.65), then the expected change in civic knowledge scores is of 61.12 points ($\gamma_b = 61.12$ (14.70), $p < 0.001$, at $\delta_{.j} = 0.65$). Conversely, if OPD scores rating dispersion is 1SD less than the average ($\overline{\delta}_{..}$ - 1SD = 0.41), then the expected change in civic knowledge scores is higher, reaching 118.03 points ($\gamma_b = 118.03$ (12.09), $p < 0.001$, at $\delta_{.j} = 0.41$).

At the beginning of this section, we have stated that Peru ICCS 2016 is an ideal example to show the advantage of the present model. Peru is one of the countries where two conditions are met: there is enough students rating variability among OPD realizations scores across schools, and its dispersion scores moderates the OPD between school estimates. These conditions are not observed in all ICCS 2016 samples. In total, three out of 24 ICCS 2016 samples share these conditions including Colombia, Peru and Italy. In the rest of the ICCS 2016 samples, where

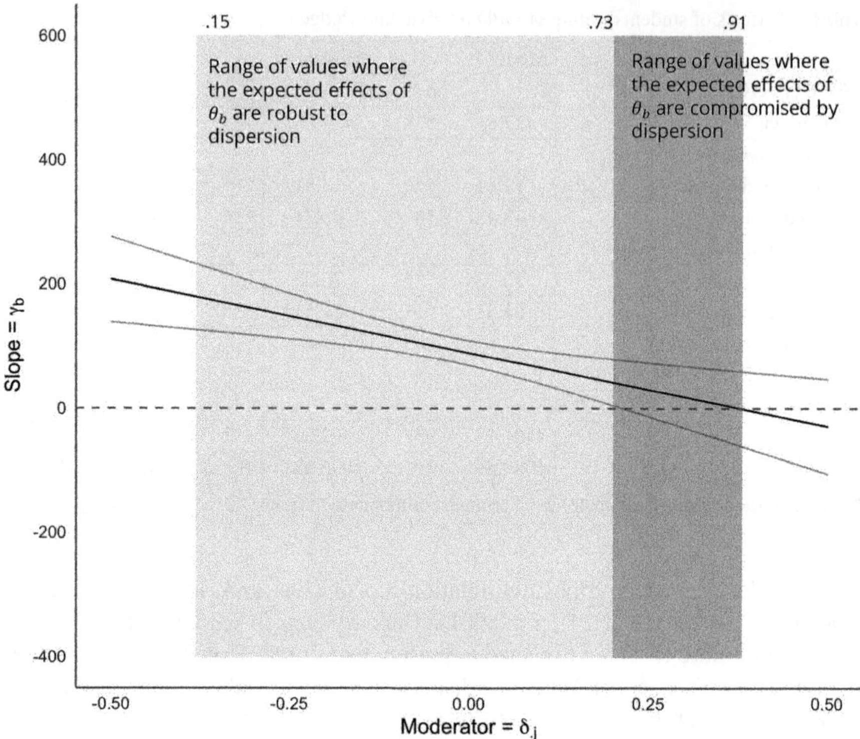

Fig. 2 Johnson-Neyman plot for γ_b conditional to $\delta_{.j} - \overline{\delta}_{..}$ scores

the moderation effect of the dispersion model is small, estimates from Model 1 and Model 3 produces similar estimates of γ_b. As such, the dispersion effect model is advantageous for only some scenarios.

The dispersion effect model permits to estimate the critical point where a lack of consensus between students from the same school compromise the estimates of a referent-shift items scale scores. In Fig. 2, we plot the expected slope of OPD school levels, at the observed values of the dispersion score. The black line represent the point estimates of γ_b at different dispersion score values. The curve lines that accompany the points estimates are the 95% confidence intervals of γ_b. The model specification has the advantage that the OPD realizations and the dispersion score are in the same scale, thus its coefficients can be interpreted in a similar manner. Between 0.73 and 0.91 of dispersion, the estimates of γ_b are compromised as its lower confidence interval crosses zero.

6 Conclusion and Discussion

In the present study, we have shown two methodological problems for reference shift scale scores. The first problem consists of relying on the compositional model specification when the relationship of interest is between schools. We illustrated this problem with the most extreme case when the within and between effects of the reflective measure scores are of the same size. The compositional model overcorrects the estimate of interest (Lüdtke et al., 2009). The present problem is easy to address by recurring to the fully disaggregated model (Rights et al., 2019), which directly retrieves the effect of interest as a between estimate. We use observed data from Italy (ICCS 2016) to illustrate this problem. If the compositional model is used, the incorrect interpretation of the between level effect could lead to wrong conclusions.

The second problem refers to students' inter-rater variability of reference-shift scale scores. These can vary significantly between groups of students from different schools and may compromise the relationship under study. Organizational literature recommends excluding groups with the low inter-rater agreement. Nevertheless, this recommendation may incur a severe loss of sample in international large scale studies (Rutkowski et al., 2010). Moreover, this recommended cut-off score is not generalizable to any grouped observations, because it depends on group size and its intraclass correlation values (Lüdtke & Robitzsch, 2009). We illustrate this problem with data from Peru (ICCS 2016), where if the recommendation is followed, there is a loss of 18% of projected schools in the sampling frame. For this problem, instead of using a cut score, we use a dispersion effect model to identify where the between school estimates of OPD are compromised, conditional to the values of lack of agreement of students' OPD ratings. With the proposed model, the relationship of interest can be retrieved while also documenting its relationship to the students' inter-rater variability.

It should be noted that dispersion scores can buffer the group attribute's relationship, as in climate strength models (Schneider et al., 2002). However, there are also examples where a lack of consensus accelerate the effect of interest (Schweig, 2016). What explains the direction of this interaction? It is an open research question. Thus, one of the limitations of the dispersion effect model, is that the direction of the effects of the dispersion scores is unknown, and might be specific to the attribute under study, and to the empirical relations of the groups under study (Schweig, 2016). In contrast, the compositional model of the between school level estimate, is always an underestimate of a reference shift scale score.

OPD is a relevant school factor involved in many civic education outcomes. However, its reflective nature is not always recognized by researchers (Carrasco & Torres Irribarra, 2018), incurring in the underestimation of its expected effects. Additionally, OPD scores are positively related to students' socioeconomic status at different degrees between countries (Carrasco et al., 2020), as such, multilevel model estimates are already underestimating its "true" effect (Castellano et al., 2014). Thus, even if the models are specified as we recommend here, its expected effects reported in the previous literature are downward bias (e.g., Carrasco & Torres Irribarra, 2018; Isac et al., 2014; Knowles & McCafferty-Wright, 2015). Moreover, is possible its effect may also be underestimated if there is an interaction with the lack of consensus among students regarding the OPD school level as we have shown here.

The approaches presented here are not applicable to OPD scores only, but to any reference-shift item scale scores. This type of measures are frequently used in education, especially in large scale assessment studies, where is common to rely on students and or teachers' responses to generate information about school level attributes. To properly accumulate knowledge about learning environment factors that uses students and teachers as informants, is imperative we use appropriate model specifications to avoid underestimations. With this type of measures is recommended to model the inter-rater variability effects, instead of removing cases based on rules of thumb. Reference-shift item scale scores should be recognized as different from latent trait type scores and treated accordingly.

Acknowledgements Research funded by the Ministerio de Educación, Gobierno de Chile and Comisión Nacional de Investigación Científica y Tecnológica CONICYT (PIA 160007), Centro de Estudios Avanzados (CJE); and Fondo Nacional de Desarrollo Científico y Tecnológico FONDECYT N° 1180667.

References

Bell, A., Jones, K., & Fairbrother, M. (2018). Understanding and misunderstanding group mean centering: A commentary on Kelley et al.'s dangerous practice. *Quality and Quantity, 52*(5), 2031–2036. https://doi.org/10.1007/s11135-017-0593-5

Caro, D. H., & Lenkeit, J. (2012). An analytical approach to study educational inequalities: 10 hypothesis tests in PIRLS 2006. *International Journal of Research & Method in Education, 35*(1), 3–30. https://doi.org/10.1080/1743727X.2012.666718

Carrasco, D., Banerjee, R., Treviño, E., & Villalobos, C. (2020). Civic knowledge and open classroom discussion: Explaining tolerance of corruption among 8th-grade students in Latin America. *Educational Psychology, 40*(2), 186–206. https://doi.org/10.1080/01443410.2019.1699907

Carrasco, D., & Torres Irribarra, D. (2018). The role of classroom discussion. In A. Sandoval-Hernández, M. M. Isac, & D. Miranda (Eds.), *Teaching tolerance in a globalized world* (pp. 87–101). https://doi.org/10.1007/978-3-319-78692-6

Castellano, K. E., Rabe-Hesketh, S., & Skrondal, A. (2014). Composition, context, and endogeneity in school and teacher comparisons. *Journal of Educational and Behavioral Statistics, 39*(5), 333–367. https://doi.org/10.3102/1076998614547576

Engelhard, G. J., & Wind, S. A. (2018). *Invariant measurement with raters and rating scales*. Routledge.

Hahn, C. L., & Tocci, C. M. (1990). Classroom climate and controversial issues discussions: A five nation study. *Theory and Research in Social Education, 18*(4), 344–362. https://doi.org/10.1080/00933104.1990.10505621

Isac, M. M., Maslowski, R., Creemers, B., & van der Werf, G. (2014). The contribution of schooling to secondary-school students' citizenship outcomes across countries. *School Effectiveness & School Improvement, 25*(January 2015), 29–63. https://doi.org/10.1080/09243453.2012.751035

Kamata, A., & Vaughn, B. K. (2011). Multilevel IRT modeling. In J. J. Hox & J. K. Roberts (Eds.), *Handbook of advanced multilevel analysis* (pp. 41–57). https://doi.org/10.4324/9780203848852.ch3

Knowles, R. T., & McCafferty-Wright, J. (2015). Connecting an open classroom climate to social movement citizenship: A study of 8th graders in Europe using IEA ICCS data. *Journal of Social Studies Research, 39*(4), 255–269. https://doi.org/10.1016/j.jssr.2015.03.002

Lang, J. W. B., Bliese, P. D., & de Voogt, A. (2018). Modeling consensus emergence in groups using longitudinal multilevel methods. *Personnel Psychology, 71*(2), 255–281. https://doi.org/10.1111/peps.12260

Lüdtke, O., & Robitzsch, A. (2009). Assessing within-group agreement: A critical examination of a random-group resampling approach. *Organizational Research Methods, 12*(3), 461–487. https://doi.org/10.1177/1094428108317406

Lüdtke, O., Robitzsch, A., Trautwein, U., & Kunter, M. (2009). Assessing the impact of learning environments: How to use student ratings of classroom or school characteristics in multilevel modeling. *Contemporary Educational Psychology, 34*(2), 120–131. https://doi.org/10.1016/j.cedpsych.2008.12.001

Lüdtke, O., Trautwein, U., Kunter, M., & Baumert, J. (2006). Reliability and agreement of student ratings of the classroom environment: A reanalysis of TIMSS data. *Learning Environments Research, 9*(3), 215–230. https://doi.org/10.1007/s10984-006-9014-8

Masters, G. N. (2016). Partial credit model. In W. J. van der Linden (Ed.), *Handbook of item response theory. Volume One. Models* (pp. 109–126). CRC Press.

Rasch, G. (1960). *Probabilistic models for some intelligence and attainment tests*. Nielsen & Lydiche.

Rights, J. D., Preacher, K. J., & Cole, D. A. (2019). The danger of conflating level-specific effects of control variables when primary interest lies in level-2 effects. *British Journal of Mathematical and Statistical Psychology, 4*, bmsp.12194. https://doi.org/10.1111/bmsp.12194

Rutkowski, L., Gonzalez, E., Joncas, M., & von Davier, M. (2010). International large-scale assessment data: Issues in secondary analysis and reporting. *Educational Researcher, 39*(2), 142–151. https://doi.org/10.3102/0013189X10363170

Schneider, B., Salvaggio, A. N., & Subirats, M. (2002). Climate strength: A new direction for climate research. *Journal of Applied Psychology, 87*(2), 220–229. https://doi.org/10.1037/0021-9010.87.2.220

Schulz, W., Carstens, R., Losito, B., & Fraillon, J. (2018). *ICCS 2016 technical report* (W. Schulz, R. Carstens, B. Losito, & J. Fraillon, Eds.). International Association for the Evaluation of Educational Achievement (IEA).

Schweig, J. D. (2016). Moving beyond means: Revealing features of the learning environment by investigating the consensus among student ratings. *Learning Environments Research, 19*(3), 441–462. https://doi.org/10.1007/s10984-016-9216-7

Torney-Purta, J. (2009). Matters for policy and practice. *American Psychologist, 64*(4), 825–837.

Woehr, D. J., Loignon, A. C., & Schmidt, P. (2015). Aggregation aggravation: The fallacy of the wrong level revisited. In C. E. Lance & R. J. Vandenberg (Eds.), *More statistical and methodological myths and urban legends* (pp. 311–326). Routledge.

A Generalizability Study of *Teach*, a Classroom Observation Tool

Diegо Luna-Bazaldua, Ezequiel Molina, and Adelle Pushparatnam

1 Introduction

1.1 Teach, a Classroom Observation Tool

Research around the world shows that teachers have a critical role in promoting student learning (Araujo et al., 2016; Azam & Kingdon, 2015; Bau & Das, 2017; Buhl-Wiggers et al., 2017; Hanushek & Rivkin, 2010). For instance, Snilstveit et al. (2016) showed in their cross-country review that out of all school-related interventions in low- and middle-income countries to improve learning, the ones that had the largest positive impacts on student learning outcomes are those that supported teachers improve the quality of their classroom instruction with appropriate training.

The first step to improve the quality of teacher-student interactions and teacher effectiveness is to measure it. However, most education systems in low- and middle-income countries do not regularly monitor teaching practices or the quality of interactions between teachers and students in the classroom, even though it consistently predicts a range of academic and socioemotional student outcomes (Burchinal et al., 2008; Cadima et al., 2010; Curby et al., 2013; Hatfield et al., 2012; Kane et al., 2011; Mashburn et al., 2008; Morris et al., 2012; Muijs et al., 2014; Rimm-Kaufman et al., 2009). Even when education systems attempt to capture teaching practices, most tools used in low- and middle-income countries fall short, as they: (i) measure either the quantity or quality of teaching practices; (ii) do not explicitly focus on teachers' efforts to develop students' socioemotional skills; (iii) use tools designed for other contexts, which may include irrelevant items or fail to

D. Luna-Bazaldua (✉) · E. Molina · A. Pushparatnam
The World Bank Group, Washington, DC, USA
e-mail: dlunabazaldua@worldbank.org; molina@worldbank.org; apushparatnam@worldbank.org

M. Wiberg et al. (eds.), *Quantitative Psychology*, Springer Proceedings in Mathematics & Statistics 353, https://doi.org/10.1007/978-3-030-74772-5_42

include important ones; and (iv) use tools that are neither evidence-based nor meet basic reliability criteria (Ladics et al., 2018).

Teach was developed to address these challenges. *Teach* is an open access classroom observation tool that provides a window into what goes on in the classroom for primary classrooms grades 1 to 6. In particular, the tool provides a common language for conceptualizing teaching in a way that is inclusive, responsive, and which facilitates whole-child development. It does so by considering not just time spent on learning but, more importantly, the quality of teacher practices. The *Teach* framework is divided into two key components: time-on-task and quality of teaching practices.

The analysis presented in this paper focuses on the second component measuring the quality of teaching practices and is organized into three primary areas: classroom culture, instruction and socioemotional skills. These areas have 9 corresponding elements that point to 28 behaviors. The behaviors are characterized as low, medium, or high, based on the evidence collected during the observation. These behavior scores are translated into a 5-point scale that quantifies teaching practices.

Previous research has provided reliability and validity evidence to support the use of *Teach* as an observation tool of instructional quality in the classroom (Molina et al., 2020). Having reliability and the impact of different sources of bias in mind, the team behind the development of this tool has focused on ensuring that the *Teach* item scores consistently reflect the teacher instructional practice and that raters have as little impact as possible in the final score. Statistical estimates show that the *Teach* items reach expected levels of internal consistency for a multidimensional tool (Molina et al., 2020). In addition, trained raters are selected to perform classroom observations only after they show high levels of inter-rater agreement of videos with respect to master codes.

1.2 Generalizability Theory Framework

Due to additional applications of the *Teach* tool, there is now the opportunity to further explore the extent to which *Teach* scores are being influenced by raters versus other sources of variation in the scores. From a psychometric perspective, the Generalizability Theory (G Theory) framework is well-suited to capture the impact of raters on the variation of *Teach* scores because its capacity to decompose multiple sources of score variation (Brennan, 1992; Cronbach et al., 1963).

Moreover, Brennan (2000) has shown how the G Theory framework can be used as a suitable psychometric approach to analyze the psychometric properties of performance assessments –like *Teach*– that involve raters (i.e., enumerators trained in the use of *Teach*) observing persons (i.e., teachers in the classroom) performing on a sample of tasks (i.e., *Teach* items). As shown by this author, when a performance observation tool has well-defined scoring rubrics and raters are trained properly, the effect of raters on the measurement tool scores is relatively small compared to the potential effects from the observed person and the task. In consequence, G Theory permits to describe the reliability of generalizations that can be made from the scores assigned to a teacher's performance on specific task to the teacher's hypothetical performance in a broad universe of admissible performance observations (Shavelson & Webb, 1991).

In G Theory, each source of score variation (e.g., raters r, persons p, and tasks t) and its levels are defined as facets. Therefore, an observed score of a measurement tool like *Teach* can be decomposed into components or facet effects (Shavelson & Webb, 1991). In this case, researchers could produce a $r \times p \times t$ design to determine how an observed score in the measurement tool (X_{rpt}) can be explained by facet effects and their possible interactions:

$$
\begin{aligned}
X_{rpt} = \; & \mu && \text{grand mean}\\
& + \mu_r - \mu && \text{rater effect}\\
& + \mu_p - \mu && \text{person effect}\\
& + \mu_t - \mu && \text{task effect}\\
& + \mu_{rp} - \mu_r - \mu_p + \mu && \text{rater} \times \text{person effect}\\
& + \mu_{rt} - \mu_r - \mu_t + \mu && \text{rater} \times \text{task effect}\\
& + \mu_{pt} - \mu_p - \mu_t + \mu && \text{person} \times \text{task effect}\\
& + X_{rpt} - \mu_{rp} - \mu_{rt} - \mu_{pt} + \mu_r + \mu_p + \mu_t - \mu && \text{residual}
\end{aligned} \tag{1}
$$

Under this study design, a random-effects model would allow to disentangle variance components $\sigma^2{*} = E^* (\mu * - \mu)$ for each effect. In this way, the G Theory framework permits to calculate the variance $\sigma^2_{X_{rpt}}$ for observer scores X_{rpt} as

$$\sigma^2_{X_{rpt}} = \sigma^2_r + \sigma^2_p + \sigma^2_t + \sigma^2_{rp} + \sigma^2_{rt} + \sigma^2_{pt} + \sigma^2_{residual} \tag{2}$$

In this way, the relative magnitude of each variance component can help to identify sources of error that could bias the observed score in the measurement tool.

With this background, to expand the documented evidence around the psychometric properties of *Teach*, the objective of the present study was to explore sources of variability in the *Teach* scores using the G Theory framework (Cronbach et al., 1963).

2 Methods

2.1 *Participants*

Data comes from various administrations of *Teach* across the world, including countries located in South Asia (SAR), Sub-Saharan Africa (SSA), East Asia (EAP), and South America (LAC). In terms of sample size by country, there were 861 elementary school classroom observations of teachers in the SSA country, 633 from the EAP country, 565 from the SAR country, and 187 from the LAC country. Depending on the local context of each country, additional sociodemographic and school information was also captured during the school visit. Most data sets included information about the school grade of the classroom observed (but in some countries, some teachers were delivering instruction in multigrade classrooms), subject of instruction (e.g., language, mathematics, science, and so on), language of instruction, and school location (e.g., rural vs. non-rural settings).

The number of observers or raters varied by country; the variation depended on the staff resources available for training and for conducting the visits to schools and observations in classrooms. A total of 12 raters participated in the classroom observations in the SAR country, 31 in the SSA country, 18 raters in the EAP country, and 5 raters in the LAC country.

2.2 *Instrument*

Teachers were observed and rated using the *Teach* observation tool. The nine items capturing the quality of teaching practices measure the extent to which the teachers created a supportive learning environment, set positive behavioral expectations, facilitated learning, checked students' understanding, provided feedback, and promoted critical thinking, autonomy, perseverance, and social & collaborative skills in students. Each item was scored on a 5-point Likert scale, with larger values indicating that the teachers demonstrated more effective behaviors related to the nine items mentioned above.

Previous research has shown evidence of the reliability (both in terms of internal consistency and inter-rater agreement) and the validity (in terms of content, cognitive processes in the response process, internal structure, and score relationship with external variables) properties of the *Teach* scores (Molina et al., 2020). In this study, the data from the SAR country produced an overall Cronbach's alpha coefficient estimate of 0.78, 0.75 for the EAP country, 0.74 for the LAC country, and 0.69 for the SSA country. The fact that these internal consistency estimates are not as high as in other standardized measures is expected due to the multidimensionality of this observation tool.

2.3 Psychometric Model and Data Analysis

The data collected in these countries was analyzed using a Generalizability model to determine sources of variance in the *Teach* scores (Cronbach et al., 1963). Data analyses were conducted and are reported separately for each country. The facets in this study were teachers' main effects (p), raters' main effects (r), and items' main effects (t). Other factors and interactions, such as the content taught during the observation and school location, were explored as part of the study, but those additional factors explained a minimal amount of score variance. Therefore, the G theory model and its corresponding variance decomposition used to analyze *Teach* observed scores is expressed as

$$\sigma^2_{X_{rpt}} = \sigma^2_r + \sigma^2_p + \sigma^2_t + \sigma^2_{residual} \tag{3}$$

The "gtheory" package (Moore, 2016) in R (R Core Team, 2019) was used to estimate the psychometric models.

3 Results

3.1 Descriptive Statistics

Descriptive statistics for each *Teach* item are presented in Table 1. Consistently across countries, teachers were rated higher in items measuring aspects linked to the classroom culture (i.e., items 1 to 3), particularly in terms of creating a supportive learning environment in the classroom. On the other side, the lowest average scores tended to be reported in areas linked to teacher's promoting social and collaborative skills among students (item 9 in SSA and EAP countries) or providing constructive feedback to students (item 5 in SAR and LAC countries).

3.2 Generalizability Study

The G theory model presented in Eq. (3) was used to calculate the impact of raters, teachers, and items on the *Teach* scores for each country separately. As shown in Table 2, results across countries consistently showed that items are the biggest source of explained total score variance (from 29% in EAP country to 45% in SAR country), followed by teachers (from 7% in SSA country to 14% in EAP country), and then raters (from 3% in EAP country to 8% in LAC country). Residual variance not explained by any of these three facets ranged from 38% to 53% percent of the total score variance in Teach.

Table 1 Descriptive statistics for the *Teach* items

Item	SAR		SSA		EAP		LAC	
	Mean	SD	Mean	SD	Mean	SD	Mean	SD
1	4.11	1.05	3.52	0.66	3.53	0.63	3.82	0.53
2	3.54	0.78	3.23	0.80	3.32	0.85	3.27	0.77
3	3.07	1.08	3.34	0.79	3.20	0.90	3.21	0.77
4	2.60	0.99	2.98	0.99	3.33	0.92	2.88	1.03
5	1.70	0.90	2.24	1.09	2.78	1.10	2.03	0.98
6	1.96	0.94	2.28	0.90	2.85	1.19	2.56	1.21
7	2.87	0.83	2.68	0.83	2.45	0.90	2.53	0.79
8	2.04	0.60	2.07	0.55	2.31	0.82	2.11	0.39
9	1.75	1.02	1.53	0.82	1.65	1.01	2.21	1.22

Note: Item "1" refers to Supportive learning environment, "2" to Positive behavioral expectations, "3" to Lesson facilitation, "4" to Checks for understanding, "5" to Feedback, "6" to Critical thinking, "7" to Autonomy, "8" to Perseverance, and "9" to Social & Collaborative skills. "SAR" refers to the country in South Asia, "SSA" to the country in Sub-Saharan Africa, "EAP" to the country in East Asia, and "LAC" to the country in Latin America

Table 2 Facet variance for the *Teach* total score

Source of variance	SAR		SSA		EAP		LAC	
	Var	%	Var	%	Var	%	Var	%
Item	0.710	45.3	0.446	38.5	0.364	29.2	0.366	30.6
Teachers	0.139	8.9	0.082	7.1	0.174	14.0	0.125	10.5
Rater	0.113	7.2	0.064	5.6	0.046	3.7	0.098	8.2
Residual	0.606	38.7	0.565	48.8	0.662	53.1	0.606	50.7

Note: "Var" refers to the variance explained by the facet and "%" to the percentage of variance explained by the Facet. "SAR" refers to the country in South Asia, "SSA" to the country in Sub-Saharan Africa, "EAP" to the country in East Asia, and "LAC" to the country in Latin America

Since there is a consistent higher proportion in variation of *Teach* scores explained by the items rather than by the raters, it can be concluded that the nine *Teach* items capture particular aspects of the teaching practice that differ much more in their average score (which is consistent with the results in Table 1) than raters differ in their average stringency when observing teachers' classroom performance.

4 Discussion

This study adds to the current research around the psychometric properties of *Teach*, a classroom observation tool that is being used around the world to help policymakers understand what teaching practices look like in a given context, and to identify areas in which teachers might need additional supports. In summary, results from this cross-country study showed *Teach* scores on each of its items are mainly influenced by the item content and the teacher performance in the classroom, with little impact by the rater on the item scores. The fact that raters represent a very small source of the item scores residual variance confirms the benefits of performing an appropriate training for the use of *Teach* before the classroom observations take place. At the same time, these results highlight the relevance of developing observation tools that measure the different aspects that constitute a high-quality teaching process.

Similar to previous research documented for other teacher observation tools (Kane & Staiger, 2012; Mashburn et al., 2014), the results here obtained show that raters play a relatively small role in the *Teach* total score variance. That is, the scores produced by the *Teach* observation tool are mostly the product of the teacher quality aspects measured by each of its items and the teacher performance, rather than the product of rater bias.

Future research will focus on examining teacher, item and rater effects in the total score variance in additional contexts; *Teach* has been used in more than 20 countries across the world at this point, so there is both opportunity and interest in identifying whether the results here presented are consistently found in other countries. Second, we will also complement the results here obtained with additional analyses on rater effects using the Many Facet Rasch Measurement models (Linacre, 1989). Third, we plan to execute longitudinal studies to determine the predictive power of *Teach* and other classroom observation tools on student performance.

Regarding future directions for the field, there is a need for more empirical evidence on the relative importance of the various elements of teaching practices (e.g. Checking for Understanding, Perseverance, Supportive Learning Environment) on student cognitive and socioemotional learning. In addition, there is a need for more research on the universality (or not) of the importance of the teaching practices that have been identified thus far in the literature.

Due to the rigorous methodology behind data collection using *Teach*, the main limitation of this study is the incapacity to determine *ex post* how much the rater training before the classroom visits decreased the potential rater bias. Results across countries show that trained raters contribute very little to the variation of *Teach* scores; nevertheless, not every classroom observation tool follows these training protocols. In the future, it will be important to compare rater bias within and between classroom observation tools. This research agenda could potentially help to improve measurement tools, which could lead to an increase in the share of the variation of students' outcomes currently explained by teaching practices, as captured by classroom observation tools.

Acknowledgments Finally, the authors would like to thank the World Bank teams, government counterparts, and partner organizations for their generosity in sharing their data from past measurement efforts. We want to thank Alice Danon for her assistance in the data management for the analyses here presented.

Appendix: Code to Estimate G Models in R Using *Teach* Data

The code in R presented here exemplifies the estimation of G model in R. The G model is estimated using the gstudy() function on the set of *Teach* items arranged in a single data column. Each *Teach* item is identified by its name. Facets explored include item name (task, *t*), rater ID (rater, *r*) and Teacher ID (person, *p*).

```
# Call libraries that will be needed for this exercise.
library(gtheory) # For generalizability models.

### 1. After calling the data to R, models are estimated.

# G Study model with main effects

### Function gstudy() comes from the 'gtheory' package.
### Command "data" identifies the data set in R environment.
### Command "formula" defines in an R formula the scores and
each of the facets to analyze. Quotation marks have to be used
to define the formula when using the gstudy() function.

Gmodel1 <- gstudy(data = Data_TR_long,
formula = "as.numeric(score) ~ (1 | teachers) +
                  (1 | rater) + (1 | item)" )
```

References

Araujo, M. C., Carneiro, P., Cruz-Aguayo, Y., & Schady, N. (2016). Teacher quality and learning outcomes in kindergarten. *The Quarterly Journal of Economics, 131*(3), 1415–1453.

Azam, M., & Kingdon, G. G. (2015). Assessing teacher quality in India. *Journal of Development Economics, 117*, 74–83.

Bau, N., & Das, J. (2017). *The misallocation of pay and productivity in the public sector: Evidence from the labor market for teachers*. The World Bank.

Brennan, R. L. (1992). Generalizability theory. *Educational Measurement: Issues and Practice, 11*(4), 27–34.

Brennan, R. L. (2000). Performance assessments from the perspective of generalizability theory. *Applied Psychological Measurement, 24*(4), 339–353.

Buhl-Wiggers, J., Kerwin, J., Smith, J., & Thornton, R. (2017). *The impact of teacher effectiveness on student learning in Africa*. Paper presented at the Centre for the Study of African Economies Conference 2017.

Burchinal, M., Howes, C., Pianta, R., Bryant, D., Early, D., Clifford, R., & Barbarin, O. (2008). Predicting child outcomes at the end of kindergarten from the quality of pre-kindergarten teacher-child interactions and instruction. *Applied Developmental Science, 12*(3), 140–153.

Cadima, J., Leal, T., & Burchinal, M. (2010). The quality of teacher-student interactions: Associations with first graders' academic and behavioral outcomes. *Journal of School Psychology, 48*(6), 457–482.

Core Team, R. (2019). *R: A language and environment for statistical computing*. R Foundation for Statistical Computing. https://www.R-project.org/

Cronbach, L. J., Nageswari, R., & Gleser, G. C. (1963). Theory of generalizability: A liberation of reliability theory. *The British Journal of Statistical Psychology, 16*, 137–163.

Curby, T. W., Brock, L. L., & Hamre, B. K. (2013). Teachers' emotional support consistency predicts children's achievement gains and social skills. *Early Education and Development, 24*(3), 292–309.

Hanushek, E. A., & Rivkin, S. G. (2010). Generalizations about using value-added measures of teacher quality. *American Economic Review, 100*(2), 267–271.

Hatfield, B. E., Hestenes, L. L., Kintner-Duffy, V. L., & O'Brien, M. (2012). Classroom emotional support predicts differences in preschool children's cortisol and alpha-amylase levels. *Early Childhood Research Quarterly, 28*(2), 347–356.

Kane, T. J., & Staiger, D. O. (2012). *Gathering feedback for teaching: Combining high-quality observations with student surveys and achievement gains*. Bill and Melinda Gates Foundation.

Kane, T. J., Taylor, E. S., Tyler, J. H., & Wooten, A. (2011). Identifying effective classroom practices using student achievement data. *Journal of Human Resources, 46*(3), 587–613.

Ladics, J., Molina, E., Wilichowski, T, and Yarrow, N. (2018). The measurement crisis: An assessment of how countries measure classroom practices. Working paper. https://riseprogramme.org/sites/default/files/inline-files/Molina.pdf.

Linacre, J. (1989). *Many-facet Rasch measurement*. MESA Press.

Mashburn, A. J., Pianta, R. C., Hamre, B. K., Downer, J. T., Barbarin, O. A., Bryant, D., Burchinal, M., Early, D. M., & Howes, C. (2008). Measures of classroom quality in prekindergarten and children's development of academic, language, and social skills. *Child Development, 79*(3), 732–749.

Mashburn, A. J., Downer, J. T., Rivers, S. E., Brackett, M. A., & Martinez, A. (2014). Improving the power of an efficacy study of a social and emotional learning program: Application of generalizability theory to the measurement of classroom-level outcomes. *Prevention Science, 15*, 146–155.

Molina, E., Fatima, S. F., Ho, A. D., Melo, C., Wilichowksi, T. M., & Pushparatnam, A. (2020). Measuring the quality of teaching practices in primary schools: Assessing the validity of the Teach classroom observation tool in Punjab, Pakistan. *Teaching and Teacher Education, 96*, 103–121. https://doi.org/10.1016/j.tate.2020.103171

Moore, C. T. (2016). *gtheory: Apply generalizability theory with R*. R package version 0.1.2. URL: https://CRAN.R-project.org/package=gtheory

Morris, P., Lloyd, C. M., Millenky, M., Leacock, N., Raver, C., & Bangser, M. (2012). *Using classroom management to improve preschoolers' social and emotional skills: Final impact and implementation findings from the Foundations of Learning Demonstration in Newark and Chicago (Report)*. MDRC.

Muijs, D., Kyriakides, L., van der Werf, G., Creemers, B., Timerley, H., & Earl, L. (2014). State of the art – Teacher effectiveness and professional learning. *School Effectiveness and School Improvement, 25*(2), 231–256.

Rimm-Kaufman, S. E., Curby, T., Grimm, K., Nathanson, L., & Brock, L. (2009). The contribution of children's self-regulation and classroom quality to children's adaptive behaviors in the kindergarten classroom. *Developmental Psychology, 45*(4), 958–972.

Shavelson, R. J., & Webb, N. M. (1991). *Generalizability theory: A primer*. Sage.

Snilstveit, B., Stevenson, J., Menon, R., Phillips, D., Gallagher, E., Geleen, M., Jobse, H., Schmidt, T., & Jimenez, E. (2016). *The impact of education programmes on learning and school participation in low- and middle-income countries: A systematic review summary report. Systematic review summary*. International Initiative for Impact Evaluation.

Index

M. Wiberg et al. (eds.), *Quantitative Psychology*, Springer Proceedings in Mathematics & Statistics 353, https://doi.org/10.1007/978-3-030-74772-5

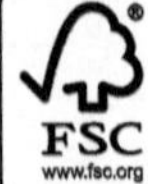

MIX
Papier aus verantwortungsvollen Quellen
Paper from responsible sources
FSC® C105338

Printed by Books on Demand, Germany